REFRACTIONS OF ISLAM IN INDIA

Bulk Sales

SAGE India offers special discounts
for purchase of books in bulk.
We also make available special imprints
and excerpts from our books on demand.

For orders and enquiries, write to us at

Marketing Department
SAGE Publications India Pvt Ltd
B1/I-1, Mohan Cooperative Industrial Area
Mathura Road, Post Bag 7
New Delhi 110044, India

E-mail us at **marketing@sagepub.in**

Get to know more about SAGE

Be invited to SAGE events, get on our mailing list.
Write today to **marketing@sagepub.in**

This book is also available as an e-book.

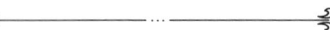

REFRACTIONS OF ISLAM IN INDIA
Situating Sufism and Yoga

Carl W. Ernst

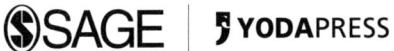

Los Angeles | London | New Delhi
Singapore | Washington DC | Melbourne

First published in 2016 by

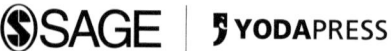

SAGE Publications India Pvt Ltd
B1/I-1 Mohan Cooperative Industrial Area
Mathura Road, New Delhi 110 044, India
www.sagepub.in

YODA Press
268 AC Vasant Kunj
New Delhi 110070
www.yodapress.co.in

SAGE Publications Inc
2455 Teller Road
Thousand Oaks, California 91320, USA

SAGE Publications Ltd
1 Oliver's Yard, 55 City Road
London EC1Y 1SP, United Kingdom

SAGE Publications Asia-Pacific Pte Ltd
3 Church Street
#10-04 Samsung Hub
Singapore 049483

Published by Vivek Mehra for SAGE Publications India Pvt Ltd, typeset in 10/13 pt Times New Roman by Zaza Eunice, Hosur, Tamil Nadu, India and printed at Chaman Enterprises, New Delhi

Library of Congress Cataloging-in-Publication Data Available

ISBN: 978-93-515-0891-5 (HB)

SAGE YODA Team: Neha Sharma, Arpita Das and Sonjuhi Negi

Contents

Preface

Publishing a volume of one's collected essays is an occasion for reconsideration of the trajectory of a scholarly career. In this case, *Refractions of Islam in India* gathers three decades of studies focusing on South Asian Sufism, and on Muslim reflections on the culture and religions of India. To my mind, and in my experience, this more than millennial tradition cannot be explained as the encounter of two separate cultures, notwithstanding the exclusivist claims underlying the partition of India from Pakistan, and the consequent acceleration of the politics of communalism. A thorough consideration of the historical and cultural dossier prior to the ascendancy of European colonialism tells a different tale; in this narration, religion was not a separate identity, but a presence suffusing the rest of life, like light refracted in amber or glass. So striking is the lack of a sense of foreignness that it takes an effort to avoid reading contemporary conflicts into these texts from centuries ago. This is not to say that there were no articulations of difference in pre-modern India; indeed, there were and are countless locations of identity defined along the lines of faith and devotion, caste and ethnicity, class and status. But the modern obsession with a binary opposition between Islam and Hinduism (or Buddhism) is remarkably inadequate to explain the rich and complex interactions that characterized much of what we now call South Asian Islam.[1]

My initial engagement with scholarship on Islam in South Asia took place after my college years; though I had been introduced to Islam in

---

[1] Barbara D. Metcalf, "Too Little and Too Much: Reflections on Muslims in the History of India," The Journal of Asian Studies, 54/4 (1995), pp. 951–967.

an introductory course by Laurence Berman at Stanford in 1969, I first encountered India in 1973, and a stop in a Bombay bookstore yielded the discovery of K. A. Nizami's *The Life and Times of Shaikh Farid-u'd-Din Ganj-i Shakar.* That densely written biography of a Sufi master of the Chishti order was my first exposure to the scholarly literature on Indian Sufism. At the same time, I became persuaded that learning Persian was a priority, at first to read the poetry of Rumi and Hafiz. That commitment led me to a doctoral program in Islamic studies at Harvard University, where I had the good fortune to study with Annemarie Schimmel, the doyenne of Sufi studies in the late twentieth century, and other outstanding professors. Arabic now claimed my time as much as Persian.

When it came time to undertake the dissertation, I was planning to do research in Iran with the help of a Fulbright-Hays doctoral fellowship, in the library attached to the shrine of Imam Reza in Mashhad. But it was the fall of 1978, and the Iranian revolution made that impossible. On the advice of Bruce Lawrence, who later became my close friend and collaborator, I went instead to Aligarh; there I studied with the outstanding historian K. A. Nizami, who introduced me to the full range of manuscript sources for the history of Islamic culture in India; he also encouraged me to think more about social history, and he insisted that I learn Urdu. The tour of libraries and archives that year provided me with a stock of materials that would take years to analyze. I now had a small library of homemade microfilms of manuscripts, along with pages of Persian and Arabic texts copied out by hand (mostly by me, though it was necessary in those days to hire a copyist occasionally). I returned to India for postdoctoral work in 1981, and spent a year doing research in Pakistan in 1986. While travel beckoned elsewhere in subsequent years, two book-length studies on South Asian Islam emerged from that period: *Eternal Garden* (1992), on the Chishti shrines of Khuldabad, and *Sufi Martyrs of Love* (2002), a comprehensive work on the Chishti Sufi order, co-authored with Bruce Lawrence. It was also during that time that I began to work seriously on the problem of Arabic and Persian texts on yoga, beginning with a research tour in Turkey in 1991.

In reflecting on this body of research, it strikes me that the salient method I have chosen time and again is to begin with a text that does not fit conventional expectations. Close readings and comparisons with parallel texts indicate the gaps that are not explained by ideologies or abstract generalizations. The texture of the text (if one may use such a phrase) is properly revealed when in effect one concentrates on seeing through its dense lexical foliage to the context beyond.

Sufi hagiography is a particularly fascinating subject, yet it offers peculiar challenges of its own. The authors of these texts extolling the virtues of the saints are often so skillful that they succeed in casting a veil of enchantment upon the reader, who then feels called upon to replicate the strategy and rhetoric of the original source. Strong analysis is necessary to resist the powerful seductions of this rich literary form. Following a diachronic historical trajectory in the biographical tradition offers the opportunity to clarify the context of the execution of Mas`ud Bakk for heresy in the fourteenth century ("From Hagiography to Martyrology"). Measuring sayings quoted in Chishti circles against canonical hadith allows the reader to gauge the extent to which rhetorical inflation of authority takes place ("The Interpretation of the Classical Sufi Tradition in India"). The question of the coherence or consistency of spiritual practice within a Sufi order, which preoccupied me and Bruce Lawrence in *Sufi Martyrs of Love*, unfolded the changing emphases within the Shattari order in response to external inquisition ("Persecution and Circumspection"). Sometimes hagiographical description provides the best examples of the intimacy and reverence that great Sufi teachers inspired in their followers ("Conversations of Sufi Saints," "The Daily Life of a Saint"). Lives of the saints can also provide surprises, as in Dara Shikoh's biography of Ahmad Sirhindi ("Lives of Sufi Saints"); while a superficial nationalist historiography places these two figures in opposite ideological camps, it is striking to see that Dara Shikoh, a Qadiri, defends the sainthood of the Naqshbandi master Ahmad Sirhindi, on the grounds that the latter performed genuine miracles.

Some sources are rich in revelations that overturn stereotypes. Such is the case with the magnificent eighteenth-century Arabic compendium by Ghulam Ali "Azad" Bilgrami, known as *Subhat al-marjan fi athat Hindustan – The Coral Rosary on Indian Antiquities*. Three of the essays in this book draw upon that extraordinary work. The first section provides astonishing details from Islamic hadith literature about the descent of Adam from Paradise to earth – landing on Sri Lanka, with powerful implications for claiming "India as a Sacred Islamic Land." The second section, an extensive series of biographies of Indian Muslim scholars, provides the baseline for "Reconfiguring South Asian Islam" when compared with nineteenth century Urdu sources (the twentieth-century extension of this topic is discussed in "Islam and Sufism in Contemporary South Asia"). Finally, the fourth section, on the types of lovers praised in Hindi poetry, presents a showcase for literary ingenuity, as Azad provides illustrations of these different lovers with examples from classical Arabic poetry and his own Arabic compositions. I invite my scholarly colleagues to take up the challenge of analyzing the complex third section, where Azad undertakes a comparative exploration of Indian and Arabic rhetorical figures.

Yet the bulk of the essays in this volume are focused on a different subject, the varying strategies and interpretive approaches taken by Muslims in their discussions of Indian religious practices, particularly those associated with yoga. This is a deep and intractable problem, inextricably entwined with the origins of Orientalism. For it was at the very moment when Sufism was discovered by Sir William Jones in the 1790s, that he simultaneously announced its dependence upon Indian mysticism – for were not all oriental religions ultimately one, in the great mysterious East? The hostility towards Islam exhibited by most early European scholars, when combined with their enthusiastic admiration of Sufism, led irresistibly to the conclusion that Sufism must be based on foreign influence. This mechanistic argument has proved to be surprisingly enduring, despite a lack of historical evidence to test it. No doubt this Orientalist legacy aroused my curiosity, leading me to undertake my first examination of the most important Arabic text on yoga, the Arabic version of the now lost *Amrtakunda* or *The Pool of Nectar.* My discovery of the complex structure of this work, including extensive quotations from the illuminationist philosopher Suhrawardi, and a narration from the Hymn of the Soul from the Gnostic Acts of Thomas, only indicated the tip of the iceberg. While this particular example of Muslim engagement with yoga turned out to be surprisingly widespread, it was far from being a significant source of the Sufi tradition. If it was no longer possible to maintain the ridiculous assertion that all of Islamic mysticism derived from Hinduism, the question remained – how was one to understand the reflections on yogic practice that are to be found in Sufi texts?

A series of articles followed on Muslim interpreters of Hinduism, looking into the Persian translation of the *Amrtakunda* ("Sufism and Yoga") as well as a historical text demonstrating the admiration of Muslim visitors for the Hindu and Buddhist caves of Ellora ("Admiring the Works of the Ancients"). More detailed studies followed on the yogic material, including a major essay attempting to survey the translations of the *Amrtakunda* into Arabic, Persian, Turkish, and Urdu ("The Islamization of Yoga"). In another programmatic article ("Muslim Studies of Hinduism?"), I attempted to lay out a program of research for studying the long history of Persian translations of Sanskrit texts, and I also proposed a model for understanding the connections between religious traditions, not through mechanical notions of influence, but in terms of active appropriation, resistance, and reinterpretation ("Situating Sufism and Yoga").

Yet many unresolved questions remained, and clues had to be followed in a whole series of separate textual explorations. These include a widely circulated work on yoga, credited to the founding figure of the Chishti order ("Two Versions of a Persian Text on Yoga and Cosmology, Attributed to Shaykh Mu`in al-Din Chishti"). The Gnostic "Hymn of the Pearl," previously unknown in Islamicate languages, was presented in a multilingual edition from the Arabic, Persian, Turkish, and Urdu translations of the *Amrtakunda* ("Fragmentary Versions of the Apocryphal 'Hymn of the Pearl'"). Encounters of Muslims with yogis were discussed ("Accounts of Yogis in Arabic and Persian Historical and Travel Texts"). A Mughal era Persian treatise on Indian philosophy, often ascribed to the poet Fayzi, was introduced and analyzed in relation to Illuminationist (*ishraqi*) thought ("Fayzi's Illuminationist Interpretation of Vedanta"). An important early Persian text, *The Fifty Verses of Kamarupa*, was explored as one of the main sources known to Muslim scholars for practices of divination by breath and summoning yogini goddesses ("Being Careful with the Goddess: Yoginis in Persian and Arabic Texts"). The earliest summary of those yoga-related practices was translated from a Persian encyclopedia ("A 14th-Century Persian Account of Breath Control and Meditation"). And a nineteenth-century Arabic treatment of yogis as a subset of the Shattari Sufi order also was presented ("Traces of Šattari Sufism and Yoga in North Africa"). Other recent articles offered a Hindu secretary's use of Islamicate philosophy to defend Vedantic metaphysics ("A Persian Philosophical Defense of Vedanta") and a broader essay on Muslim thinkers' engagement with Indian religions in terms of universalist perspectives ("The Limits of Universalism in Islamic Thought: The Case of Indian Religions"). All these articles used specific examples of documented interactions of Muslim intellectuals with Hindu themes and practices, setting up an archive that complicates any abstract generalizations about Islam and Hinduism.

The articles included here are in general reproduced as they were written, with minor editing and correction. Yet they are far from being the last word on the subject of Islam in South Asia. Attentive readers will notice that I have been promising to release my edition and translation of the Arabic translation of *The Pool of Nectar* for well over twenty years, but it has not yet been delivered. There are plenty of excuses for that delay, mainly based on the need to unravel the immensely complex threads of the literary transmission of yogic teachings in Sufi circles. Recent discoveries, including some generously communicated to me by Kazuyo Sakaki, have altered the picture I initially sketched of this intricate literary problem. In recent years, the formation of the international scholarly project known as Perso-Indica (http://www.perso-indica.net/), aimed at tracking and analyzing the vast translation movement from Sanskrit into Persian, has also made possible a much more sophisticated approach to this inter-cultural activity. The new tools and perspectives provided by this project have enabled me to move beyond the Orientalist obsession with "origins," focusing instead on cultural translation as a form of reception history. I hope to provide readers with some new analyses of Muslim interaction with the religions of India in the near future.

The pleasant duty remains to thank the many colleagues without whose assistance these studies would never have seen the light of day. I particularly want to thank Arpita Das, publisher of Yoda Press, who proposed this publication in the first place; and then several UNC doctoral students, including Brian Coussens for valuable editing, Micah Hughes for handling permissions, and Matthew Lynch for indexing. Let me also express here my gratitude to the many friends and scholars who have encouraged this work over the years, notably David Gilmartin, the late John Richards, Zia Inayat Khan, Omid Safi, Munis Faruqui, Nalini Delvoye, F. Canguzel Zulfikar, Supriya Gandhi, Muzaffar Alam,

Fabrizio Speziale, Francis Robinson, Charlotte de Blois, the late Samina Quraeshi, Eva Orthmann, Scott Kugle, David White, James Mallinson, Sunil Kumar, Mohamed Tavakoli-Targhi, and Debra Diamond. Above all, I want to thank my friend and collaborator, Bruce Lawrence, for the irreplaceable conversations that have sustained an intellectual project over more than three decades; this volume is dedicated to him.

Carl W. Ernst
Chapel Hill NC
25 January 2016

Acknowledgments

Permission is gratefully acknowledged for the reprint of these articles and book chapters, as indicated below.

"From Hagiography to Martyrology: Conflicting Testimonies to a Sufi Martyr of the Delhi Sultanate." *History of Religions* XXIV (May, 1985), pp. 308–27. Reprinted with permission of University of Chicago Press.

"India as a Sacred Islamic Land," "Lives of Sufi Saints," and "Conversations of Sufi Saints." In *Religions of India in Practice*, ed. Donald S. Lopez, Jr., Princeton Readings in Religions, 1 (Princeton University Press, 1995), pp. 556–64, pp. 495–512, pp. 513–17. Reprinted with permission of Princeton University Press.

"The Interpretation of the Classical Sufi Tradition in India: The Shama'il al-atqiya' of Rukn al-Din Kashani." *Sufi* 22 (1994), pp. 5–10. Reprinted with permission of the editor.

"Persecution and Circumspection in the Shattari Sufi Order." In *Islamic Mysticism Contested: Thirteen Centuries of Controversies & Polemics*, ed. Fred De Jong and Berndt Radtke, Islamic History and Civilization: Studies and Texts, 29 (Leiden: Brill, 1999), pp. 416–35. Reprinted with permission from Koninklijke Brill NV.

"The Daily Life of a Saint, Ahmad Sirhindi (d. 1624), by Badr al-Din Sirhindi," in *Islam in South Asia in Practice*, ed. Barbara D. Metcalf (Princeton: Princeton University Press, 2009), pp. 158–65. Reprinted with permission of Princeton University Press.

East 30/3 (2010), pp. 156–64. Copyright 2010, Duke University Press. Reprinted by permission.

"The Limits of Universalism in Islamic Thought: The Case of Indian Religions." *Muslim World* 101 (January 2011), pp. 1–19. Reprinted with permission from John Wiley and Sons.

"A Fourteenth-Century Persian Account of Breath Control and Meditation." In *Yoga in Practice*, ed. David Gordon White, Princeton Readings in Religions (Princeton: Princeton University Press, 2011), pp. 133–39. Reprinted with permission of Princeton University Press.

PART 1
Sufism and Islam in South Asia

1

From Hagiography to Martyrology

Conflicting Testimonies to a Sufi Martyr of the Delhi Sultanate*

Martyrdom is the final resort of the weak against the powerful. It is an act of truth performed without regard for one's life. As Cardinal Danielou observed, "Martyrdom is ... the archetypal form of conflict with evil, the summit of Christian sanctity through conformation to Christ, and ... the official proclamation of the Gospel to the accredited representatives of the earthly city."[1] The Islamic world has also had martyrs who resisted tyranny and injustice at any cost, from Muhammad's grandson Husayn to the self-sacrificing warriors who sought paradise through battle. Just as the Christian world created a formidable literature on martyrdom, so too there are traditions of Islamic martyrology. Important insights into the nature and development of this mode of sacred biography can be gained by analyzing the total literacy tradition that has grown up around a martyr, in century on century of religious reflection. The case of Mas`ud Bakk, a Sufi mystic put to death in India in the late fourteenth century by Firuz Shah Tughluq, is a striking example of the growth of

---

* Portions of the research for this article were supported by a Fulbright-Hays grant for doctoral dissertation research abroad (1978–79) and a senior research fellowship from the American Institute of Indian Studies (1981–82).
[1] Jean Danielou, *The Lord of History: Reflections on the Inner Meaning of History*, trans. Nigel Abercrombie (Chicago: Henry Regnery, 1958), p. 13.

a martyrology. Sufi biographers initially avoided any reference to the execution of this man and presented instead Mas`ud's most admirable qualities to form a portrait consistent with the normative paradigms of moderate Sufism. Later hagiographers gradually inserted references to Mas`ud's martyrdom into his biography, until eventually his trial and execution became the subject of a dramatic martyrology. The transformation of Mas`ud Bakk's biography was strongly influenced by the model of al-Husayn ibn Mansur al-Hallaj (d. 922), the early Sufi martyr of Baghdad; Hallaj, with his ecstatic utterances, had become a symbol of the intoxicated saint and martyr, in contrast to the standard Islamic hagiographic paradigm, based on adherence to legal and ethical norms. The way in which the hagiographies gradually accepted the image of the martyr reveals a tension between paradigms in the Sufi biographical tradition and, incidentally, contrasts with the historical interests of the court and legal circles; it demonstrates, in addition, the extraordinary influence of the model of Hallaj on Sufi martyrology.

HAGIOGRAPHY AND MARTYROLOGY IN ISLAMIC HISTORIOGRAPHY

In attempting to describe the different modes of biography in Islamic historiography, it will be helpful to adopt some of the genre categories that have been so well developed by the Bollandists and their successors in the study of the biographies of Christian saints and martyrs.[2] The *vita* or hagiography is the record of an exemplary life, held up as a model for the imitation of the faithful. The *passio* or martyrology, on the other hand, is the dramatic account of conflict with secular authorities, resulting in persecution, trial, and death; this death is not a defeat, however, but a testimony to indestructible faith in God and often brings about the downfall of the martyr's persecutors. Both types of Christian biography are in

---

[2] Rene Aigrain, *L'Hagiographie: Ses sources, ses methodes, son histoire* (Paris: Bloud & Gay, 1953); Hippolyte Delehaye, *The Legends of the Saints*, trans. Donald Attwater (New York: Fordham University Press, 1962), and *Les Passions des martyrs et les genres littéraires* (Brussels: Société des Bollandistes, 1921); Peter Brown, *The Cult of the Saints: Its Rise and Function in Latin Christianity* (Chicago: University of Chicago Press, 1980); Charles F. Altmann, "Two Types of Opposition and the Structure of Latin Saints' Lives," *Medievalia et Humanistica*, n.s., no. 6, *Medieval Hagiography and Romance* (Cambridge: Cambridge University Press, 1975), pp. 1–11.

some sense imitations of the life of Jesus but with different emphases; the hagiography stresses attaining the highest degree of virtue while the martyrology focuses on the direct opposition between good and evil. Christian martyrology is historically the predecessor of hagiography and ultimately derives from the liturgies associated with the feasts of the martyrs and the stories that were to be read out (*legenda*) on those occasions. It was only after the Christianization of the Roman Empire that hagiography began to evolve into a separate genre, as a suitable model for imitation in a Christian society.

The various forms of Islamic biographical literature are also essentially paradigmatic, and their roots, naturally enough, are to be found in the study of the life of the Prophet Muhammad. The life of the Prophet or *Sira* by Ibn Ishaq (d. 768) is the earliest surviving example of this genre. Its construction includes various elements of biblical legend, Arab oral epic, and accounts of the military actions (*maghazi*) of the Prophet, but the most distinctive aspect of the *Sira* is its reliance on hadith, the oral reports of the sayings and deeds of the Prophet.[3] Since the Prophet's life was exemplary, hadith took on a paradigmatic aspect from the very beginning. Other biographical writings were conceived of as ancillary to the life of Muhammad. The first biographical dictionary arranged by "classes" or generations (*tabaqat*) was Ibn Sa`d's (d. 844–45) work on the companions of the Prophet; this compilation was oriented toward the study of these men as transmitters of hadith.[4]

The function of Islamic biographical literature is thus essentially paradigmatic; its basic unit of evidence, the hadith, was the source for the *sunna* or Prophetic example, which all the faithful were called on to imitate. Thus the hadith-based Prophetic biography, as well as its supplements, was designed to serve as the basis for legal and ethical norms. Works devoted to the lives of jurists and religious scholars

---

[3] W. Montgomery Watt, "The Materials Used by Ibn Ishaq," in *Historians of the Middle East*, ed. Bernard Lewis and P. M. Holt, Historical Writing on the Peoples of Asia (London: Oxford University Press, 1962); this whole volume is of great value for the study of Islamic historiography. Ibn Ishaq's work, as edited by Ibn Hisham (d. 834), has been translated by Alfred Guillaume, *The Life of Muhammad* (1955; repr., Oxford: Oxford University Press, 1974). Compare also G. Levi della Vida, "Sira," in *Shorter Encyclopaedia of Islam*, ed. H. A. R. Gibb and J. H. Kramers (Leiden: E. J. Brill; London: Luzac & Co., 1961), pp. 547–49.

[4] Hamilton A. R. Gibb, "Ta'rikh," *The Encyclopaedia of Islam, Supplement* (Leiden: E. J. Brill, 1938), pp. 233–45.

demonstrated the continuous history of the custodians of revelation and served to ensure the transmission of religious norms. At the same time, secular dynastic history grew parallel with religious tradition, usually presenting historical events to serve as warnings for moral edification (and, incidentally, to flatter royal patrons). Secular annals differed from the oral method of hadith by employing written documents to produce continuous narrative in imitation of the Iranian and Hellenistic dynastic chroniclers. Nonetheless, even universal histories, like the great *History of the Prophets and Kings* by al-Tabari (d. 923), were still considered adjuncts to the study of Qur'an and hadith. The biographical mode continued to dominate local histories, also, so that the massive *History of Baghdad* by al-Khatib al-Baghdadi (d. 1071) is basically a long series of biographies of both secular and religious figures.[5]

From the very beginning, Sufi biographical writing was strongly focused on the Prophetic paradigm and the hadith methodology. The earliest known Arabic hagiography was the *Classes of the Sufis* of `Abd al-Rahman al-Sulami (d. 1021), which contains 999 biographies arranged by generations (as in Ibn Sa`d's work mentioned above). The dependence of this work on the hadith methodology is striking. Most of the entries begin with a hadith of the Prophet transmitted by the Sufi in question, followed by a series of the Sufi's own mystical sayings.[6] Sulami's objective was not narrative biography but the illumination of each saint's "words, character, and life-story, as a guide to his path [*tariqa*], his inner state, and his knowledge."[7] This was followed by the encyclopedic *Ornament of the Saints* of Abu Nu`aym al-Isfahani (d. 1038), in 10 volumes, which contained an important narrative

---

[5] An excellent guide to Islamic historiographical sources is Jean Sauvaget's *Introduction to the History of the Muslim East: A Bibliographical Guide*, based on the 2nd ed. as recast by Claude Cahen (Berkeley: University of California Press, 1965), chap. 3, "Narrative Sources."

[6] For Sufi reliance on the Prophetic example, see Tor Andrae, *Die Person Muhammeds in Lehre und Glauben seiner Gemeinde*, Archives d'Etudes Orientales 16 (Stockholm: Kungl. Boktryckeriet, P. A. Norstedt & Soner, 1918), esp. pp. 213–28; Earle Waugh, "Following the Beloved: Muhammad as Model in the Sufi Tradition," in *The Biographical Process: Studies in the History and Psychology of Religion*, ed. Frank E. Reynolds and Donald Capps, Religion and Reason 2 (The Hague: Mouton Publishers, 1976).

[7] Abu `Abd al-Rahman Muhammad b. al-Husain b. Muhammad b. Musa al-Sulami, *Kitab tabaqat al-sufiyya* [sic], ed. Johannes Pedersen (Leiden: E. J. Brill, 1960), p. 5.

element to fill out the doctrinal picture.[8] At this early stage, however, narrative was clearly subordinate to the essential spiritual message. It was only with such master storytellers as the Persian Farid al-Din 'Attar (d. ca. 1220) and the Egyptian al-Yafi'i (d. 1367) that story began to take precedence over doctrinal paradigm, so that we find the luxurious florescence of a truly legendary corpus of hagiography.[9] In both Persian and Arabic, the Sufi hagiography continued in the paradigmatic mode while also incorporating important narrative elements.[10]

Typical of the best Indian Sufi hagiographies is 'Abd al-Haqq Muhaddith Dihlawi's *Tales of the Great Ones*, completed in 1591. Its paradigmatic focus on the Prophetic model is made clear in the author's introduction. He says that since sainthood is a continuation of the Prophetic mission, it is, by this analogy, great beyond all estimation. Thus, the best form of devotion is keeping the company of the saints, or else hearing about the deeds of the saintly, because this will bring about great spiritual concentration (*himmat*) and many other blessings.[11] 'Abd al-Haqq strenuously applied the methods of hadith study to both written and oral sources and said that his work is based on "trustworthy transmitters regarding whose truthfulness there is a clear preference, but it is especially concerned with using the type of close scrutiny, accrediting, testing, and proving, required of the efforts of writers of history

---

[8] Raif Georges Khoury, "Importance et authenticité des textes de *Hilyat al-awliya' wa-tabaqat al-asfiya'* d'Abu Nu'aym al-Isbahani (336 430/948–1038)," *Studia Islamica* 46 (1976): 73–113.

[9] Farid al-Din 'Attar, *Muslim Saints and Mystics: Episodes from the Tadhkirat Auliya'* [Memorial of the saints], trans. A. J. Arberry, Persian Heritage Series, no. 1 (London: Routledge & Kegan Paul, 1966); Hellmut Ritter, *Das Meer der Seele: Mensch, Gott, und Welt in den Geschichten des Fariduddin 'Attar* (Leiden: E. J. Brill, 1955). V. Vacca traces some comparisons between Yafi'i's writings and Christian saints' lives in "Piccoli appunti di agiografia araba," in *A Francesco Gabrieli* (Rome: Dott. Giovanni Bardi, 1964). A number of the Islamic stories have clear precedents in the religious fiction of Hellenistic Christianity.

[10] The vast Persian hagiographical literature is described in C. A. Storey, *Persian Literature: A Bio-bibliographical Survey*, 2 vols. (London: Luzac & Co., 1927–71), 1:923–1067; cf. Annemarie Schimmel, *Mystical Dimensions of Islam* (Chapel Hill: University of North Carolina Press, 1975), pp. 85ff.

[11] 'Abd al-Haqq Muhaddith Dihlawi al-Bukhari, *Akhbar al-akhyar fi asrar al-abrar*, ed. Muhammad 'Abd al-Ahad (Delhi: Matba'-i Mujtaba'i, 1332), pp. 5–7; cf. the similar introduction by 'Attar, *Muslim Saints and Mystics*, trans. Arberry, pp. 11–12, which stresses the "words" of the saints, though the narrative element is dominant throughout the text.

and auditors of hadith reports; it is written down just as it was heard."[12] One strength of a hagiography such as *Tales of the Great Ones* is that it is likely to mirror contemporary traditions without adding the author's own conceits and inventions, although selectivity and, occasionally, suppression of controversial material occurred in these works.[13] The inferior works suffer more or less from padding with ornate and inflated prose style and are less critical of miracle stories.

The concept of martyrdom occurs very early in the Islamic tradition and gave rise to several different kinds of martyrology. Originally, the Arabic term *shahid* was used in the Qur'an to mean "witness," one who sees as well as one who testifies. Among the early Muslims there were several who suffered persecution or death for their faith.[14] Many of these would be remembered as *ghazis* or holy warriors who died in God's cause. But it was above all among the Shi`is that a sense of martyrdom arose, in the wake of the undeniably severe persecutions inflicted on the imams descended from the Prophet. The beginnings of a martyrological literature on the "killing" (*maqtal*) of the imam can be traced to such origins.[15] Later on, however, even in Sunni Islam, the concept of martyrdom became generalized enough to make a "martyr" of anyone who died for the faith, whether in battle with the infidels or while engaged in pious and holy deeds.[16] Shi`ism even developed an elaborate lamentation poetry and popular passion plays for use in the emotionally charged Muharram celebrations, in memory of the martyrdom of Husayn. This contrasts

---

[12] `Abd al-Haqq, *Akhbar al-akhyar*, p. 8. For `Abd al-Haqq's impressive hadith scholarship, see Khaliq Ahmad Nizami, *Hayat-i Shaykh `Abd al-Haqq Muhaddith Dihlawi*, Silsila-i Nadwat al-Musannifin, 54 (Delhi: Nadwat al-Musannifin, 1953), pp. 164–76, 198–205, 283–86.

[13] For an example of such selectivity, see Fedwa Malti Douglas, "Controversy and Its Effects in the Biographical Tradition of al-Khatib al-Baghdadi," *Studia Islamica* 46 (1976): 115–32.

[14] A. J. Wensinck, "Khubaib," *Shorter Encyclopaedia of Islam*, p. 257.

[15] James A. Bellamy, "Sources of Ibn Abi-'l-Dunya's *Kitab Maqtal Amir al-Mu'minin `Ali*," *Journal of the American Oriental Society* 104 (1984): 3–19; stories of the martyrdom of Husayn are summarized by Mahmoud Ayoub, *Redemptive Suffering in Islam: A Study of the Devotional Aspects of `Ashura' in Twelver Shi`ism*, Religion and Society 10 (The Hague: Mouton Publishers, 1978), esp. pp. 93–139.

[16] W. Bjorkman, "Shahīd," *Shorter Encyclopaedia of Islam*, pp. 515–16; M. J. Kister, "The 'Kitab al-Mihan', a Book on Muslim Martyrology," *Journal of Semitic Studies* 20 (1975): 210–18.

with the Christian martyrs' liturgies, which were initially the central literary form and only later developed into paradigmatic hagiography. Islamic historiography reverses the relationship between *passio* and *vita*. The Islamic martyrologies are later and derive their authority from the norms established by the Prophet and the imams.

For Sufis, it was above all Hallaj who served as the model of the martyr. Hallaj actively courted martyrdom at the hands of his fellow Muslims. He cried, "Kill me, my trustworthy friends, for in my killing is my life."[17] The French scholar Louis Massignon devoted over 50 years to the study of Hallaj, "the mystical martyr of Islam," as he subtitled his great monograph *La Passion de Husayn ibn Mansur Hallaj*.[18] In a review of the first edition of Massignon's book, Hans Heinrich Schäder concluded: "He [Hallaj] is the martyr of Islam, for he took the final and unalloyed consequence of the most deeply embedded tendencies in the Islamic religion toward personal appropriation and confirmation of the divine manifestation, the consequence of perfect loving surrender to the unity of the divine being—not in order to win holiness in secret, for oneself alone, but to preach it, to live in it, and to die for it."[19] In the second volume of *The Passion*, Massignon has charted out the main lines of the amazingly wide influence of the name and example of Hallaj in the Islamic world. Among the many whom Hallaj influenced are a significant number of Sufis who were put to death by local authorities. In their understanding, and to many of their contemporaries, the example of Hallaj was never far away.[20] His life established a pattern of proclamation of mystical union by the phrase *ana al-haqq* (I am the Truth), instruction

---

[17] Husayn ibn Mansur Hallaj [sic], *Akhbar al-Hallaj. Recueil d'oraisons et exhortations du martyr mystique de l'Islam Husayn ibn Mansur Hallaj*, ed. and trans. Louis Massignon and Paul Kraus, 3rd ed. (Paris: Librairie philosophique J. Vrin, 1957), no. 50.

[18] Louis Massignon, *La Passion de Husayn Ibn Mansur Hallaj, martyr mystique de l'Islam exécuté à Baghdad le 26 mars 922: Etude d'histoire religieuse*, new ed., 4 vols. (Paris: Gallimard, 1975); *The Passion of al-Hallāj: Mystic and Martyr of Islam*, trans. Herbert W. Mason, 4 vols. (Princeton, N.J.: Princeton University Press, 1982).

[19] H. H. Schäder, *Der Islam*, vol. 15 (1926), quoted by Annemarie Schimmel, *Al-Halladsch. Märtyrer der Gottesliebe* (Cologne: Jacob Hegner, 1968), p. 15; cf. Schimmel, *Mystical Dimensions of Islam*, pp. 62–77.

[20] These names include Hallaj's son Mansur, ʿAyn al-Qudat al-Hamadani in Iran, Shihab al-Din al-Suhrawardi al-Maqtul in Syria, Nesimi in Turkey, Ibn Sabʿin in Andalusia, Sarmad in Mughal India, and others.

of disciples and ecstatic preaching in public, and seeking death before the law as a sacrifice to the divine beloved.

Sufi martyrology was, however, a controversial subject. Hallaj's eccentric behavior and audacity caused many leading Sufis to disown or ignore him, at least in public, for some time after his death. It was felt that lesser souls might construe Hallaj's internally directed spirituality as a license to escape the responsibilities of the external religious law; antinomianism and libertinism could be the unintended result of publicizing his example among the undisciplined masses. Yet it is likely that the Sufis cultivated their own form of martyrology in private, for we know of several no longer extant books on the perse-cution of the Sufis that circulated in the twelfth century.[21] The public norms characteristic of hagiography were not always compatible with the explosive possibilities suggested by martyrology. The ethical and legal ideals of hagiography were bound up with a social system whose presuppositions were questioned by martyrs; thus many moderate Sufi writers attempted to avoid the conflict between *vita* and *passio* by simply not mentioning the execution of Hallaj or by quoting his writings anonymously.

Although Hallaj's spiritual state and cruel death earned him the respect of many moderate Sufis, nonetheless, his position remained ambiguous. There was substantial support for the view that his execution was required because he had revealed the secret of divine lordship. As the Persian poet Hafiz put it, "That friend by whom the gibbet's peak was ennobled—his crime was this, that he made secrets public."[22] The eminent North Indian Sufi Sharaf al-Din Maneri (d. 1380) was of this opinion; he quoted with approval the view of the great Sufi theologian Abu Hamid al-Ghazali (d. 1111) that "the killing of him who has explained the divine unity is better than the resurrection of ten others."[23] Yet Maneri, like Ghazali,

---

[21] On the problem of persecution, see my *Words of Ecstasy in Sufism*, SUNY Series in Islamic Spirituality 2 (Albany: State University of New York Press, 1984), esp. pt. 3.

[22] Khwaja Shams al-Din Muhammad Hafiz Shirazi, *Diwan* (Tehran: Shirkat Offset, n.d.), p. 111, no. 142 (Qazwini ed.).

[23] Abu Hamid al-Ghazali, *Ihya' `ulum al-din* (Cairo: Dar al-Shu`ab, n.d.), pt. 1.61, quoted (with some typographical errors) in Sharaf al-Din Yahya Maneri, *Maktubat-i jawabi* (Cawnpore: Newal Kishore, 1910), no. 15, pp. 21–22.

recognized the validity of Hallaj's spiritual attainments; the difficulty, they felt, lay in the probability of ordinary people's misinterpreting his example, and this problem was best avoided by not discussing the martyr's fate in public. It is easy to see how tension could arise between the models of normative hagiography and enthusiastic martyrology in the case of someone like Hallaj. The natural instinct of the traditional Islamic scholar, oriented toward the hadith-based Prophetic paradigm, would be to minimize the sensational and potentially revolutionary implications of martyrdom.

Nevertheless, India possessed at an early date an enthusiastic martyrology that was permeated with the Hallajian model. As Annemarie Schimmel has pointed out, the folklore and vernacular songs of north-west India are full of references to Mansur (Hallaj) and his fate.[24] Hallaj also occupied an important place in the high literary tradition of Persian writing in India. An eloquent example of this interest in Hallaj is furnished by Qadi Hamid al-Din Nagawri (d. 1244), a close companion of the Chishti leader Qutb al-Din Bakhtiyar Awshi (near whose tomb Mas'ud Bakk would be buried). In his *Treatise on Love*, he has given an impressive eulogy of Hallaj and *ana al-haqq*:

> If you listen with the ear of the soul, every moment the cry of *ana al-haqq* is rising in all things; there is no cry in the world but this. Yet, in the spiritual state of Mansur [Hallaj], when his tongue entered into speech, so much meaning was expressed, that when the saintly lord Husayn Mansur Hallaj— God's mercy on him—was torn to pieces and burned and his ashes thrown to the wind, nevertheless [his remains] voiced [?] and spread [?] this cry, and thus it became well known. But that cry was not from Mansur: "I am I, God" [*inni ana allah*, cf. Qur. 20:12] came forth from the bush, and the bush was not really there. What wonder, then, if it came forth from Mansur, and Mansur was not really there?[25]

---

[24] Schimmel, *Mystical Dimensions of Islam*, p. 75.
[25] Qadi Hamid al-Din Nagawri, *'Ishqiya*, MS 21/192 Farsiya, Habib Ganj Collection, Maulana Azad Library, Aligarh Muslim University, Aligarh, fol. 143b: cf. Nagawri's *Tawali' al-shumus* MS 21/41 Farsiya, Habib Ganj Collection, Maulana Azad Library, Aligarh Muslim University, fols. 10a, 63b–64a. For Nagawri's interest in Hallaj, see further Bruce B. Lawrence, "The *Lawa'ih* of Qadi Hamid al-Din Nagauri," *Indo-Iranica* 20 (1975): 34–53. I am grateful to Bruce Lawrence for sharing his insights with me on this subject.

The Qadi's celebration of the martyrdom of Hallaj and the cosmic chanting of *ana al-haqq* is modeled precisely after the remarkable portrait of Hallaj given by Farid al-Din `Attar, whose brilliant narrative ability has already been mentioned.[26] This passage is clear evidence that the theory of Hallaj's martyrdom developed by `Attar was well known in Indian Sufi circles in the early thirteenth century.

The influence of the martyrdom of Hallaj on Indian Sufism reveals itself further in the writing of Sayyid Mir Mah of Bahraich, a Sufi who flourished during the reign of Firuz Shah. His account is especially interesting since Mir Mah lived near the tomb of the warrior-saint (*ghazi*) Salar Mas`ud in Bahraich, in an environment saturated with the symbolism of holy war and martyrdom.[27] He narrates that once a Hindu army raided Bahraich, killing several Sufis in the hospice and wounding Mir Mah himself. In setting the stage for describing this incident, Mir Mah has given a litany on the martyrdoms suffered by the prophets and saints, beginning with Adam; the sufferings of these holy ones began when God ("the Sultan of love") revealed Himself to them:

> Adam the pure, on the day when the Sultan of love showed His face, was cast out of paradise and placed in the world as a stranger.... [Noah, Jonah, Abraham, etc. are described.] ... The Prophet of God Muhammad, on the day when He [God] showed his face, migrated from Mecca to Medina; and likewise Husayn Mansur that time when they put him on the gibbet, and `Ayn al-Qudat Hamadani that time when he was in the fire, alas, they burned him. And [so it was] that day the Sultan of love showed his face to the author of this book, in the region of Bahraich.[28]

The importance of the Sufi martyrs can be gauged by the fact that this list includes 10 major prophets and only two Sufis, Hallaj and `Ayn al-Qudat (`Ayn al-Qudat Hamadani, d. 1131, was another famous Sufi martyr in the Hallajian tradition). The coupling of these two names points to `Ayn al-Qudat as another major source from which Indian Sufis knew of

---

[26] See `Attar's *Muslim Saints and Mystics*, pp. 264–71, on Hallaj. Compare further Schimmel, *Mystical Dimensions of Islam*, p. 74; Massignon, *Passion*, 2:382–84.

[27] K. A. Nizami, "Ghazi Miyan," *Encyclopaedia of Islam* (1965), 2:1047–48. For the warrior-saints of India, see the suggestive remarks of Richard M. Eaton, *Sufis of Bijapur* (Princeton, N.J.: Princeton University Press, 1977), pp. 22–37.

[28] Sayyid Mir Mah Bahraichi, *Risalat al-matlub fi `ishq al-mahbub*, in `Abd al-Rahman Chishti, *Mir'at al-asrar*, MS 676, H.L. 204A–B, Khudabakhsh Oriental Public Library, Patna, fols. 459b–460a; cf. Storey, *Persian Literature*, 1:1005.

Hallaj.[29] Mir Mah's ranking of the Sufi martyrs Hallaj and `Ayn al-Qudat with the prophets as exemplars for his own suffering shows that he held them in very high respect indeed.

Alongside these enthusiastic admirers of Hallaj's martyrdom there were, to be sure, some cautionary voices among Indian Sufis. This more restrained attitude in public is evident in the advice of Husam al-Din Manikpuri (d. 1418), a Chishti in Bengal who maintained that Hallaj and `Ayn al-Qudat were not good models for novices to follow.[30] In the same way, a Sufi attached to the court of Firuz Shah, Jalal al-Din Bukhari, said that Hallaj's execution was justified both externally as punishment for an affront to the religious law and internally as deliberate self-sacrifice.[31] Although the more ecstatic Sufis greatly and uncritically admired the example of Hallaj, others tempered their private approval of Hallaj with an ambivalence toward the concrete re-enactment of the sacrifice of martyrdom. In the biographical tradition surrounding Mas`ud Bakk, a Sufi martyr who admired and quoted both Hallaj and `Ayn al-Qudat, it will not be surprising to find a tension between hagiographical and martyrological modes of representation.

THE MAKING OF A MARTYR

Mas`ud Bakk[32] was one of the most striking figures in early Indian Sufism. According to most accounts, he was born in the region of Bukhara in

---

[29] Compare Schimmel, *Mystical Dimensions of Islam*, pp. 295–96, 348; Nizami, *Some Aspects of Religion and Politics in India during the Thirteenth Century*, 2nd ed., I.A.D. Religio-Philosophy Series 2 (Delhi: Idarah-i Adabiyat-i Delli, 1978), pp. 198, 273; Massignon, *Passion*, 2:176–78; 4:67, no. 1116a.

[30] Husam al-Din Manikpuri, *Anis al-`ashiqin*, MS 29767 Farsiya Tasawwuf, Sub-hanullah Collection, Maulana Azad Library, Aligarh Muslim University, fols. 53b–54a.

[31] Jalal al-Din Bukhari Makhdum-i Jahaniyan, *Khulasat al-alfaz bahr al-`ulum*, MS 1209 Persian, Asiatic Society, Calcutta, fols. 71b–72a.

[32] Bakk is said to be the name of a town in the vicinity of Bukhara, and although grammatically this should imply a surname of "Bakki," it is an acceptable archaism to write "Mas`ud Bakk," along the lines of "Ahmad Jam" (omitting the suffixed -i of *idafa* in spoken Persian). The alternative reading of Mas`ud's name is "Mas`ud Beg." "Beg" being a title among the Turkish nobility. There is no evidence, however, that this title was applied to Mas`ud, and his name is always made to rhyme (in *saj`*) with words ending in *-ak*. Metrically it must end in a double consonant since in the concluding poem of his *Diwan* his name must be scanned as "Mas`ud Bakk-i Ahmad-i Mahmud Nakhshabi"; cf. A. Sprenger, *A Catalogue of the Arabic, Persian and Hindustany Manuscripts of the Libraries of the King of Oudh*, vol. 1, *Persian and Hindustany Poetry* (Calcutta: Baptist Mission Press, 1854), p. 486.

Transoxania, where he belonged to a princely house; later he migrated to India and is said to have been a close relative of the Sultan, Firuz Shah. It was probably during the chaotic last year of Firuz Shah's reign (1387) that Mas'ud was put to death.[33] Soon after his arrival in India, Mas'ud was attracted to the Chishti order, which, since its introduction in India at the end of the twelfth century, was well on its way toward becoming the most popular Sufi order in the subcontinent. Affiliation with the Chishtis would have been rather unusual for someone having connections with the court since the Chishtis were notable for their refusal to accept royal patronage and interference.[34] The contemporary documentation of Mas'ud's life is very sketchy, aside from his own literary works.[35] Mas'ud Bakk's writings were very popular among later generations of

---

[33] Bruce B. Lawrence, *Notes from a Distant Flute: The Extant Literature of Pre-Mughal Indian Sufism* (Tehran: Imperial Iranian Academy of Philosophy, 1978), pp. 47–49. It is hard to imagine the conditions for the execution of heretics in 800/1397, the more commonly mentioned date for Mas'ud's death. At that time there was no central authority in Delhi, only warring factions and a complete breakdown of order. It was this shambles of imperial Delhi that Timur sacked the following year. Compare Banarsi Prasad Saksena, "Firuz Shah Tughluq," and Mohammed Habib, "Successors of Firuz Shah Tughluq," in *The Delhi Sultanat (A.D. 1206–1526)*, ed. Mohammed Habib and Khaliq Ahmad Nizami, vol. 5 of *A Comprehensive History of India* (Delhi: People's Publishing House, Indian Historical Congress, 1970), pp. 618–19, 624–25.

[34] K. A. Nizami, "Čishtiyya," *Encyclopaedia of Islam*, 2:50–56.

[35] These include a collection of poetry, *Nur al-Yaqin*, which has been edited by Syed 'Abdul Shakoor Qadr, "Edition of Diwan-i Mas'ud Bek" (PhD diss., Nagpur University, 1972); this edition has not been available to me. In addition, Mas'ud is the author of two speculative treatises: *Mir'at al-'arifin*, ed. Abu Rija' Muhammad 'Abd al-Qadir (Hyderabad: Matba'-i Mufid, 1310/1892), and *Umm al-saha'if fi 'ayn al-ma'arif*, MSS 202, 1444 Tasawwuf Farsi, Andhra Pradesh Oriental Manuscripts Library and Research Institute, Hyderabad. Since this article is concerned primarily with the biographical tradition, I am not going to discuss here the internal evidence from his writings for historical purposes (*Umm al-saha'if* is to be identified with the lost *Tamhidat* mentioned by 'Abd al-Haqq since its organization is closely modeled on 'Ayn al-Qudat's work of the same name). The letter purportedly written by Mas'ud Bakk to another Chishti Saint, Gisu Daraz (d. 1422) was probably written by the latter since it reflects the views of Gisu Daraz exactly. Compare Sayyid Muhammad al-Husayni Gisu Daraz, *Maktubat*, ed. Sayyid 'Ata' Husayn (Hyderabad, 1362), pp. 124–33; Syed Shah Khusro Hussaini, "Sayyid Muhammad al-Husayni-i Gisudiraz (721/1321–824/1422): On Sufism" (master's thesis, Institute of Islamic Studies, McGill University, 1976), p. 69, n. 75; 85. The Rawa 'ih or *'Ishq nama* ("Fragrances" or "The Book of Love") attributed to Mas'ud Bakk (MS 276 Farsiya Tasawwuf, Maulana Azad Library, Aligarh Muslim University) is a sixteenth-century forgery; the *incipit* is copied verbatim from that of Mas'ud's authentic work, *Mir'at al-'arifin*.

Indian Sufis, some of whom went to the extent of making talismans out of his writings, and his death anniversary was regularly observed along with those of other major saints.[36] The first unambiguous historical reference to Mas`ud Bakk is in the biography of a Chishti saint of the next century, `Abd al-Quddus Gangohi (1456–1537). Unexpectedly entering a Sufi hospice, he noticed another Sufi hastily conceal a book—the *Diwan* of Mas`ud Bakk's poetry—for fear that a jurist would see him reading it.[37] As it turned out, these fears were groundless, for `Abd al-Quddus later became devoted to the work of Mas`ud Bakk and quoted his poetry frequently in his own writings.[38] Still, it is an interesting indication that, nearly a century after the death of Mas`ud Bakk, his works were controversial enough for someone to fear being caught reading them. At the same time, this incident is a sign of the strong appreciation of Mas`ud's writings in Sufi circles. Royal connoisseurs of poetry appreciated Mas`ud's verses, too; Sultan Sikandar Lodi (r. 1489–1517) had one of Mas`ud's poems inscribed in a royal tomb in Delhi in 1494, and the same poem was imitated by his Hindu court poet Brahmin.[39]

It was only in the Mughal period, however, that a complete biographical notice of Mas`ud Bakk finally appeared in `Abd al-Haqq's *Tales of the Great Ones*, and even this able author remained vague about the matter of Mas`ud's death. The fact that such a popular Sufi as Mas`ud Bakk was not included in biographical works until two centuries after his death (and even then with considerable delicacy) is further evidence for his controversial position until that time. Here is `Abd al Haqq's narrative:

---

[36] Khalifa Khwishagi Chishti (Ghulam Mu`in al-Din `Abd Allah), *Ma`arij al-wilaya*, MS in personal collection of K. A. Nizami, Aligarh, p. 604; cf. Storey, *Persian Literature*, 1:1101; Muhammad Najib Qadiri Naguri, *Kitab al-a`ras* (Agra, 1300/1883), p. 206 (17 Muharram). I am much indebted to K. A. Nizami for his kindness in allowing me access to his magnificent collection and for his assistance with sources cited in this essay.

[37] I`jaz al-Haqq Quddusi, *Shaykh `Abd al-Quddus Gangohi awr un ki ta`limat* (Karachi: Academy of Educational Research, All Pakistan Educational Conference, 1961), pp. 179–80. This incident probably took place around 1475.

[38] Simon Digby, "`Abd al-Quddus Gangohi (1456–1537 A.D.): The Personality and Attitudes of a Medieval Indian Sufi," *Medieval India: A Miscellany* 3 (1975): 52.

[39] Digby, "`Abd al-Quddus Gangohi," p. 52, n. 228; Simon Digby, "The Tomb of Buhlul Lodi," *Bulletin of the School of Oriental and African Studies* 38, no. 3 (1975): 560–61; `Abd al-Qadir ibn Muluk Shah Bada'uni, *Muntakhab al-tawarikh*, ed. Ahmad `Ali (Calcutta: College Press, 1868), 1:323.

Mas'ud Bakk was a relative of Sultan Firuz; his original name was Shir Khan. Once he wore the dress of the wealthy and the powerful, but suddenly one of the divine raptures overwhelmed him, and he entered into the service of the dervishes and the circle of their society. He became a disciple of Shaykh Rukn al-Din ibn Shaykh Shahab al-Din Imam. He was in the extremity of intoxication, one of those intoxicated with the wine of unity, who smash their glasses in the wine-house of reality. He spoke intoxicated words; no one in the Chishti order had ever revealed the secrets of reality so blatantly or acted so intoxicated as he. They say that his tears were so hot that if they fell on one's hand it would be burned. He wrote many works on the science of Sufism and unification. He had one work named *Tamhidat*, based on the *Tamhidat* of 'Ayn al-Qudat Hamadani; many subtle realities are contained therein. And he has a *Diwan* of poems, odes and lyrics, and the remaining portion of his sayings are there. He has also written responses to most of the odes and poems of Amir Khusraw. Although in regard to some of the events of his spiritual path he was not noticed as a poet, some of his intoxicated poetical sayings have been in circulation. He has another work entitled *Mir'at al-'arifin* [*The Mirror of the Gnostics*], for he says, "We became the archetype of the prophet Muhammad, since every heart is in the prophetic archetype" [i.e., the title alludes to Muhammad as the mirror in which the perfected mystics see themselves]. His grave is in the tomb of his master, near the place of Khwaja Qutb al-Din in Ladosarai [Mehrauli, south of Delhi]. He has gone to rest in the manner of an ascetic and a poor man [*mujarradana wa-gharibana khufta ast*].[40]

The account begins with a typical conversion story, but there is a strong characterization of Mas'ud in terms of his predominant quality of intoxication, reinforced by the example of his burning tears; although ecstasy is frequently met with in the hagiographies, Mas'ud Bakk was quite unusual in this respect. The amount of his writings is also impressive and attests to his scholarship; he was in the first generation of Chishtis to engage in extensive literary production. 'Abd al-Haqq is not entirely eulogistic, though, since he discreetly observes that Mas'ud was not always a first-rate poet. The concluding sentence of the biography is

---

[40] 'Abd al-Haqq, *Akhbar al-akhyar*, pp. 168–69. An almost identical but much more prolix account is given in the slightly later *Akhbar al-asfiya'* of 'Abd al-Samad ibn Afdal Muhammad ibn Yusuf Ansari, a nephew of the Mughul wazir Abu al-Fadl, writing in 160, MS 668, Khudabakhsh Oriental Public Library, Patna, no. 57, fols. 51b–52a: cf. Storey, *Persian Literature*, 1:983.

rather tantalizing in its lack of detail; however, the precision of the rest of the account is not in harmony with such a banal generality. `Abd al-Haqq's account is clearly a *vita*, emphasizing those qualities of Mas`ud's most suitable for imitation. Mas`ud's repentance from the court life was especially to be admired, in accord with the Chishtis' traditional repudiation of royal authority. But `Abd al-Haqq reserved special praise for Mas`ud's treatise *The Mirror of the Gnostics*, from which he excerpted a full chapter; he regarded this as a praiseworthy mystical work precisely because it illustrated the universal qualities of the Prophet Muhammad.[41]

In spite of the skillful portrayal by `Abd al-Haqq, the traditional *vita* of Mas`ud Bakk would soon turn into a martyr's *passio*. The gap in `Abd al-Haqq's account was filled 25 years later by one of his favorite disciples, Muhammad Sadiq, in a hagiographical work called *Words of the Sincere* (written in 1614). After quoting literally from his master's account, Sadiq went on to add the following: "In short, he [Mas`ud] was unique in his time in the sect of passion and love, and the religious scholars of the day were completely at odds with him; just as it is said, he went to his death by their juristic decision, like Husayn Mansur [al-Hallaj]." Sadiq here for the first time describes Mas`ud Bakk's death as a trial and execution. The only circumstantial detail in this report is a comparison with the fate of Hallaj, which is rendered vague by its anonymity of source. Sadiq amplified further on this account in a later work devoted to the lives of poets, saints, and scholars of the generations after Timur, the *Classes of Shahjahan* (1636–37). After quoting again literally from the account in *Tales of the Great Ones*, Sadiq included the following appendix: "And they say that the religious scholars of the day hated him, as the saying goes, 'A man hates what he does not understand.' In the year 800 [1397], having approved a juristic decision for his execution, they hung him from the gibbet, just like Husayn Mansur [al-Hallaj]—may God be pleased with them both! After he died they burned him."[42] This version adds two features also found in the story of the martyrdom of

---

[41] Another famous hadith scholar, `Ali al-Muttaqi (d. 1567), also praised Mas`ud Bakk's *Mir'at al-`arifin*, in his *al-Jawahir al-thamina*, MS 231 Tasawwuf Farsi, Andhra Pradesh Oriental Research Institute Library.

[42] Muhammad Sadiq Hamadani, *Kalimat al-sadiqin*, MS 671, H.L. 202, Khudabakhsh Oriental Public Library, Patna, fol. 60b (cf. Storey, *Persian Literature*, 1:985), and *Tabaqat-i shahjahani*, MS 22/46/1 Farsiya, Maulana Azad Library, Aligarh Muslim University, Aligarh, p. 28 (cf. Storey, *Persian Literature*, 1:1171).

Hallaj (gibbet, burning of the body) but adds further to the vagueness by using a proverb to explain the persecution of Mas'ud. For some reason 'Abd al-Haqq chose to avoid discussing the circumstances of Mas'ud Bakk's death, but he must have been aware of these two accounts, written during his own lifetime by one of his disciples. Evidently the public had come to identify Mas'ud Bakk as an archetypal Hallajian martyr, and it was this controversial reputation that caused Indian Sufis to speak of him in a gingerly fashion. Sadiq, however, has transformed his master's paradigmatic hagiography into a martyrology by linking Mas'ud's fate with that of Hallaj.

Later hagiographers paid 'Abd al-Haqq the tribute of quoting his biography of Mas'ud Bakk in full, but usually with a few atmospheric touches suggestive of martyrdom. In 1613, Muhammad Ghawthi in his *Rose Garden of the Pious* described Mas'ud Bakk as "the Mansur of the age," that is, a Hallajian martyr.[43] 'Abd Allah Khwishagi, in the *Ascensions of Sainthood* (1683), made an interesting and fortuitous slip in the entry devoted to Mas'ud's master Rukn al-Din. Although he elsewhere recorded Mas'ud's traditional epithet as being *maqbul Allah*, "he who is acceptable to God," in this instance, by the addition of a single dot, he dubbed him *maqtul Allah*, "he who has been killed by God." After this inspired mistake, it is also worth noticing how Khwishagi effortlessly managed to bring the name of Hallaj into conjunction with that of Mas'ud by judicious quotation of Persian verses alluding to Hallaj's martyrdom.[44] In 1712, the story of Mas'ud Bakk's execution was told once more by Muhammad Bulaq, again with the suggestive comparison to Hallaj.[45]

It was not until the early nineteenth century, though, that a detailed narrative of the causes and circumstances of this execution was given. Sometime after 1815, Muhammad Gul Ahmadpuri, a Chishti master who maintained a large academy in the Punjab, dictated a supplement to an earlier hagiography, and in this he evidently included much oral tradition. Ahmadpuri's account is as follows:

---

[43] Muhammad Ghawthi, *Gulzar-i abrar*, Urdu translation by Fadl Ahmad Jewari, *Adhkar-i abrar* (Lahore: Islamic Book Foundation, 1395), pp. 491–92, 214.

[44] Khwishagi, *Ma'arij al-wilaya*, p. 604.

[45] Muhammad Bulaq, *Rawdat al-aqtab*, cited by K. A. Nizami, *Salatin-i Dihli ki madhhabi rujhanat*, Silsila-i Nadwat al-Musannifin-i Dihli 67 (Delhi: Nadwat-al Musannifin, 1377/ 1958), p. 413. On Bulaq's work, see Storey, *Persian Literature*, 1:1014.

It is related…that one day the revered Mas`ud Bakk was carrying a pair of sandals for his master. A religious scholar met him on the road and asked, "Whose shoe have you lifted up [that is to say, on your head]?" He replied, "I have lifted up the shoe of God Most High." The externalist religious scholars reached a unanimous decision; beneath the Firuzabad fort on the riverbank, they martyred that revered man. Having torn his blessed limbs to pieces, they cast him into the river. After the occurrence of this event, although the believers cast nets into the river's water, they found no trace of him. After much doubt, they found him, all limbs united and re-formed into a body, in the private room of the revered Nizam al-Din Awliya' [d. 1325] in Kilokri [an old suburb of Delhi near the Jumna]. Raising him up from that place, they buried him in the tomb of his masters, near the station of Qutb al-Islam Bakhtiyar Awshi in Ladosarai.

When this news reached [Mas`ud's master Rukn al-Din], he asked the judge for what reason they had martyred him. The judge said, "He affirmed that God Most High has a foot." [Mas`ud's] master said, "… Had you asked him whether the shoe of God Most High was for the personal use of God Most High?"

He [Rukn al-Din] continued, saying, "'To God belong all things in heaven and on earth' [Qur. 2.284], so the shoe undoubtedly belongs to God Most High!" He said that the judge was unable to reply, so then the revered master was stirred and said, "You black-face!" At once the face of the judge became black, and he was ruined.[46]

In modern times, at any rate, this has become the standard version of the story of Mas`ud Bakk.[47]

---

[46] Muhammad Gul Ahmadpuri, *Takmila-i siyar al-awliya'*, MS in personal collection of K. A. Nizami, Aligarh, fol. 18b. The sentence marked with a question mark I have read as follows: *kih idafat bara-yi adna sirr-i nisbat-i durust ast.* In the immediately following sentence I read *shuma pursida budid* for *shuma pursida bud.* For Ahmadpuri, see Storey, *Persian Literature*, 1:1037. Ten years earlier in Hyderabad, Ghulam `Ali Shah Musawi presented this story in nearly identical words, in a massive hagiography of Deccan Sufis entitled *Mishkat-i nubuwwat*, MS 194 Tadhkira Farsi, Andhra Pradesh Government Oriental Manuscripts Library, Hyderabad, fol. 369b. Ahmadpuri's work is more complete, though, and is presumably based on some as yet undiscovered hagiography known to Muhammad `Aqil.

[47] A. Rashid, *Society and Culture in Medieval India (1206–1556 A.D.)* (Calcutta: Firma K. L. Mukhopadhyay, 1969), p. 23, who gives no source. The same account was repeated to me by Rashid's teacher, S. H. Askari of Patna University, in a conversation in Patna, July 1979. I am grateful to S. H. Askari for sharing his insights with me on this subject.

It is remarkable that it took four centuries for a fully detailed account of Mas'ud Bakk's trial and execution to emerge, yet there are reasons that tend to give credence to these late written versions. Mas'ud's excessive veneration for his master's sandals could easily have triggered political repercussions, as can be seen from an incident that occurred several decades previously, involving Shaykh Fakhr al-Din Zarradi (d. 1347) and Sultan Muhammad ibn Tughluq (d. 1351). When the Sultan summoned the leading Sufis of Delhi to demand their support in preaching a holy war against the infidels of the south, the Chishti masters were uncooperative. He tried to intimidate one of Fakhr al-Din's disciples, who was holding his master's shoes under his arms as a servant would (the disciple had just stepped forward to intercept the Sultan's gifts to Fakhr al-Din since he knew that Fakhr al-Din would refuse the gifts and thus arouse the wrath of the capricious king). When the Sultan questioned the disciple's right to do this, the disciple stoutly replied, "To honour him I put his shoes on my head, so what is it to you that I keep them under my arm, and myself hold his robe and silver?" The Sultan, enraged, shouted, "Leave off these beliefs of infidelity [*i'tiqad-ha-yi kufr-amiz*] or I will kill you!" The disciple replied that he would welcome such martyrdom for his master's sake, and the Sultan, finding that his intimidation had failed, desisted.[48] Now obviously it was not just the veneration of the master's shoes that caused the Sultan to threaten punishment, but it did provide the excuse for him to accuse the disciple of religious unorthodoxy.

The real issue for the Sultan was his power and authority, and persecution and religiously based charges were invoked whenever they assisted his program.[49] Prostration on the ground, though contrary to generally accepted Islamic legal decisions, was customary in the court of Firuz Shah, where the wazir would touch his head on the ground three times before greeting the Sultan. Up to the time of Nasir al-Din Mahmud

---

[48] Mir Khurd (Sayyid Muhammad ibn Mubarak 'Alawi Kirmani), *Siyar al-Awliya' fi Mahabbat al-Haqq Jalla wa-'Ala'* (1302/ 1885; repr., Islamabad: Markaz-i Tahqiqat-i Farsi-i Iran wa-Pakistan; Lahore: Mu'assasa-i Intisharat-i Islami, 1398/1975), pp. 281–83; an abridged version is given by 'Abd al-Haqq, *Akhbar al-akhyar*, pp. 91–92. Mir Khurd states that he heard this directly from the disciple, Qutb al-Din Dabir.

[49] Muzaffar Shams Balkhi, a professor in one of Firuz Shah's colleges, commented on the Sultan's tendency to use the law to support his own whims, in his *Maktubat*, no. 163, trans. S. H. Askari, *Maktub Literature as a Source of Socio-political History: The Maktubat of a Sufi Firdausi Order of Bihar—a Case Study*, Khuda Bakhsh Annual Lecture Series 6 (Patna: Mahboob Husain for Khuda Bakhsh Library, 1976).

Chiragh-i Dihli (d. 1356), the Chishti Sufis had practiced full prostration before the master, but thereafter only kissing of the feet since prostration (as in the ritual prayer) is only lawful before God.[50] It is scarcely possible to overestimate the importance of such symbolic actions as prostration and reverence for shoes. If a Sufi, such as Fakhr al-Din's disciple or Mas`ud Bakk, placed his master's sandals on his head, this in effect meant that the authority of the king, or of any other mortal, was of no consequence whatsoever. This was of course a terrible affront to the Sultan. If Mas`ud also uttered the ecstatic conclusion that his master was to him as God, that would only have furnished the king with an excuse to raise an appropriate theological accusation. It is understandable that the Sultan might have reacted violently against an independent and unorthodox Sufi, particularly one who (like Mas`ud Bakk?) was a member of the royal family and hence doubly a rival for authority.

In other words, although there is no way to confirm the very late account of Ahmadpuri, and although it may have been influenced by other stories, it is psychologically an absolutely accurate portrayal of the relationship of the independent Sufi toward the authority of the king and the jurists. The judge's remark about God having a foot is also a typical literal-minded misunderstanding. When Mas`ud said that he bore the sandals of God, he meant to glorify his master as one who had attained union with God, not to assert that God has feet. Yet, it is entirely believable that an unimaginative judge, thinking in terms of the old handbooks of heresy, could have supposed Mas`ud to have asserted that God has a foot (this would constitute the classical heresy of *tashbih* or assimilating God to a created being).[51] In addition, the description of Mas`ud's body being torn to pieces by a mob seems quite plausible when compared with

[50] Mahdi Husayn, *Tughluq Dynasty* (Calcutta: Thacker Spink & Co., 1963), p. 652; Nasir al-Din Chiragh-i Dihli, Khayr al-Majalis, comp. Hamid Qalandar, ed. Khaliq Ahmad Nizami, Publication of the Department of History, Muslim University, no. 5, Studies in Indo-Muslim Mysticism 1 (Aligarh: Muslim University, Department of History, [1959]), p. 157; see "Introduction," p. 29, n. 5. I have seen only one instance of a contemporary legal text condemning this court practice in Sharaf Muhammad al-`Attari, *Fawa'id-i Firuz Shahi*, MS JF 287 Fiqh, Maulana Azad Library, Aligarh Muslim University, fol. 249a. It would be interesting to know the Sultan's reaction to this work that he commissioned.

[51] An account of Firuz Shah's inquisition includes lengthy descriptions of standard heresies from the classical theological handbook, the *Tamhidat* of Abu Shakur al-Salimi (d. ca. 1077); cf. the anonymous *Sirat-i Firuz Shahi*, MS 167, Sarkar Collection, National Library, Calcutta, pp. 129–47 (this is a copy of MS 540, Khudabakhsh Oriental Public Library, Patna, fols. 63a–72b).

an incident that Firuz Shah recorded in his triumphal inscription in the Firuzabad mosque of old Delhi. A man claiming to be the awaited messiah or *mahdi* was declared an infidel by the jurists, and torn limb from limb by a mob.[52] Therefore, one cannot rule out the possibility that, a few years later, Mas`ud Bakk was killed in a similar manner.

Mas`ud Bakk's biographical journey toward martyrology is not an isolated case in Indian Sufi hagiography; an even more remarkable example of martyrdom's attractive imagery can be seen in the case of two men best described as eccentrics, Ahmad Bihari and his associate `Izz of Kako, two would-be Sufis of Bihar. The most eminent Sufis of the day, such as Gisu Daraz and the successors of Sharaf al-Din Maneri, regarded these men as insane or pathologically deluded.[53] They had publicly insulted the Prophet Muhammad, and the Sultan swiftly put them to death.[54] Yet because these two had been put to death for bizarre religious opinions, uncritical biographers classified them as martyrs. An astonishing scenario unfolded in several Indian hagiographies, in which Sharaf al-Din Maneri cursed the city of Delhi because of Firuz Shah's impious persecution of these "saints," and the devastating invasion of Timur in 1398 was the divine punishment for the execution of these martyrs.[55] This story perfectly fulfills the requirements of the *passio*, with a trial, execution, and wreaking of divine vengeance on the tyrant. It also shows

---

[52] Firuz Shah Tughluq, *Futuhat-i Firuz Shahi*, ed. Shaikh Abdur Rashid (Aligarh: Muslim University, Department of History, 1954), pp. 7–8.

[53] Gisu Daraz, *Jawami` al-kalim*, comp. Sayyid Muhammad Akbar Husayni (Hyderabad: Intizami Press, 1356/1937), pp. 157–58; Husayn Mu`izz Balkhi (d. 1440), *Ganj-i la yakhfa*, MS H.L. 3979, Khudabakhsh Oriental Public Library, *majlis* 49, fol. 8lb; Ahmad Langar Darya Balkhi (d. 1486), *Mu'nis al-qulub*, pp. 134–35, cited by A. Rashid, *Society and Culture in Medieval India*, p. 42, n. 160.

[54] Firuz Shah Tughluq, p. 7. This passage has usually been interpreted to mean that Ahmad Bihari and his associate were "confined and punished with chains," so Sir H. M. Elliot, *The History of India as Told by Its Own Historians: The Muhammadan Period*, ed. John Dowson (Allahabad: Kitab Mahal Private, n.d.), 3:378. But the men were already in chains before the trial, so the phrase *bi-qayd-u-zanjir siyasat farmudim* must be interpreted in its historical sense: under Muhammad ibn Tughluq, *siyasat*, "punishment," had become a euphemism for execution; see Mahdi Husayn, *Tughluq Dynasty*, pp. 348–55; Nizami, *Salatin-i Dihli ki madhhabi rujhanat*, p. 425.

[55] Shu`ayb Firdawsi, *Manaqib al-asfiya'* (Calcutta: Nur al-Afaq, 1313/1895), pp. 129–30; `Abd al-Rahman Chishti, *Mir'at al-asrar*, fol. 464a. This material is discussed by Paul Jackson, "The Life and Teaching of a Fourteenth-Century Sufi Saint of Bihar (Sharafuddin Ahmad Maneri)" (PhD diss., Patna University, 1979), pp. 140–41; I would like to thank Paul Jackson for his valuable communications on this subject.

how certain characteristics came to be associated with martyrdom, such as giving expression to outrageous views in public. If, however, contemporary Sufis (and the Sultan!) were right in seeing these men as deranged pretenders, then in this instance the growth of a martyrology has been made possible by imagination alone through a story that flies in the face of known facts. Significantly, Gisu Daraz observed that Ahmad Bihari used to say things like the ecstatic sayings of Hallaj and `Ayn al-Qudat, but the imitation seems to have been only superficial. In this instance, the same process of growth in martyrological legend has taken place, which makes it like the story of Mas`ud Bakk but with a far less solid foundation.

Ahmadpuri's story of Mas`ud Bakk's death represents the triumph of martyrology over the standard hagiography of `Abd al-Haqq's account. The miraculous restoration of Mas`ud's body is an eloquent testimony to his saintliness, especially since it was discovered in the room of Nizam al-Din Awliya', one of the most revered figures among the early Chishti masters. The miracle also serves as a reproof to the royal power that unjustly had him put to death with judicial approval. Just as in life Mas`ud had left royalty behind and sought the society of saints, so in death his remains were cast from the Sultan's citadel and discovered in the room of a master. It is perhaps not accidental that Mas`ud Bakk is not mentioned by any of the royal chroniclers of the Tughluq era or by any of the jurists who wrote numerous legal works under Firuz Shah's commission. Mas`ud had renounced the authority to which they were bound and thus removed himself from their purview. Even the later literary historians who mentioned Mas`ud's poetry avoided referring to his death.[56] The emergence of this martyrological complex occurred at just the time when the royal authority of the Mughals had irrevocably faded away.[57] The accommodations that medieval Sufis made with the throne were no longer necessary. Although the hadith-oriented Islamic establishment

---

[56] Taqi Awhadi (ca. 1615), `Arafat al-`Ashiqin, MS 209 Tadhkira Farsi, Andhra Pradesh Government Oriental Manuscripts Library, Hyderabad, under the letter *M*, fols. 378aff. (cf. Storey, *Persian Literature*, 1:810); Ilahi Hamadani (d. 1654), *Khazina-i ganj-i Ilahi* (cited by Sprenger, *Catalogue of the Arabic, Persian and Hindustany Manuscripts*, pp. 66–67, 84; I have not seen this, but according to Sprenger, it is partially based on Taqi Awhadi); Rida-Quli Hidayat, *Riyad al-`arifin* (Tehran: Kitabkhana-i Mahdiya, 1316), pp. 221–22.

[57] I owe this observation to Richard Eaton of the University of Arizona, who kindly commented on an earlier draft of this essay.

was still very much alive in the academies of Muslim learning, it did not hold a monopoly over the aspirations of Indian Muslims. Martyrology may have succeeded at this time because of its ability to appease the uncertainties of the post-Mughal period and to demonstrate the infallible power of the spirit over all opposition. Yet, regardless of the reason for its success at this time, the portrayal of Mas`ud Bakk as a martyr still retains its appeal. Rather than solving a problem of history, it raises new questions, as do all martyrologies, about the authority of a secular power over independent spirituality, and it affirms the eternal worth of the martyr's sacrifice.

2

Forgotten Sources on Islam in India

INDIA AS A SACRED ISLAMIC LAND

Modern political nationalism in the South Asian subcontinent partitioned formerly British India into two nations, Pakistan and India, along religious lines. This political division postulates, according to some, an essential opposition between India and the Islamic tradition. Before modern times, however, this political construction did not exist. Muslims have lived in South Asia from the first Islamic century, as a result of raids and conquest on the northwest frontiers of Sind and the Punjab and from trading colonies established all around the coasts of India on the route to the Spice Islands. India from a very early period occupied an important position in Islamic cosmology. Accounts in hadith reports (sayings attributed to the Prophet Muhammad) relate that India (more precisely, Ceylon) was the site of Adam's descent to earth after his expulsion from paradise. The first Indian Muslim to give notable literary expression to these stories was the poet Amir Khusraw Dihlawi (d. 1325), who referred repeatedly to Adam's descent to India in his Persian epic *The Eight Paradises*; there he set forth seven poetical arguments demonstrating that India is indeed paradise on earth. On the mountaintop in Sri Lanka called Adam's Peak, pilgrims of different religions still pay homage to the massive footprint variously ascribed to Adam, Shiva, or the Buddha.

The most exhaustive presentation of India as a sacred Islamic land is the work of Ghulam `Ali of Bilgram, better known by his pen name Azad. Azad (1704–86) was a prolific author of poetry in both Persian and Arabic; his Arabic odes in praise of the Prophet Muhammad earned him the epithet "the Hassan of India" (after Hassan ibn Thabit, d. 674, an Arab poet who eulogized Muhammad). Azad wrote biographical works on officials of the Mughal Empire and the Deccan as well as a hagiography devoted to the saints of Khuldabad, the western Indian town where he himself was buried. Azad summarized the symbolic significance of Adam's descent to Ceylon in a remarkable Arabic treatise, *Subhat al-marjan fi athar Hindustan* (*The Coral Rosary of Indian Antiquities*), which he completed in 1764. It is a work in four parts, dealing with 1) the references to India in the sayings of the Prophet Muhammad; 2) biographies of eminent Indian Muslim scholars; 3) rhetorical figures in Arabic and Sanskrit; and 4) lovers and love poetry in the Islamic and Hindu traditions. It is from the first of these four parts, entitled *The Ambergris Fragrance*, that the following selections are taken. From the numerous accounts that he culled from disparate classical Arabic sources, Azad concluded that Adam's Peak is the second holiest place on earth next to Mecca; India was the site of the first revelation, the first mosque on earth, and the place from which pilgrimage to Mecca was first performed. Using the Sufi mystical concept of Muhammad's primordial prophetic nature, Azad described India as the place where the eternal light of Muhammad first manifested in Adam, while Arabia is where it found its final expression in the physical form of the Prophet. The black stone of Mecca descended with Adam, the staff of Moses grew from a myrtle that Adam planted on the peak, and all perfumes and craft tools derive from Adam's descent to India. The modern editor of Azad's work dismisses these traditions as unreliable in terms of hadith criticism, due to their "weak" sources and transmitters; they are, moreover, "semi-historical, based on legends."

While these objections to Azad's collection of hadith are perhaps valid from a reformist point of view, they fail to explain the symbolic significance of Azad's portrait of a sacred Islamic land of India. Azad was perfectly aware of the strictures of hadith criticism about unreliable reporters. He had studied hadith in Medina with the celebrated Indian scholar Muhammad Hayat al-Sindi, who trained an entire generation of scholars and Sufis in the study of hadith. As a historian, Azad sought out eyewitness reports from travelers, describing contemporary pilgrimage to Adam's footprint under the friendly eyes of Ceylon's "Hindu" (actually Buddhist) rulers. Azad's purpose in writing this admittedly novel treatise was not, however, to produce a standard work of hadith studies; he wanted instead to describe "the land of India, which God made the realm of vicegerency (*dar al-khilafa*) and singled out with this distinction." Since it was in India that Adam first exercised the authority that God gave humanity over the earth, it had the unique status of being the first place on earth where human vicegerency (*khilafa*, also "caliphate") was established. Azad even made a connection between the location of the famous Black Stone on the east corner of the Ka`ba in Mecca and the eastern orientation of Hindu temples in India. Ingeniously, Azad concluded that, since Adam was in all essential respects an Indian, so all of his descendants are Indians too.

Azad described India's sacredness by reference to the highest scriptural authorities in Islam, the Qur'an and the sayings of Muhammad, scrupulously citing his sources and keeping his own commentary separate. His work points up the importance of Arabic as an Indian classical language, even in relatively recent times. The centuries of Islamic sources on which Azad drew illustrate an important point that runs counter to current political dogma: for Muslims, India has been a sacred land as long as they can remember.

The Coral Rosary of Indian Antiquities
Part One: The Ambergris Fragrance[1]

Now, no one has woven a treatise in this fashion before, nor could any disposition attain the like of it, so may God Most High aid his trusting and imploring servant with the writing of it—the poor man, Ghulam `Ali, al-Husayni by clan [descended from the Prophet's grandson Husayn], al-Wasiti by origin [from the Iraqi town of Wasit], and al-Bilgrami by birth [from the northern Indian town of Bilgram]—may God work his grace privately and publicly. He included in it what mention of India he found in the great commentaries on the Qur'an and the noble hadith sayings of the Prophet; he entitled it *The Ambergris Fragrance, on what has*

---

[1] This selection is translated from Ghulam `Ali Azad al-Bilgrami, *Subhat al-marjan fi athar Hindustan*, ed. Muhammad Fadl al-Rahman al-Nadwi al-Siwani, 2 vols. (Aligarh: Jami`at `Aligarh al-Islamiyya, 1976–80), pp. 7–57, abridged.

come down from the Chief of Men [the Prophet Muhammad] concern-ing India, hoping from the Lordly Presence and the merciful threshold that its breezes would perfume the horizons and its fragrances scent the coasts. For He is the Protector, the One whose aid is sought, the One who is worthy of forbearance and beneficence.

Know (may God Most High aid you!) that when God (who is glorious) decreed in pre-eternity the power of his Names, his Attributes, and the mirrors of His Lights and Manifestations, He called creatures into being and manifested the Realities until he ended at the uttermost locus of mani-festation. The most perfect of these, which radiates with His noble form, and is adorned with the jewels of His primordial Attributes, is the human race. Its Creator then made the victor of men, Adam (on whom be peace). God chose him as a vicegerent for His sacred threshold and an adornment for His transcendent throne. He taught him the sacred names and com-manded the angelic spirits to bow down before him. Then, He caused him to descend from heaven to earth, on the land of India, which He made the realm of vicegerency and distinguished with this excellence. So this vicegerent sat on the seat of nobility, and his decrees rule until the Day of Judgment. The divine sciences spread, the hidden secrets manifested, and abundant blessings and manifold distinctions were bestowed on the region of India.

But Adam's time is far removed, and his ages are long gone, and noth-ing is found of his sayings in Islamic books save a little bit, and his affair is as the affair of the drop of the heavenly fountain Salsabil. Then, we did not learn of any existing traces, except for a certain number of subjects, due to the lack of materials. Among them is the point that the land of India was honored with the descent of the vicegerent of God, his Pure One [Adam] (on whom be peace). And therefore Serendip [the ancient name of Ceylon] is known as "the realm of vicegerency." And no one before me has applied this term to it, though it was well-deserved, for God Most High inspired me to do so.

The Master Jalal al-Din al-Suyuti [d. 1505] (may God Most High have mercy on him), in *The Strung Pearl*, commenting on *sura* 46 of the Qur'an, citing Ibn Abi Hatim from `Ali [nephew of Muhammad, d. 661] (may God be pleased with him), said that [the Prophet Muhammad] said, "'The best of valleys for humanity are the valley of Mecca and the valley where Adam descended in India.'"

I say, this compares the best spot in India with the land of "the secure town" [i.e., Mecca] (Qur. 95.3), may God ennoble it until the Day of Judgment. And one of the implications of the comparison is the descent of one of the pair, that is, Adam, at Serendip, and the descent of the other, that is, Eve, at Jidda [in Arabia]. Adam (on whom be peace) named the place he descended "the holy mount," and he heard there the voices of the angels. He saw them honoring the throne of God Most High, and he found there the scents of heaven and its perfume, as is found (God Most High willing) in the report of Ibn Sa`d [d. 845], from Ibn `Abbas [d. 688] (may God be pleased with them both).

The Master `Ali al-Rumi (May God Most High have mercy on him) said, in his book *Discourses of the Ancients and Conversations of the Moderns*, "The first place where the springs of wisdom gushed forth was India, and then the Meccan sanctuary, on the tongue of the first teacher unto humanity, Adam the Pure (God's blessings and peace be upon him, and on all the prophets)." The Master mentions this in his commentary, and he says also in his *Discourses*, "The first place where books were made and where the springs of wisdom gushed forth was India . . . and [Adam] performed pilgrimage to Mecca more than once, on foot. Then, he emigrated to the noble sanctuary of Mecca, due to its nobility, and he preferred it to all other countries. He was the first to emigrate due to the nobility of a place or location. And emigration is the custom of the prophets and messengers (God's blessings and peace be upon them all)."

The Imam al-Zahid [d. 1125] said in his Qur'anic commentary, quoting Ibn `Abbas (God be pleased with them both), "Adam descended to Serendip in India, placing his right hand upon the left; and Eve descended in Jidda. And from Serendip to Jidda it is seven hundred leagues." And in *The History of Jerusalem*: "When Adam descended to Serendip, he performed the prostration of thanks and the attestation of the created signs, and his head touched the stone of the temple [at the Dome of the Rock in Jerusalem], for it is the loftiest place on the face of the earth, and the path to ascension to heaven is from it."

In addition, there is the footprint of Adam. The Master `Ali al-Rumi said in his *Discourses*: "The first place where Adam descended was the mountain called Rahun on an Indian island in the kingdom of Serendip in the place called Dujna, upon which is his footprint (peace be upon him). On the footprint is a luminosity that dazzles the eyes, which none can endure to see. The length of his footprint in the rock is seventy spans, and on the mountain there is a light like dazzling lightning. There is no doubt that it rains there every day and washes his footprint. From this mountain, Adam traveled to the seacoast in a single step, though it is a journey of two days."

In the days when I was writing this book, a trustworthy traveler came to "the realm of victories," Arcot, which is a well-known town among the important cities in Karnataka, not far from "the realm of vicegerency," Serendip (may God water it with downpours of rain!). That traveler came from Serendip after having spent three months there. He told me, "I made pilgrimage to the footprint of Adam (peace be upon him), and I circumambulated that place." A group of Madari dervishes had lived there for some time, attending the sacred footprint and accepting donations made to it. They have a leader to whom they are related, Shaykh Badi` al-Din Qutb al-Madar (may God illuminate his tomb), one of the greatest and most famous saints of India. He died 18 Jumadi I, 838 [20 December 1434], according to tradition. His tomb is in the village of Makanpur, a day's journey from the city of Kannauj, which is mentioned in *The Ocean* [a famous dictionary]. The rulers of Ceylon today are Hindus who revere the blessed footprint and honor its pilgrims.

Another point is the acceptance of the repentance of Adam (peace be upon him) and his learning the [divine] words in India. It has been mentioned in the *Testament of Adam* (peace be upon him), "So repentance descended upon me on this earth," as the hadith goes. And al-Tabari [the Persian historian, d. 923] said in his *History*, "After three hundred years, 'Adam learned from his Lord the (divine) words, and he repented' (Qur. 2.37), and Gabriel came with good tidings, so he wept on that mountain for a year in gratitude and joy. Herbs grew from his tears on that mountain, and a perfume is carried to this day from India to the horizons."

Another point is the return of Adam (peace be upon him) from the sanctuary of Mecca (may God increase its honor and dignity) to India, and his choice of it as a homeland. Al-Tabari said in his *History*, "When Adam finished the pilgrimage, he departed with Eve for the mountain of India where he had descended from heaven; then, he performed pilgrimage after that for forty years. Whenever he completed a pilgrimage, every year, he departed for India." He also said in his *History*, "Then, he built for himself a house in India, and God conferred the land of India upon him and gave him its beasts, both wild and tame, and its birds. And He made the rain fall and the plants grow, and He tamed animals for him, some for food, some for riding, and some for bearing loads." . . . I say, I deduce from this that the affection of Adam (peace be upon him) was for India since he returned to it and chose it for a homeland.

Another point is the sealing of the Covenant on Mt. Dujna, according to a tradition. Al-Suyuti said, citing Ibn Jurayj [d. 768] and Ibn al-Mundhir, from Ibn `Abbas (may God be pleased with them), "Adam (peace be upon him) descended on Mt. Dujna, and God stroked his back and extracted every soul that he would create until the Day of Judgment. Then, he said, 'Am I not your Lord?' And they said, 'Yes' (Qur. 7.172). And on that day 'the pen dried up' for that which he has created, up to the Day of Judgment." I say, among the souls who came forth on the Day of the Covenant from Adam's back were the prophets (peace and blessings be upon them), as related in a long hadith ascribed to the Prophet by Abu Hurayra [d. 676] (may God be pleased with him). And al-Suyuti has related in his Qur'an commentary, "Adam said, 'Lord! Who are these people whom I see revealing light?' He said, 'These are the prophets from your offspring.'" So it appears that the Day of the Covenant honored the land of Mt. Dujna [i.e., India] with the presence of a sufficiency of prophets and messengers (the blessings and peace of God upon them all). Another point is the rising of the sun of prophecy for the first time from the region of India since the first of the prophets was Adam (peace be upon him).

Another point is the loftiest and most sublime of miracles—may God inspire me with His beauty of expression, the reins of which no one's hand has grasped. Al-Suyuti said, citing Ibn `Umar al-`Adani from Ibn `Abbas (peace be upon them), "[Muhammad, scion of] the Quraysh tribe, was a light in the hands of God Most High, two thousand years before He created Adam. That light praised Him, and the angels recited His praise. And when God created Adam, He placed that light in his loins." The Messenger of God (God bless him and grant him peace) said, "He caused me to descend to earth in the loins of Adam and put me in the loins of Noah and cast me into the loins of Abraham. Then, God continued to transfer me from the noble loins and pure wombs until he brought me forth from my parents, who had never encountered fornication."

So it is proved that India is the place of the dawning of the Muhammadan Light, and the origin of this eternal effusion. And Arabia is its end and goal, the locus of manifestation of his elemental existence and illumination (God bless him and grant him peace). Thus, India suffices in honor and excellence. How excellent was Ka`b ibn Zuhayr [d. after 632] (peace be upon him), when he said [regarding Muhammad], "The Messenger is a light illuminating God's drawn swords of Indian steel."

Another point is the descent of the Holy Spirit on Adam (peace be upon him) for the first time, in India. And another point is that the call to prayer of the monotheistic community was first called and the drum of Muhammadan fortune first struck in this land.

Another point is the descent of the Black Stone for the first time in India. Al-Suyuti said, citing al-Azraqi, from Ibn `Abbas (peace be upon him), "Adam descended from heaven carrying the Black Stone under one arm, and it was one of the sapphires of heaven. If God had not dimmed its brightness, no one could have endured seeing it," as the hadith says. And al-Suyuti said, citing al-Bayhaqi in *The Proofs*, from al-Sindi, "Adam left heaven with the Stone in his hand and a leaf in his other hand. The leaf propagated in India, and from it are derived all of the perfumes that you see. But the Stone was a white sapphire full of light. When Abraham built the House [i.e., the Ka`bah], he reached the place [reserved] for the Stone and said to Ishmael, 'Bring me a stone for me to place here.' And he brought him a stone from the mountain, but he asked for another. Time after time, he rejected the stone, not being pleased with what he brought. So he himself went again, and Gabriel (peace be upon him) came with a stone from India, which Adam had brought from heaven, so he [Abraham] placed it there. And when Ishmael came, he said, 'Who brought you this?' He said, 'Someone who is livelier than you.'"

I say, I once attained the felicity of visiting the Sacred Precinct and the Noble House (may God increase it in honor and glory). I found its four corners facing the four directions of the world and its walls facing the four intermediate directions. The corner of the Black Stone faces the east, which is the direction of prayer of the people of India, and the direction of their worship. Now it is known that this corner is one of the sapphires of heaven. This is the noblest of the corners and the bezel in the seal-ring of faith, the right hand of God, by which He greets His servants and those who accept Him, who have sworn obedience to God and His Messenger. It has eyes, a tongue, and lips to bear witness to those who accept Him in truth, for it is the repository of the covenants of humanity.

It is honor sufficient to it that the Messenger of God (God bless him and grant him peace) lifted it up with his hand and kissed it with his lips.

And another point is the cup of Adam (peace be upon him). In *The Treasury of Wonders* is a long tale of Alexander the Great, when he journeyed to the land of India. There the king of India sent a message to Alexander about his wonderful gifts, among which was a cup from which his entire army could drink, which was the cup of Adam (peace be upon him), made from heavenly jewels.

There are other diverse matters. Al-Suyuti said, citing Ibn Abi Hatim, from Qutada that [the Prophet] said, "It was said to me that the earth is twenty-four thousand leagues, of which twelve thousand are the land of India, eight thousand are China, three thousand are the West, and one thousand are Arabia."

Al-Suyuti said, citing Ibn Abi Hatim and Abu al-Shaykh, in *The Greatness*, from `Abd Allah ibn `Amr ibn al-`As (may God be pleased with them), that [the Prophet] said, "The world was formed in five forms, in the form of a bird, with its head, breast, wings, and tail. Medina, Mecca, and the Yemen are the head. The breast is Egypt and Syria. The right wing is Iraq, and beyond Iraq the people called Waq, and beyond Waq the people called Waqwaq, and beyond that are people known only to God. The left wing is Sind, and beyond Sind is India, and beyond India is a people called Nasak, and beyond Nasak is a people called Mansak, and beyond that are people known only to God. And the tail is from Dhat al-Hama to the setting sun, and the evil part of the bird is the tail."

In the *Life of the Prophet* of al-Halabi in the eighth chapter, al-Nasa'ı and al-Tabarani transmitted by a sound chain from Thawban, the client of the Messenger (God bless him and grant him peace), that the Prophet said (God bless him and grant him peace), "There are two bands from my community that God Most High will protect from hellfire: the band that engages India in holy war and the band that will be with Jesus son of Mary."

In the *Book of Proclamation on the Conditions of the Hour*, by Sayyid Muhammad al-Barzanji al-Madani, on the mention of the Messiah (may God Most High be pleased with him): "Then, the land will be guided by the Messiah, and it will accustom itself to him. All the kings of the land will enter into obedience to him. He will send a mission to India and conquer it, and he will bring the kings of India in chains; their treasures will be conveyed to the Sacred House and made into an adornment for the Sacred House."

This is what I know of the mention of India in the noble scripture and the solid books. The completion of this book took place on Sunday, the twenty-first of Sha`ban, 1163 [26 July 1750], at "the realm of victories," Arcot (may God protect it from calamities).

Postscript. After writing this book, a group of people from Bukhara and Samarqand objected that India is a land that is the object of divine wrath because God (glory be to Him) caused Adam (peace be upon him) to descend while in a state of wrath. But I said to them, "God made Eve descend to Jidda, which is of the land of Mecca, which is the noblest of places. If one examines it closely, one will learn that their descent from heaven to earth was caused externally by their eating from the forbidden tree and internally by something else, namely, the decree of the Unitary Presence that it manifest its characteristics on the tribunal of existence and bring forth its Manifestations to the assembly of visibility. Yes, if Adam (peace be upon him) had not descended there, who would have brought beauty to this desolation through civilization, and who would have displayed the special wonders of the human race? It is no secret that the children of Adam are all Indians because their father Adam (peace be upon him) was an Indian; he dwelled to the end of his life in India and brought his children there. After they reached maturity, they spread from India through the seven climes."

> The Creator promised Adam His light
>
> shining like a burning star.
>
> India is our father's descent and station—
>
> a true story with a firm foundation.
>
> The earth of India's land shines in its beginning,
>
> from the light of Muhammad: the best of distinctions.

LIVES OF SUFI SAINTS

The Life of Sayyid Muhammad ibn Ja`far al-Makki

The concept of sainthood in Islamic history may be considered one of the fundamental religious categories that has guided the development and structure of Islamic society. Hagiography, the writing of lives of the saints, has accordingly been one of the most prominent forms of Islamic religious literature. The hagiographer chooses exemplary figures from among the "friends of God" (*awliya'*, pl. of *wali*), and the resulting portrait is designed to mirror for the faithful the qualities of the perfect human being. Sainthood is one of the basic principles of Sufism, the mystical tradition of Islam, and lives of the saints were first written down in large collections in Arabic at the end of the tenth century C.E., when the Sufi movement had become highly visible in Islamic society in the Arab countries and Iran. In India, large biographical dictionaries of saints began to be written in Persian in the late sixteenth century, under the patronage of the Mughal emperors. The selection that follows is from one of the best of these hagiographies, *Notices of the Noblest Concerning the Secrets of the Sanctified*, by `Abd al-Haqq Muhaddith Dihlawi (d. 1642). It concerns a Sufi saint from the fifteenth century, Sayyid Muhammad ibn Ja`far al-Makki. After providing brief notes regarding the training, writings, and life of his subject, `Abd al-Haqq gives extensive excerpts from the writings of al-Makki's letters to a friend, which had been written in 1421 and collected under the title *The Sea of Meanings*. These excerpts elucidate two topics: the nature of sainthood and mystical experience.

Traditions going back to hadith reports from the Prophet Muhammad affirm that there is a special class of servants of God, usually numbered as 356 (but here counted as 357), upon whom the maintenance of the world rests, though they remain unknown to the world. These include the "Substitutes" (*abdal*), the "Pegs" (*awtad*), the "Solitaries" (*afrad*), and the supreme figure of the hierarchy, the "Axis" of the world (*qutb*). Al-Makki not only describes these figures but also claims to have met them personally in his mystical experiences (it is noteworthy that his biographer seems to take these claims with a grain of salt). Like many Sufi authors, al-Makki relates the qualities of the members of the spiritual hierarchy to the supreme religious personalities of Islam, the Prophet Muhammad and, to a lesser extent, his son-in-law and cousin, `Ali.

Al-Makki comments on various figures from the Sufi tradition, both from India and from beyond. He describes two famous Sufi saints, `Abd al-Qadir Jilani (d. 1166) and Nizam al-Din Awliya' Bada'oni (d. 1325) as having attained the highest possible station, that of being the beloved of God; Nizam al-Din, whose tomb is in Delhi, was the teacher of al-Makki's teacher. Al-Makki reports that this was confirmed to him personally by the deathless master Khidr, who has initiated many well-known Sufis.

He also takes up the controversial topic of the ecstatic sayings of the early Sufis Hallaj (executed in Baghdad in 922) and Bayazid Bistami (d. 874); Hallaj was renowned for having said "I am the Truth," while Bayazid was famous for saying "Glory be to Me! How great is My Majesty!" Although to some these sayings sounded like blasphemous pretension to divinity, Sufi tradition saw here the annihilation of the individual ego and the manifestation of God directly through the tongue of a mortal. Al-Makki complicates the discussion by reporting that the renowned Andalusian Sufi Ibn 'Arabi (d. 1240) saw Hallaj's saying as a manifestation of the divine Essence. Al-Makki argues that this is impossible, since a complete effacement of the self in the divine Essence would prevent the concept of "I" from ever arising. Using a theological distinction common in Islamic thought, he maintains that the Essence is utterly transcendent, but that it is possible for the divine Attributes, Acts, or Influences to manifest in a human being, since these Attributes (known best as the divine names in the Qur'an) are the medium through which God relates to the created world. The most peculiar aspect of this discussion is the fact that Ibn 'Arabi never held this position regarding Hallaj but, instead, took a view similar to al-Makki's; who al-Makki's source was and how the issue became confused remain obscure.

The final passage concerns a meditation retreat that al-Makki under-took under the direction of an otherwise unknown Sufi who maintained a hospice in Egypt; al-Makki arrived there from India by levitation. The experiences that are described here put al-Makki on a higher level of mystical experience than the early Sufis whose sayings he has criti-cized. Al-Makki informs us that he has attained the manifestation of the Essence and has truly gone beyond his ego.

Notices of the Noblest Concerning the Secrets of the Sanctified

The Life of Sayyid Muhammad ibn Ja`far al-Makki[2]

Sayyid Muhammad ibn Ja`far al-Makki al-Husayni was one of the greatest of the designated successors of Shaykh Nasir al-Din Mahmud [d. 1356]; in unity and unification he has a lofty station. He is among

---

[2] The selections are translated from `Abd al-Haqq Muhaddith Dihlawi al-Bukhari, *Akhbar al-akhyar fi asrar al-abrar*, ed. Muhammad `Abd al-Ahad (Delhi: Matba`-i Mujtaba'i, 1332/1913–14), pp. 136–39, with corrections from Muhammad ibn Nasir al-Din Ja`far al-Makki al-Husayni, *Bahr al-ma`ani*, MS 1235 Persian, Asiatic Society, Calcutta, fols. 86a–b, 98b–101b.

the Solitaries of the saints. Regarding that which he himself has written about his internal and external states, the intellect is amazed. If all of this is without taint of obscurantism and is purely what it appears to mean, then he is one of the Perfect Ones of the age (may God sanctify his conscience).

He has a book entitled *The Sea of Meanings* in which are explained many realities of unity and sciences of the Sufis and secrets of gnosis. He speaks with intoxication, and he has other books: *The Subtleties of Meanings* and *The Realities of Meanings*, which he promises to write, but God knows if they have been written or not. He has other books: a treatise explaining the Spirit, and a treatise called *The Five Points*, and *The Sea of Relationships*, in which is an explanation of the family of the Prophet Muhammad, showing his relation to his ancestors. He makes many claims, but he has verified by experience the internal states that he explains.

He had a long life, from the time of Sultan Muhammad ibn Tughluq [d. 1351] to the time of Sultan Buhlul [reigned 1451–89], his years exceeding one hundred. His forefathers are of the Sharifs of Mecca, having come to Delhi and established themselves in Sirhind. Now his tomb is in the same city. He says in *The Sea of Meanings*: "For a period of sixty years I remained in external knowledge, pursuing the acquisition of excellence, and I was heedless of the Eternal Beloved and the Eternal Goal. For thirty years I have been seeing that which is shown, and I have been hearing that which the ear hears. Beloved! The range of the thoughts of the externalists and their barren intellects are impediments; and if not, I shall sct off in the trappings of ceaselessness to the desert of eternity! The little that I say, Beloved, is that which has not been heard. That which I from the wordless promise of 'and he has the Mother of the Book' (Qur. 39.13) is put into words, and it is unknown to humanity. It is thirty-three years since I have repented of what humanity says, and no object has been attained from what I say."

In that book he explains about the Substitutes and Pegs and Axes and Solitaries and the other men of God, and he has distinguished and differentiated their members, names, ranks, ages, states, and divisions, beyond which nothing could be conceived, and he has said, "I have had conversation with all of them and have been blessed by each, and I have contemplated all of their stations." And he says, "There are 357 different Substitutes, and I conversed with them on the mountain at the source of the Nile, where they were dwelling, living on the gum of trees and the locusts of the deserts."

And he also says, "O Beloved! There is no number to the society of Solitaries. They are many and are veiled from the sight of humanity, although the Chief Axis and some of the Axes know them and see them. Wherever the perfect Solitaries are, who are the manifestations of the aspect of the singularity of `Ali (God ennoble his countenance), they advance on the path. They find a rank by the Heart of the Prophet (and `Ali, God ennoble his countenance, found a rank by the Spirit of the Prophet). When from the heart vessels of the Prophet they advance on the path, they arrive to the True Axis, and from the station of the True Axis to the station of Beloved, which is unity.

"O Beloved! In the station of the Axis, out of all the saints, two have attained the station of Beloved, which no one else like them has attained. Who are those two, Beloved? The first is Shaykh al-Din `Abd al-Qadir Jilani, the second Shaykh Nizam al-Din Bada'oni; both were vessels of the Spirit of Muhammad. Beloved! You have considered well; nothing comes from my pen that has not been witnessed. Beloved! One day I was in the company of the Revered Khidr in a boat on the Nile in Egypt, and some words were spoken of the contemplation of the unending. Khidr also said that Shaykh al-Din `Abd al-Qadir Jilani and Shaykh Nizam al-Din Bada'oni were in the station of Beloved."

And he also says, "O Beloved! Nineteen years I was sober, and twenty-one years I was intoxicated to the extent that I knew nothing, but I was in the neighborhood of Shaykh Ya`qub who was the Axis of the region. He told me of these twenty-one years of mine, so it was known that I was intoxicated for twenty-one years. And after this time, by the grace of the master in his solitariness, it is some years since I descended from the state of intoxication.

> I am a single pearl; I sat down alone
>
> for in myself I have many lights from singleness;
>
> if I am not Moses (Musa), I am still a songbird (*musi*),
>
> for there is a musician within my breast

"O Beloved! Ibn al-`Arabi [d. 1240], author of *The Bezels*, writes that in Mansur Hallaj [c. 922] was the manifestation of the Essence and that he held the station of Solitaries. But I say that if the manifestation of the

Essence had been in Mansur Hallaj, he never would have said 'I am the Truth' nor would another [Bayazid Bistami, d. 874] have uttered 'Glory be to Me' because the manifestation of the Essence is effacement—and what does the effaced know of 'who am I?' and 'what am I?' so that he would say 'I am the Truth' and 'Glory be to me'? 'He who knows God is dumb' in the manifestation of Essence 'and becomes eloquent' in the manifestation of Attributes. In the manifestation of Attributes and Acts and Words, it is right, Beloved, when the dervish is totally absorbed in the manifestation of Attributes. Then, he sees himself by the glory of one of His Attributes, that is: the essence of the possible existence becomes absorbed by the light of the glory of the Attributes into the Attributes of the Necessary Existence; and that Attribute enters, as a Necessary Existence, into the temporal, and utterly ravishes away the being of the possible existence. When this Attribute [one of the divine names, as 'Truth,' 'Grace,' 'Wrath,' etc.] has ravished someone in this way, it enters into his speech, and he says 'Glory be to Me' and 'I am the Truth' and 'Truly God is speaking by the tongue of `Umar.' What shall I do? Ibn al-`Arabi is no longer living. I would have said to him what I said here, and he would have heard that which is certain.

"My words are not the measure of *The Sea of Meanings*. Who can bear it? Where are there still words? God willing, one day I shall write of that Beloved. Beloved! When by the grace of the 'Solitary of Reality,' Shaykh Nasir al-Din Mahmud [his master], there was advancement on the path of wayfaring, from the manifestation of Attributes to the manifestation of Essence—which is the station of solitariness—I descended in a veiled condition. In a dream I saw the 'Solitary of Reality' repeating a silent chant; I entered and pressed the face of supplication in the dust. On his blessed tongue came the words, 'You royal falcon of the field of the world of divinity, and pure one come from the world of power, and player in the worlds of the angels and humanity!' After that a longing flickered across my eyes, and he said, 'This longing is for the light of the glory of the Essence.' This dream happened in the year 811 [1407 C.E.].

"When night came, I was levitated from the town of Khatlan [in Afghanistan] and entered Egypt. I was honored with kissing the feet of Shaykh Awhad Simnani, who at that time was Axis of the world. He also praised me by the same words that 'the Solitary of Reality' had praised me with. He was in his cell, and told me to take one corner. In the room were two men, a Sufi and a student. I did the sunset prayers levitating and performed evening prayers in the company of the Axis of the world, Shaykh Awhad Simnani. After that, for two-thirds of the night I read the Qur'an through three times completely and sixteen of its thirty sections in addition. I looked down and my heart had become light, and it encompassed the great throne [of God], and the great throne became as a mustard seed in my sight. Then, I looked at myself, and the very hairs of my person became images, and I looked at each image, and I saw that it was the image of myself. Then, the images began to be obliterated, and then I looked and all the worlds, the heavens, and the souls began to take on an indescribable condition, and all the manifestations of Attributes and Actions and Influences began to be obliterated. Beloved! This is the very obliteration into obliteration!

"Just then, in the twinkling of an eye, I travelled through seven hundred thousand worlds of manifestations. Then, by an unmediated Word, I heard the command: 'O my servant! My Glory is a veil on my Beauty, and my Beauty is the light of my Glory, and you are between my Glory and my Beauty!' After the Word, I was ennobled by the manifestation of the Essence, the nature of which is only attainable by witnessing. From that time I descended into the world of divinity, which is the place of solitariness. After the manifestation of the Essence, on the seventeenth day, I entered the world of sobriety; I was still dwelling in the cell of Shaykh Awhad Simnani.

> I became drunk with Him, by the wine of longing,
>
> my being became lost in His;
>
> our existence became nonexistent in His existence—
>
> everything but Him was scorned.
>
> When I became perfectly detached from existence,
>
> neither name nor reality remained to me.
>
> When Muhammad became annihilated from being,
>
> who else could he see? There was no other!

"Then, Beloved! After the manifestation of the Essence in the cell of Shaykh Awhad Simnani, I lost my senses, and on the seventeenth day, the Shaykh himself came into the cell and kissed me on the forehead. If the shaykh had not been fully aware of my condition, the very companions of my cell would have enshrouded me as a dead man for burial. Then, I returned to the world of sobriety. This was because of the beginning of manifestation: for some time thereafter, wherever I looked I saw a light that was always with me; this image is the 'hangover' of the station of solitariness, which grasps all Creation on the level of nobility. And all this was from the blessed words of 'the Solitary of Reality' (God sanctify his secret!). For one day 'the king of the verifiers,' the great prince Ja`far Nasir (who is my father) was seated in the presence of my master, who said, 'Amir Ja`far Muhammad is the royal falcon of the field of divinity; he will be influenced by the blessings of over three hundred and seventy saints, the Axes and the Solitaries, and he will be ennobled by these blessings.' And on that day, I was in the presence of the master Mawlana Shams al-Din Yahya [fourteenth century], disciple of Nizam al-Din Awliya' (God sanctify his secret!), reading digests. Praise be to God, Lord of Creation. Beloved! When I was united to this station, I brought these verses to speech:

> Now I say, I don't know who I am;
>
> this slave is not the Creator; then, what am I?
>
> Slavery was obliterated, but no freedom remained;
>
> no atom of happiness or misery remained in my heart.
>
> I was without quality or direction;
>
> I am a gnostic, but I have no gnosis.
>
> I don't know whether you are I or I am you;
>
> I was annihilated in you, duality became lost.

"Beloved! For the lost one, whence comes this speech? Whoever speaks, speaks of the manifestation of the Attributes. In the manifestation of the Attributes, there is speech. When I want to write something about that Beloved, I have become sobered from the manifestation of the eternal Essence. That is the reason; otherwise, what does this Beloved have to do with these words? One should ask that Beloved in prayer that he hold this beggar in the world of sobriety so that I may put the wordless library into words for that Beloved. Beloved! You have considered well and have said goodbye to the house of humanity. Beloved!

Enter bravely, for in this path, scent and color have no worth.

Arise as the whole from existence; don't fall in the narrow path.

Tie a Magian belt around your waist; then, go chant in the temples.

Know of a truth, that in the two worlds, in your path, the only trap is you.

This noble letter was completed on the last of Shawwal, 824 [October 27, 1421]."

The Life of Burhan al-Din Gharib

Another kind of sacred biography is the eulogistic praise of a saint by devotees who are interested in the power of the saint as an intercessor with God. This kind of hagiography is not so much concerned with teachings as with demonstrations of power, often in the form of miracles. Retrospective portraits of saints by later devotees stress prophecies of their coming, attributed to famous early Sufis, and they often emphasize the establishment of the center that later becomes the focus of pilgrimage to the saint's tomb. Frequent also is an admixture of political considerations, based on the desire of kings to borrow legitimacy from the saints by becoming patrons of their shrines.

In the selection that follows, an anonymous author describes the life of Burhan al-Din Gharib (d. 1337), a master of the Chishti Sufi order. It is noteworthy that the author does indicate that the text, *The Victory of the Saints*, was composed in the city of Burhanpur in western India in 1620 and that it was dedicated to the Mughal governor 'Abd al-Rahim Khan-i Khanan (d. 1627) and the emperor Jahangir (d. 1627); this occurred, coincidentally, during a siege of Burhanpur by the forces of the Deccan kingdom of Ahmadnagar. Since the tomb of Burhan al-Din Gharib lay in Ahmadnagar territory, in the town of Khuldabad near Daulatabad fort, it is tempting to conclude that the commissioning of this hagiography by the Mughal governor was at least in part an assertion of

Mughal sovereignty over the Deccan, which is here called the dominion of Burhan al-Din Gharib. The emperor Akbar's conquest of Burhanpur in 1601 appears to be the fulfillment of Burhan al-Din Gharib's prophecy nearly three centuries earlier, and it implicitly places the Mughals in the position of being patrons and rulers over the Deccan as well. The emphasis on the saints as agents of conversion to Islam fits in with the imperialistic ambitions of the Mughals and other rulers and is wholly lacking in Sufi texts of the fourteenth century. The interpenetration of political and religious symbolism is also indicated by the use of the title "Sultan" to describe Burhan al-Din Gharib.

This biography begins by describing a miraculous encounter in which the great saint of Delhi, Nizam al-Din Awliya' (d. 1325), is given a boon by heaven, that whomsoever he entrusts with any dominion will retain it forever. According to this concept, every major saint is responsible for a particular territory around his shrine and has supreme spiritual and temporal authority there. Then, the text tells how Nizam al-Din sent his chief successors to various parts of India to assume their dominions. The main concern now is how Burhan al-Din Gharib is assigned the Deccan (the southern region of India, south of the Tapti River down to the Tungabhadra, roughly comprising the present states of Maharashtra, Karnataka, and Andhra Pradesh). The Deccan had previously been in the care of Burhan al-Din Gharib's brother Muntajib al-Din, but through a hint of Nizam al-Din, it is revealed that he has just passed away. When Burhan al-Din Gharib expresses his anguish at parting from his master, Nizam al-Din sends along his sandals as symbols of his authority as well as a company of seven hundred (or fourteen hundred) of his disciples. Burhan al-Din Gharib then heads for Daulatabad but halts to pray on the site of a future city, Burhanpur, that would be named after him. His holiness and prayers are invoked as the basis for the foundation of the city, the establishment of his tomb-shrine, and for the presence of later Chishti saints in the region of Burhanpur, such as Shah Nu'man (d. 1476–77). The saint's prophecy about Akbar uses traditional local Indian imagery of fertility and power, showing the king discovering the form of an elephant in a massive stone in the Tapti River; Akbar then caused the stone to be carved in that shape (the elephant stone was still being worshiped by Hindus in the seventeenth century, according to European travelers).

Of the actual religious behavior and teaching of the saint, only a fraction remains. The biographer falsely ascribes "many writings" to the saint, though extensive works by Burhan al-Din Gharib's disciples refute this. The biography concludes only by observing that the saint was celibate and that he taught many disciples (both points confirmed by other sources). This hagiography is of less value for the actual life of the saint than as an indication of the religious and political concerns of later generations, for whom the saint acts as a source of authority.[3]

The Life of Burhan al-Din Gharib[4]

In praise of the revered sultan of the gnostics, the Axis of the wayfarers, the cream of the companions of reality, the exemplar of the lords of the path, the sun of the sphere of excellence and perfection, the revealer of the secrets of majesty and beauty, who is raised up on the pillars of unity and stability, Sultan Burhan al-Din Faruqi al-Chishti. He was one of the worthy successors of the revered sultan of the masters, Nizam al-Din Awliya'. He was, for a time, in the company of the latter and reached the degree of perfection in meditation, piety, asceticism, and God-fearing. He has many writings in the science of spiritual realities and wayfaring, and he is the master of the dominion of the entire Deccan.

One day, the sultan of the Sufis, the lamp of the Chishtis, Master Nizam al-Din Awliya' was in the state of joy and expansion, in the intoxicated feast of select divine manifestations of the Essence and royal Attributes, which is the encompassing sea of divine illuminations. He was totally immersed in the sea of annihilation, drowned and absorbed in God, when suddenly a loving voice from the Divine Presence reached his conscious hearing, saying, "Nizam al-Din, ask for whatever desire you have, for it will be given to you, and request whatever object you have, for it will appear from the hidden veil into the manifest world." Since the state of absorption overpowered him, he remained silent. A second time also the voice gave the same cry, but the master did not attend to it and did not turn his face from the prayer-direction of his absorption, and because of

---

[3] For further reading, see Carl W. Ernst, *Eternal Garden: Mysticism, History, and Politics at a South Asian Sufi Center*, SUNY Series in Muslim Spirituality in South Asia (Albany: State University of New York Press, 1992).
[4] This translation is from an anonymous manuscript, "Fath al-awliya'," in the collection of the Committee Khuddamin Dargahjat Rauza Kalan, Khuldabad, pp. 18–25. No other copies of this document are known.

that state, he did not raise his head from the form of the treasury-*seraglio* of unity. Then, a third time, the voice conveyed the good news of acceptance to his blessed ears, saying, "Nizam al-Din, you are a marvel to be without desire, for from the limitless bounties of the Divine Presence and the sublime sources of lordly grace, you hold yourself back." The master arose, full of the well of meditation and vision, and pressed the face of indigence in the earth of weakness and helplessness.

He lifted up the hand of prayer, hopeful of answer to the threshold of majesty, and said, "My God and Lord, let anyone to whom Nizam gives dominion hold it safely until the resurrection, and give no change or alteration in that path." The prayer of the master was chosen to be answered in the court of God, whose existence witnesses and comprehends all existences. After a few days, having commanded each of his successors, who are perfect and unsurpassed in the realm of asceticism and discipline, to reside in a city and a dominion, he dispatched them. For example, in the environs of Gujarat, he put the exemplar of those who attain union and the prayer-direction of the people of the inner path, Master Husam al-Din [d. 1329] safely in as master of the domain; in the realm of Delhi, he honored the Axis of Axes, the knower the secrets of reality, the announcer of the illuminations of the religious law, Master Nasir al-Din Mahmud Chiragh-i Dihli [d. 1356]; in the realm of the Deccan, he gave the portion to the master of religion, knower of principle and application, master of chivalry and piety, Muntajib al-Din [d. 1309?]; and in the domain of Malwa, he appointed the standard of master of religion, Master Wajih al-Din Yusuf [fourteenth century]. Likewise, he appointed each one of them over every clime and domain, and each one over a realm and district. This was because God has made the prophetic faith and Muhammadan proof eternal until the resurrection, and as long as they remain externally alive, they will call creation to the faith of Muhammad the Chosen (God bless him and grant him peace) and convey every seeker of God to his desire. After they leave the station of impermanence for the palace of eternity, until "the day when the hour [of judgment] arrives" (Qur. 31.12), every later saint that appears in these territories is from their giving grace and their internal assistance. Every rebel and sinner who has been of the community of our revered Prophet Muhammad the Messenger (God bless him and grant him peace) is taken into the divine mercy and forgiven through the concentration of their saintly spirits.

It is related that one day Master Nizam al-Din Awliya' (may God sanctify his conscience) was performing ablutions, and Sultan Burhan al-Din (may God sanctify his conscience) was present in the fortunate assembly, rendering the customary service, pouring water from a vessel he held in his hand. The master [Nizam al-Din] glanced at the sultan [Burhan al-Din Gharib] affectionately and asked, "Was Master Muntajib al-Din your elder or younger brother?" The sultan knew by his prescience for certain and realized by the indication of his master and had intelligence by his cardiognosy and wit that the master just mentioned had been joined to the mercy of God. The next day he prepared materials for the third-day funeral observance and attended the noble gathering. Several of the lovers wondered and asked the sultan the meaning of this. He said, "When the revered master's blessed tongue asked whether my brother Muntajib al-Din was elder or younger, by prescience I knew for certain that my brother had passed away because the word 'was' indicated the past tense." After that, before the whole assembly, Nizam al-Din Awliya' (may God sanctify his conscience) said to him, "I have made you the leader in place of Muntajib al-Din; I have made you his successor. You should go to Daulatabad."

The sultan obediently accepted the pearl-like words of the master and put the seal of silence on his lips, but in his thoughts, from the pain of separation from the master, a great grief and bitter pain appeared. From this condition, pain and perturbation began to beat in waves upon him. From both of his eyes tears ran as from the springs of rivers, and weeping overwhelmed him. The meaning of his condition could not fit into the capacity of mere words. At this point the master came and examined his condition and enquired of him the cause of his consternation. He replied, "I will be separated from these sandals." The master replied, "The master will be your companion," meaning, "Take the sandals as your companions." The sultan obediently placed the noble sandals on his head and pressed his blessed forehead to the grace-bestowing threshold. From the pain of separation, the fear of loneliness, and the dread of trouble, however, he reached a point such that despite all his perfect self-possession and control of the reins of will, the halter of disturbance slipped out of the grasp of his will, and from his extreme sadness and regret and his great terror and pains, losing sight of his own aspirations, he could not set foot outside his master's hospice.

They say that a second time Master Nizam al-Din Awliya' (may God sanctify his conscience) became aware of his condition, and his luminous eye perceived that no amount of preaching could make the heart grasp the hem of patience. To his spiritual son he said, "What is the cause of the delay in your leaving?" With weakness and humility, he replied, "I shall be separated from the eternal assembly of the laws of God." When he saw and witnessed his painful, lamenting, and burning cry, then by way of generosity and affection, he gave the whole assembly, with all the noble successors and disciplined disciples, to the sultan, saying, "The master will be your companion." Some say the successors and disciples were seven hundred, and others hold that there were fourteen hundred who came in the company of the sultan. Among the successors, one was Amir Hasan [d. after 1329], the second Master Kamal Khujandi, the third Master Jam, the fourth Master Fakhr al-Din, the fifth Master Nasir al-Din Chiragh-i Dihli, and other masters. At the time of farewell, he honored him with five guidances. The first was the cloaks of service that were entrusted to him in the traditional way from the time of Master `Uthman Harwani [d. 1211] and from Master Mu`in al-Din Chishti [d. 1236] and others, which had been intended for Mawlana Da'ud-i Husayn Shirazi, known as Master Zayn al-Din [d. 1369], for they would reach the latter, just as these events will be explained in the section on Master Zayn al-Din. The second guidance was... [illegible]. Third, "Do not abandon the communal Friday prayer." Fourth, "Do not forget to inquire after the condition of my master's daughter who dwells here." Fifth, "Always remain celibate."

After hearing the five points, he headed toward Daulatabad, and in the year 720 [1320 C.E.; actually 1329], he reached Daulatabad. They say that the sultan, after completing several stages in a few days, reached the land of this city [Burhanpur]. It was a very pleasant and delightful place, and he saw an inhabited village. Longing for it to be established [as a city] took root that day in his luminous mind. He spread a cloth to stand on by the bank of the Tapti River. The sultan stood and made ablutions and performed communal prayer on the stone in the middle of the river that they call the "elephant stone." Entering into intimate conversation with God, the holy and exalted Creator, he asked that in this place a town by the name of Burhanpur become inhabited. This became a prayer chosen to be granted, inasmuch as the news of blessing in respect of the habitation of this region reached from the hidden world into his ear. When he was praying the midnight prayers and was absorbed in recollection of God in the middle of the night, he summoned one of the knowers of His secrets [an angel]. Regarding what he said, the power of God opened up his heart to its destiny; an inhabited city appeared to his vision so that the beholder became astonished at its habitation.

After the dawn prayer, he was said to leave for Daulatabad. The best time of all the days in the environs of that region was illuminated by the vision of that graceful one. Since the groups of scholars and notables residing together there obtained perfect delight and inclusive participation in his pure and eternal authority and his abundantly blessed company, after a few days, some of the dear ones received his permission to depart and returned to Nizam al-Din Awliya' (may God sanctify his conscience). And some remained in the service of the sultan, and today the tombs of the lovers are famous and well known, near his blessed shrine.

After some years, Shah Nu'man [d. 1476-77] was residing down below the Asir fort [near Burhanpur]. The influence of his [Burhan al-Din Gharib's] prayers was manifest. This desert and desolation had become inhabited, and its fortune had been sustained by Burhan al-Din Awliya'.

When the revered nester in the divine throne, the crown-bestower on the face of the earth, the victorious by the grace of God, the eternal king Jalal al-Din Muhammad Akbar Padshah [d. 1605], in the year 1008 [1600 C.E.; actually 1601], honored the region of Burhanpur and conquered the fortress of Asir, at that time he made that stone called the "elephant stone" into the shape of an elephant and made a statue from its internal meaning which had lacked external thought so that it would remain forever the chief memento (of his conquest).

It is related that one day the mother of the sultan ordered him to get married. This presented a great difficulty to the sultan, for the advice of his master was to remain celibate and his mother's pleasure lay in his getting married. That very day he vowed to fast, and he said, "I am fasting. Whenever I break my fast, I will do whatever I am ordered." And he formed the intention to fast for several years. As time went on, the weakness of his body reached such a point that at the time of kneeling and prostration, his brain was disturbed. Then, his mother passed away, and the sultan did not maintain his asceticism [but remained celibate].

For some time, he bestowed knowledge of truth and divine gnosis on the people of that place, and he brought plenty of people to the universal goal and the essential object and conveyed the basis of divine gnosis. In the year 738 [1337 C.E.], the bird of his spirit took flight from the defile of humanity, and in Daulatabad, he built his angelic nest. His blessed shrine, which is full of grace and the first spirit, is located two miles from the fort of Daulatabad.

The Miracles of Ahmad Sirhindi

One of the most controversial religious figures in Mughal India was Ahmad Kabuli Sirhindi (1562–1624). He was initially a successful scholar attached to the court of the emperor Akbar (d. 1605) and was associated with the prime minister Abu al-Fazl (Abul Fazl, d. 1601). He underwent a great change, however, when he was initiated into the Naqshbandi Sufi order under the guidance of the Central Asian master Baqi Billah Billah (d. 1603). As the excerpt below shows, Sirhindi gained notoriety from appearing to claim, in one of his widely circulated epistles, that he was spiritually superior to one of the companions of the Prophet Muhammad, Abu Bakr. Eventually, criticism of Sirhindi's claims led Emperor Jahangir to imprison him in 1619 for a year, and the controversies continued through the nineteenth century both in India and in Arabia.

In the twentieth century, Muslim nationalists gave Sirhindi a new role as defender of Islam against the heresies of the emperor Akbar. This is based primarily on a few selected passages in his writings that are critical of Akbar and Abu al-Fazl and that show a markedly hostile attitude to Hindus in the Mughal bureaucracy. These remarks took on new significance in the polemical climate of religious nationalism, which now tried to read Indian history as an eternal conflict between Islam and Hinduism. The same attitude places the Mughal prince Dara Shikuh on the side of his great-grandfather Akbar because of Dara's interest in translating Sanskrit religious texts (such as the *Upanisads*) into Persian. Curiously, this political judgment is shared by Hindu fundamentalists, but in their view, one simply reverses the evaluation so that Sirhindi becomes an evil fanatic, while Akbar and Dara become tolerant liberals.

The extract given below is the description of Sirhindi from Dara Shikuh's well-known biographical work on Sufi saints, *The Ship of the*

Saints, which was written in 1640. Contrary to the political interpretation just mentioned, Dara does not find Sirhindi to be an opponent, nor does the latter's attitude toward Hindus seem to be of interest. Instead, Dara is concerned to defend Sirhindi from criticism. The defense of Sirhindi as a saint is based on the direct testimony of Dara's spiritual master, Miyan Mir (d. 1635) of Lahore, who personally observed Sirhindi's miraculous ability to read unspoken thoughts. When Miyan Mir met Sirhindi, he decided to test Sirhindi by thinking of three questions for him to answer. The first question related to the charge that he claimed superiority to Abu Bakr. The second question was the accusation that Sirhindi's master Baqi Billah had begun to teach without authorization from his own master Khwajagi Amkunagi (d. 1599–1600); this was a charge made against a newcomer by disgruntled older disciples. The third question was Sirhindi's opinion of the man who initially questioned Baqi Billah's credentials, Khawand Mahmud (d. 1642–43). Sirhindi passed the test. He spontaneously produced the controversial letter (the eleventh in his collected epistles) and showed it to Miyan Mir, who found it blameless. He related how Khawand Mahmud questioned Baqi Billah's authorization to teach and told how he himself refuted it and persuaded Khawand Mahmud of the truth. Finally, Sirhindi smoothed over any dispute with Khawand Mahmud by praising him and attributing any problems to the latter's followers. The text is of particular interest because it shows how different Dara's perception of Sirhindi was from the modem political view of them both.[5]

The Ship of Saints[6]

The revered Ahmad Kabuli al-Sirhindi was a descendant of the revered Commander of the Faithful `Umar Faruq [d. 644]. He was a Hanafi in his legal school [follower of Abu Hanafi, d. 767] and lived in Sirhind. He was a disciple of Master Baqi in the Naqshbandi order, who was disciple of the learned Khwajagi Amkunagi, who was a disciple of his father, the learned Dervish Muhammad. He also had obtained authorization to

---

[5] For further reading, see Yohanan Friedmann, *Shaykh Ahmad Sirhindi: An Outline of His Thought and a Study of His Image in the Eyes of Posterity* (Montreal: McGill-Queen's University Press, 1971).

[6] This selection is translated from Dara Shikuh, *Safinat al-awliya'*, ed. Mr. Beale (Agra: Matba`-i Madrasa-i Agrah, 1853), pp. 339–41.

guide others from modern Qadiri and Chishti masters. He was a master of meditation, asceticism, miracles, and writing. Toward the end of his life, some accused the shaykh of saying, "My rank is higher than that of the rightly-guided caliphs [Abu Bakr et al.]," but this is pure slander and defamation by opponents of the shaykh.

I myself have heard from the protector of dominion and leadership, the possessor of excellences and perfections, who is conscious of realities and gnosis, the most excellent of the age, my teacher, my learned one, my instructor, the revered Mirak Shaykh ibn Shaykh Fasih al-Din [that is, Miyan Mir], who said, "Once we happened to pass through Sirhind, and somehow there was an opportunity to meet with Shaykh Ahmad. In the midst of the talk, it occurred to me that if the shaykh can perform miracles, he should do three things: first, recall for me what people have said about him; second, explain what I have heard about Master Baqi his master taking a disciple without authorization from the learned Khwajagi Amkunagi: third, whether he believed in Master Khawand Mahmud.

"After I had been sitting before the shaykh a time, he gave me a piece of paper he had beneath his cushion and told me to read it. After I saw all of it, he said 'Something has happened because of this.' I said, 'From this itself nothing has happened; everything in here is fine.' Again, after a time he said, 'The same is true of what happened to me; the rest is lies.'

"Then, after a time, he said, 'One day, Master Khawand Mahmud had come here and said, "Master Baqi did not have a clear authorization from his master, since one day the learned Khwajagi Amkunagi was eating watermelon and, having himself cut it in pieces, gave it into the hands of bystanders and disciples, but he did not give it to Master Baqi." Those present said, "The Master [Baqi Billah] is here too," but the learned Khwajagi Amkunagi said, "We have given him watermelon in the right way." From this Master Baqi became conceited, thinking, "He has authorized me to give guidance."'"

"'I [Sirhindi] said, "This is not so, for we have never heard such words from our master or others; rather, Master Baqi used to deny it, saying, 'This act was never done by me, and I cannot be responsible for it. The learned Khwajagi [actually] said, "We gave authorization and you ought to do this work."' At this time some of the older men [present during the conversation between Khawand Mahmud and Sirhindi] also said, "We were present in the assembly, when the learned Khwajagi gave authorization for guidance to Master Baqi." Master Khawand Mahmud then admitted, "We have listened to error."'

"Then, Shaykh Ahmad said, 'Do you believe what you have heard from the disciples of Master Khawand Mahmud? The master is not like that, and I do not believe that of him.'"

All three doubts had passed through the thoughts of my revered teacher [Miyan Mir], and the shaykh [Ahmad Sirhindi] answered them. His death took place in the year 1034 [1624 C.E.], and the length of his life was sixty-three years. His tomb is in Sirhind.

A Woman Saint: Bibi Jamal Khatun

As in other sectors of Islamic culture, women played an important, though less public, role than men in Islamic mysticism. Among the early Sufis in Iran and Iraq were a number of prominent women, and during the growth of Sufi orders, women participated as patrons and disciples of Sufi masters. The following extract concerns Bibi Jamal Khatun (d. 1647), also known as Bibi Jiv, the sister of the Sufi leader Miyan Jiv or Miyan Mir (d. 1635). This passage occurs in *The Peace of the Saints* which Dara Shikuh (author of the previous selection) wrote between 1640 and 1642 as a biography of Miyan Jiv and his disciples.

Dara Shikuh, himself a disciple of Miyan Jiv, knew Bibi Jamal Khatun and held her in great respect. As a sign of his esteem, he placed her biography immediately after that of her brother, before the notices of Miyan Jiv's other disciples; large biographical works, such as Dara's own *The Ship of the Saints*, typically put the biographies of female mystics together as an appendix. Dara describes her saintly virtues in somewhat stereotyped and formulaic terms, comparing her to the famous early woman Sufi, Rabi'a (d. 801) of Basra. This selection, typically, emphasizes her miracles as a sign of her spirituality.

Bibi Jamal Khatun is an example of a woman who independently pursues a spiritual path in a way that includes but goes beyond the normal social role of family life. Her mother Bibi Fatima had been widowed at an early age and had returned to live and study with her father, Qazi Qazin, a renowned Sufi of Sind (in southern Pakistan). Although she trained all her five sons and two daughters in Sufi practice, Miyan Jiv was the one who had the strongest mystical vocation, and all his brothers and sisters later became his disciples and followed his "path" (*tariqa*) or spiritual method. Bibi Jamal Khatun was nonetheless outstanding even in this spiritually talented family, as shown by the vision in which she saw her brother predict the date of his death.

Although Bibi Jamal Khatun married, Dara Shikuh treats it as an unimportant event, to the extent that he fails to mention her husband's name. Evidently she had no children, and after six years of marriage, she lived apart from her husband, who must have died or divorced her four years later. The choice of celibacy was her conscious decision to seek a closer relation to God; her later life was passed primarily in prayer and meditation, and she never left her home in Sivastan in Sind.

The miracles ascribed to Bibi Jamal Khatun stress her attainment of mystical states. The episode of the fish, which became luminous after her gaze fell on it when she emerged from a powerful trance, illustrates the concept of mystical experience as the contemplation of light; the light not only filled the soul of the saint but also spilled over onto an ordinary object like a fish, which was preserved as a holy relic and source of blessing. Her other miracles also concern household items, like the chicken and the wheat that can feed any number of guests and the transformation of oil into milk; her blessings also produce sons. Despite her relative isolation, she evidently had many visitors who sought her help. Her contact with Jalal Khamush, a recently deceased saint, shows how the invisible hierarchy was consulted by ordinary people; they referred problems to her, the most eminent living Sufi in the district, and she in turn invoked God's blessings on someone with higher spiritual status so that he would convey divine assistance to the petitioner. The fact that Jalal Khamush was dead in no way impaired his ability to act as an intercessor with God.

Five years after completing the book, Dara Shikuh appended a postscript giving the date of Bibi Jamal Khatun's death.

The Peace of the Saints[7]

Memorial of the Felicitous Conditions Surrounding the Revered Bibi Jamal Khatun (may God prolong the blessings of her noble breaths).

She is the sister of the revered Miyan Jiv (may God sanctify his conscience), and she is the daughter by whose existence the noble

---

[7] This selection is translated from Muhammad Dara Shikuh, *Sakinat al-awliya'*, ed. Muhammad Jalali Na'ini (Tehran, 1344/1965), pp. 129–31.

mother of the revered Miyan Jiv was ennobled. Today, in the year 1050 (1640–41), she is still living. The revered Bibi Jiv mastered lofty states and stages, austerities, and exertions, and in renunciation and detachment she is unique. She is the Rabi'a of her time, and many miracles and wonders manifested from her and continue to do so.

In the beginning of her spiritual career, she entered into the path of spiritual exercises under the guidance of her illustrious mother and father. After that, the revered Miyan Jiv sent word to her, through the intermediary of his brother Qazi Tahir, to occupy herself with his path. Thereafter, Bibi was occupied in this path.

In accordance with fate conformable to the religious law, she became joined to one of the nobly born and a legal bond was made between them, and for a space of 10 years, she was his spouse. Altogether six years passed that they were bed-fellows. After that, a divine longing and love won the victory over her in respect to married life, and maintaining complete aloofness, she kept herself separate in her room. She has two maid-servants who are at her service in the day, who prepare water for ablutions and other necessities. At night, she is alone in that room, occupied with the remembrance of God. In these days absorption prevails over her. And from the time that the revered Miyan Jiv left his homeland, she did not come to see him, nor did the revered Miyan Jiv go to see her, but there was mutual inquiry, and the revered Miyan Jiv frequently praised her.

It is said that one day a fish was brought into Bibi's house when she was absorbed in ecstasy. When she came back from that state, she opened her eyes; her blessed gaze, from which a light emanated, fell on that fish. From the influence of this glance, a luminosity appeared on that fish and remained. After that, Bibi Jiv said, "This fish has become holy, and when you preserve it among your possessions, much blessing will be evident in it." Until now, that fish exists in the house of one of her relatives, and its blessings are evident.

Muhammad Amin, nephew of the revered Miyan Jiv, said, "I heard Bibi say, 'When the time of the revered Miyan Jiv's passing approached, in the angelic world he met me and said, "On such-and-such a day in such-and-such a month, I shall be a traveler in the realm of eternity. Knowing me to be present, occupy yourself with the remembrance of God."'"

Another story is that often, by the grace of the spirits of the saints, she was cooking a certain amount of food when many people came together. She asked to have a rooster brought, and the first time, saying, "In the name of God, the Merciful, the Compassionate," with her own hand she slaughtered it to make a bit of food, and after that, she would have someone else do the slaughtering. Whatever number of people were present, all were completely satisfied.

They say that, one day, for some reason, milk was required and was not to be met with anywhere. This request was conveyed to Bibi Jiv, who asked for a bottle of oil, put her own blessed hand on it, and commanded, "Take milk, as much as you require." They saw that the bottle was full of milk. They got as much milk as they wanted.

And it is said that in the house of Amir Khan, the judge of Tatta, there were several daughters. The family of Amir Khan, going in attendance on Bibi Jiv, made many supplications and lamentations, asking for a son. Bibi Jiv said, "After this there will be sons." From the blessing of her saying, five sons were born, one after another.

They say that once Bibi Jiv cast a quantity of two maunds (about two kilograms) of wheat into the wheat-vessel with her own blessed hand. From the blessings of her hand, for a year the whole expense of the house was taken from that, and the wheat remained in the same condition.

They say that in those regions there had been a noble named Jalal Khamush, who had perfect renunciation and detachment, from whom Bibi Jiv also had benefited internally. Whenever a difficulty befell anyone or a need became pressing, they would refer it to the revered Bibi Jiv. Then, Bibi Jiv would go to the grave of Shaykh Jalal Khamush and spiritually turn to him. The problem of that person would be solved in accordance with her prayer.

The noble age of Bibi Jiv Khatun is in excess of sixty and she dwells in her own abode in Sivastan, and she has never left that place for any other.

Her miracles are more numerous than one could list, but for the sake of blessing this piece of information was written after the composition of this book: her demise took place on Tuesday the twenty-seventh of Rabi` the First in the year 1057 (2 May 1647).

CONVERSATIONS OF SUFI SAINTS

The primary medium through which the Sufi masters communicated their teachings in India was oral instruction. Although most Sufis studied Islamic law, theology, and mysticism in Arabic and Persian, the early masters of the most popular Indian Sufi order, the Chishtis, did not themselves write. Several of them were, however, surrounded by disciples of a literary bent, who decided to record their masters' teaching in a diary form. The pioneer of this new literary form was Amir Hasan Dihlawi (d. after 1329), a famous poet at the Delhi court. From 1307 until 1322, he recorded the conversations of his teacher, Nizam al-Din Awliya' (d. 1325), whenever he was able to visit Delhi. His compilation, *Morals for the Heart*, became extremely popular as a summary of the master's teaching, and subsequent generations of Sufis likewise had disciples record their discourses (*malfuzat*) in writing.[8]

In this way, one of Nizam al-Din's chief successors, Shaykh Nasir al-Din Mahmud Chiragh-i Dihli (d. 1356) is known to us through the vivid diary of his sayings recorded in 1354 by his disciple Hamid Qalandar (belonging to the unconventional "qalandar" type of Sufi). This text, entitled *The Best of Assemblies*, was in part personally corrected by the shaykh, who pruned down the verbose style of his disciple, making it into a beautiful example of clear and simple Persian prose. Unlike formal treatises on mysticism, it conveys the dynamic give-and-take of living conversation and personal interaction. This selection is the thirty-sixth assembly, given in full, followed by a brief excerpt from the twelfth assembly. Chiragh-i Dihli is shown here as a Sufi who has fully imbibed the canonical tradition of the Qur'an and the hadith sayings of the Prophet Muhammad, which he uses as the basis for his homilies. We also see him receiving a "man of the world," who has sought the saint's supernatural aid in some unspecified difficulty. As soon as the man comes in, the saint observes, without being told, that the man's difficulty has been solved. Chiragh-i Dihli uses the incident, however, to point out the hidden benefits of afflictions sent by God, who tolerates the ephemeral success of evildoers like Pharaoh. This leads him, a celibate, to reflect on the distractions inherent in earthly possessions and family life, which disturb the meditations of the mystic. In all cases he recommends "recollection of God" (*dhikr*), meditation on the names of God, which is one of the principal spiritual methods of classical Sufism. Of particular interest is his skillful adaptation of the story of Moses and the idolater to the Indian environment; a similar story had been told by the Persian poets Rumi and Sa'di but without any reference to India. Here, Chiragh-i Dihli has the

---

[8] For further reading, see Hasan Dihlawi, *Morals for the Heart*, trans. Bruce B. Lawrence (New York: Paulist Press, 1992).

idolater address the idol in Hindi, and the story of the idolater's renunciation of paganism and his forgiving acceptance by God brings the audience to tears. The master concludes with some words about the divine mercy. This is a typical example of how Sufi tradition forged in Iraq and Iran came to be adapted to the situation of South Asia.

The brief excerpt from the twelfth assembly is a remark about the importance of breath control in meditation. It is significant because of the casual mention of Hindu yogis, whose technique is acknowledged to be fundamentally similar to that of the Sufis, regardless of their doctrinal differences.

The Conversations of Nasir al-Din Mahmud Chiragh-i Dihli[9]

The Thirty-sixth Assembly

Good fortune and happiness! The happiness of speech [with the master] was facilitated. The master (God remember him to the good) had mentioned some useful point, and eminent learned men were seated [in attendance]. He kindly told me to come sit closer. Then, he began to speak. I [still] did not hear, so he repeated his remarks, saying, "A man came into the presence of the Messenger of God (God bless him and grant him peace) and said, 'Counsel me, Messenger of God.' The Messenger of God said, 'He who works an atom's weight of good will see its reward. And he who works an atom's weight of evil will see its reward.' The man said, 'That suffices me, Messenger of God.' He replied, 'The man has understood.' That is, he will do as he has heard."

Then, a man came in to see the master. He was an eminent man of the world, just and renowned, and having sought the master's help, he was released [from his difficulty] by the blessing of the thought of the master. As soon as he entered, the master brightened up and said, 'Welcome! How wonderful! Sit down, for you were released." He said, "By the blessing of the thought of the master, last night I was released." Then, the master said, "When a thorn pricks one's foot or an ant bites one, one should know that it is the reward of one's action, as God says in the holy Qur'an: 'And the affliction that befalls you is acquired by your own

[9] The selections are translated from Nasir al-Din Mahmud Chiragh-i Dihli, *Khayr al-majalis*, compiled by Hamid Qalandar, ed. Khaliq Ahmad Nizami, Publication of the Department of History, Muslim University, no. 5, Studies in Indo-Muslim Mysticism 1 (Aligarh: Muslim University, Department of History, [1959]), pp. 120–25,59–60.

hands' (Qur. 42.30)." Then, he said, "What is affliction? An occurrence that is disliked. In general, the word 'affliction' (*musibat*) is that which people dislike. But the words 'occurrence' (*isabat*) and 'befell' (*asaba*) have been mentioned in reports of the Prophet also. God says, 'Whatever of good befalls you is from God' (Qur. 4.79)." Then, he said, "The word 'affliction,' for a disliked occurrence, is acknowledged as a legitimate category." Again he said, "When something disliked occurs, the sins one has committed are forgiven on that account because one is awakened thereby and turns back toward God, and sorrowing repentance is brought about. One's errors are forgiven on that account."

Then, he said, "Whatever injury and affliction God sends is one's guide to happiness. But the person who has been granted a long life and has many worldly goods is sent no difficulties, and he falls short in his devotions; this is 'being led on,' and 'being led on' is very near to punishment. God says: 'Step by step we lead them on from whence they know not' (Qur. 7.182)." Then, he said, "Pharaoh never had a headache. Throughout the long life he had, he claimed that he was God but never had a headache."

Then, he said, "The Master of the Law has called possessions and children a trial. 'Your possessions and children are a trial' (Qur. 8.28)." He said, "They are a trial because you want to be occupied in devotions in the corner of the house for a time. The children come and pull on your garment, saying, 'This devotion of yours is no good to us! Go, get something for us to eat!' Because of children you abandon your devotions to God. Then, you come out and become worried and distracted. Thus are children a trial. Wealth is also a trial because as long as there is no wealth, you are occupied with God. When wealth comes, one gets to thinking of pretty girls and longs for enjoyment and delight. Thus, wealth is also a trial."

"But if one does not spend on oneself that which God has given him, what does one do? One spends it for the sake of God, such as in giving to dervishes, visiting the sick, building mosques, and doing other good deeds. When one turns the corrupt tool of wealth into good deeds, it is not a trial."

Then, he said, "Be involved in whatever work you do, speak, and do the world's business. But never let your tongue be empty of the remembrance of God for one minute. Whether standing, sitting, or tumbling in

His path, you should remember God," and he recited this verse: "'Those who remember God standing and sitting and on their sides' (Qur. 3.191). When your tongue is busy remembering God, it is to be hoped that it will remove all the sorrows of the world from your heart and make you sorrowless." Then, he said, "What happiness is there beyond this, that in the corner of your house, or in the mosque, or in a shrine, you are occupied with the remembrance of God and are not occupied with human devils? Who are the human devils? They are the ones who hold you back from the remembrance of God when you wish to be occupied in remembrance of God, for God is seated beside you. It is said in the divine sayings, 'I am seated beside him who remembers me,' and God reminds us in the Qur'an, 'Remember me, and I will remember you' (Qur. 2.152). When you hold back from remembering God, your companions are devils. God says, 'He who turns away from the remembrance of the Merciful, We assign to him a devil' (Qur. 43.36), or 'We entrust [to him a devil].' And when you are occupied in remembrance of God, who will be your companion?" At this point he turned both eyes up toward heaven and said, "God will be. See what God has said: 'I am seated beside him who remembers me.'" Then, he said, "This is the saying of Abu Bakr al-Tamistani [d. 954] (God have mercy on him); the Shaykh of Shaykhs [i.e., Abu Hafs `Umar Shihab al-Din al-Suhravardi, d. 1234] (God sanctify his soul) has said in the `Awarif that Abu Bakr al-Tamistani (God have mercy on him) said, 'Keep the company of God, and if you are unable, keep the company of those who keep the company of God, in order that the blessing of their company may unite you with the company of God.'

After that he told the following story. "In the age of the prophet Moses (God's prayer and peace be upon him), there was an idolater among the Israelites, who had practiced idolatry four hundred years. He had not ceased for a day in these four hundred years, and he did not raise his head from the foot of the idol, nor did he pray for any necessity during these four hundred years. One day, he got a fever, and he placed his head on the idol's foot and said, '*Tu mera gusa'in, tun mera kartar, mujh is tap tahin chura.*' In Persian, that is, he said to the idol, 'You are my God, you are my Creator, release me from this fever!' He said this in the Indian language, just as it is written. However much he spoke to the idol, what answer comes from stone? No answer came. His fever increased. He got up and kicked it, saying, '*Tu mera kartar nahin!*' That is, 'You are not my Creator!' He went out and saw a mosque before him. He put his head inside the mosque and said once, 'O God of Moses!' From four directions, the cry came, 'I am here, my servant! I am here, my servant!' This was heard seventy times, without interruption. He was astonished, saying 'For four hundred years I have not raised my head from the foot of the idol, and I never prayed for any necessity. Today, I pray for one, but the idol did not supply my necessity. He gave no reply, no matter how much I implored him. A single time I called out in the name of the God of Moses, and seventy times I heard, "I am here, my servant!" I am His servant! So much of my life has been wasted!' Then, he prayed for what he needed: 'O God of Moses, remove this fever from me!' At once, the fever left him."

"Afterward he went before Moses, saying, 'O Moses! If one has practiced idolatry for four hundred years and, during these four hundred years, not once lifted one's head from the foot of the idol but afterwards turns back to your God, will your God make peace with him or not?' Moses (on whom be peace) was wrathful. When he heard that someone had practiced idolatry for four hundred years and never once lifted his head from the idol's foot, the expression of wrath was plain on Moses' face, the idolater grew afraid and fled from Moses, and every moment he was looking back and thinking, with trust in the mercy of God, that he would call him back. At that moment, a revelation occurred: 'O Moses! Receive my servant, and tell him, "What of four hundred years? If you practice idolatry for four thousand years and despair of the idol in time of need, then just once cry out in our name; mercy is from us. I reply without interruption seventy times, and every necessity that you pray for I provide."' Moses ran barefoot, saying, 'Come! For your repentance has been accepted, and your faith has been found acceptable! It is decreed, even so: "If for four hundred years, nay! If for four thousand years you practice idolatry and never once lift your head from the idol's foot and then despair of him and come to us and just once cry out, then seventy times without interruption I will reply, and every necessity that you pray for I will provide to your desire."''"

The master told this story, and those who were present wept with loud cries and exclamations. A clamor arose, and I became upset from weeping. He said something that I did not follow. I composed myself and listened. He was saying, "God is kind and merciful. He has said,

'My mercy is quicker than my wrath.' Since mercy is quicker, wrath is delayed." After that he said, "He gives life, he bestows the blessing of faith, and he distributes sustenance. God says, 'Though you reckon the blessings of God you will not count them' (Qur. 14.34). Do not forget a God such as this. He did not exclude an infidel who had practiced idolatry for four hundred years; if a Muslim repents, he is merciful and kind; he accepts it." After that he recited this verse, "'Truly God does not forgive that one should associate partners with him, and he forgives all else besides that to whomsoever he wishes' (Qur. 4,48)." And praise be to God, Lord of Creation.

From the Twelfth Assembly

He said, "The essence of this matter is restraint of breath, that is, the Sufi ought to hold his breath during meditation. As long as he holds his breath, his interior is concentrated, and when he releases his breath, the interior is distracted, and it destroys his momentary state."... Then, he said, "Therefore the Sufi is he whose breath is counted. The adept is the master of breath; this has but a single meaning. The accomplished yogis, who are called *siddha* in Indian language, breathe counted breaths."

3

The Interpretation of the Classical Sufi Tradition in India

The *Shama'il al-atqiya'* of Rukn al-Din Kashani

INTRODUCTION

The notion of tradition, the transmission of culture over generations, assumes adherence to earlier models of thought or behavior. In literary traditions, and especially in religious traditions with a strong emphasis on scripture, particular texts are elevated to an authoritative position and are treated as classics. In the currents of Islamic mysticism that we subsume under the term "Sufism," a series of texts written in Arabic and Persian from the ninth through the thirteenth centuries have often been treated as forming the "classical" literature of Sufism. Of course, this terminology often carries with it a common (and unspoken) presupposition about the nature of history and culture; a "classical" period is equivalent to a "golden age" that is inevitably followed by a "decline" and even a "degeneration." Scholars lament the lack of "originality" in authors from later ages; the classics, it seems, form a pinnacle in comparison with which all else is found wanting.

Many have disputed the philosophies of history elaborated by Spengler and Toynbee on the grounds that the biological analogy for the rise and fall of civilizations can be easily falsified by detailed historical analysis and by changing the focus of arbitrary units of comparison.[1] Nonetheless, the "classicism and decline" model has long exercised a fascination over students of Islamic culture. It is especially odd to notice that the "decline" of Islamic civilization was an unquestioned axiom accepted by Orientalists and fundamentalists alike—in both cases, the colonization of much of the Muslim world and the consequent loss of political power by Muslims were interpreted as the judgment of history (or God) upon a civilization that had become inadequate.

If we do not intend to support, however, the agendas of either colonialism or fundamentalism, then the notion of "classicism and decline" is distinctly unhelpful in the study of a tradition like Sufism.[2] Sufi authors in what Hodgson called the "late middle period" of Islamic history certainly participated in a complicated literary culture with a high degree of reference.[3] But the rigid concept of a fixed text does not appear to have exercised the same tyranny over these medieval authors as it does over modern scholars. What we may call oral transmission and flexible concepts of quotation were hard to separate from fixed and literal modes of textual citation.[4]

FLEXIBLE TRANSMISSION OF CLASSICAL SUFI TEXTS

To demonstrate the referential complexity of later Sufi texts, I would like to examine a case in which a Sufi of the "post-classical" period makes a synthetic representation of the entire Sufi tradition, drawing on authorities from the Qur'an and the Prophet Muhammad up to his own day. The author in question is Rukn al-Din Dabir Kashani (d. after 738/1337), a disciple of the Indian Chishti master Burhan al-Din Gharib (d. 738/1337).

---

[1] Oswald Spengler, *The Decline of the West*, 2 vols. (New York: Knopf, 1961); Arnold Toynbee, *A Study of History* (New York: Barnes & Noble Books, 1995).

[2] This notion of classicism and decline underlies the threefold scheme advanced by J. Spencer Trimingham to describe the development of Sufism. J. S. Trimingham, *The Sufi Orders in Islam* (Oxford: Oxford University Press, 1971).

[3] Marshall G. S. Hodgson, *The Venture of Islam: Conscience and History in a World Civilization*, 3 vols. (Chicago: University of Chicago Press, 1978).

[4] For an example of this flexible mode of textual transmission, see C. W. Ernst, "The Man without Attributes: Ibn `Arabi's Interpretation of Abu Yazid al-Bistami," *Journal of the Muhiyiddin Ibn `Arabi Society* 13 (1993): 1–19.

Rukn al-Din wrote two Persian texts that are of great importance for understanding the development of Chishti Sufism in India: one, *Nafa'is al-anfas*, was a collection of the discourses (*malfuzat*) of his teacher in diary form, but the second work, the encyclopedic *Shama'il al-atqiya'*, is the one that concerns us here. This latter is a large collection (455 pages in rare lithograph edition) of teachings current in Sufi circles in the Delhi Sultanate during the fourteenth century. It is well-suited to help us see how Indian Chishtis viewed their predecessors in the Sufi tradition because Rukn al-Din has carefully documented every point under discussion with quotations either from the "classical" sources of Sufism or from recent authorities in Indian Sufism. At the beginning of the work he has given a bibliographical list of all his sources, including about seventy-five works on the standard Islamic religious sciences (Qur'anic exegesis, hadith, theology, and law), about one hundred twenty-five books on Sufism, and another fifty sources of oral traditions. The two-hundred-odd sources cited by Rukn al-Din (some of which are no longer extant) are almost equally spread out over the seven Islamic centuries preceding him. I have reproduced and annotated this "Sufi bookshelf" in an appendix to my book *Eternal Garden*.[5] In what follows, I would like to take the analysis a step further by examining the use of classical Sufi sources in *Shama'il al-atqiya'*. This may be done in two ways: first, by comparing Kashani's quotations from classical Sufi writings with the texts as we know them from recent printed editions in order to establish Rukn al-Din's editorial methods; second, by analyzing the content of the materials that he quotes from Indian Sufis in order to determine what is distinctive about the Indian development of Sufism. I have chosen for comparison and analysis the fourth, fifth, and sixth chapters of *Shama'il al-atqiya'*, which cover the crucial topics of spiritual mastery, succession to the authority of the master, and sainthood.[6]

When quoting from classical Persian sources, Kashani takes a relatively liberal approach to citation, picking out short phrases and longer sentences as needed, but the comments that he adds may take off

---

[5] C. W. Ernst, *Eternal Garden: Mysticism, History, and Politics at a South Asian Sufi Center*, SUNY Series in Muslim Spirituality in South Asia (Albany: State University of New York Press, 1992), App. A, pp. 251–63; cf. also pp. 75–76, 79.

[6] Rukn al-Din Kashani, *Shama'il al-atqiya'*, Persian lithograph ed. by Sayyid `Ata' Husayn, Silsila-yi Isha`at al-`Ulum 85 (Hyderabad: Matbu`at Ashraf Press, 1928–29), pp. 25–42.

in a rather different direction than that intended in the original text. An example is the discussion of specific techniques of teaching disciples at different levels. Kashani quotes a Persian translation of `Umar al-Suhrawardi's (d. 632/1234) *`Awarif al-ma`arif* to define the role of the Sufi master in calling people to God using the Persian term *da`wat*:

> *Da`wat* means to call someone toward something and towards someone, and it is of several types: by wisdom, by preaching, and by disputation, as God Most High said, "Call to the path of your Lord with wisdom and fine preaching, and dispute with them by means of that which is best" (Qur. 16:125); that is, "O Muhammad, by whatever means his carnal soul dominates his heart, call him with a fine preaching." This is directed toward the pious ones (*abrar*), by recalling heaven and hell. "And for anyone whose heart dominates his carnal soul, call him with wisdom." This was directed toward the wayfarers and seekers of the Real, who are hopeful of finding internal purity, gnosis, unity, and nearness. This is by hint, and it is a gift. "Say: This is my way; I call toward God with insight, I and whosoever follows me" (Qur. 12:108) is the secret of this meaning.[7]

The thrust of Kashani's comments lies in distinguishing the ordinary pious believer, who is best taught by preaching on the afterlife, from the spiritual seekers who are called by wisdom to inner experience. Kashani achieves this by intermediate glosses that identify particular terms in the Qur'anic verse with radically distinct religious types. The corresponding passage in the Arabic original of Suhrawardi's *`Awarif* is considerably different. It occurs in the chapter on the bestowal of the initiatic robe (*khirqa*) and treats the Qur'anic verse as the basis for a general outline of the kinds of meditation and ritual that are appropriate to different kinds of disciples, without linking specific Sufi practices to the Qur'an by exegesis:

> God Most High said, "Call to the path of your Lord with wisdom and fine preaching, and dispute with them by means of that which is best" (Qur. 16:125). So wisdom is a level (*rutba*) of invitation, as are likewise preaching and disputation… Thus the master knows who is in the position of the pious (*al-abrar*) and who is in the position of the proximate ones (*al-muqarribin*), for whom prolonged recollection (dhikr) is appropriate, for

---

[7] Kashani, *Shama'il al-atqiya'*, p. 27; Ernst, *Eternal Garden*, pp. 159–160.

whom prolonged ritual prayer is appropriate, and who is subject to desire in rough or easy circumstances; he breaks the disciple's habit, brings him out of the constraint of his carnal desire, nourishes him with his volition, clothing him in a garb and form that are appropriate....[8]

While both passages take off from the same Qur'anic verse to enlarge on the problem of teaching disciples at different levels, there is barely a verbal echo of the Arabic original in the Persian "translation" (just the single reference to "the pious"). Without further information, it is not possible to identify which of the many Persian translations of the *Awarif* has been consulted by Kashani; this passage does not appear to occur at all in the well-known Persian translation by Mu`izz al-Din Kashani.[9] There may have been more than one stage in the transformation of Suhrawardi's text before it reached the Indian Deccan. Kashani's version seems to represent a greater emphasis on esotericism as a principle, while Suhrawardi's text is more of a repertory of appropriate techniques. There are a number of other cases where Kashani cites earlier Sufi authors such as Qushayri or `Ayn al-Qudat Hamadani with similar transformations and additions.[10] Another example is the way he deals with the topic of sainthood, using the important discussion of that topic in `Ali Hujwiri's *Kashf al-mahjub* ("Revelation of the Veiled"), composed in Persian before 1070. Hujwiri refers to the well-known distinction between the two Arabic vocalizations *walaya* (Persian *valayat*) and *wilaya* (Persian *vilayat*) to bring out different aspects of the concept of sainthood, and he discusses at length their theological implications. Kashani chooses to ignore these theoretical distinctions, concentrating instead on the practical implications of sainthood. In the first instance, Hujwiri cites a Qur'anic parable on the worldly results of ascribing partners to God: "God's saying, 'In this case, *walaya* belongs to God, Who is the Truth; He is best for

---

[8] S. Abu Hafs `Umar al-Suhrawardi, *`Awarif al-ma`arif*, ed. `Abd al-Halim Mahmud and Mahmud ibn al-Sharif (Cairo: Matbu`at al-Sa`ada, n.d.), 1:257–58.

[9] Mu`izz al-Din Kashani, *Misbah al-hidaya: tarjuma-yi `awarif* (Lucknow: Nawal Kishor, 1322/1904).

[10] For example, Kashani, *Shama'il al-atqiya'*, p. 33, quotes (with significant additions) `Ayn al-Qudat Hamadani, *Tamhidat*, ed. `Afif `Usayran (Tehran: Kitabkhana-yi Manuchihri, 1962), p. 11; Kashani, *Shama'il al-atqiya'*, p. 41 quotes Hamadani, *Tamhidat*, pp. 44–45. In the section on *sama`*, Kashani has apparently added a reference to dancing to a quotation from Qushayri; cf. Ernst, *Eternal Gardens*, p. 152.

reward and best for consequence' (Qur. 18:44)—*valayat* means lordship (*rububiyat*), and it means love (*mahabbat*)."[11]

In reproducing this statement, Kashani changes the order of clauses and abridges them, adding the following comment by way of a gloss: "That is, 'We shall, with our servants on the day of resurrection, fulfill both lordship and love.'"[12] Rukn al-Din's gloss introduces two elements that were not present in Hujwiri's comments: the saints as instruments of God's will and their role with respect to humanity at the resurrection. In defining the second vocalization of the term, Kashani quotes Hujwiri as follows: "*Vilayat* means rule."[13] Then, he goes on to comment, "That is, the master of *vilayat* orders the servants of God to obedience, worship, God-fearing, and asceticism, brings them out from external disobediences and internal flaws, and finds it necessary to protect them from contemptible practices, rebelliousness, and the corruption of faith."[14] This is a considerable expansion of a one-word definition. What is noteworthy about these citations and comments is that Kashani has paid little attention to the theological and metaphysical framework that Hujwiri used to clarify and justify, for instance, the views of Hakim Tirmidhi on the nature of sainthood. Instead, Kashani has taken only the most basic etymological statements of Hujwiri and used them as a jumping-off point for comments on the practical nature of sainthood, here defined as intercession for the believers at the resurrection and preaching right thought and behavior to them in this life.

There are occasions when Kashani quotes extensively from a Sufi text but subtly elevates the significance of it by ascribing the author's views to God or the Prophet. This occurs in the last quotation from Hujwiri in the section on sainthood, where three passages are quoted with liberal paraphrasing. The first passage is a hadith on the saints: "Their faces are luminous, and they sit on thrones of light; they are not afraid when men are afraid, nor do they grieve when men grieve." Kashani repeats that, but then he skips Hujwiri's quotation of the oft quoted Qur'anic verse,

---

[11] `Ali b. `Uthman Hujwiri, *Kashf al-mahjub*, ed. `Ali Qawim (Islamabad: Markaz-i Tahqiqat-i Farsi-yi Iran u Pakistan, 1398/1978), p. 189, abridged. The translation is from R. A. Nicholson, *The Kashf al-majub: The Oldest Persian Treatise on Sufism*, E. J. W. Gibb Memorial Series 17 (London: Luzac and Company, Ltd., 1976), pp. 210–11.

[12] Kashani, *Shama'il al-atqiya'*, p. 35.

[13] Hujwiri, *Kashf al-mahjub*, p. 189; trans. Nicholson, *The Kashf al-majub*, p. 210.

[14] Kashani, *Shama'il al-atqiya'*, p. 36.

"The friends of God, they have no fear nor do they sorrow" (Qur. 10:62); he also omits a hadith from the Prophet warning against offending the saints:

> The Prophet (God bless him and grant him peace) said, "God said, 'One who injures a friend of mine considers war with me permissible.'" This means that you should know that God (the great and glorious) has friends whom he has selected for his friendship and *wilayat*. They are the rulers of his kingdom whom he has chosen and made the target of the manifestation of his action. He has selected them for various charismatic miracles and kept them pure of the evils of nature. He has freed them from following their carnal self and desire, so that their concentration is only on him, and they are intimate with none but him.[15]

The second statement that Kashani quotes from Hujwiri is actually Hujwiri's comment on the omitted hadith, but Kashani introduces it instead as what God has said on the subject of saints; now Hujwiri's third-person comment, though still in Persian, has been transformed into a first-person account by God, in effect a new hadith *qudsi* (the phrases quoted from Hujwiri are in italics): "God Most High has said regarding them, 'I have servants who *are the rulers* of My *kingdom*, and I *have kept them pure of the evils of nature; they are intimate with none but Me.*'"[16]

A third comment by Hujwiri goes as follows: "They [the saints] existed before us in past centuries, and they now exist, and after this they will exist until the resurrection because the Lord Most High has honored this community over all other communities and has guaranteed it, [saying,] 'I will protect the religious law (*shari`at*) of Muhammad.'"[17] This comment of Hujwiri's is actually introduced by Kashani as a hadith, and in his abridged version, it runs as follows: "The Messenger, on whom be peace, said, '*They existed before us, and they now exist, and they will exist until the resurrection.*' [Kashani comments:] These words are an honor for the community of Muhammad (God bless him and give him peace), that they [the saints] will exist until the resurrection."[18] Kashani has raised Hujwiri's statement about the eternal presence of the saints

---

[15] Hujwiri, *Kashf al-mahjub*, p. 190; trans. Nicholson, *The Kashf al-majub*, p. 212.
[16] Kashani, *Shama'il al-atqiya'*, pp. 41–42.
[17] Hujwiri, *Kashf al-mahjub*, p. 190; cf. trans. Nicholson, *The Kashf al-majub*, p. 213. Nicholson translates *shari`at* as "religion."
[18] Kashani, *Shama'il al-atqiya'*, p. 42.

into a prophetic dictum, although in its own context Hujwiri's statement takes the form of a theological argument against the Mu'tazila and the anthropomorphists (*al-hashwiyya*). In addition, where Hujwiri deduced the ongoing presence of the saints from God's promise to preserve the religious law, which he defined as a special honor granted to the Muslim community, Kashani has left out the reference to the *shari'at* altogether, simply assuming that the saints are the honor promised by the alleged hadith. By telescoping some of Hujwiri's remarks and by describing other passages as quotations from God and the Prophet, Kashani has given sainthood a much more authoritative status with respect to its scriptural support.

TEACHINGS OF THE CHISHTIS

Now when we look at Kashani's own writings in this section and his references to recent masters in the Chishti order, we can see that some original developments have taken place in Sufi thinking on the fundamental topics of the nature of mastery, successorship, and sainthood. We can take as an example an extended passage from Kashani's own commentary on the Qur'an, *Rumuz al-walihin* (*Ciphers of the Maddened Lovers*), which exists only in quotations embedded in the text of *Shama'il al-atqiya'*. This passage presents a portrait of the perfect Sufi master as one who encompasses the qualities of the highest angels.

> The perfect master and teacher is that one who is both lover and beloved, both the seeker and the sought, both the impassioned and the impassioning, both the perfect and the perfected, both the enraptured wayfarer and the wayfaring enraptured one, both the astonished and the absorbed. His way is sometimes intoxicated and sometimes sober, at times absorbed and at times effaced. The master is the guide and exemplar. The teacher must have the qualities of the four proximate angels [i.e., trust, mercy, death, and wrath].
>
> The first attribute is Gabriel's. "Gabriel is the trusted one of God in the realm of revelation." Thus the master also must be trusted with secret revelation, until the permission of God is obtained and he completely fulfills his charge for the disciples. The master should be the bearer of the words of God, for "Gabriel bears the word and is not a beast of burden for the prophets." That is, he does not give out the secrets and enigmas of the divine word that he carries without the permission of God. The master should be a friend of the prophets by calling and guiding, for "Gabriel is the helper of the prophets and saints." The master should be the destroyer

of God's enemies so that he repels the evil of the religious and worldly enemies of his disciples and slays the disciple's "soul commanding [evil]" [cf. Qur. 12:53], for "Gabriel is the encompasser of God's enemies."

The second attribute is Michael's, for "Michael is the angel of mercy and creation by the bounty of God." The master should bring his disciples with special mercy to the presence of God and illuminate his disciples inwardly and outwardly with the lights of worship and gnosis from his compassion and bounty, and God will have pity on them. He asks for help for his devoted and obedient disciples, so they truly remain firm in outward and inward worship.

The third attribute is Israfil's, for "Israfil bears the canopy of God and is the master of the trumpet and waits for the command of God." The master also should in the beginning remove base qualities from the disciples' hearts, and in the end, the praiseworthy qualities, so their gaze will not fall upon that. At the first call that Lord Israfil blows all will die, and at the second call all will come to life. The master should also by right have the attribute of "He gives life and death" (Qur. 2:258) by God's permission; that is, with one breath, he brings the hearts of disciples to life with the light of love and gnosis of God, and with another breath, he slays the disciples' "souls commanding [evil]" with the influence of the wrath of majesty and beauty so that the carnal desires and dark veils are delayed and repelled. And the master is constantly awaiting the command of God. He should communicate to his disciples whatever hidden inclinations descend upon the heart of the master.

The fourth attribute is Azrael's, for "Azrael seizes the spirits." The master should also be chosen by the wrath of majesty so that he seizes the life of anyone on whom he looks with wrath. That is, in the midst of his spirit the holy illuminations appear as a veil. He annihilates the bodies of some. This is the influence of the wrath of majesty.[19]

This description is a sophisticated synthesis, using the ideal qualities of the angels to describe the attributes of the Sufi master. Like the quotations from classical Sufi authorities, this description attests to a subtle elevation of the status of the Sufi master to a plane above ordinary humanity.

Kashani then takes up the question of appointing a successor or vicegerent (*khalifa*), the key principle of continuity in Sufism that permitted the orders to present themselves as an unbroken chain of succession from the Prophet Muhammad. Here we see how Kashani

---

[19] The descriptions of the angels in quotation marks are in Arabic, but I have not identified the source. *Rumuz-i walihin* in Kashani, *Shama'il al-atqiya'*, pp. 29–30.

models the chain of Sufi masters on the first successors to the Prophet, who were given the title of Caliph (*khalifa*) as his vicegerents, leading the Muslim community in his place.

The meaning of vicegerency (*khilafat*), i.e., a vicegerent (*khalifa*), is to appoint someone in one's place or on one's own behalf. In the case of prayer, if the imam is in a state of ritual impurity, he chooses someone to set the example in his place, and himself goes to his ablutions. But real vicegerency belonged to Lord Adam. As God said, "I am placing a vicegerent on the earth" (Qur. 2:30). Then it came to Lord David, for "O David, We make you a vicegerent on the earth, so judge between the people" (Qur. 38:26). Then it came to the revered Prophet: "I am the vicegerent of God." Then it came to the Commander of the Faithful Abu Bakr, as the Prophet said, "Abu Bakr, I am the vicegerent of God and you are my vicegerent after me." Then it came to other companions, as the Prophet said, "The vicegerency is for thirty years after me."[20] The other prophets were adorned with the mantle of prophecy and miracles, not with vicegerency.

From this fundamental vicegerency, Kashani deduces its separation into the temporal power of rulers and the spiritual power of the saints.

Afterwards that vicegerency was of two types: one the external vicegerency that came to sultans, governors, and judges, for "The sultans are the vicegerents of the Seal of the Prophets, and the governors and judges are the vicegerents of the sultans." The second is internal vicegerency, which came to God's masters and the absolute teachers so that they could lead and guide God's creatures toward God. As God said, "He will appoint them as vicegerents on the earth as he appointed those before them as vicegerents" (Qur. 24:55). That is, necessarily the masters choose vicegerents just as the four original vicegerents chose each other as vicegerent, and after them the followers, and after them the followers of the followers, and so on. The masters and teachers will be the revivers of the exemplary customs (*sunan*) of the Prophet until the Resurrection. As the Prophet said, "He who revives my example (*sunna*) is my vicegerent and the vicegerent of the prophets before me."[21]

---

[20] Cf. A. J. Wensinck, *Concordances et Indices de la Tradition Musulmane* (Leiden: E. J. Brill, 1992), 2:70, citing Ibn Hanbal. None of the other hadith texts cited by Kashani are from the canonical collections, and it would be an interesting project to trace the sources on which he draws.

[21] *Rumuz-i walihin* in Kashani, *Shama'il al-atqiya'*, pp. 32–33.

From this discussion one can see how the Sufi masters are unambiguously presented as the legitimate successors to the Prophet Muhammad in terms of both spiritual guidance and implementation of Islamic law.

The high status given to the Sufi master is especially evident in passages where Kashani cites the sayings of the Chishti shaykhs. The power of the master, according to Kashani's master Burhan al-Din, is extraordinary. It consists not merely in the ability to attain states of nearness to God, but by that very nearness, the master has the power to bring disciples across the vast spaces of the intermediate stages of existence to the very threshold of divinity.

> It is appropriate for mastery, and proper for leading and guiding some-one, that, having traversed the three worlds, he attains the fourth. Those three worlds are humanity (*nasut*), the angelic realm (*malakut*), and power (*jabarut*). The fourth world is divinity (*lahut*).… In traversing these three stations, one must frequently turn away from the whisperings of the carnal soul and the misguiding attacks of demons, and there is fear of polytheism and the disaster of unbelief. The devil has made the boast, "I shall mislead all of them" (Qur. 15:39), in these three stations. The true master and abso-lute guide should take the disciple past this frightening precipice and peril-ous event, and take them to the fourth station, which is the world of divinity, for this is the placeless place of the pure essence of God Most High.[22]

Burhan al-Din takes it for granted that spiritual progress is inconceivable without the guidance of a perfect master. Repeating a theme that is well known in early Sufism, Kashani also quotes the early master Qutb al-Din Bakhtiyar Kaki (d. 633/1235) to the effect that the shaykh must have the ability to discern the prospective disciple's heart in the Preserved Tablet, otherwise, their relationship is doomed.[23]

---

[22] Burhan al-Din Gharib (*al-shaykh al-muhaqqiq*), in Kashani, *Shama'il al-atqiya'*, p. 31.
[23] *Fawa'id al-salikin* (purportedly the *malfuzat* of Mu`in al-Din Chishti, recorded by Qutb al-Din Bakhtiyar Kaki), in Kashani, *Shama'il al-atqiya'*, p. 31. This passage could not be located in the 36-page Urdu version of *Fawa'id al-salikin*, bound together with seven other *malfuzat* texts as Qutb al-Din Bakhtiyar Kaki, *Hasht bihisht* (Lahore: Allah Wale ki Qawmi Dukan, n. d.). This "retrospective" text is quoted seven times in *Shama'il al-atqiya'*, mostly in reference to Sufi practice; cf. Ernst, *Eternal Garden*, p. 79, with n. 342. On the impor-tance of the master seeing the disciple in the Preserved Tablet, see A. Schimmel, *Mystical Dimensions of Islam* (Chapel Hill: University of North Carolina, 1975), p. 101.

The remarks just cited pertain to the reflections of the Indian Chishtis on the general subjects of mastery and sainthood. On these subjects, it seems legitimate to conclude that they placed a greater emphasis on the transcendental status and indispensable role of the master than did their predecessors in Iran two or three centuries earlier. In practice, the concrete example of the Sufi master in the Chishti tradition depended absolutely on the legitimate transmission of authority. Without the formal naming of the successor in a vicegerency document (*khilafat-nama*) and the explicit bequest of the regalia of the Chishti masters, it is impossible for anyone to claim the position of a spiritual master. Kashani gives the example of the transmission that took place on the death of his teacher Burhan al-Din Gharib, which was still fresh in his mind when he completed *Shama'il al-atqiya* ':

> It is a basic rule that one whom the real master names as vicegerent, on whom he bestows his prayer mat, staff, prayer carpet, and rosary, and whom he appoints to say thanks to God after setting forth the meal in front of him, he teaches him the knowledge of the prayer carpet so that he may be worthy to sit on the prayer carpet. He [the master] advises his personal attendant that, after the master's death, on the third day, that person should be brought the robe of mastery and vicegerency before all the Muslims, scholars, masters, and all present in the assembly, since the revered master has given him the vicegerency and apportioned to him his own place so that he may invite the servants of God to the road of the religious law and the spiritual path. Just so, after the passing of the revered Pole of Guidance, the Shaykh al-Islam, the Sultan of the gnostics, Burhan al-Haqq wa l'Haqiqa wa l-Yaqin [i.e., Burhan al Din Gharib], the one singled out for the proximity of the lovers and known by the appellation of "the Poor" (*al-gharib*), may God be pleased with him, the answerer—then that personal attendant of comprehensive piety and perfect uprightness, Kaka Shad Bakht (God sanctify his dear conscience), having brought together the revered Shaykh al-Islam Zayn al-Din and Sayyid Nasir al-Din in accordance with the testament of the revered and blessed master, on the third day, along with the imams, scholars, masters of the covenant, the group of Sufis, Khans, great nobles, and famous and renowned people, he kissed the hands of the two and congratulated them. He read out in front of everyone the vicegerentship-letters that had been found, and by their sincerity, their vicegerentship was established with perfect reliability and grounding.

> One to whom the real master does not give these conditions, and who (nonetheless) gives the hand of master to the servants of God and takes disciples, is one who leads astray; whatever gift is placed in his name is unlawful, and if he claims miracles and sainthood, there is fear that his faith has gone.[24]

---

[24] Kashani, *Shama'il al-atqiya'*, pp. 34–35; cf. Ernst, *Eternal Garden*, p. 135, with n. 204.

The ritual aspect of the transmission of spiritual authority has become highly formalized, with the need to pass on various ritual objects (prayer mat, staff, prayer carpet and rosary) from a master to his successor. By its very nature, the reliance on such tangible objects as signs of legitimacy led to disputes focusing on the question of who had, in fact, received the authentic relics.[25] Although the cloak (*khirqa*) had considerable importance in earlier Persian Sufism, there is little evidence in the "classical" texts of the initiatic importance of so many ritual objects.[26] It appears that there have been ritual accretions in Indian Sufism, adding to and focusing the authority of the shaykh through the concrete symbols of sainthood. The specific characteristics of the Indian Chishti masters, as enshrined in their regalia, served to make the order distinctive and shape its transmission over generations.

CONCLUSION

The references to the classical Sufi tradition in *Shama'il al-atqiya'* are not just a series of library citations. They are a very personal meditation of Sufi teaching. They would be meaningless apart from Rukn al-Din Kashani's discipleship to Burhan al-Din Gharib. Although he refers to his sources as written texts, over one-fifth of his sources are oral, and the written texts themselves are viewed only insofar as they are given life and transmitted by an actual teacher.[27] Further evolution of the meanings of this text can doubtless be found in its seventeenth-century translation into Dakhani Urdu and in a new translation into modern Hindi that is presently being completed by a scholar at Marathwada University.[28] It is ironic that the modern editor of the Hyderabad lithograph states that he found it necessary to correct the manuscripts that he consulted for the

---

[25] S. Digby, "*Tabarrukat* and Succession among the Great Chishti Shaykhs," in *Delhi Though the Ages: Essays in Urban History, Culture and Society*, ed. R. E. Frykenberg (Delhi: Oxford University Press, 1986), pp. 63–103.

[26] For the Sufi cloak, see R. Gramlich, *Die schiitischen Derwischorden Persiens*, vol. 2, *Glaube and Lehre*, Abhandlungen für die Kunde des Morgenlandes 36/2–4 (Wiesbaden: Franz Steiner, 1976), pp. 172–173.

[27] Ernst, *Eternal Garden*, p. 76.

[28] To the references in Ernst, *Eternal Garden*, p. 304 n. 329, should be added Rukn al-Din `Imad, *Intkhab-i Shama'il al-atqiya'*, Dakhani Urdu transl. from Persian by Miran Ya`qub, edited and abridged by Badi' Hussayni (Hyderabad: Shu`ba-yi Urdu, `Uthmaniyya University, 1967).

many mistakes that he found in the citation of Sufi classics, and he states that he has rectified these throughout. We have found, to the contrary, that Kashani regularly revises his texts to stress the importance of the Sufi saints with even greater emphasis than do his sources, and he even shifts significant remarks of authors like Hujwiri to a scriptural status by ascribing them to God or the Prophet. The elasticity of texts and authors in the oral tradition should remind us that translation can have more than one meaning. Originally, the term from which our word "translation" comes meant the transfer of a saint's body from one location to another. Words, like persons, derive their meaning from contexts. Rather than measure "copyist's errors" against a purified "original text," we should perhaps be more sensitive to the multiple extended meanings that a text can take on in new "translations."

In terms of the subject of spiritual mastery and sainthood, the writings of Kashani himself and the sayings of his master Burhan al-Din Gharib and his predecessors in the Chishti order emphasize several distinctive aspects. First, mastery and sainthood are in total continuity with the core of Islamic tradition going back to Adam, the early Israelite prophets, the Prophet Muhammad, and his vicegerents. Mastery is not only prophetic but also angelic in character, as we are told in the section on the qualities of the four angels. Second, it requires profound abilities to guide those who seek to be taught: one must be able to read the primordial nature of a prospective disciple and to take the disciple beyond the intermediate stages of the spirit to the realm of divinity. Third, the authority of the master has been emphasized by ritual extensions in the ritual transmission of regalia to authorized successors. These themes hardly constitute a "degeneration" from the model of the classical Sufi tradition. They further develop the model of mastery and sainthood that was outlined by the early Sufis. If we can dispense with the unspoken reasons that motivate classicism and the nostalgia for the golden age, we may better be able to grasp the subtle hermeneutic with which later Sufis revivified and quickened their textual classics, thus making them relevant to their own master-disciple relationships.

4

Persecution and Circumspection in the Shattari Sufi Order

What happens to a Sufi order when one of its foremost leaders is persecuted and charged with heresy? This question, which may be framed with respect to a number of Sufi leaders over the course of Islamic history, has a special interest in connection with the Shattari Sufi order. This group, which was established in the South Asian sub-continent in the late fifteenth century, had a colorful history that was closely intertwined with the political fortunes of the dynasties of northern India. Its membership spread to western India and the Deccan, and then, via the Hejaz, it was exported to Southeast Asia. The Shattari order was known especially for its emphasis on meditative techniques, and this gave it a characteristic style. Most Sufi orders defined themselves by initiatic lineages that went through Junayd, the Baghdadian master of "sober" Sufism. In contrast, the Shattaris derived their authority from chains of transmission that went to the Khorasanian ecstatic, Bayazid Bistami. The extent and impact of the Shattari order has not yet been adequately assessed; most of the texts that detail the history of the order are unpublished.[1] Little scholarly work has been directed to this topic; a few articles written several decades ago focused on Shattari activity in northern India, and some work has also been done on Shattaris in the

---

[1] An exception is the Arabic translation of the Persian meditation manual by Muhammad ibn Khatir al-Din ibn Khwaja al-`Attar [Muhammad Ghawth], *al-Jawahir al-Khams*, ed. Ahmad ibn al-`Abbas, 2nd ed., 2 vols. (Egypt: Muhammad Rif`at `Amir, 1393/1973).

Deccan.[2] A single dissertation, written in Aligarh in 1963, has attempted a reconstruction of the history of the Shattaris.[3] Biographical sources for the Shattaris are relatively abundant, however, and so an initial effort can be made here to analyze their reaction to the problem of persecution.[4] The material used for this study suggests that persecution of the Shattari leader Muhammad Ghawth was based upon ecstatic statements that he made regarding his spiritual status. As in other cases of this kind, going back to the trial of al-Hallaj, the exact circumstances of the persecution are hedged around with hagiographical interpretations that make it hard to evaluate precisely, although it is clear that political considerations are always relevant in cases of religious persecution.[5] Also comparable to the case of al-Hallaj is the encouragement of a climate

---

[2] See Khaliq Ahmed Nizami, "The Shattari Saints and Their Attitude towards the State," *Medieval India Quarterly* 3 (1950): 56–70; Syed Hasan Askari, "A Fifteenth Century Shuttari Sufi Saint of North Bihar," *Proceedings of the 13th Indian History Congress* (1950): 148–57; M. M. Haq, "The Shuttari Order of Sufism in India and Its Exponents in Bengal and Bihar," *Journal of the Asiatic Society of Pakistan* 16 (1971): 167–75; Richard M. Eaton, *Sufis of Bijapur 1300–1700: Social Roles of Sufis in Medieval India* (Princeton University Press, 1978); Muhammad Yousuf Kokan, *Arabic and Persian in the Carnatic 1710–1969* (Madras: Hafiza House, 1974); id., "Sufi Presence in South India," in *Islam in India: Studies and Commentaries*, ed. Christian W. Troll, vol. 2, *Religion and Religious Education* (Delhi: Vikas Publishing House Pvt. Ltd., 1985), pp. 73–85; Saiyid Athar Abbas Rizvi, *A History of Sufism in India*, 2 vols. (New Delhi: Munshiram Manoharlal Publishers Pvt. Ltd., 1983), 2:151–73.

[3] Qazi Moinuddin Ahmad, "History of the Shattari Silsilah," (PhD diss., Aligarh, 1963). Regrettably, many of the manuscripts listed in this study are no longer in existence.

[4] The sources include a biography of Muhammad Ghawth by Fazl Allah Shattari, *Manaqib-i Ghawthiyya*, Urdu trans. Muhammad Zahir al-Haqq (Agra: Abu al-Ma`ali Steam Press, 1933). This rare lithograph, consulted at the University of the Punjab in Lahore, has been translated from a Persian MS in the khanqah of Shaykh Wajih al-Din `Alawi in Ahmedabad, which apparently covered the life of Muhammad Ghawth up to 941/1534–35, the remainder being added by the translator on the basis of "well-known books" (p. 80). A standard hagiography of the Mughal period with considerable material on the Shattaris is Muhammad Ghawthi Mandawi, *Adhkar-i abrar, Urdu tarjuma-i gulzar-i abrar*, trans. Fazl Ahmad Jewari (1326/1908; repr., Lahore: Islamic Book Foundation, 1395/1975); the original Persian text has never been printed, and I cite it according to the Urdu translation except for a few sections for which I had access to manuscripts. Another source that is indispensable for this topic is the detailed modern hagiography by Sayyid Muhammad Muti` Allah Rashid Burhanpuri, *Burhanpur ke Sindhi awliya', al-ma`ruf ba-tadhkira-i awliya-yi Sindh* (Karachi: Sindhi Adabi Board, 1957). For later Shattaris in Arabia, see F. Wüstenfeld, "Die Çufiten in Süd-Arabien im XI. (XVII.) Jahrhundert," *Nachrichten von der Gesellschaft der Wissenschaftern zu Göttingen, Philologisch-historische Klasse*, 30/1 (1883).

[5] See my *Words of Ecstasy in Sufism*, SUNY Series in Islam (Albany: State University of New York Press, 1985), and my "From Hagiography to Martyrology: Conflicting Testimonies to a Sufi Martyr of the Delhi Sultanate," *History of Religions* 24 (1985): 308–27.

of circumspection in the wake of persecution. Conspicuous conformity with shari`a-based norms of behavior characterized Shattari activity in the generations following upon Muhammad Ghawth, just as it did for tenth-century Sufis after the execution of al-Hallaj. Perhaps because multiple initiation into different Sufi orders was a norm from an early period for Shattari masters, the criticism of Muhammad Ghawth encouraged them to maintain, at least publicly, a more conservative profile that might be viewed as "the Qadiri option." This kind of self-censorship reached its apparent limit in the case of the Shattari master Burhan al-Din Raz-i Ilahi. He is said to have turned some disciples over to a shari`a court for execution because they ecstatically identified their master as God. Subsequently, we look in vain for any Shattari Sufis who emulate publicly the ecstatic claims of Muhammad Ghawth. In this case, persecution may have actually succeeded in suppressing the most extravagant claims of ecstatic Sufism.

THE PERSECUTION OF
MUHAMMAD GHAWTH

Shaykh Muhammad Ghawth Gwaliyari is believed to have been born 7 Rajab 907/16 January 1502, and he died on 14 Ramadan 970/7 May 1563.[6] In his youth, he spent about 13 years meditating and practicing asceticism in the lonely fortress of Chunar (now in eastern U.P.). He witnessed the conquest of the great fort of Gwalior by Sultan Ibrahim Lodi (probably around 925/1520), after he had been advised in a vision to move to that location.[7] Although he was approached with gifts by Ibrahim Lodi, Muhammad Ghawth was critical of the sultan because the latter had imprisoned a number of powerful nobles, and friendship between the two became impossible; the result of the saint's displeasure was that the Mughals defeated the Lodi forces at Panipat in 932/1526.[8] That same year Muhammad Ghawth, who was living in Gwalior, interceded with the emperor Babur on behalf of Tatar Khan, the rebellious

---

[6] Fazl Allah, *Manaqib-i Ghawthiyya*, p. 76.
[7] Fazl Allah, *Manaqib-i Ghawthiyya*, p. 33; Khwajah Nizamuddin Ahmad, *The Tabaqat-i-Akbari*, trans. B. De, Bibliotheca Indica 300 (1911; repr., Calcutta: Asiatic Society, 1973), 1: 401–2.
[8] Fazl Allah, *Manaqib-i Ghawthiyya*, pp. 40–41, 44.

governor of Gwalior.[9] Further dealings with the Mughals on the part of Muhammad Ghawth included pleading the case of another rebellious noble, Rahim Dad, in 936/1530.[10] In another case the following year, the saint cursed a rebel named Bayazid the Afghan, who had devastated a nearby town, and within a few days, the malefactor was executed by Babur.[11] Muhammad Ghawth's elder brother Shaykh P'hul (or Bahlul), another Shattari master, became the chief Sufi adviser to Babur's successor Humayun at this time. So closely intertwined did P'hul become in politics that he lost his life in the service of Humayun, when he was executed in Bengal by the rebellious Mirza Hindal. With such close relations to the Mughals, it is not surprising to learn that Humayun's defeat by Sher Shah Suri in 947/1540 led to problems for Muhammad Ghawth, resulting in his departure for Gujarat that same year. His exile in Gujarat would last over 16 years, until the restoration of Humayun.[12]

Hagiographers indicate that the first hint of persecution had arisen on the part of advisers to Sher Shah.[13] A disciple named `Ali Sher Bangali simply observed that Muhammad Ghawth "had seen the internal evil of the Sur Afghans."[14] A later hagiographer, `Abd Allah Khwishagi, writing in 1096/1685, specified that Sher Shah's advisers had objected to a treatise in which Muhammad Ghawth described his ascension (*mi`raj*) into heaven along the lines of the famous ascension of Abu Yazid al-Bistami; the audacious claims that the shaykh made about his encounters with God and numerous prophets and saints were apparently viewed as serious enough to deserve capital punishment.[15] Although here and elsewhere the offending treatise is called simply *Risala-i mi`rajiyya* (or *The*

---

[9] Fazl Allah, *Manaqib-i Ghawthiyya*, pp. 42, 58–61; this is far more circumstantial than the laconic account in Zahiru'd-din Muhammad Babur Padshah Ghazi, *Babur-nama (Memoirs of Babur)*, trans. Annette Susannah Beveridge (New Delhi: Oriental Books Reprint Corporation, 1979 [1922]), pp. 539–40.

[10] Babur, *Babur-nama*, pp. 688, n. 2, 690.

[11] Fazl Allah, *Manaqib-i Ghawthiyya*, p. 43; Babur, *Babur-nama*, p. 677.

[12] Fazl Allah, *Manaqib-i Ghawthiyya*, p. 66, states that the exile was 18 years. He also notes that Muhammad Ghawth built a mosque in Ahmedabad dated 963/1556.

[13] Fazl Allah, *Manaqib-i Ghawthiyya*, p. 65.

[14] Ghawthi, *Adhkar-i abrar*, p. 309.

[15] Rizvi, *History of Sufism*, 2:157–58, quoting `Abd Allah Khwishagi Qasuri, *Ma`arij al-wilayat*, MS Adhar collection, Punjab University Library, fol. 543a. For Khwishagi and his hagiography, see Muhammad Iqbal Mujaddidi, *Ahwal u athar-i `Abd Allah Khwishagi Qusuri*, Silsila-i Matbu`at-i Dar al-Mu'arrikhin 3 (Lahore: Muhammad Shams al-Din, 1391/1972), pp. 80ff.

Treatise on Ascension), the correct title is *Awrad-i ghawthiyya* (*Litanies of the Ghawth*), and it is available in two manuscripts in Calcutta.[16] While much of the text is devoted to explaining the characteristic Shattari meditation techniques and the initiatic genealogies in which the author was confirmed, the lengthy closing portion indeed contains a remarkable account of the spiritual training of Muhammad Ghawth by his master Shaykh Zuhur Hajji Hudur, culminating in a detailed description of his ascension experience.[17] We do not know precisely what actions the Suri regime took against the shaykh, but his prudent departure for Gujarat temporarily put him out of danger.

The second phase of the persecution of Muhammad Ghawth began after his arrival in the kingdom of Gujarat. When he reached the city of Ahmedabad, problems began. The scene was described in vague though dramatic terms by his disciple ʿAli Sher Bangali:

> Here some short-sighted scholars and ignorant dervishes began to search for an excuse for their enmity toward him. By linking him with expressions they neither knew nor understood, they only succeeded by this means in making his pure and luminous heart more illuminated. Staying in that place was unpleasant for him. On a certain occasion good tidings came from heaven, that the reason for emigration [to Gujarat] has vanished, and the occasion for opposition has arisen. Hearing this, he departed for Gwalior.[18]

A modern hagiographer, the editor of Fazl Allah, is somewhat more circumstantial:

> During the time of his stay in Gujarat, certain incidents took place, the story of which event has, like it or not, apparently been well told. The reason for this can be described as follows. He had expressed himself with ecstatic sayings (shathiyyat), that is, spiritual realities in the style of his lofty imagination, in extremely clear words. The understanding of these was considerably beyond the masses, and beginning with those ignorant folk, such a quantity of hostility was generated that the religious scholars, the learned, and even the sultan of the age were necessarily included.[19]

---

[16] Muhammad Ghawth, *Awrad-i ghawthiyya*, MS 446 Curzon Persian and MS 1252 Persian, both in the Asiatic Society, Calcutta.

[17] Muhammad Ghawth, *Awrad-i ghawthiyya*, MS 1252, fols. 107–30.

[18] Ghawthi, *Adhkar-i abrar*, p. 309.

[19] Fazl Allah, *Manaqib-i Ghawthiyya*, p. 65.

Both of these accounts fall into the vagueness of stock hagiographical narrative; all that they do is to connect Muhammad Ghawth with unknown accusers and to portray him as a model mystic. Ghawthi reports that some of the local scholars became opposed to Muhammad Ghawth, leading one of them to send his son to spy on the shaykh.

> Since the short-sighted people of Gujarat were infatuated with his reputation, therefore through envy and lack of insight they began to turn against Ghawth al-Awliya'. Among them Shaykh `Abd al-Muqtadir Banbani sent his younger son confidentially into the Ghawthiyya Khanqah with instructions to be present at all times, in order to take note of the words and deeds of Ghawth al-Awliya' that were objectionable, and to convey those deeds to his superiors for their consideration. It is said that this spy one day said [to Muhammad Ghawth], "This least of disciples has been hopeful of instruction for some time." The answer came [from the shaykh], "The goal of wayfaring is advancement. God willing, you can work in the faqirs' kitchen; this will produce the influence of instruction." Finally, after a few days, a strong attraction overcame him, and his eyes saw reality, so that in all states and in all stations he repeated this phrase continually, "When this is the state of the hypocrite, what do you say to the person who lays his secret at the threshold of this perfect saint?"[20]

Thus, the saint's spiritual power foiled this underhanded attempt to undermine his position, as the would-be spy became a disciple. Muhammad Ghawth appears to have thrived in Gujarat, and we find reference to his presence at different times in the cities of Broach (950/1543–44) and Ahmedabad (951/1544–45) [21] One of his last actions there was to build a mosque, which is dated by a commemorative verse to 963/1556.[22]

It was left for a secular chronicler, the Mughal courtier Bada'oni, to give a fully detailed narrative of the controversy in Gujarat, in which Muhammad Ghawth was accused by the notable scholar `Ali al-Muttaqi (885–975/1480–1567). In this controversy, the shaykh was defended by another scholar, Wajih al-Din `Alawi, who, in the course of the dispute, ended by becoming a Shattari disciple.

---

[20] Ghawthi, *Adhkar-i abrar*, p. 288.
[21] Ghawthi, *Adhkar-i abrar*, pp. 362, 427.
[22] Fazl Allah, *Manaqib-i Ghawthiyya*, p. 66.

When Shaykh Muhammad Ghawth went from Hindustan to Gujarat, in the reign of Sultan Mahmud of Gujarat, Shaykh `Ali al-Muttaqi, one of the greatest Shaykhs, most influential religious leaders and greatest sages of that time, wrote a *fatwa* for the execution of Shaykh Muhammad Ghawth, and the Sultan abrogated it at the instance of Miyan Wajih al-Din. When Miyan Wajih al-Din went on the first occasion to the Shaykh's house he was powerfully attracted by his face, and tore up the *fatwa*, and Shaykh `Ali came, beside himself (with rage), to the Miyan's house, and rent his clothes and said, "Why do you assent to the spread of heresy, and to a schism in the faith?" He answered, "We follow the letter and the Shaykh the spirit. Our understanding cannot reach his perfections and (even), as far as the letter of the law goes, no exception, by which he could be pronounced blameworthy, can be taken to him." And this was the cause of the great faith which the Sultans and rulers of Gujarat had in Shaykh Muhammad Ghawth, and of his deliverance from that position of peril. (The Miyan) from that time repeatedly said in assemblies, "One ought to obey the letter of the law after the manner of Shaykh `Ali al-Muttaqi, and the spirit after the manner of my spiritual guide" (i.e., Shaykh Muhammad Ghawth).[23]

In this version, we are not told what was the precise cause of `Ali al-Muttaqi's wrath, but a new dramatic twist is furnished by Wajih al-Din `Alawi's decision to become a follower of Muhammad Ghawth. In other respects, this narrative echoes other famous persecutions from Sufi hagiography, such as the abstention of Ibn Surayj from judging the case of al-Hallaj or `Attar's mythical portrait of Junayd's response to the final trial of al-Hallaj.[24] A later Shattari text, `Aqil Khan Razi's *Thamarat al-hayat* (1053/1643–44), also relates another incident in which `Ali al-Muttaqi while in Ahmedabad suspiciously inquired about a copy of Ibn `Arabi's *Fusus al-hikam* that was being read by Shaykh Lashkar Muhammad `Arif, a disciple of Muhammad Ghawth. When Shaykh Lashkar briefly

---

[23] `Abdu-'l-Qadir ibn-i-Mulukshah al-Badaoni, *Muntakhabu-'t-tawarikh*, trans. Wolseley Haig, Biblioteca Indica 97 (Calcutta: The Asiatic Society of Bengal), 3:71–72 (text, 3:44), with slight spelling changes. This account, from the article devoted to Wajih al-Din `Alawi, contrasts with the absence of any mention of persecution in the separate notice given by Bada'oni to Muhammad Ghawth: "After the rebellion in India, when Sher Shah began to oppress Shaykh Muhammad, he betook himself to Gujarat where also he brought princes and rulers under the yoke of subjection to him and belief in his teaching, so that all alike were ready to do him service" (ibid., 3:8; text, 3:5).

[24] See Ernst, *Words of Ecstasy*, pp. 102–3, 131.

responded with the essence of Ibn 'Arabi's teaching on the divine unity, 'Ali al-Muttaqi was satisfied with his answer, and he respectfully told his own disciples that this kind of man was worthy of the knowledge of divine realities.[25]

A question arises, however, concerning 'Ali al-Muttaqi's participation in this inquisition. He had been favored with the attention of the sultan of Gujarat, Bahadur Shah (r. 932–43/1526–37), though he was reluctant to accept gifts from the latter. Some of 'Ali al-Muttaqi's biographers report that he departed from Gujarat when Humayun's armies first began their invasions of that territory in 941/1534 and that, after his arrival in the Hejaz, he remained there for the next 30 years.[26] Others say that he left India for Arabia later on, in 953/1546–47.[27] The curious thing is that only Bada'oni refers to 'Ali al-Muttaqi's role in the affair. 'Ali al-Muttaqi's principal biographer, 'Abd al-Haqq Muhaddith, does not seem to mention 'Ali al-Muttaqi in connection with the persecution of Muhammad Ghawth, either in the brief notice devoted to 'Ali al-Muttaqi in the comprehensive dictionary of saints, *Akhbar al-akhyar*, or in the monographic biography of 'Ali al-Muttaqi and his successor 'Abd al-Wahhab al-Muttaqi, *Zad al-muttaqin*.[28] A history of Gujarat completed in 1022/1613, the *Mir'at-i Sikandari*, simply lists the names of 'Ali al-Muttaqi and Muhammad Ghawth together, as famous religious figures of the reign of Sultan Mahmud (r. 943–61/1537–54), without indicating that there was any conflict between the two.[29] Ghawthi mentions the participation of Wajih al-Din 'Alawi and Hamid Lar in defending Muhammad Ghawth with "answers both traditional and rational," but he fails to name any of the shaykh's persecutors.[30] 'Ali al-Muttaqi is said to have returned temporarily to Gujarat during the reign of Mahmud, which would have enabled him to confront Muhammad Ghawth.[31] From an *ijaza* document

---

[25] 'Aqil Khan Razi, *Thamarat al-hayat*, MS 1278 Persian, ASB, Calcutta, fols. 61b–62a.

[26] M. Hidayat Hosain, "al-Mutta²i al-Hindi," EI², 7: 800–1.

[27] Ghawthi, *Adhkar-i abrar*, p. 402.

[28] 'Abd al-Haqq Muhaddith Dihlawi al-Bukhari, *Akhbar al-akhyar fi asrar al-abrar*, ed. Muhammad 'Abd al-Ahad (Delhi: Matba'-i Mujtaba'i, 1332/1913–14), pp. 257–69; the unpublished *Zad al-muttaqin* is summarized by Rizvi, *History of Sufism*, 2:319–27.

[29] Edward Clive Bayley, *The History of India as told by its own Historians: The Local Muhammadan Dynasties—Gujarát*, ed. Nagendra Singh (repr., New Delhi: S. Chand & Co., 1970), p. 441.

[30] Ghawthi, *Adhkar-i abrar*, p. 345.

[31] Rizvi, *History of Sufism*, 2:321.

signed by `Ali al-Muttaqi, it is established that he was back in Mecca by 961/1554, so the incident of persecution would have to have taken place by then.[32] We can compare `Abd al-Haqq's reticence on this subject to his reluctance to discuss the martyrdom of the early Chishti Sufi Mas`ud Bakk, a subject that was broached more openly by `Abd al-Haqq's disciple Muhammad Sadiq.[33] `Abd al-Haqq's discreet silence can probably best be explained in terms of his strategy as a hagiographer interested in emphasizing shar`i norms.

In any case, after the years of exile in Gujarat, Muhammad Ghawth finally returned to northern India after 963/1556, when Humayun briefly reasserted his authority and Akbar was crowned emperor after Humayun's untimely death.[34] Muhammad Ghawth was received with general acclaim in Delhi and Agra. When he approached Akbar for an interview in 966/1558–59 in Agra, according to Bada'oni, he immediately aroused the enmity of the chief *sadr* (official in charge of charitable trusts), a Suhrawardi Sufi named Shaykh Gada'i. Bada'oni interpreted this enmity as entirely based on Shaykh Gada'i's professional jealousy. In any case, this set the stage for the third phase of persecution of the Shattari master. Due to Shaykh Gada'i's promptings, the regent Bayram Khan introduced in court with ridicule the claims Muhammad Ghawth had made about his ascension, once again evidently in allusion to *Awrad-i ghawthiyya*.[35] The shaykh retired in some discomfiture to Gwalior, which had recently been reconquered by the Mughals from Sher Shah's forces. He could be comforted, however, by the immense revenues that had been designated for his support, doubtless with the approval of Akbar.[36] Muhammad Ghawth had a final meeting with Akbar when the latter came hunting

---

[32] `Ali al-Muttaqi, Arabic *ijazat nama* in Shadhiliyya, Madyaniyya, and Qadiriyya orders; MS 52 Arabic, acc. no. 239, Jamia Millia Islamiyya, New Delhi, fol. 247a, dated 18 Sha`ban 961/19 July 1554 in Mecca.

[33] See Ernst, "From Hagiography to Martyrology" for details.

[34] Ghawthi, *Adhkar-i abrar*, p. 298, says this occurred in 963/1556; Bada'oni (*Muntakhabu-'t-tawarikh*, 3:8 [text, 3:5]) says that Muhammad Ghawth's departure from Gujarat for Agra occurred in 966/1558–59 and that he witnessed the shaykh riding amid a great throng of people in Agra's bazaar. This roughly agrees with the statement of Fazl Allah (*Manaqib-i Ghawthiyya*, p. 66), that Muhammad Ghawth spent 18 years in Gujarat.

[35] Bada'oni, *Muntakhabu-'t-tawarikh*, 2:28–29 (text, 2:34–35); Sukumar Ray, *Bairam Khan*, ed. M. H. A. Beg (Karachi: Institute of Central and West Asian Studies, 1992), pp. 175–77.

[36] Bada'oni (*Muntakhabu-'t-tawarikh*, 2:28–29 [text, 2:34–35]) estimates the shaykh's income at 100,000 rupees, a huge sum.

in the region of Gwalior and had his curiosity aroused by tales of the fine cattle kept by the shaykh. At this meeting, Muhammad Ghawth took the hand of the young king in the ritual of Sufi initiation, offering to become his spiritual guide. Akbar treated this as a joke, however, and his minister Abu al-Fazl regarded the shaykh and his pretensions with scorn.[37] Muhammad Ghawth remained in Gwalior, training disciples in Shattari exercises, until his death in 970/1563.

From the details summarized above, several points emerge with considerable force. First, although some accounts are vague about what actually aroused the opposition to Muhammad Ghawth, his ascension experience has been cited as the text that scholars regarded with suspicion in all three reported instances of persecution, first by the Suri regime, then by the sultan of Gujarat, and later by the regent of Akbar. Second, in all these cases the fortunes of Muhammad Ghawth were dependent on his close personal relationship with the Mughal rulers; all commentators, whether friendly or hostile to the shaykh, agree that he had an extraordinary influence over many political figures. His persecution by Sher Shah is clearly understandable as directed against a Mughal supporter, while his principal accuser in Gujarat, 'Ali al-Muttaqi, had been allied with a Gujarati sultan opposed to the Mughals. In the last instance, it appears that Akbar's good-natured regard for the brother of one of his father's spiritual advisers saved Muhammad Ghawth from the hostility of Shaykh Gada'i and Bayram Khan. Third, while Muhammad Ghawth was threatened in all these instances, he was an extremely influential and powerful man, and he emerged unscathed from the attempts of his opponents. His brother Shaykh P'hul only lost his life because he fell afoul of a purely political quarrel. Fourth, the persecution of Muhammad Ghawth was an unusual event in that none of the rulers or scholars who opposed the Shattari master was opposed to Sufism in principle. The Suris, the Gujarati sultans, and the Mughals were all generous patrons of Sufism. Muhammad Ghawth's critic 'Ali al-Muttaqi had in his childhood been initiated into the Chishti order, and later on, while studying hadith in Arabia, he had also been initiated into the Qadiri, Shadhili, and Madyani orders. Nor was 'Ali al-Muttaqi hostile to ecstatic Sufism on principle. Through his Chishti master Baha' al-Din Shah Bajan, 'Ali al-Muttaqi

---

[37] *The Akbar Nama of Abu-l-Fazl*, trans. H. Beveridge (Delhi: Ess Ess Publications, 1977), 2:133–35 (text, 2:88–89).

had a connection with the Chishti martyr Mas'ud Bakk, whose writings he frequently quoted, even translating one work by Mas'ud Bakk from Persian into Arabic.[38] He thus can hardly be characterized as an opponent of Sufism, although he was a spirited critic of the Mahdawi movement. Thus, if we wish to understand the "anti-Sufi" issue in the case of Muhammad Ghawth, it must be sought in his ascension narrative, which will be discussed further below. For the moment, let me suggest that the kernel of unacceptable statement lies in the claims of Muhammad Ghawth to have gone even beyond the level of Bayazid Bistami.

CIRCUMSPECTION IN THE LATER SHATTARI ORDER

We search in vain for any immediate effects of the persecution upon Muhammad Ghawth himself, in terms of any kind of alteration of his teachings. When Humayun wrote to express his concern about the troubles Muhammad Ghawth was undergoing as an exile, the shaykh shrugged them off as unimportant in his reply.[39] Although Muhammad Ghawth revised his meditation handbook *Jawahir-i khams* at the request of his disciples in 956/1549, correcting all known copies in the process, this appears to have been unrelated to any external political concern.[40] Khwishagi suggested that the initial persecution (under the Suri regime) was aimed at the ascension narrative in *Awrad-i ghawthiyya*, and he further maintained that Muhammad Ghawth later adopted a conciliatory stance regarding this controversial text, which he clarified by saying that his ascension was only in spirit and not bodily like that of the Prophet.[41] In what appears to be a version of the same story, Ghulam Sarwar (who

---

[38] See the biography of 'Ali al-Muttaqi in *Nuzhat al-khawatir*, 4:234–44. 'Ali al-Muttaqi quotes Mas'ud Bakk in his *Jawami' al-kalim fil mawa'iz wal-hikam*, also known as *al-Jawahir al-thamina*, a miscellany with quotations from Ansari, Sa'di, Husayni Sadat, Mas'ud Bakk, and others; cf. MS 1254 Persian, Asiatic Society, Calcutta. 'Ali al-Muttaqi translated the *Minhaj al-'arifin* [i.e., *Mir'at al-'arifin*] of Malik-zada Mas'ud [Bakk] into Arabic under the title *al-Nash al-wafi lil-qalb al-shafi*, MS Punjab University, Lahore, Sherani 3923/871/6, cat. II, 262, no. 1452.

[39] Ghawthi, *Adhkar-i abrar*, pp. 292–94.

[40] Some have suggested (Haq, "The Shuttari Order," p. 174; Nizami, "The Shattari Saints," p. 59) that the *Jawahir-i khams* came in for severe criticism by religious scholars, but this appears to be a confusion with *Awrad-i ghawthiyya*.

[41] Khwishagi, *Ma'arij al-wilayat*, fol. 553b, in Rizvi, *History of Sufism*, 2:158.

often cites Khwishagi) in 1280/1864–65 wrote that Wajih al-Din 'Alawi advised Muhammad Ghawth to take a variable position, according to whether the scholars were against him or not; if they supported him, he should maintain that his ascension veritably occurred during wakefulness, but if they opposed him, he should say that it took place during a dream.[42] Against this view suggesting a *taqiyya*-like dissimulation, we may note the observation found in one source that Muhammad Ghawth wrote *Awrad-i ghawthiyya* at age 43, three years after his arrival in Gujarat; in that case, the problems that the shaykh had with Sher Shah had nothing to do with the ascension treatise. If this is correct, it suggests that the report of Khwishagi about the Suri persecution of Muhammad Ghawth may have erroneously read back the controversy over *Awrad-i ghawthiyya* into an earlier, purely political persecution.[43]

Nonetheless, among the successors of Muhammad Ghawth, a distinctly conservative shari'a-oriented pattern became the norm. While most early Shattari writings by Muhammad Ghawth and his contemporaries are collections of esoteric meditation practices, later Shattari Sufis, particularly those located in the city of Burhanpur, increasingly focused on obligatory shari'a worship and Qur'anic and hadith studies. This conservative trend was already evident in Wajih al-Din 'Alawi (1504–89), the jurist who preserved Muhammad Ghawth from persecution in Gujarat and then became his disciple. Wajih al-Din's Sufi writings learnedly expound Sufi metaphysics in contrast to Ash'ari theology, but he pointedly avoids or mutes controversial topics in these discussions. For example, his mystical treatise *al-Haqiqat al-Muhammadiyya* makes an ingenious distinction between the legislative and gnostic aspects of prophecy, but Wajih al-Din is quick to assert that prophecy is always superior to sainthood, thus avoiding any heretical suggestion that would denigrate the Prophet. One of his sources for this doctrine, interestingly enough, is Bayazid Bistami, to whom the name of Ibn 'Arabi is also joined.[44] Making the point about the superiority of prophecy establishes his conservative credentials while, at the same time, he marks the

---

[42] Ghulam Sarwar, *Khazinat al-asfiya'*, pp. 333–34.

[43] Fazl Allah, *Manaqib-i Ghawthiyya*, p. 76.

[44] Wajih al-Din 'Alawi, *al-Risala al-musamma bil-haqiqat al-Muhammadiyya*, ed. with Urdu trans. Muhammad Zubayr Ghulam Nabi Qurayshi (Ahmadabad: Sarkhej Rawda Committee, 1385/1966), pp. 29–30.

centrality of the saint (Bayazid) who is the pivotal figure in the standard Shattari lineage. It should be recalled that Bayazid's ecstatic sayings that seemed to infringe on the status of the Prophet had previously been sanitized by popularizers of Sufism such as `Attar.

The contrast between Muhammad Ghawth and his more conservative disciples may be seen in an incident that took place when he met Tahir Muhammad Muhaddith, a pious scholar who later became a devoted disciple. "His glass is so pure and fine," remarked the shaykh. "How wonderful it would be to fill it with wine!" This scandalized the scholar, who was not yet accustomed to hearing Sufis use the name of "the mother of iniquities," though he eventually got used to it.[45] After spending some time in Berar, Tahir Muhammad (d. 1004/1595–96) settled in Burhanpur in 982/1574–75, where he composed works based on the classical Sufi writings of Qushayri, Makki, and Ghazali, along with digests and indices of works on hadith.[46] Only one of his writings hints at ecstatic sayings; his *Riyad al-salihin* contains three sections: the first contains explanations of hadith, the second comments on the sayings of Sufi masters (including `Abd al-Qadir Jilani, Ghazali, Abu Talib Makki, Shihab al-Din Suhrawardi, and, curiously enough, `Ali al-Muttaqi), and the third deals with the expressions and allusions of "the masters of unification and ecstasy, the people of love and gnosis" (such as Ibn `Arabi, `Ayn al-Qudat Hamadani, Sadr al-Din Qunawi, "and other followers of *wahdat al-wujud*").[47] Although the last section appears to be potentially controversial, it becomes clear from comparison with other Shattari works that articulation of the *wujudi* metaphysics associated with Ibn `Arabi was standard among nearly all Shattari authors. Evidently, in India, the views of Ibn `Arabi were not regarded as problematic at this time.

Another disciple of Muhammad Ghawth was Lashkar Muhammad `Arif (d. 993/1585), who came from a warrior clan; he guided Sufis for many years in Ahmedabad before coming to Burhanpur at the end of his life. Shaykh Lashkar exhibited a degree of piety toward the Prophet Muhammad that was remarkable. He stated that it is easy to reach God but quite difficult to reach the level of the Prophet. The reason is that one

---

[45] Rashid, *Burhanpur*, pp. 5–6, citing *Kashf al-haqa'iq*, fol. 3.
[46] Ghawthi, *Adhkar-i abrar*, pp. 426–33, enumerating eight writings, with a long excerpt from a Qushayri-style *tafsir* on pp. 427–32.
[47] Ghawthi, *Adhkar-i abrar*, p. 433.

must attain the most perfect of all attributes to come close to the Prophet, but God manifests in all degrees of creation and is therefore more easily accessible.[48] Shaykh Lashkar was the subject of a lengthy debate among his followers concerning an anecdote told by his saintly daughter Bibi Rasti. This daughter is also known as Bubu Rasti, and it is after her that the Burhanpur neighborhood of Rastipura is named. In a gathering that took place in 1013/1605, which included several leading Sufis and the Mughal minister ʿAbd al-Rahim Khan-i Khanan, she described how her father reached an indescribable state, which he later revealed was the station of Bayazid Bistami.[49] It was only by God's grace, he told her once he recovered his senses, that he did not repeat the famous utterance of Bayazid, "Glory be to me" (*subhani*). He reflected that it is better to say, "Glory be to him" (*subhanahu*), or some variation, to avoid the error of lese-majesté committed by Bayazid. Muhammad Ghawthi, author of *Gulzar-i abrar*, was quite cognizant of the delicacy of this situation. He himself offered a more nuanced interpretation:

> When the Sufi with the aid of annihilation in the journey of ascension removes the created garment of the body and enters the divine dress, and his goal becomes his own transcendence, then at that time there is need for interpreting and explaining his verbal utterance of "Glory be to him." And if he utters the cry of "Glory be to me," that is not improper, since that is in fact his goal. Therefore, on account of the superiority of saying "Glory be to him," both explanations apply.[50]

This tentative approval of the "Bayazidian rank" was first put forward by the chief disciple of Shaykh Lashkar, ʿIsa Jund Allah. Using Ibn ʿArabi's *Fusus* as a model, ʿIsa would have taken al-Hallaj to a higher state than the qualification with divinity that led to his ecstatic utterance, "I am the Real"; that higher state (reminiscent of Shaykh Ahmad Sirhindi's criticism of Ibn ʿArabi) was qualification with created existence.[51] Both in the report of the debate over Shaykh Lashkar's Bayazidian *temptatio*,

---

[48] Ghawthi, *Adhkar-i abrar*, p. 362.

[49] Khan-i Khanan and his son Darab Khan also attended the lectures of Bibi Rasti on Sufi classics such as ʿIraqi's *Lamaʿat*; see Rashid, *Burhanpur*, p. 51.

[50] Ghawthi, *Adhkar-i abrar*, p. 364.

[51] Ghawthi, *Adhkar-i abrar*, pp. 365–66; this section quotes extensively from the section on Noah in Ibn ʿArabi's *Fusus al-hikam*.

and in the highly ambivalent reflections by `Isa, we can see a reluctance
to approve of ecstatic states without grounding them in approved
metaphysical theories.

Shaykh `Isa Jund Allah (d. 1031/1622), a nephew of Tahir
Muhammad, was generally an irenic soul. He wrote primarily on meditation techniques employing the Arabic names of God, plus a couple of
treatises commenting on the metaphysics of *wahdat al-wujud*.[52] When a
dispute over hadith between religious scholars threatened to erupt into
a heresy accusation, he persuaded `Abd al-Rahim Khan-i Khanan to
send the heresy-hunting scholar on pilgrimage to Mecca.[53] Nonetheless,
such was the harmonious atmosphere established by the Faruqi kings in
Burhanpur prior to the Mughal conquest that `Isa, like many other local
Sufis, supported the Faruqis against Akbar. But the Mughals finally succeeded in taking the Faruqi fortress of Asir by stratagem and treason in
1010/1601. Consequently, Akbar planned to exile `Isa to Agra for a time,
along with other dissident Sufis, on the pretext of requesting him to give
spiritual instruction to the army; fortunately, the prayers of the shaykh
were answered and he did not have to suffer this ordeal for long.[54] This
seems to have been a fairly mild persecution, if we can call it that, and it
was a political affair unrelated to Sufism per se.

The trend toward greater shar`i conservatism continued with Shaykh
`Isa's children. `Isa's son Baba Fath Muhammad Muhaddith is known
primarily for his devotional writings on ritual prayer. When `Isa's future
successor in Burhanpur, Burhan al-Din Raz-i Ilahi, came to `Isa seek-
ing instruction, he was offered two choices: a letter of introduction to
the *sadr* if he sought money and land, or study with Fath Muhammad if
he sought religious learning; since Raz-i Ilahi sought knowledge of the
names of God, he remained with `Isa.[55] Fath Muhammad wrote over a
dozen treatises on ritual prayer and meditation, along with some short
summaries of *wahdat al-wujud* in the form of creeds. He also wrote on
the determination of the correct direction of Mecca from Burhanpur for

---

[52] Rashid, *Burhanpur*, pp. 63–73, provides a list of works, with a short treatise entitled
Risala-i daqiqa on pp. 74–80.

[53] Rashid, *Burhanpur*, pp. 45–46.

[54] Rashid, *Burhanpur*, pp. 55–57, 106–7. On the report of `Isa's disciple and *malfuzat*
recorder Farhi, these dissident Sufis were put under the authority of Shaykh Ahmad
Sirhindi's successor, Mir Muhammad Nu`man Naqshbandi.

[55] Rashid, *Burhanpur*, p. 41, citing *Rawa'ih al-anfas*, p. 13.

purposes of ritual prayer.[56] These are only a few examples of the later Shattari order after Muhammad Ghawth. Richard Eaton has remarked, with reference to Wajih al-Din `Alawi and his disciple Sibghat Allah (the translator of the *Jawahir-i khams* into Arabic), that these later Shattaris exhibit the characteristics of the "scholastic" and the "puritanical reformist" rather than the extravagant ecstatic.[57] While these terms may have to be modified to some extent when it is possible to give a fuller account of the teachings of these Sufis, the basic contrast seems to be correct.

Does this move to shar`i conservatism constitute a response to persecution? Evidence drawn from the life of Burhan al-Din Raz-i Ilahi (d. 1083/1673) suggests that this was in fact the case. This shaykh was drawn into the succession struggle between two claimants to the Mughal throne, Dara Shikuh and Awrangzib. Raz-i Ilahi was by temperament a strict ascetic and a conservative scholar. He was also opposed to performance of flute music if it led to dancing.[58] His writings consist of a credal commentary (*Sharh-i amantu billah*), a testament, and several collections of discourses recorded by disciples. He was very reluctant to form any connection with members of the court. When the noble Shayista Khan once joined the shaykh at Friday prayers, Raz-i Ilahi retired afterward to perform his prayers over again, remarking to a disciple that the presence of a noble (*amir*) in effect made his prayers nugatory.[59] So when Awrangzib came to the retreat of Raz-i Ilahi disguised as an ordinary person, accompanied by the legal scholar Shaykh Nizam (compiler of the legal work *al-Fatawa al-`Alamgiriyya*), Raz-i Ilahi was reluctant to acknowledge him in any way. There are two conflicting accounts of the outcome of this meeting. According to the historian Khwafi Khan, Awrangzib requested the aid of the saint in his struggle against Dara Shikuh, on the grounds that the latter had said that Islam was the same as infidelity (*kufr*). In this version, Raz-i Ilahi gave the prince a blessing, and Shaykh Nizam predicted victory for Awrangzib. Another historian, Ma`muri, reports instead that the shaykh refused to become a partisan in the succession dispute.[60] One is tempted to speculate that Khwafi Khan

[56] Rashid, *Burhanpur*, pp. 70, 118–42, with a short *mathnawi* poem presented on pp. 143–50.
[57] Eaton, *Sufis of Bijapur*, pp. 60, 206.
[58] Rashid, *Burhanpur*, pp. 322–23.
[59] Rashid, *Burhanpur*, p. 296.
[60] Anees Jahan Syed, *Aurangzeb in Muntakhab-al Lubab* (Bombay: Somaiya Publications Pvt. Ltd., 1977), p. 83, with n. 11.

stretched the story to fit a royal historiography. In any case, if Raz-i Ilahi was approached by Awrangzib to take sides on an ostensibly religious issue, it may well have sensitized him to the problems of persecution. The most striking example of his conservatism occurred when one of his disciples, Shaykh Nur Ramz-i Ilahi, began to shout aloud the phrase, "Burhan is God Most Great," and others joined in the chant. According to Khwafi Khan, the shaykh warned the disciples to desist, and when they continued, he handed them over to the qadi for execution.[61] This would indeed be an internalization of the persecution initially visited upon Muhammad Ghawth, but in this case, it was much more successful than the persecution of the earlier saint. Here the spiritual status of the saint was not proclaimed by the saint himself but by his disciples. Unlike the case of the ambiguity of Shaykh Lashkar about his own "Bayazidian rank," here Raz-i Ilahi rejected outright the suggestion of his disciples that he was identical with God. A verse by the shaykh seems to recall this incident: "Burhan is the proof of God, yet he is nothing but an intercessor of the beloved; I saw that the master is the outer form of God, and God is his inner form."[62] Local narrative sees Raz-i Ilahi as strictly conforming with the expectations of sanctity in his encounter with Awrangzib. It is popularly believed in Burhanpur that the tomb of Raz-i Ilahi was built by order of Awrangzib, and that the sum for the base of the tomb was taken from the emperor's earnings from the sale of his knitted hats and copies of the Qur'an; since the dome, however, was to be built with funds taken from the imperial treasury, the saint rejected that donation as contrary to Islamic law, and the present dome was accordingly financed otherwise.[63]

What is especially curious is that very little evidence survives in Shattari writings regarding the original persecution of Muhammad Ghawth. At one time a document describing the accusations against Muhammad Ghawth was reported to be in the Pir Muhammad Shah library in Ahmedabad, but the current custodians have no record of it. In an extended commentary on this question, Muhammad Zubayr Qureshi remarks that there is an account of the persecution of Muhammad

---

[61] K. A. Nizami, "Sufi Movement in the Deccan," in *History of Medieval Deccan (1295–1724)*, ed. H. K. Sherwani and P. M. Joshi, 2 vols. (Hyderabad: The Government of Andhra Pradesh, 1973–74), 2:194, quoting *Muntakhab al-lubab*, 2:554.

[62] Rashid, *Burhanpur*, p. 333.

[63] Rashid, *Burhanpur*, pp. 354–56.

Ghawth and the role of `Ali al-Muttaqi in a hagiography entitled *Mukhbir al-awliya'*, but it is not yet clear if this contains any material not already known from other sources.[64] Qureshi observes that the disciples of Muhammad Ghawth wrote many works preserved in manuscript, "Yet no one refers to the encounter of Muhammad Ghawth Gwaliari [with his accusers]. They observe discreet silence. It is strange."[65] If the suggestions made above are correct, it seems that Shattari masters subsequent to Muhammad Ghawth preferred to forget altogether about his persecution. It was an unpleasant episode, and they did not wish to revive it as a martyrology.

CONCLUSIONS

What was controversial enough to lead to the persecution of Muhammad Ghawth? I have proposed above that it was the claim of attaining a spiritual state beyond that of Bayazid Bistami that provoked outrage. Naturally political conditions also needed to be such that persecution of a Sufi saint was worth the trouble it might otherwise cause for a ruler. The Mughal struggles with other Indian dynasties furnished the political occasion for such persecution. A brief comparison with other cases within the Sufi tradition affords several instances where the status of Bayazid Bistami became the standard against which mystics measured their experiences. The biographies of Ruzbihan Baqli of Shiraz (d. 606/1209) record only a single instance of judicial doubt regarding his many striking spiritual claims. This doubt arose when a scholar found the passage in Ruzbihan's autobiographical work *Kashf al-asrar* where Ruzbihan described himself sitting on a mountain top, clinking glasses with God and tossing roses down to the plain where Bayazid Bistami and other Sufi saints looked on enviously. The scholar's doubts were removed, however, when Bayazid Bistami appeared to him in a dream to confirm the truth of Ruzbihan's vision.[66] Another notable example of using Bayazid Bistami as a mystical standard to be exceeded is Ibn

---

[64] This title, ascribed to Mawdud Lala Chishti, is noticed by Storey in a single Bombay MS (Mulla Firuz 14), but Qurayshi knows of another copy in a Chishti shrine in Ahmedabad. C. A. Storey, *Persian Literature: A Bio-bibliographical Survey*, 2 vols. (London: Luzac & Co., 1927–71), 1:1059, no. 55.

[65] Personal communication, letter dated 13 February 1995.

[66] See my *Ruzbihan Baqli: Mysticism and the Rhetoric of Sainthood in Persian Sufism*, Curzon Sufi Series 4 (London: Curzon Press, 1996).

`Arabi, who viewed Bistami with intense ambivalence; while he con-
sidered some of Bistami's formulations to be evidence of a supremely
advanced state, he also criticized the boasting (*fakhr*) that is inherent in
ecstatic expressions (*shathiyyat*), in this way putting himself in a position superior to that of Bistami.[67] To take a case slightly after the time
of Muhammad Ghawth, we may consider Shaykh Ahmad Sirhindi, who
explicitly claimed a spiritual status that exceeded both Abu Yazid and Ibn
`Arabi, observing that their claims were based on improperly interpreted
experiences that his own teachings clarified; his critics in turn charged
him with arrogance. In addition, his apparent claim to exceed the rank
of Companions of the Prophet such as Abu Bakr was pretext enough to
cause Sirhindi to be imprisoned by the Mughal emperor Jahangir.[68] The
basic principle that caused offense in these claims is that the ecstatic
vaults over the "horizontal" authenticity afforded by historical tradition
through approved Sufi lineages. With direct access to God as its own
verification, "vertical" authenticity can dispense with the validation of
historical tradition. That is the ultimate challenge offered to established
religion by ecstatic Sufis.

A search for other causes for the persecution of Muhammad Ghawth
fails to provide convincing alternatives. The Shattari order, as we have
seen, was very insistent about the performance of normal shar`i ritual,
and in this respect, it did not differ from most of the established Sufi
orders. The philosophy of Ibn `Arabi, though perhaps restricted to circles
of capable students, was retained as the basic theoretical framework for
mystical Islam by nearly all the Shattari masters.

Some may suggest that the interest of Muhammad Ghawth in yoga
was controversial since he is known to have translated the Arabic version of a hatha yoga treatise into Persian under the title *Bahr al-hayat*.
There is, however, no evidence to suggest that anyone made objections
to yogic practice on religious grounds during the lifetime of Muhammad
Ghawth. The net effect of the yogic practices discussed in Shattari texts

---

[67] See my "The Man without Attributes: Ibn `Arabi's Interpretation of Abu Yazid
al-Bistami." *Journal of the Muhiyiddin Ibn `Arabi Society* 13 (1993): 1–18.

[68] Yohanan Friedmann, *Shaykh Ahmad Sirhindi: An Outline of His Thought and a Study
of His Image in the Eyes of Posterity* (Montreal: McGill-Queen's University Press, 1971),
pp. 28, 60, 88, 62–68, 94–96; Ghulam `Ali Azad Bilgrami, *Subhat al-marjan fi athar
Hindustan*, ed. Muhammad Fazl al-Rahman al-Nadwi al-Siwani (Aligarh: Jami`at Aligarh
al-Islamiyya, 1972), 1:131–37.

had little relevance to any Hindu theology. The disciples of Muhammad Ghawth were agreed that his treatment of yogic disciplines had basically Islamicized them.[69] Succeeding generations of Shattaris continued developing specialized meditations that owed little to any integral yogic tradition. In the recollections of Raz-i Ilahi, there remains little residue of the intense interest in yoga characteristic of Muhammad Ghawth. The only incident that Raz-i Ilahi relates concerning yoga is a story in which Muhammad Ghawth was bitten on the thigh by a snake; such was the saint's power that the snake immediately died. A yogi who observed this event recognized the shaykh as a perfected *siddha*.[70] This anecdote retains nothing of yogic practice, but simply perpetuates the hagiographic formula in which Sufis outperform yogis in thaumaturgy. Similarly, Shaykh `Isa once told a disciple to seek his next master by visualization, whether he appeared to be a proper Sufi shaykh, a wild qalandar, or a yogi.[71] Here the yogi functions simply as a stock comparison, to signify that which is least conventional for Sufi disciples; `Isa would even approve of a disciple studying with a yogi if that would help the disciple advance.

The early Shattaris may have been aware of the potential tendency of their ecstatic approach to strain relations with the historical traditions of Islam. The tendency to provide a legitimizing multiple lineage for Shattari masters is found already in biographical accounts of the founder of the Indian branch of the order, `Abd Allah Shattari (d. 832/1428–29), who is credited with Qadiri and Kubrawi initiations.[72] Likewise Baha' al-Din Ansari (d. 921/1515) was known as a Qadiri with a Shattari affiliation (*mashrab*).[73] Muhammad Ghawth himself claimed 14 separate initiations in different Sufi orders. As a tentative observation concerning this phenomenon, I would propose that multiple initiation was a way of maximizing historical validation by tradition, by claiming as many possible avenues of contact with the founding figures of Sufism. The fact that this might be achieved by purely internal Uwaysi contacts is the homage that spontaneous ecstasy pays to historical tradition. In any case, a review of the history of the Shattari order in the century after

---

[69] For a full discussion, see my *The Pool of Nectar: An Islamic Interpretation of Yoga* (SUNY Press, forthcoming).

[70] Rashid, *Burhanpur*, pp. 313–14, citing *Rawa'ih al-anfas*, p. 380.

[71] Rashid, *Burhanpur*, p. 46.

[72] *Nuzhat al-khawatir*, 3:100–1, citing *Majma` al-abrar* and *Gulzar-i abrar*.

[73] `Abd al-Haqq, *Akhbar al-akhyar*, p. 198.

Muhammad Ghawth provides a striking portrait of retreat from the bold claims of spiritual ecstasy. In the aftermath of repeated criticism and persecution of their chief organizer, later Shattari masters modulated the natural tendency of ecstatic experience and muted the urge to engage in boasting contests with the founding figures of mysticism. Persecution is always a political act, and its power can be internalized to the point of self-censorship. The circumspection of the later Shattaris would seem to be evidence of the power of persecution to modify public behavior.

5

The Daily Life of a Saint, Ahmad Sirhindi (d. 1624), by Badr al-Din Sirhindi

One of the most prominent features of Islam in South Asia is the Sufi tradition, especially as embodied in the major Sufi orders. Among these, the Naqshbandi order is distinctive for its rigorous practices and well known for its charismatic leaders. Originating in Central Asia, the Naqshbandi lineage had a history of strong involvement in politics. In terms of Sufi practice, the Naqshbandis were known for insisting on the silent recollection (*dhikr*) of the names of God and for a resolute avoidance of music.

Of all the leaders of the Naqshbandi order, one of the most important was Shaykh Ahmad Sirhindi (1574–1624), whose metaphysical and mystical teachings are preserved in his large collection of letters, the *Maktubat*. Sirhindi became controversial for certain claims that he made regarding his spiritual status, which according to some came close to disrespect for the Prophet Muhammad. The emperor Jahangir briefly imprisoned him, and his letters were proscribed by Aurangzeb. Nevertheless, his followers regarded him as the "renewer of the second millennium," and granted him near-messianic status as he reasserted the centrality of Islamic law and ritual practice in the lives of Muslims. In recent times, Sirhindi has been viewed as a reformer whose ideas prefigure modern notions of religious identity, such as the formation of Pakistan as an Islamic state; these interpretations considerably exaggerate the importance of a few political remarks by Sirhindi (such as his antipathy for Shi'is and for non-Muslims), which were rather peripheral to his central religious concerns.

The passage translated here is taken from a contemporary hagiography dedicated to Sirhindi and his successors, composed and completed around 1643 by Sirhindi's disciple Badr al-Din Sirhindi. It comprises the fifth section of the book, on the spiritual practices of Sirhindi. It is preceded by sections on his mystical genealogy, predictions of his advent, and his unique characteristics, and it is followed by chapters defending him against his critics, recording his sayings and his miracles, and offering short accounts of his descendants and successors.

The emphasis throughout this selection is on Sirhindi as the epitome and embodiment of the authentic practice of the example (*sunna*) of the Prophet Muhammad in every possible detail. His daily routine is nothing less than an exhaustive account of the performance of the five obligatory ritual prayers of Islam, along with the supererogatory ("extra credit") prayers that were so commonly observed in Sufi circles. Minute details are provided about his behavior with respect to ritual ablutions before prayer, sleep, eating, the toilet, etc., extending to such details as the toothbrush (*miswak*) recommended in pious Muslim practice as an emulation of a habit of the Prophet. The Qur'an is present throughout, frequently recited during ritual prayer, and continually invoked in additional meditations. Sirhindi acts as imam and leads his followers in ritual prayer. He is also presented as rejecting certain customary practices that he views as incompatible with the strict teachings of the Hanafi school of law, which was dominant in Central Asia and South Asia. This rhetorical insistence on Sirhindi as the defining figure of correct Islamic practice was also integral to the later Naqshbandi defense of Sirhindi against his critics.

Sufi practices are invoked throughout this hagiographical portrait, although in an unobtrusive fashion. Sirhindi is depicted as leading a circle of recollection (*dhikr*), where disciples would chant the names of God or Arabic formulas such as the Muslim profession of faith. Although he is shown as experiencing extraordinary spiritual states, his strength of character is such that he makes no physical display or reaction whatsoever. He is naturally ascetic and only indulges in food in order to comply with the example of the Prophet. His recitation of the Qur'an and his performance of prayer are awe-inspiring to his disciples, but he makes no attempt to embellish his recitation of the Qur'an with musical emphasis. He is surrounded by disciples, both novices and adepts, whom he counsels on the basis of his profound mystical insights; he can also act directly on their inner states through his power of concentration (*tawajjuh*), a faculty particularly cultivated by Naqshbandi masters. He is regarded as the personification of correct behavior.

Taken as a whole, this excerpt is a good example of a hagiographical presentation that aims at enhancing the sanctity of its saintly subject in terms of the core ritual practices of Islam.

FROM BADR AL-DIN SIRHINDI'S
HAZARAT AL-QUDS [SACRED PRESENCES][1]

Midnight Purifications

His practice in both cold and hot weather, both away and at home, was that, after midnight, he awakened and recited the prescribed invocations of that hour. After that, he went to the toilet, first putting his left foot in the toilet area and, after that, the right foot, and then reciting the prescribed prayer of that hour. After he was done with the toilet, he stood on his left foot and then cleaned himself with earth and water according to prophetic custom. Then, he performed ablutions, sat facing the direction of prayer, asking someone's assistance in ablutions. With a ewer in the left hand, he first poured water on the right hand and then on the left. After that he washed both hands together and the spaces between the fingers from the palm of the hand outward. While rinsing, he employed a toothbrush, brushing three times on the right, three times on the left, and three times on the top; if he did more than that, it was to care for the gums, beginning from the upper teeth of the right side, then the lower teeth of the same side, then the upper teeth on the left side, and after that the lower teeth of that side. In every ablution, he employed the toothbrush, and when he was finished, as this writer has witnessed, he placed the toothbrush above his ear and frequently also entrusted it to the attendant. His companions kept their toothbrushes in a fold of their turbans.

---

[1] The selections I have translated here are from the Persian work compiled by Badr al-Din Sirhindi [d. 1648], *Hazarat al-quds [Sacred Presences]* (Lahore: Mahkama-i Awqaf, 1971), pp. 80–92.

He then spat out the rinse water and three times rinsed his mouth and nostrils with fresh water. He slowly poured water on his blessed face with perfect gentleness from the top of his forehead. He gave a slight precedence to passing his right hand over his right cheek before passing the left hand over the left cheek so that he could begin with the right. When washing his blessed face, he pushed his turban to one side so that part of his head would be exposed, and he washed it from that side. The amount of water that he poured on his blessed face was such that the drops never splashed on his robe or his body. Every time he let all the drops fall from his hand to his face so that none of it dripped on his robe.

After that he washed the arms up to the elbow three times, each time repeatedly wiping his right hand upward so that not a drop remained, and likewise with the left hand. He poured water on the fingers, and the water for wiping that he took in his right hand, he conveyed to the left hand, scattering it far away so the drops would not splash on the ground and reach his robe. He wiped his whole head from the front to the back, and he wiped the top of the head with the inside of his right-hand fingers and the sides of the head with the palms of both hands, bringing them from the back to the front. Then, with the same water, he wiped the inside of the ear with the index finger and the outside with the thumb. Then, with the back of the hand, he wiped the neck. He repeated the washing of the right and left feet three times, washing the ankle part of the leg, rubbing the hand upward every time so that it nearly became dry. He observed the customary prayers prescribed for the time of performing a full body ablution.

Late Night Prayers (Supererogatory)

After completing ablutions, he also recited customary prayers, but he did not clean the body with a robe after ablutions. Then, he put on a fine clean robe, and with a splendid and dignified bearing, he headed to ritual prayer. He performed two minimum cycles of ritual prayer, and he did the rest of the late night prayer with lengthy recitations from the Qur'an. Usually he recited two or three portions of the 30 equal portions of the Qur'an. Sometimes, he went from midnight to dawn in a single cycle of prayer. When the attendant called, saying that dawn had arrived, he performed a second cycle of ritual prayer in the minimum fashion and said the peace. Most of the time, he performed up to 12 cycles of ritual prayer, more or less, according to the needs of the hour. After every double prayer, in submission and humility, he became absorbed in meditation, and when he was done, he prayed for forgiveness and performed other prayers and blessings, a hundred times. He meditated until dawn, or else recited the profession of faith, and a little before dawn, in accordance with the traditional example of the Prophet (prayers, blessings, and salutations upon its source), he would go to sleep, thus realizing the saying, "Keep late night vigil between two times of sleep."

Dawn Prayer (Obligatory)

Before dawn he would awaken and, after performing a new ablution, would follow custom in his house. After that, he would stretch out facing the direction of prayer with his right hand propped under the right side of his chin, but later he would stop stretching out. After that, he performed the obligatory dawn prayer in the mosque with a large crowd, at the first light and the last twilight. He himself acted as imam, reciting the Qur'an at length and in detail. After completing ritual prayer, he recited some customary prayers, and then turning to the people, or the left, or the right, lifted up his hands in voluntary prayer.

Morning Prayer (Supererogatory)

After the voluntary prayer, he drew both hands across his face, and he then sat in the circle of recollection with his companions and performed this internal practice until the sun rose up a spear's length. Within the circle, they sometimes also listened to the Qur'an from one who had memorized it. Then, he performed two cycles of the morning prayer with lengthy recitations. Then, he performed two minimum cycles of prayer, after which he recited the prayer of seeking guidance and the completion of the customary appointed prayers.

Advising Disciples

Then, he went into seclusion and, according to the requirements of his spiritual state, was absorbed in recitation of the holy Qur'an or, sometimes, the recitation of the profession of faith. Sometimes, he summoned his disciples separately, asking each one questions about his spiritual state, and, in accordance with that state, gave guidance to each. There were many whose hidden spiritual states he explained, regarding both present and future, and he clarified them in detail. He trained them and made them aware of the divine names, the spiritual stations, the ecstasies, and the visitations.

Sometimes, he summoned his advanced disciples, explained his own chosen secrets, and unveiled to them divine knowledge. He ordinarily tried to conceal those secrets with all his heart, but when he was explaining this divine knowledge, it was perceptible that he was encountering and receiving the spiritual state (of those secrets and that divine knowledge). There were many who, when they heard this sublime divine knowledge from his pearl-scattering tongue, in gazing upon him at that very instant themselves, experienced that divine knowledge. Most of the time that this revered one spent with his companions and others was in silence. His companions, from their extreme awe and wonder at him, did not even have the power to breathe. His control was at such a level that, in spite of the onslaught and frequency of numerous kinds of enrapturing visitations, no external sign of the rapture of that revered one ever appeared. He was never seen to be agitated, to exclaim, to shout, or to cry out, except on very rare occasions. Occasionally, he wiped away a tear or was close to weeping, and sometimes, in the midst of explaining divine realities, his face became flushed.

Mealtime

To return to the topic of discussion, when the morning became advanced, he performed two cycles of the morning prayer, though at times from necessity he performed four. He then took food, and while eating, he could be seen most of the time to be dividing food for the dervishes, his family, the attendants, and guests. During this time he would sometimes pick up a morsel with three fingers, and sometimes, reaching for a plate, he would put some food in his mouth and taste it. At that time, it was well known that he scarcely needed any food, and he only ate because eating is the prophetic tradition; prophets have not dispensed with that. At the time of eating, his manner of sitting was by the path of the prophetic tradition: sometimes he pulled up both knees, and sometimes he put the right foot on the left foot and the right knee on the left knee. After finishing with food, he recited the customary prayers of that hour, but he did not, according to popular practice, recite the Opening [*fatiha*, the first chapter of the Qur'an] after eating for that is not in accordance with the prophetic example.

Forenoon Prayer (Supererogatory) and Noon Prayer (Obligatory)

After eating, for an hour, he took a siesta, in accordance with the prophetic example. Then, when shadows disappeared at noon and the muezzin gave the call to prayer, the muezzin's words, "God is most great," and the awakening of that revered saint took place simultaneously. Immediately, with firmness and dispatch, he stood up on the ground; he never varied from this routine. While listening to the call to prayer, he repeated every word, except that during the two invitations ("Come to prayer" and "Come to salvation"), he recited the prayer, "There is no might or power save in God." After he was done listening to the call to prayer, he recited a voluntary prayer, and when that was done, he got up, performed ablutions, put on a clean robe, and came to the mosque. First, he performed two cycles of ritual prayer in salutation of the mosque, and after that, he performed the four prescribed cycles of the forenoon ritual prayer with lengthy recitations from the Qur'an. After that, he performed the four prescribed cycles of ritual prayer set for noontime. Then, he recited the standing glorification of God, led prayers as imam, and recited from the Qur'an at length and in detail. After the completion of the required duties, he arose, performing no other prayers except, "God! You are peace, and peace is from you. You have blessed us, glorious and generous one." He performed the two other prescribed ritual prayers set for that time. Then, he performed the four cycles of ritual prayer that are in addition to the prescribed ones, and he recited the invocations that are customary after the obligatory ones. Then, he sat down facing the people and had his companions form a circle. One who had memorized the Qur'an recited it, while he with his disciples sat attentively in meditation.

Afternoon Prayer (Obligatory)

When that was completed, he completed one or two elementary lessons until the time of mid-afternoon arrived. He arose to perform fresh ablutions. After the return of two-thirds of the original shadow, at the beginning of the time of afternoon prayer, he came to the mosque and performed two cycles of the prayer of salutation to the mosque and four cycles of prescribed ritual prayer. Then, he led prayer as imam and performed the obligatory afternoon prayer with a large crowd. After that he recited the invocations that are customary after the obligatory ones. Then, he sat down facing the people and had his companions form a circle. One who had memorized the Qur'an recited it, and that revered one and his companions were absorbed in it. During this time, he was internally concentrating on their spiritual states, and he exerted his concentration for their advancement. Sometimes, he performed other virtuous actions.

Sunset Prayer (Obligatory)

After that, he first performed the ritual prayer of sunset. After the obligatory rituals, he performed the two cycles of prescribed ritual prayer set for that time, with neither delay nor haste. Then, he recited six cycles of ritual prayer, with three repetitions of the peace and lengthy readings from the Qur'an. Most of the readings that had been read during the prayer of the penitents, or mid-morning prayer, i.e., the Event [Qur. 56], and Sincerity [Qur. 112], as well as others, were read now also.

Evening Prayer (Obligatory)

He then came to the mosque for the evening prayer after "the departure of the whitening of the horizon," (which, according to "the greatest imam," Abu Hanifa, is an expression for twilight and an agreed-upon time). First, he recited two cycles of ritual prayer or of salutation of the mosque, and after that, he performed four cycles of prescribed ritual prayer. After that, he performed four cycles of obligatory ritual prayer in congregation, performing no other prayers except, "God! You are peace," etc. Then, he arose and performed two cycles of prescribed ritual prayer set for that time and four additional recommended cycles of ritual prayer. Then, he offered special voluntary prayers. After that, he recited Prostration [Qur. 32], and sometimes, in the four cycles of ritual prayer after the obligatory ones, he recited Prostration, the Blessed [Qur. 67], Unbelievers [Qur. 109], and Sincerity. Sometimes, in the four cycles of ritual prayer, he recited all four books that begin with "Say," and in the special voluntary prayers, he recited praise of the divine name, Unbelievers, and Sincerity. He then combined the two standing prayers of the Hanafi and Shafi'i schools of law, which the Hanafis combine and consider good. After the special voluntary prayer, he recited the beginning of two cycles of ritual prayer, reciting from Earthquake [Qur. 99] and Unbelievers. But, at the end, he left off the two cycles of ritual prayer, saying that there is disagreement about them. The prostration that is usually observed after the special voluntary prayer was not performed by that revered one, for the legal scholars have agreed that it is objectionable. Sometimes, he performed the special voluntary prayer at the beginning of the evening and, sometimes, at the end. After the late-night prayer, he repeated it, for according to the saying of the Prophet (peace be upon him), a single night does not have two special voluntary prayers. After that, at the time of sleeping, having recited books, verses, praises, and prescribed prayers, he stretched himself out in a long arbor so that he faced the direction of prayer and his right hand was beneath his face. And the righteous sleep of that revered one was completely in the presence of meditation, union, and witnessing the divine beauty.

How wonderful are the degrees of the sleep that is better than wakefulness!

When reciting the Qur'an, during prayer or at other times, he had a way of reciting that you would swear actually conveyed the meaning within each word. On listening to his recitation, it would suddenly become apparent to listeners that the secrets of the Qur'an were pouring forth upon that one who was brought near to the glorious God. Most of the people who had not entered the circle of his disciples said that this revered one recited the Qur'an in such a manner that one would say that the words came forth from his heart. But he never attempted to recite in a musical style. During the long prayers of Ramadan, we saw few listeners who did not succumb to sleep, but when they heard that revered one recite the Qur'an, most of them were standing up, and they were never affected by sleep.

That revered one had disciples, masters of spiritual states, whom he had guided as students in his presence. Before they reached the level of perfection and the capacity to perfect others, he gave them permission to teach the spiritual path so that, by saving people from the whirlpool of error, they could guide them towards God (glory be to Him). But because of their lack of perfection, he repeatedly and emphatically explained to them that they should never imagine themselves to be perfect, for they would fall into consternation and the path of their advancement would be blocked. Of all the paths of the masters, he considered the lofty path of the Naqshbandis to be the best, for he said that this path is identical with the path of the holy companions of the Prophet, so he held this lineage to be superior to other lineages.

This lowly one [i.e., Badr al-Din Sirhindi], prior to entry into the group of servants of that imam who is the source of concentration, several times went to his mosque, and I saw him performing prayer. Involuntarily, I left my place, for I knew that he was talking face to face with the Leader of Creation (i.e., Muhammad, may God bless him and grant him peace) and that he saw that revered Prophet (may God bless him and grant him peace) performing prayer; he himself was performing prayer according to that example. Otherwise, this lowly one has seen religious scholars and masters, but I have never seen this kind of prayer from anyone.

He had perfect morals, humility, compassion for God's creatures, acceptance, and submission. His relatives suffered much from corrupt rulers, but with submission and acceptance, he paid them no attention. Whenever an important person came to see him, he arose respectfully and gave a place to the visitor at the head of the assembly, speaking to him according to the man's measure. He never showed respect to infidels, even if they were politically powerful and prominent. It was his custom that he was first to greet anyone, and it is not known if anyone ever succeeded in being first to greet him. He exerted himself with extreme compassion in protection of the rights of the people, and whenever the news of someone's death reached him, he took it as a warning and expressed his regret. He said words of consolation and attended funeral prayers, reciting prayers for assistance.

FURTHER READING

A good biographical study is available in Yohanan Friedmann, *Shaykh Ahmad Sirhindi: An Outline of His Thought and a Study of His Image in the Eyes of Posterity* (Montreal and London: McGill-Queens University Press, 1971).

6

Islam and Sufism in Contemporary South Asia

Sometime during his rule over Pakistan during the 1980s, then-President General Zia ul-Haq was reputedly asked to address a conference dedicated to the topic of South Asian Islam. Upon his arrival (three hours late as usual), he stepped to the microphone and announced, "There is no such thing as South Asian Islam. There is only one true Islam, based on the Qur'an and the Prophet Muhammad." This declaration undoubtedly put a damper on the conference. It was based on the notion that religion has no history or location but that it is essentially related only to unchanging scripture and founder figures. The Hindu fundamentalist groups who urged on the destruction of the Babri Masjid in Ayodhya in 1992 would certainly have welcomed this statement from General Zia since, in their view, it would confirm the notion that Islam is essentially foreign to India.

This view of Islamic identity as purely scriptural and unrelated to history is what I would describe as a kind of "Protestant" version of Islam, which has been supported and spread in recent times by the reformist and fundamentalist groups associated with Salafi and Wahhabi perspectives. This Protestant model of religion has also been widely accepted by ideologues from other religious traditions because of its extraordinary political effectiveness, and so non-Muslim opponents of Islam readily employ what is clearly a fundamentalist interpretation of Islam.[1] It is in order to historicize this essentialist understanding of religion that scholars

---

[1] Carl W. Ernst, *Following Muhammad: Rethinking Islam in the Contemporary World*, Islamic Civilization and Muslim Networks 1 (Chapel Hill, NC: University of North Carolina Press, 2003).

since Marshall Hodgson have used the term "Islamicate" to indicate the larger non-religious and cultural complex, often associated with the presence of Islamic religion, which has characterized many societies and has included extensive participation by non-Muslims.[2] Striking the historical and cultural balance suggested by the term "Islamicate" is therefore of considerable importance in providing a scholarly understanding of the role of Islam in any society. If we wish to have a better view of the distinctive factors that might constitute South Asian Islam, we will have to look elsewhere than in the bastions of Islamic fundamentalism (although they do, ironically, constitute an important strand of Islam in South Asia). Such an approach is not new; one may consider, for example, the memorable if idiosyncratic approach to Iranian Islam established by Henry Corbin, focusing on Sufism, Shi`ism, and Illuminationist philosophy as the keys to the distinctive genius of Persia.[3] Equally, one might propose a typological and historically focused exploration of the varieties of Islam in North Africa, Central Asia, China, Turkey, or the Gulf. Admittedly, one can run the risk of succumbing to the romance of local nationalism, but that temptation is best fended off by employing some of the comparative and critical resources of the social and human sciences.

There are several ways in which one may approach this geographic specification of an Islamic culture in the South Asian subcontinent. Bruce Lawrence has demonstrated two such approaches in a pair of thought-provoking though conceptually very different articles written for encyclopedias. In one of these, "Islam in South Asia," he adopted a peripheral approach and looked at the most far-flung regions of the subcontinent (including Bengal and Kerala) to provide an off-centered perspective.[4] In the other, "The Eastward Journey of Muslim Kingship," he presented a vivid narrative of the imperial institutions of the Mughals

---

[2] Marshall G. S. Hodgson, *The Venture of Islam: Conscience and History in a World Civilization*, 3 vols. (Chicago: University of Chicago Press, 1978).

[3] Henry Corbin, *En Islam iranien, aspects spirituels et philosophiques*, 4 vols. (Paris: Gallimard, 1971).

[4] Bruce B. Lawrence, "Islam in South Asia," in *The Oxford Encyclopaedia of the Modern Islamic World*, ed. John Esposito (New York: Oxford University Press, 1995), 2:278–84. Lawrence notes that this presentation was designed to offset the "vast and numbingly circular literature on Islam in South Asia" that asserts a depressing teleology of decline centered on the colonial experience.

as a lens through which to view the formation of Muslim society.[5] Another and much more extensive cultural treatment was Annemarie Schimmel's volume on *Islam in the Indian Subcontinent*, which is indeed a classic in its comprehensiveness and its remarkable command over the sources.[6] While those academic presentations have their own charm, the approach I would like to take at the moment is rather different, being complementary to the personal journey of one South Asian Muslim woman, Samina Quraeshi. Such a personal perspective as hers is admittedly subjective and centered on particular sets of experiences. In particular, she speaks to the deep spiritual appeal of the major centers of Sufism in the central and northwestern heartlands of South Asia. She invokes the rural landscapes of the Punjab and the Gangetic plain, as well as the ancient cities of Lahore and Delhi. While this vision does not exhaust by any means the astonishing complexities of the culture of South Asian Muslims, it does bring into play traditions of great importance for the understanding of South Asian Islam.

The sense of a distinctive destiny for South Asian Islam is not new. As early as the thirteenth century, the historian Minhaj-i Siraj saw Muslim India as the bulwark of Islam, and indeed, its central redoubt in the aftermath of the catastrophe of the Mongol invasion of the Middle East and the overthrow of the caliphate in 1258. Muslim rulers, not only in the Delhi Sultanate but also in outlying kingdoms, maintained the symbolism of the caliphate in their own coinage for over a century after this blow to notions of Islamic sovereignty. The persistence of the imperial idea of the caliphate in such a fictional mode, as Toynbee would have put it, was at the same time a powerful assertion by Indo-Muslim rulers of their role in preserving that Islamic legacy.[7] Certain rulers shored up the Turkish-Central Asian concept of world-imperial rule with patronage of Islamic law, as in the case of Sultan Firuz Shah ibn Tughluq; in the late fourteenth century, he proclaimed his renunciation of non-shari`a

---

[5] Bruce B. Lawrence, "The Eastward Journey of Muslim Kingship: South and Southeast Asia," in *The Oxford History of Islam*, ed. John Esposito (New York: Oxford University Press, 1999).

[6] Annemarie Schimmel, *Islam in the Indian Subcontinent*, Handbuch der Orientalistik, Zweite Abteilung: Indien 4:3 (Leiden-Köln: E. J. Brill, 1980). See also Annemarie Schimmel, *The Empire of the Great Mughals: History, Art and Culture* (London: Reaktion Books, 2004).

[7] Arnold Toynbee, *A Study of History* (New York: Barnes & Noble Books, 1995).

instruments of government and methods of taxation, while at the same time sponsoring numerous scholarly works on the Hanafi teachings of Islamic law. In a similar fashion, the late Mughal emperor Aurangzeb appealed to Islamic symbols and institutions in his sponsorship of collections of legal *responsa* (the famous *Fatawa-i `Alamgiri*) and by introducing Islamic touches to the edifice of the Mongol and Persian monarchy constructed by his forebears Akbar, Jahangir, and Shahjahan (though the portrait of his "orthodox" posture and anti-Hindu iconoclasm has been considerably exaggerated).

Yet, as Samina Quraeshi makes clear, the institute of kingship cannot be seen as the real locus of the culture of South Asian Muslims, despite the romantic fascination of its tales of courtly intrigue and power. To get to the heart of India's role in the Muslim cosmos, one has to go back considerably further. This powerful insight was deployed at length in a late Arabic masterwork of the Indian poet and scholar Ghulam `Ali Azad Bilgrami (d. 1786), who pointed out in his *Coral Rosary of Indian Traditions* that India plays a central role in the most canonical of Islamic sources, the hadith sayings of the Prophet Muhammad. As abundantly illustrated, for instance, in the massive *History of the Prophets and Kings* by al-Tabari (d. 923), India was the site of one of the primordial dramas in the cosmology of Islam, i.e., the descent of Adam from paradise to earth.[8] It was on a mountain-top in the great island of Serendib, as the Arabs called it—Ceylon, or modern Sri Lanka—that Adam first set foot on earth; the spot today is known appropriately as Adam's Peak, though the massive footprint enshrined there is also revered as Buddha's or Shiva's by devotees from Buddhist and Hindu backgrounds. But for Muslims, it has been a sacred spot for centuries. Consider the report of the famous traveler Ibn Battuta in the early fourteenth century:

> The mountain of Sarandib [Adam's Peak] is one of the highest in the world. We saw it from the sea when we were nine days' journey away, and when we climbed it we saw the clouds below us, shutting out our view of its base. On it there are many evergreen trees and flowers of various

---

[8] *The History of al-Tabari*, vol. 1, *General Introduction and From the Creation to the Flood*, trans. Franz Rosenthal (Albany : State University of New York Press, 1988); Carl W. Ernst, trans., "India as a Sacred Islamic Land," in *Religions of India in Practice*, ed. Donald S. Lopez, Jr., Princeton Readings in Religions 1 (Princeton University Press, 1995), pp. 556–63.

colours, including a red rose as big as the palm of a hand. There are two tracks on the mountain leading to the Foot, one called Baba track and the other Mama track, meaning Adam and Eve. The Mama track is easy and is the route by which the pilgrims return, but anyone who goes by that way is not considered by them to have made the pilgrimage at all. The Baba track is difficult and stiff climbing. Former generations cut a sort of stairway on the mountain, and fixed iron stanchions on it, to which they attached chains for climbers to hold on by. There are ten such chains, two at the foot of the hill by the "threshold," seven successive chains farther on, and the tenth is the "Chain of the Profession of Faith," so-called because when one reaches it and looks down to the foot of the hill, he is seized by apprehensions and recites the profession of faith ("there is no god but God, and Mohammed is His messenger!") for fear of falling. When you climb past this chain you find a rough track. From the tenth chain to the grotto of Khidr is seven miles; this grotto lies in a wide plateau, and nearby it is a spring full of fish, but no one catches them. Close to this there are two tanks cut in the rock on either side of the path. At the grotto of Khidr the pilgrims leave their belongings and ascend thence for two miles to the summit of the mountain where the Foot is.

The blessed Footprint, the Foot of our father Adam, is on a lofty black rock in a wide plateau. The blessed Foot sank into the rock far enough to leave its impression hollowed out. It is eleven spans long. In ancient days the Chinese came here and cut out of the rock the mark of the great toe and the adjoining parts. They put this in a temple at Zaytun, where it is visited by men from the farthest parts of the land. In the rock where the Foot is there are nine holes cut out, in which the infidel pilgrims place offerings of gold, precious stones, and jewels. You can see the dervishes, after they reach the grotto of Khidr, racing one another to take what there is in these holes. We, for our part, found nothing in them but a few stones and a little gold, which we gave to the guide. It is customary for the Pilgrims to stay at the grotto of Khidr for three days, visiting the Foot every morning in evening, and we followed this practice. When the three days were over we returned to the Mama track, halting at a number of villages on the mountain. At the foot of the mountain there is an ancient tree whose leaves never fall, situated in a place that cannot be got at. I have never met anyone who has seen its leaves.[9]

I cite this report at length so one can get the flavor of the experience of this Muslim judge from Morocco as he approached the Indian shrine of Adam's footprint. The atmosphere is rich in mythical overtones, with

---

[9] Ibn Battuta, *Travels in Asia and Africa 1325–1354*, trans. H. A. R. Gibb (New York: Robert M. McBride & Company, 1929), pp. 258–59.

gendered approaches for pilgrims and a liminal grotto dedicated to the deathless prophet Khizr, which still attracts dervishes and other devotees today.[10] Four centuries after Ibn Battuta, Azad Bilgrami commented on the popularity of the site, its Sufi attendants, and the friendly "Hindu" ruler (actually a Theravada Buddhist) who welcomed Muslim visitors. More importantly, for Azad, India was, next to Mecca and Medina, the holiest spot in the world for Muslims: it was the site of the first hajj pilgrimage (as Adam left India seeking Eve, who had landed in Jedda), the place where all arts, sciences, and rarities had been first revealed on earth, and the locus of the first manifestation of Muhammad's spiritual reality through Adam. In short, concluded Bilgrami, since we are all children of Adam, we are all in fact Indians.

And even in the realm of the formal traditions of Arabic-Islamic scholarship, Bilgrami maintained that it had primarily been the non-Arabs—Persians, Turks, and, of course, Indians—who had done the most to advance the arts and sciences, particularly through the medium of Arabic. While he acknowledged that the Muslims of India had primarily focused their attention on the lives of the Sufi saints, for whom they held such affection (we shall return to this momentarily), he provided his own account of biographies of Islamic scholars nourished in al-Hind (as the Arabs called the subcontinent). What is most interesting about this eighteenth-century portrait, written shortly before the successful onslaught of British colonial rule, is the breadth of intellectual perspective reflected in the lives of South Asian Muslim scholars. While Qur'anic studies and particularly Prophetic hadith among the Islamic religious sciences were favored by the Indians, these scholars had strong linkages to the Sufi orders, and many were seriously engaged with the philosophical traditions going back to the ancient Greeks. Moreover, they were deeply immersed in the humanistic tradition of Arabic and Persian poetry. Further, Bilgrami himself demonstrated a thorough mastery of Indian literary traditions, which he described in the latter parts of the *Coral Rosary* by providing extensive specimens of Arabic poetry to demonstrate the figures of Indian rhetoric and the different types of lovers enumerated in Indian lore. The cosmopolitanism and civility exemplified by

---

[10] See the rich textual and visual documentation of the Khizr shrine near Adam's Peak (and its parallel Hindu and Buddhist interpretations) available online at the Kathirkamam web site, http://kataragama.org/islamic.htm.

Bilgrami were undoubtedly sustained, both intellectually and materially, by the networks of Indian Sufi centers that were constructed around the tombs of the saints.[11]

So, in what way can it be said that the Sufi saints provide a defining influence for South Asian Islam? One might take as an emblem of this phenomenon a song made famous in the repertoire of the celebrated Qawwali singer, the late Nusrat Fateh Ali Khan, which celebrates the lineage of the great Chishti saints of the thirteenth and fourteenth centuries. With powerful rhythm and emphasis, the refrain is enunciated: "God, Muhammad, the Four Friends (*Allah Muhammad chahar yar*): Hajji, Khwajah, Qutb, Farid." This is a clear reference to the Chishti saints Hajji `Uthman Harwani (d. 1211), Khwajah Mu`in al-Din Chishti (d. 1236), Qutb al-Din Bakhtiyar Kaki (d. 1235), and Farid al-Din Ganj-i Shakkar (d. 1265). Their very names encapsulate a sacred geography. `Uthman Harwani was the last Chishti master to reside in the Afghan town of Chisht, while his successors oversaw the transfer of the order to India; Mu`in al-Din's tomb is in Ajmer in Rajasthan, Qutb al-Din's tomb is in the south of Delhi, while Farid al-Din's shrine lies in Pakpattan in the Pakistan Punjab. These sacred centers still attract multitudes today, with visitors ranging from elite Sufi disciples to ordinary people of all walks of life. To give but one example of an elite seeker of solace from these saints, one may consider Jahanara, the Mughal princess, daughter of Shahjahan and sister to both Dara Shikuh and Aurangzeb. She used her scholarly bent to author biographies of her mentor, the Qadiri shaykh Mullah Shah, and of Mu`in al-Din Chishti. Her modest tomb is in the precincts of the shrine of Farid al-Din's successor, Shaykh Nizam al-Din Awliya' (d. 1325), in Delhi, where her plain tombstone reads: "Let no one cover my shrine with anything but greenery, for grass is enough as the grave-cover for the poor." Countless ordinary folk also attend the shrines of the saints, particularly at the festival of the death-anniversary (`urs), when benefits both spiritual and material may be sought. The intercession of the saints for divine favor has, however, been challenged in modern times by those who favor the

---

[11] For further details on Bilgrami's work, see my article, "Indian Islam: Reconfiguration of the Relation between Religion and World in Sufism and Reformist Islam since the 18th Century" (paper presented at the conference on "Religion and Civil society—Germany, Great Britain and India in the 19th century," Berlin, 10–13 May 2006).

austere approach of Salafi or Wahhabi reformism or the missionary zeal of the Tablighi Jama'at.

Yet it is remarkable to consider the extent to which the Sufi saints have elicited passionate and loyal followings among non-Muslims. The classic case is probably the aforementioned Farid al-Din Ganj-i Shakkar, one of the key figures in the Chishti Sufi lineage. While he was thoroughly educated in the scholarly languages of Arabic and Persian, his mother tongue was evidently an early form of Punjabi (only described as Hindawi or "Indian language" in the Persian texts). He and other Sufis born in India habitually composed poetry in their native dialect, although in his case these occasional verses attained immortality when they became enshrined in the sacred scripture of the Sikhs, the Guru Granth Sahib. Despite the skepticism of colonial British scholars like MacAuliffe, the authenticity of the Farid verses in the Guru Granth Sahib seems to be confirmed by manuscript evidence in fourteenth-century Chishti writings from the Deccan.[12] In the realm of religious practice, the presence of Hindus, Sikhs, Christians, and others at major Sufi shrines is a well-attested social phenomenon that shows no sign of disappearing, despite the criticism of purists on all sides. Just to cite one example, the tomb of Shahul Hamid, a famous sixteenth-century saint of South India, was constructed in his honor by the Hindu king Maharaja Pratap Singh (there is also a smaller version of it on the Malaysian island of Penang, built by Indian immigrants). There are numerous spaces in the South Asian subcontinent (like the shrine of Adam's Peak) where the presence of Sufi saints affords multiple clienteles the possibility of constructing their own relationships with sainthood.

But the role of the Sufi saints as intermediaries and arbiters of human destiny has been seriously challenged in recent years, most notably by those textually-based movements that seek doctrinal purity and religious authenticity in a return to the imagined origins of their religion. This kind of fundamentalism is of course found not only among Muslims but also in Hindu circles. It is important to recognize the relatively recent origin of these movements, despite their appeal to ancient authority. The advent of British colonialism and the elimination of native elites spelled the demise of the institutions of higher education that had fostered the

---

[12] Carl W. Ernst, *Eternal Garden: Mysticism, History, and Politics at a South Asian Sufi Center*, 2nd ed. (New Delhi: Oxford University Press, 2005), pp. 166–68.

cosmopolitanism documented by Azad Bilgrami. After the abortive 1857 Indian revolt against the British, new forms of Muslim piety arose, like the Deoband academy, which focused its curriculum on the hadith sayings of the Prophet Muhammad as the source for judgments on every imaginable question of behavior and religious teaching. What was new in Deoband was, in a sense, modern and technical—print technology replacing the manuscript for dissemination of knowledge in a bureaucratic educational regime modeled on British precedents. In a sense, it was a retrenchment that focused on sacred texts to the exclusion of all else, though couched in a modern medium. Yet, it was also an explicit rejection of the culture of the British overlords.

In recent years, it has become fashionable to portray the madrasa academies as one-dimensional sources of fanaticism. Much of this is based upon the role of Deoband-related schools located in refugee camps on Pakistan's North-West Frontier, which played a mobilizing role in organizing jihad in collaboration with the Taliban. Breathless journalists continue to file reports on these academic centers as the sources of anti-Americanism, wishfully seeking to isolate what is seen as the irrational source of violent activity. In reality, the situation is much more complex. It is still possible for Deoband theologians to be well versed in their Rajput genealogies according to the great Hindu epic, the Mahabharata.[13] And, as a recent author has indicated, the experience of going through these madrasas can vary quite dramatically from one institution to another.[14]

But perhaps the most important decisive variable for the Indian subcontinent has been the factor of nationalism. Often couched in terms that meld religion with ethnic or linguistic identity, this has become such a potent force that it often threatens to overwhelm everything else in its path. The Partition of British India in 1947 into India and Pakistan along roughly religious lines had devastating effects on the populations subjected to territorial transfer, including the deaths of as many as two million people. Its sequel was the similarly catastrophic breakup of Pakistan in the

---

[13] Shail Mayaram, "Rethinking Meo Identity: Cultural Faultline, Syncretism, Hybridity or Liminality?", *Comparative Studies of South Asia, Africa and the Middle East* 17, no. 2 (1997): 35–44 .

[14] Ebrahim Moosa, "Inside the Madrasa: A Personal History," *Boston Review* 32, no. 1 (2007), http://bostonreview.net/moosa-inside-madrasa.

1971 Bangladesh war of independence, whose tale of tragic violence has never been fully told. The Islamic Republic of Pakistan has been subject to numerous contradictions in the attempt to enunciate its identity as either a land for Muslims or alternatively as an Islamic state.

The tensions of this paradox were made clear to me one evening at a typical dinner party in Islamabad when a senior Pakistani diplomat confided to me a parable in which he compared the birth of Pakistan and its sense of identity to the ritual recitation of the call to prayer (*azan*) to a newborn infant. Pakistan at its birth, he told me, heard two azans recited into its ears. One of these azans was secular and nationalist. It said, "You are a nation, you have geographic boundaries, a history based on the land, with languages and a culture that are your very own, and you must defend them." The other azan was religious. It said, "You are a Muslim; your religion is Islam; and it is your destiny to follow the divine will by implementing that religious vision." Was Pakistan to be a state to safeguard the interests of Muslims, or was it to be an Islamic state? Both of these azans spoke to the inner character of Pakistan, but there has always been a gap between them, which the Pakistan of history has never been able to bridge.

This parable deftly encapsulates the dilemma faced by Pakistanis attempting to define their national identity. Are they a distinctive nation with their own local traditions based upon culture, history, and ethnicity? Or, is their identity essentially religious, predicated upon timeless principles derived from sacred scripture, transcending history and locality? Both perspectives have their ardent supporters, and it is the negotiation between them that determines the ongoing political discourse of Pakistan today. Since the beginning of the Pakistan movement in the 1940s, the slogan has constantly unfurled on banners, *Pakistan ka ma`na kya? La ilaha illa allah, Muhammad rasul allah*: "What is the meaning of Pakistan? 'There is no god but God, and Muhammad is the messenger of God.'" As a sentiment asserting the identity of Pakistan with Islam, it may have seemed admirable, but the slogan left out any reference to the culture or history of the region, which is precisely what differentiates Pakistan from other Muslim countries such as, say, Algeria or Egypt. In fact, the only thing about this slogan that is particularly Pakistani is the Urdu phrase that raises the question of identity; the Arabic answer that asserts this to be universal Islam is poignant in its transcendence of the actual situation of Pakistan. This kind of abstraction may have occasioned the dry remark attributed to Pushtun politician Wali Khan, who put national identity into the longer-term perspective of religion and ethnicity: "We have been Pakistanis for forty years, we have been Muslims for fourteen hundred years, but we have been Pathans for four thousand years."

Particularly since the terrorist attacks of 11 September, 2001, and the beginning of the US-led "war on terrorism," Islamic identity everywhere has become complicated by nationalism, anticolonial ideologies of resistance, and the security aims of the nation-state. Here I would like to trace briefly some of the ways in which Pakistanis have interpreted their Islamic identity, focusing on conflicting interpretations of founder figures Jinnah and Iqbal. While it would be politically inconceivable for any Pakistani leader to abandon Islamic identity, in the post-September 11th period, Pakistan's president, General Pervez Musharraf, was clearly steering a course away from the Islamization policies of his predecessors. Yet, the inability of the state to control sectarian factionalism, and its ambivalence about dealing with jihadist networks, remain formidable if not insoluble problems.

For Pakistan, the debate on national identity most frequently takes the form of argument about the true intentions of the two founding fathers, the Muslim League leader Quaid-e-Azam Muhammad ʿAli Jinnah and the poet-philosopher Muhammad Iqbal. The letters to the editor columns of Pakistani newspapers are frequently filled with salvos citing chapter and verse from various documents, resolutions, and speeches of Jinnah to shore up a particular interpretation of the true nature of the Pakistani state. The historical thinness of the dossier makes this material difficult to use as a satisfactory basis for national identity. How can the separate ethnic groups of Sind, Punjab, Baluchistan, and North-West Frontier Province be made to feel that their ambitions and identities are perfectly enfolded by the formulations of a leader who died shortly after the birth of the nation? Jinnah's relatively non-religious upbringing and his ambiguous statements about religion make it difficult to accommodate his vision to any form of Islamic identity. Nevertheless, it is equally difficult to label the leader of the Pakistan movement as a secularist because of the absence of any identifiable public demand for secularism in the Pakistan movement.[15]

---

[15] It is still worth reading the thoughtful comments of Wilfred Cantwell Smith on the Pakistani concept of an Islamic state, in *Islam in Modern History* (New York: The New American Library, 1957), pp. 208–56.

Debates over Jinnah's attitudes toward religion and politics have continued ever since his untimely death, barely a year after Pakistan gained independence in 1947.[16] Commentators, both in India and Pakistan, are still rehashing the political history of the Indian freedom movement from the 1920s onward. The evaluation of actors such as Nehru, Gandhi, Patel, Azad, and many others has been endlessly refashioned and repackaged in books, the news media, and in officially approved history textbooks. Pakistanis have felt that their side of the story has been given short shrift, particularly because of the canonization of Gandhi through a series of glowing portrayals culminating in Richard Attenborough's film *Gandhi*, in which Jinnah comes off as a very negative figure. In response, Pakistani anthropologist Akbar Ahmed produced a counter-film on Jinnah in 1998, portraying him as a great and liberal-minded statesman; despite controversies about financing, authorship of the script, and casting (Jinnah was played by horror-film actor Christopher Lee), this film is probably the most publicly available portrayal of Jinnah as the founder of a non-fundamentalist Pakistan.[17]

Although poet and philosopher Muhammad Iqbal (d. 1938) died before the creation of Pakistan, he is unambiguously regarded as the intellectual father of the country because of his advocacy of a separate homeland for Indian Muslims, something he discussed in correspondence with Jinnah. His complex literary legacy, in Persian and Urdu poetry and in English prose, is the subject of more admiration than analysis within Pakistan. His critical engagement with contemporary European philosophy (Bergson, Nietzsche, Whitehead) and with Middle Eastern and European literature (Dante, Rumi, Hafez, Ghalib) does not yield a single clear and simple interpretation, however. As a result, his poetry is quoted in defense of every imaginable position on the political spectrum.[18]

---

[16] Akbar S. Ahmed, *Jinnah, Pakistan and Islamic Identity: The Search for Saladin* (London: Routledge, 1997), especially pp. 193–202.

[17] See the BBC article on the film opening. *BBC News*, "World: South Asia Troubled Jinnah Movie Opens," September 26, 1998, http://news.bbc.co.uk/hi/english/world/south_asia/newsid_180000/180736.stm.

[18] For a representative collection of articles, see Hafeez Malik, ed., *Iqbal: Poet-Philosopher of Pakistan* (New York: Columbia University Press, 1971).

An illuminating example of the debate over Jinnah and Iqbal is provided in a series of discussions between Pakistani liberals, conservatives, and Islamists held in 1998, sponsored by the Institute of Policy Studies in Islamabad, a fundamentalist think tank.[19] One of the invited speakers was Aitzaz Ahsan, a Pakistani senator and prominent leader of the People's Party of Pakistan. Ahsan is well known for his anti-fundamentalist book *The Indus Saga*, which portrays Pakistan's national identity as a liberal and tolerant culture based upon local roots and Central Asian heritage.[20] Ahsan, like everyone else, has focused upon the critical speech that Jinnah delivered on 11 August 1947, at the very moment when Pakistan was gaining its independence. Here are some critical passages from that speech:

> I cannot emphasize it too much. We should begin to work in that spirit and in course of time all these angularities of the majority and minority communities, the Hindu community and the Muslim community, because even as regards Muslims you have Pathans, Punjabis, Shias, Sunnis and so on, and among the Hindus you have Brahmins, Vashnavas, Khatris, also Bengalis, Madrasis and so on, will vanish. Indeed if you ask me, this has been the biggest hindrance in the way of India to attain the freedom and independence and but for this we would have been free people long long ago. No power can hold another nation, and specially a nation of 400 million souls in subjection; nobody could have conquered you, and even if it had happened, nobody could have continued its hold on you for any length of time, but for this.

> Therefore, we must learn a lesson from this. You are free; you are free to go to your temples, you are free to go to your mosques or to any other place or worship in this State of Pakistan. You may belong to any religion or caste or creed that has nothing to do with the business of the State.

> As you know, history shows that in England, conditions, some time ago, were much worse than those prevailing in India today. The Roman Catholics and the Protestants persecuted each other. Even now there are

---

[19] Tarik Jan, ed., *Pakistan between Secularism and Islam: Ideology, Issues & Conflict* (Islamabad: Institute of Policy Studies, 1998), pp. 51–155. Further articles on the subject are available at the website of this organization http://www.ips.org.pk/.
[20] Aitzaz Ahsan, *The Indus Saga and the Making of Pakistan* (Karachi: Oxford University Press, 1996); Carl W. Ernst, "Local Cultural Nationalism as Anti-Fundamentalist Strategy in Pakistan," *Comparative Studies of South Asia, Africa, and the Middle East* 16 (1996): 68–76.

some States in existence where there are discriminations made and bars imposed against a particular class. Thank God, we are not starting in those days. We are starting in the days where there is no discrimination, no distinction between one community and another, no discrimination between one caste or creed and another. We are starting with this fundamental principle that we are all citizens and equal citizens of one State. The people of England in course of time had to face the realities of the situation and had to discharge the responsibilities and burdens placed upon them by the government of their country and they went through that fire step by step. Today, you might say with justice that Roman Catholics and Protestants do not exist; what exists now is that every man is a citizen, an equal citizen of Great Britain and they are all members of the Nation.

Now I think we should keep that in front of us as our ideal and you will find that in course of time Hindus would cease to be Hindus and Muslims would cease to be Muslims, not in the religious sense, because that is the personal faith of each individual, but in the political sense as citizens of the State.[21]

A very lively debate followed the presentation of Aitzaz Ahsan, in which he was accused of misrepresenting both Jinnah and Iqbal by selective quotations out of context (needless to say, his opponents used exactly the same techniques). The antagonistic atmosphere may be gauged by the fact that one respondent angrily demanded to know whether Ahsan considered himself a Muslim. It is doubtful whether anyone walked away from this discussion with altered views on the question of Jinnah and Iqbal. Nevertheless, it is clear that quotations from these two authorities continue to be touchstones for major ideological divisions within Pakistan today.

What seems to me ironic about this debate is the extent to which Jinnah's language about avoiding sectarian violence has been tragically betrayed and undermined in recent years. Militias of a Salafi inspiration (reputedly encouraged by the martial law government during the 1980s) have assassinated Shi`i leaders and stimulated the formation of rival Shi`i militias. The fissiparous formation of rival groups along

---

[21] The text of this address is available at http://www.pakistani.org/pakistan/legislation/constituent_address_11aug1947.html.

ideological lines is further exacerbated by tribal tensions. But the most disastrous influence on the region has been the corrosive effects of weapons, money, and drugs unleashed by decades of the Afghan war and then the jihadi irregulars formerly sponsored by the CIA. Now proponents of Islamic ideology, who once opposed the creation of Pakistan as un-Islamic nationalism, have been ceded considerable political leverage by a succession of military governments and weak elected rulers who lacked political legitimacy. As a result, merely uttering the word "Islam" is enough to bring conversation to a halt, and ideologues have not failed to take advantage of the power that their claim to represent Islam confers.

The rise of monolithic interpretations of Islam is ironic, however, because Islam has never meant one thing, nor will it in the future. History reveals multiple interpretive authorities clustered around core texts and practices, with variations manifest in local traditions. Modern communications, together with the new concept of Islam as an anticolonial ideology, have made it appealing to invoke the idea of Muslim unity. Dissident views are discouraged as fractures in the universal community of Muslims. Distinctive local practices are frowned upon as deviations from a homogeneous norm. Yet who is entitled to decide what Islam is, once and for all?

At the same time that globalizing communications have opened up the possibility of a monolithic Islamist discourse, previously unheard voices are now being heard. Among the new developments is a re-evaluation of tradition by feminists, including Islamist women. While it will be tempting for development-minded Euro-American feminists to view their own trajectory as the only possible model for Muslim women, they will need to resist that assumption if they wish to hear the actual voices of their Muslim sisters. We are likewise now able to hear the voices of Muslim minority groups, including those who have been dismissed as sectarian heretics. Countries like Pakistan that define themselves as Islamic states are wrestling with the questions of the rights of women and the rights of religious minorities, as human rights issues. These debates about pluralism will answer not only to local constituencies but also to international scrutiny through the media.

Who has the authority to define Islam? The pragmatic pluralism of historical times and places works against the will to power that would reduce Islam to a single voice, like that of General Zia in his rejection of the concept of South Asian Islam. Yet it will be a challenging task for South Asian Muslims to re-imagine their Islam beyond the narrow range of intimidating and authoritarian positions that have taken the stage in recent years. Here Samina Quraeshi proposes, not a rigid definition, but a multiple, locally inflected vision of Islam in South Asia that is enriched by art and which takes account of both feminine and masculine perspectives. The poverty of recent ideology can be offset by tapping the richness of an imagination based on the historical depth of culture. It is in this sense that I hope that readers will benefit from the perspectives which this book presents on the complex Islamic culture that has been grounded in South Asia.

7

Reconfiguring South Asian Islam

From the 18th to the 19th Century*

What does it mean to define or inflect Islam in terms of a regional identity? Region and locality clearly have a definitive role in creating particular cultural expressions of any religious tradition, including Islam. The tendency to ascribe a default Arab identity for all Muslims is unrealistic; the Arabian peninsula is, after all, only one of many cultural situations that refract Islamic religious texts and doctrines into different regional contexts.[1] Then again, focusing on one particular region such as South Asia may end up postulating unchanging and essential character-istics of a particular region as a location of Islamic culture, regardless of change over time. An even more typical error is to view the history of religion in a particular region in terms of teleological political outcomes of local identity. Perhaps the most common narrative concerning South Asia defines the region in terms of religious identities that culminate in the formation of modern nation states; thus, India is seen as a Hindu state, while Pakistan and Bangladesh uneasily aspire to be the Islamic equivalents. Ascribing a definitive identity to South Asian Islam begs

* An earlier version of this paper was presented at the conference on "Religion and Civil society—Germany, Great Britain, and India in the 19th century," at the Wissenschaftszentrum Berlin, 10–13 May 2006.
[1] Bruce B. Lawrence, "Islamicate Civilization: The View from Asia," in *Teaching Islam*, ed. Brannon Wheeler (New York: Oxford University Press, 2003), pp. 61–76.

the question of historical change, particularly with respect to massive transformations such as the experience of European colonialism.

An alternative way of approaching this problem is to examine a region like South Asia diachronically, by examining notable figures from the periods just before and after the onset of European colonial rule over the South Asian subcontinent. A convenient medium to explore for this purpose is biographical literature, which tends to portray its subjects in terms of ideals widely accepted in society. The two cases proposed for study here—the eighteenth-century scholar, Azad Bilgrami, and the nineteenth-century reformist Sufi, Hajji Imdad Allah—share many common characteristics, including literary skills, training in the Islamic sciences, and engagement with Sufi networks. But in a number of key respects, they lived in altogether different worlds. Since the bulk of recent scholarship on Islamic culture in South Asia has focused on the colonial and postcolonial eras, I would like to emphasize here the period just prior to European colonialism, precisely because it has been to a great extent eclipsed and forgotten. Bilgrami's biographical dictionary of Indian Muslim scholars furnishes an extensive baseline for the pre-colonial period, and I will try to summarize its leading characteristics in the remarks that follow. Two biographies of Hajji Imdad Allah from the colonial and postcolonial periods provide a remarkable contrast suggestive of the new cultural dynamics that followed from British domination and its sequels. The narrowing of intellectual perspectives that were sacrificed with the loss of Muslim power and patronage was countered by a broadening of the social base through new religious institutions.

The first example to consider is the eighteenth-century Indian Muslim scholar and poet, Ghulam `Ali "Azad" Bilgrami (1704–86), a scion of an important family from North India who traveled widely in the Middle East before he established himself in the Deccan.[2] Bilgrami was one of the last Indian Muslim scholars to express himself at length in Arabic as well as in Persian; he was an accomplished poet in both languages. His Persian works include three notable anthologies of poetry as well as a hagiography devoted to Sufis of the Deccan. In a strikingly original Arabic treatise entitled *The Coral Rosary of Indian Traditions* (written

---

[2] A. S. Bazmee Ansari, "Azad Bilgrami," *Encyclopaedia of Islam* (Leiden: EJ Brill, 1960), 1:808a–b; C. A. Storey, *Persian Literature: A Bio-bibliographical Survey* (London: Luzac & Company, Ltd., 1972), 1:855–67.

in 1763–64), Bilgrami provided a snapshot of his concept of the world, seen from the perspective of an Indian Muslim.[3] What was Bilgrami's concept of Islam in South Asia? This book presents a vision of the world in which Arabia is the ritual center, but where networks of religious scholarship and humanistic culture are firmly based in India. Bilgrami's world definitely included local political rulers whose sphere of power and patronage was important. But the key elements in his intellectual formation, as nourished by contemporary social organizations, ranged through a variety of disciplines, including the study of authoritative Islamic religious texts, logical and philosophical treatises, the humanistic traditions of Arabic and Persian poetry, plus the rich resources of non-Muslim Indian ("Hindu") literature and aesthetics.[4] All this activity was sustained by charitable foundations (*waqf*), especially those associated with the Sufi orders.

Bilgrami's notion of civility and culture is worth examining as an example of pragmatic pluralism that soon would go out of fashion. When one briefly considers comparable Indian Muslim figures from the height of the colonial period at the end of the nineteenth century, the contrast is stark. An overall assessment of the impacts of British colonial rule on Indian Islam is beyond the scope of this essay.[5] But a comparison between Bilgrami and a leading figure of Indo-Muslim culture from the nineteenth century indicates major changes. In India, as in other regions, colonialism led to the breakup of scholarly networks previously supported by Muslim patronage, with a consequent abandonment of the higher curriculum of philosophical study and a deliberate rejection of cultural practices that were considered overly Hinduized in favor of a focus on authoritative Islamic texts. Such is arguably the case with the second figure under discussion here, Hajji Imdad Allah (d. 1899), the renowned Sufi and religious scholar whose students became the founders

---

[3] Ghulam `Ali Azad al-Bilgrami, *Subhat al-marjan fi athar Hindustan*, ed. Muhammad Fadl al-Rahman al-Nadwi al-Siwani, 2 vols. (Aligarh: Jami`at `Aligarh al-Islamiyya, 1976–80). The curious may have access to some pages from this rare publication online at http://www.unc.edu/courses/2006spring/reli/179/001/.

[4] On the difficulties of defining Hinduism, see David N. Lorenzen, *Who Invented Hinduism? Essays on Religion in History* (New Delhi: Yoda Press, 2006).

[5] The scope of the problem is indicated by Barbara D. Metcalf, *Islamic Contestations: Essays on Muslims in India and Pakistan* (New Delhi: Oxford University press, 2006).

of the reformist academy of Deoband in 1867.[6] While his successors may have moved further in the direction of authoritarian reformism than he anticipated, Imdad Allah continued to play a guiding role in the biographies that they devoted to his memory. A contrast between Bilgrami's biographies of his contemporaries and the narratives of Imdad Allah written by his successors is suggestive of the changing landscape of cultural possibilities for Muslims in the transition from precolonial to colonial India. Hajji Imdad Allah's biographers showed no interest in any non-religious intellectual disciplines nor in any poetic references to Hindu culture; they were initially interested in his credentials in core Islamic religious texts and saintly virtues, though later on they became absorbed in his heroic leadership in jihad against the British infidels. From the eighteenth to nineteenth century, the concept of Muslim culture in South Asia shifted from a local inflection of universalist Islamicate learning under aristocratic patronage to a defensive posture of authenticity articulated by a new class of religious scholars under the pressure of foreign colonial rule. While this comparison is not symmetrical—I am comparing Bilgrami's biographies of his contemporaries with accounts of Imdad Allah by his successors—the striking thing is how difficult it would have been to find any equivalent for Imdad Allah among his eighteenth-century predecessors.

For a survey of Islamic learning in South Asia in the eighteenth century, it is hard to improve upon *The Coral Rosary*, a composite work that Bilgrami wrote separately in four parts, later combined together. The first part is devoted to the statements of the Prophet Muhammad (hadith) regarding the sanctity of India as the place where Adam landed on Earth after his expulsion from Paradise.[7] The second part, from which I draw primarily in this essay, is a biographical dictionary containing accounts of 45 Indian Muslim scholars who wrote in Arabic, ranging

---

[6] For Hajji Imdad Allah and the Deoband school, see Barbara D. Metcalf, *Islamic Revival in British India: Deoband 1860–1900* (New York: Oxford University Press, 2004).

[7] I have translated excerpts from this section in "India as a Sacred Islamic Land," in *Religions of India in Practice*, ed. Donald S. Lopez, Jr., Princeton Readings in Religions 1 (Princeton University Press, 1995), pp. 556–64. There, I translated the title of the text as *The Coral Rosary of Indian Antiquities*, but "traditions" is probably better than "antiquities" as a rendering of the original Arabic term *athar* in terms of its pre-modern meaning. For comparable material from an early Islamic source on Adam's descent to India, see *The History of al-Tabari: General Introduction and from the Creation to the Flood*, trans. Franz Rosenthal (Albany: State University of New York Press, 1989).

from the eighth century to the author's own day. The third and fourth parts are concerned with prosody and the categories of lovers found in Indian literature, illustrated in part by Arabic verses of the author's own composition. Bilgrami subsequently translated the third and fourth parts into Persian, substituting examples of Persian poetry to complete this comparative study of Arabic, Persian, and Indic rhetoric and poetics.[8]

While each of the four sections of *The Coral Rosary* is important for Bilgrami's concept of Indian Muslim culture, the second biographical section is of particular significance in the way it presents the Arabic Islamic intellectual tradition as received by the author. Part two begins abruptly with a lengthy quotation from the Ottoman bibliographer Katib Chelebi (d. 1657), taken from his immense survey of Arabic writings, the *Kashf al-Zunun*.[9] The brunt of this passage, which is clearly marked by the technical vocabulary of the famous North African historian Ibn Khaldun, is a diatribe on the lack of artistic and scientific contributions by the Arabs, whose nomadic existence has led them to concentrate their genius exclusively in the realm of eloquence, especially poetry. Thus he laments the fact that the Arabs of his day know little of books because of their concentration on their immediate needs, and he ascribes the very development of scholarship—largely by non-Arabs—to the fear of the loss of Islamic sacred texts and the need to transmit them to future generations. So it is primarily the non-Arabs (especially the Persians) who are responsible for preserving the Arabic literature of Islam because of their civilized habits and their cultivation of the arts and crafts. Thus the chief masters of Arabic grammar, hadith, Qur'an, Islamic law, and, in short, all intellectual disciplines were non-Arabs. Bilgrami concurs with this judgment, and he celebrates the creativity of the non-Arabs in all fields of intellectual endeavor. He furthermore observes that the height

---

[8] Mir Ghulam `Ali Azad Bilgrami, *Ghazalan al-Hind: Mutala`a-i Tatbiqi-i Balaghat-i Hindi va Parsi*, ed. Sirus Shamisa (Tehran: Sada-yi Mu`asir, 1382/2004). The title of this printed edition is a mistake for *Ghizlan al-Hind* (Gazelles of India), which is a chronogram for the year of the book's composition (1178/1764–65).

[9] This extraordinary compilation is, remarkably, available in a bilingual Arabic-Latin edition. See Kâtip Çelebi, *Lexicon bibliographicum et encyclopaedicum…ad codicum Vindobonensium Parisiensium et Berolinensis fidem primum edidit Latine vertit et commentario indicibusque instruxit Gustavus Fluegel*, Arabic text with Latin trans. by Gustav Lebrecht Fluegel, 7 vols. (Leipzig: Published for the Oriental Translation Fund of Great Britain and Ireland, 1835–58).

of intellectual achievement in the Islamic sciences has been in the lands of Iran, Central Asia, and India.

> Fortunate are the non-Arabs, who are the riders of the racetrack of the sciences and the knights of the battlefield of terms and concepts; they pour from the jugs of wisdom the purest of wine, and they attain from the secrets of the sciences that which lies in the Pleiades.... When Islam approached India through Iran and Turan [Central Asia], and its perfect light unveiled the curtain of darkness from these lands, the Islamic sciences originated first of all in those lands, and the branches of this blessed tree flourished there.[10]

This is far from the situation we observe since the twentieth century, when linguistic nationalism and notions of Arab authenticity have become the norm. Indeed, the relatively recent ascent of the Arabs to a cultural pinnacle may be an anomaly as far as these Indian and Ottoman intellectuals are concerned.[11]

Bilgrami then describes the advent of Islam in the Indian subcontinent beginning in the first Islamic century, with the Arab conquest of Sind in 710, the Ghaznavid conquest of the tenth, century and the establishment of the Delhi Sultanate in the twelfth century, dwelling on the dominion of Muslim rulers as nearly synonymous with Islam itself. But then, he remarks, despite the presence of outstanding Islamic scholars and writers, their story has not yet been told because the Indians have been nearly exclusively concerned with the lives and teachings of the Sufi saints. In this way they have neglected the lives of Muslim religious scholars, but this deficiency is precisely what Bilgrami's book is designed to remedy.[12] While most of the subjects described in this biographical section are closer to the author's own time, he begins with a member of the first Arab military expedition to Sind, a certain Rabi` ibn Sabih (d. 776–77), who has been described as "the first one to write [books] in Islam." Whatever the merits of that historical claim, the argument for the superiority of

---

[10] Bilgrami, *Subhat al-marjan*, 1:60–61.

[11] For the modern tendency to equate the Arabic language with Islamic authenticity, see A. Kevin Reinhart, "Fundamentalism and the Transparency of the Arabic Qur'an," in *Rethinking Islamic Studies: From Orientalism to Cosmopolitanism*, ed. Carl W. Ernst and Richard C. Martin (Columbia, SC: University of South Carolina Press, 2010), pp. 97–113.

[12] Bilgrami, *Subhat al-marjan*, 1:58–63.

non-Arabs, made by an Indian author with support from an Ottoman scholar, is not a new phenomenon.[13] This belongs to the well-established tradition of ethnic contestation known as the Shu'ubiyya, which includes numerous literary efforts to demonstrate the virtues of non-Arabs over Arabs by using the medium of classical Arabic.[14] Bilgrami's purpose is more than simple patriotism, however, since he makes the claim for Indian Muslim achievement in the name of Islamic universalism. In other words, it is not simply the case for him that Indian Muslims are more clever than other Muslims. He views India as a unique repository of Islamic values. In this respect, he echoes claims made by earlier writers going back to the days of the Delhi Sultanate, like Minhaj-i Siraj (d. after 1260), who wrote that, during the Mongol era, "the kingdom of Hindustan . . . became the focus of the people of Islam, and the orbit of the possessors of religion."[15] It may be added that, while Bilgrami's audience may have been in good part other Indian Muslim scholars, he clearly had in mind a broader transregional readership. As he records at the end of the first part of *The Coral Rosary*, certain scholars of Bukhara and Samarqand registered objections to the centrality of India in the first draft of his presentation, arguing that India was rather the object of divine wrath; but he effectively refuted them—since Adam first landed in India, therefore all of his descendents are Indians![16]

While Bilgrami's concept of Indo-Muslim culture doubtless can be ascertained throughout this series of biographies, the last half of this section is of special interest since nearly all of the figures mentioned there overlap with the lifetime of Bilgrami himself (and he concludes with his own biography). The political environment of India during the early eighteenth century was still in theory that of the Mughal Empire, which technically held hegemony over most of the Indian subcontinent, despite a massive decentralization that in effect meant independence for a number of regions, including Bengal and the Deccan. Thus, the author's

---

[13] On the claims concerning Rabi' ibn Sabih, see Yohanan Friedmann, "The Beginnings of Islamic Learning in Sind—A Reconsideration," *Bulletin of the School of Oriental and African Studies* 37 (1974): 659–64.

[14] S. Enderwitz, "Shu'ubiyya," *Encyclopaedia of Islam*, 9:513b–516a.

[15] Minhaj-i Siraj-i Juzjani, quoted in Carl W. Ernst, *Eternal Garden: Mysticism, History, and Politics in the South Asian Sufi Center* (Albany, NY: State University of New York Press, 1992), p. 25.

[16] Bilgrami, *Subhat al-marjan*, 1:56–57.

grandfather 'Abd al-Jalil Bilgrami (d. 1725) received a bureaucratic appointment from the court of the Mughal emperor Farrukhsiyar (r. 1713–19), a position that was inherited by his son Sayyid Muhammad (Azad Bilgrami's uncle). The grandfather had also written Arabic pan-egyric poems in honor of political figures such as the Barhi Sayyids, as well as a congratulatory poem for the victory of the emperor Aurangzeb in Satara in 1699.[17] Azad Bilgrami had visited and studied with his grandfather in the capital Shahjahanabad (Delhi) in 1721–22, and then later stayed with his uncle Sayyid Muhammad for several years while the latter held administrative posts in the towns of Bhakkar and Sistan (Sind), even serving as deputy for two years (1730–32) while the uncle took leave in the family home in Bilgram.

But the political networks cited here extended outside of the Mughal realm in northern India. So we hear of the fortunes of the philosopher Sayyid 'Ali Dashtaki of Shiraz (d. 1705), who was born in Medina, escaped political turmoil in the Deccan kingdom of Golkonda, and received an imperial appointment from Aurangzeb, for whom he served as a military governor and treasurer before departing to perform the Shi'i pilgrimage and retire to Iran.[18] Likewise, in the biography of the hadith scholar 'Abd Allah al-Basri (d. 1726), a resident of Mecca, there is a detailed description of the floods that took place in 1630, requiring an extensive renovation of the holy shrines by the Ottoman Sultan Murad IV.[19]

Bilgrami himself, however, is at some pains to dissociate himself from close proximity to political power. Although, by his own account, Bilgrami was a close friend of Nasir Jang, the second Nizam of Hyderabad, until the latter's murder in 1750, Bilgrami stipulates that the two lines of poetry he dedicated to the Nizam were the only verses that he ever composed for the rich and powerful. He further maintains that, despite the urgings of many people, he refused to take an official government position, though he may well have had some kind of stipend.[20]

The political sphere is for Bilgrami only a background, however, for the intellectual attainments that are the principal subject of his

---

[17] Ibid., 1:208–9.
[18] Ibid., 1:217–23.
[19] Ibid., 1:250–54.
[20] Ibid., 1:305–8.

narrative. He spends considerable time documenting the contributions of Indian scholars to the central textual traditions of Islam, particularly hadith. There are specialists in the Qur'an as well, such as Nur al-Din al-Ahmadabadi (d. 1742), among whose 150 writings are rhymed commentaries on the first two suras of the Qur'an amounting to over 40,000 verses.[21] But it is clearly hadith that forms the preferred field of religious study. This becomes evident in the biography of Muhammad Hayyat al-Sindi (d. 1750), a famous scholar who trained numerous outstanding figures in this field of study, including the eminent Indian thinker Shah Wali Allah (d. 1762).[22] Bilgrami studied hadith with al-Sindi in Medina in 1738, becoming one of many Indians participating in the network of pilgrimage and scholarship between Arabia and India.[23] It is evident that hadith study was a key element of the ethical and devotional practices that formed the backbone of the intellectual and religious networks of many Muslims during this era. Bilgrami also had a great deal of respect for 'Abd Allah al-Basri, whom he describes as the renewer of hadith studies in Mecca; he was said to have completed two full recitations of the famous *Sahih* of al-Bukhari in Mecca in 1709 at the age of 72. 'Abd Allah's commentary on the latter text was preserved in a valuable autographedmanuscript owned by an Indian scholar named Muhammad As'ad, who sent it for protection with the rest of his books to a library in Aurangabad (quite possibly the library associated with the Sufi retreat of Shah Musafir where Bilgrami later resided for seven years). Muhammad As'ad was unfortunately killed along with the third Nizam, Muzaffar Jang, in a battle in 1752, and Bilgrami said the prayers at his funeral.[24] Scholars like Bilgrami took hadith for granted as a central and important field of study, and they commonly used it for reference and to clinch arguments, as Bilgrami did when he justified the use of his name Ghulam 'Ali ("the slave/devotee of 'Ali") to his old teacher Muhammad Hayyat al-Sindi, when the latter had doubts about the idolatrous implications of the name.[25]

---

[21] Ibid., 1:241.

[22] John Voll, "Muhammad Hayyat al-Sindi and Muhammad ibn 'Abd al-Wahhab, an Analysis of an Intellectual Group in 18th-Century Medina," *Bulletin of the School of Oriental and African Studies* 38 (1975): 32–39.

[23] Bilgrami, *Subhat al-marjan*, 1:244–47.

[24] Ibid., 1:250–56.

[25] Ibid., 1:248–49.

Nevertheless, sacred Islamic texts were far from being the exclusive focus of study among these Muslim intellectuals in eighteenth-century India. There was in India a rich tradition of the study of logic and philosophy, drawing upon the heritage of Aristotelian and Platonic thought as mediated by Avicenna (d. 1037) and the Persian thinkers of the school of Isfahan in Safavid Iran. Most of the authors discussed by Bilgrami wrote commentaries on standard works in the rational sciences as well as in religious fields. An outstanding example was Mulla Mahmud al-Faruqi of Jaunpur (d. 1652); Bilgrami quotes at length from Mahmud-i Jaunpuri's treatise refuting the doctrine of temporal origination proposed by the Iranian philosopher Mir Damad (d. 1616).[26] There are also commentators on the metaphysical works of Mulla Sadra of Shiraz (d. 1640), such as Nizam al-Din ibn Qutb al-Din (d. 1748), whom Bilgrami met in Lucknow.[27] In addition, we find philosophically-minded legal thinkers like Muhibb Allah Bihari (d. 1707), appointed as the supreme judge in India by the emperor Aurangzeb; his original writings are especially noted for integrating logic into the principles of Islamic jurisprudence.[28] Bilgrami spends considerable time also in the account of his friend Qamar al-Din Aurangabadi (1711–79), whose father was a disciple of a prominent Naqshbandi Sufi. It seems typical of his training that he studied the intellectual and religious sciences first, before learning the Qur'an. His principal work on the metaphysics of existence, *Mazhar al-Nur*, takes off from a debate between Avicenna and his student Bahmanyar on the question of whether God's continuous creation of the universe means that entities are indeed the same over time; it is quoted at length by Bilgrami, along with a commentary on it written by Qamar al-Din's son Nur al-Huda.[29] Natural sciences were also part of the philosophical curriculum; a cousin of Bilgrami's, Sayyid Muhammad Yusuf Bilgrami, is singled out for his knowledge of astronomy, which he demonstrated when an incompetent navigator brought a ship bound for Bombay to Sri Lanka by mistake.[30] Bilgrami relates these philosophical and scientific accomplishments as a matter of course; there was no need for him to justify the compatibility

---

[26] Ibid., 1:145–62.

[27] Ibid., 1:242.

[28] Ibid., 1:197–99.

[29] Ibid., 1:262–98. When Bahmanyar challenges the notion that entities are the same over time, Ibn Sina caustically remarks that if that is the case, who is it that continues to argue this point?

[30] Ibid., 1:251.

of rational sciences with traditional religious disciplines in the relatively open intellectual climate that sustained these enterprises.

The religious and philosophical traditions were in turn complemented in these circles by the belletristic study of Arabic and Persian literature. This is evident in the very texture of *The Coral Rosary*, which regularly shifts into the rhyming ornate prose (*saj'*) that is considered a hallmark of literary Arabic style. Many biographies record the completion of a standard sequence that includes lexicography, biography, metrics, and poetry, often capped ceremonially by recitation of a Fatiha (*sura* 1 of the Qur'an) to mark completion of the course of study. There are frequent digressions of Arabic poetry, including quotations from classical masters such as al-Hariri and al-Mutanabbi, not to mention Bilgrami's own poetry. Bilgrami's grandfather ʿAbd al-Jalil was noted for his anthology of selections from the classic *al-Mustatraf*.[31] One of the favorite recreations of Bilgrami is the chronogram (*ta'rikh*), an artifice made possible by the fact that each letter of the Arabic alphabet has a numerical value according to the ancient *abjad* or *hisab al-jummal* system. This means that clever writers can compose phrases or verses, the sum of whose letters will yield numerological equivalents indicating a particular year.[32] Bilgrami lavishes considerable skill and effort on this device, which provides the reader with a refined literary aesthetic of time, life, and death, not to mention a corrective to slips of the pen in transcribing numerical dates.[33] As

---

[31] Ibid., 1:223. This is the well-known collection of Arabic literature, *al-Mustatraf fi kull fann mustazraf*, by the Egyptian scholar Baha' al-Din Muhammad al-Ibshihi (d. ca. 1446); see "al-Ibshihi," *Encyclopaedia of Islam*, 3:1005a–1006a.

[32] See the *Encyclopaedia of Islam* articles "Abdjad," 1:97a, "Hisab al-Djummal," 3:468a; "Ta'rikh. III," 10:301b.

[33] This omnipresent feature of Islamicate historiography had a late colonial continuation in the Persian compilation *Miftah al-tawarikh* ("The Key to Chronograms") by Thomas William Beale, composed in 1849; see Sir H. M. Elliot, *The History of India as told by its own Historians, The Muhammadan Period*, ed. John Dowson (1867–77; repr., Allahabad: Kitab Mahal, n.d.), 8:441–44. On the basis of those poetic devices, an English epitome was created: *An Oriental Biographical Dictionary, founded on materials collected by the late Thomas William Beale*, ed. Henry George Keene (London: W. H. Allen & Co., Limited, 1894), which, however, in providing dates dispensed with the poetic chronograms themselves on the grounds that "when the result has been produced [it] is not of much more use than the scaffolding of a building when the building is complete" (p. vii). Beale's collection has, however, come in for its share of criticism; Robert Skelton complains of "his normal practice of contriving at least one error per entry" ("Shaykh Phul and the Origins of Bundi Painting," in *Chhavi-2: Rai Krishnadasa Felicitation Volume* [Benares: Bharat Kala Bhavan, 1981], p. 125, n. 18).

an example, his departure for the pilgrimage to Mecca is memorialized by the phrase "a good journey" (*safar khayr*), which yields the date in question, 1150/1737.[34] He records lengthy and learned commentaries by scholars adjudicating the question of whether one should count the numerical value of the written form of a letter or its spoken form.[35] He demonstrates a method of composing chronograms using circular diagrams to facilitate addition.[36] A characteristic example of the attachment these scholars felt to the chronogram is the story of `Abd Allah al-Basri, who amazingly heard the chronogram of his own death while still living. This happened because Bilgrami was trying to write a chronogram for the death of his teacher Muhammad Hayyat al-Sindi, but the formulation that he came up with (which he shared with `Abd Allah) was excessive by one year. When `Abd Allah al-Basri died the following year, Bilgrami was able to dedicate the same chronogram to him instead.[37] It is fitting indeed that, for the death of Bilgrami, a suitable chronogram was composed yielding the date 1200/1786; it needs no translation (*ah! Ghulam `Ali Azad!*).[38]

For the moment, I will not go much further into Bilgrami's engagement with the literatures of India, but it suffices to say that, as with most Indian Muslims, his mother tongue was one of the regional languages that have become the modern languages of South Asia, doubtless a form of what today is called Hindi. His detailed Arabic commentary on Indian prosody and the poetics of love was part of a long tradition of Indological study by Muslims in the subcontinent, going all the way back to al-Biruni and al-Shahrastani.[39] This was a locally based cosmopolitanism, or cultural pluralism, that was fully compatible with the broader concept of *adab*, the urbane and cultured learning fostered in the early Arab caliphate, which is practically synonymous with the humanistic study of literature in Arabic and Persian. Moreover, it is worth noting that Bilgrami's chief disciple in Persian literature was a Hindu scholar, Lachhmi Narayan

---

[34] Bilgrami, *Subhat al-marjan*, 1:300.

[35] Ibid., 1:247–48.

[36] Ibid., 2:268–74; id., *Ghizlan al-Hind*, pp. 108–12.

[37] Bilgrami, *Subhat al-marjan*, 1:256. The chronogram in question was *qada nahbahu `alim majid*, "a distinguished scholar has expired" (1164/1751). Al-Sindi died in 1163/1750.

[38] Bilgrami, editor's introduction in English, *Subhat al-marjan*, 1:7.

[39] Carl W. Ernst, "Muslim Studies of Hinduism? A Reconsideration of Persian and Arabic Translations from Sanskrit," *Iranian Studies* 36 (2003): 173–95.

"Shafiq" Awrangabadi (1745–ca. 1808).[40] The latter was of course one of many non-Muslim Indian authors who mastered Persian, often to enter the bureaucracy of the Mughal empire and other Islamicate regimes, but there were a significant number of Persian poets among them.[41] Mohammed Arkoun looks to the humanism of Arab intellectuals of the tenth century as a time of aspiration for what the philosopher al-Farabi called the "Virtuous City," in a process of building civic culture.[42] It may be suggested that, in late Mughal India, intellectuals like Bilgrami shared comparable ideals.

From a social perspective, it is evident that the intellectuals described by Bilgrami belonged to networks of scholarship that were to some extent structured by family relationships, while at the same time they were sustained by patronage of local rulers. The long-range travel that included pilgrimage and scholarly study in the Arabian Peninsula must also have been linked to the Indian Ocean trade. Some of the academic achievements chronicled by Bilgrami were undoubtedly accomplished with the support of charitable endowments, which permanently alienated land, property, and wealth from the taxing authority of the monarchy. India does not offer the extensive archival documentation of charitable trusts that is available for the Ottoman Empire, probably because of the combined effects of climate, destructive insects, and political turmoil. Nor does Bilgrami provide any details on the financial support of scholarly circles on the part of rulers and other individuals. But from a circumstantial point of view it is noteworthy that, after completing his pilgrimage to Arabia, Bilgrami returned to India and spent seven years in residence at the famous Sufi shrine established in Aurangabad by Shah Musafir, known today as the Panchakki ("waterwheel"). This is an extensive establishment featuring large tanks of water supplied by a network of canals that were constructed by followers of the Central Asian Sufi who established this center some decades prior to Bilgrami's arrival.[43]

[40] Storey, *Persian Literature*, 1:476–78, and references cited in the index, 1:1416.

[41] Stefano Pellò, "Hindu Persian Poets," *Encyclopedia Iranica* (http://www.iranica.com/articles/hindu-persian-poets).

[42] Mohammed Arkoun, "Locating Civil Society in Islamic Context," in *Civil Society in the Muslim World: Contemporary Perspectives*, ed. Amyn B. Sajoo (London: I.B. Tauris Publishers, 2002), p. 51.

[43] Nile Green, "Auspicious Foundations: The Patronage of Sufi Institutions in the Late Mughal and Early Asaf Jah Deccan," *South Asian Studies* 20 (2004): 71–98.

It was clearly a center of Sufi activity and scholarship, and there are indications that the library there was of extremely high quality, as it must have been to attract a scholar like Bilgrami (this library was reputedly appropriated by the Nizam and must therefore form part of the formidable Asafiyya collection in Hyderabad). The shrine must also have provided other important local services, as indicated by the presence of a very practical waterwheel for grinding grain.

The other sustaining dimension for the scholarly networks described by Bilgrami is Sufism. While Bilgrami attempted to distinguish his biographical account of Indian Muslim scholars from the generality of lives of saints produced in South Asia, it is remarkable to see how frequently the Islamic religious scholarship and philosophical studies of these figures are framed by initiation into a Sufi order. This not only included the master-disciple relationships and spiritual training that is characteristic of the inner circles of the Sufi orders, but also academic study and commentary on the more metaphysical writings of the Sufi tradition, in particular the works of Ibn ʿArabi. Bilgrami himself is the author of a Persian hagiography (*Rawzat al-awliya'*) devoted to the Sufi saints of the Deccan, which he composed in 1740.[44] He was buried outside of the town of Khuldabad, which is a major regional center of pilgrimage particularly for the Chishti Sufi order.[45] While Bilgrami does not spend much time describing inner spiritual disciplines, Sufism unquestionably provides a central framework for the formation of character and ethical training in this precolonial Indian Muslim environment. His status was probably that of a pious devotee who fully accepted the guidance of Sufi teachers, though he did not live the detached life of an elite Sufi disciple.

Bilgrami in his survey of Indian Muslim culture paid no attention to Europeans whatever, although he had recorded their military and political presence in India in his other writings. Recent research has indicated that the relationship between Indo-Muslim and European intellectuals of the eighteenth century contained far more engagement and interaction

---

[44] Ernst, *Eternal Garden*, esp. pp. xix–xx, 91, 138.
[45] For a photograph of the threshold of Bilgrami's tomb, see Carl W. Ernst, "Khuldabad: Dargahs of Shaykh Burhanuddin Gharib and Shaykh Zaynuddin Shirazi," in *Dargahs: Abodes of the Saints*, ed. Mumtaz Currim and George Michell, special issue of *Marg* 56, no. 1 (2004): 104–19, fig. 13.

than was previously thought.[46] Nevertheless, one can certainly find other examples of contemporary Indian Muslim scholars who did not take Europeans too seriously on the cultural level. As an example, the Naqshbandi Sufi leader Mirza Mazhar Jan-i Janan (d. 1799) once wrote a letter to his disciples intended to curb their conceit, on the topic, "Any Sufi Disciple Who Does Not Consider Himself Worse Than a Frankish Infidel Is in Fact Worse Than a Frankish Infidel." So it is possible that Bilgrami did not see Europeans as a challenge to the intellectual universe of Indian Muslims; he could have viewed them primarily as foreign mercenary forces, whose presence would have no lasting consequence. Alternatively, it may be that Bilgrami deliberately avoided referring to the Europeans in an encyclopedic work that was intended to preserve traditional culture against their potential threat. In the very twilight of Bilgrami's life, however, at the age of 85, he did have contact with officials of the British East India Company, who referred to him with great respect as they mined his poetic anthologies for historical information at the dawn of the era of Orientalism.[47] But the Europeans cannot be said to play any significant role in Bilgrami's picture of Indian Islamic culture.

When we turn our attention a century later to examine the impact of British colonial rule, the figure of Hajji Imdad Allah provides an apposite comparison for Bilgrami, as a Muslim intellectual steeped in both the scholarly and mystical traditions.[48] While this comparison must be brief, it is worthwhile to observe the contrast between the two figures. While all of Hajji Imdad Allah's followers acknowledge his engagement with Sufism, in the sources examined here, it is recast in a reformist mold and placed in a political context of anticolonial resistance. The following

---

[46] Mohamad Tavakoli-Targhi, *Refashioning Iran: Orientalism, Occidentalism, and Historiography* (New York: Palgrave, 2001).

[47] Henry Vansittart, "History of Asof Jah," *The Asiatick Miscellany* 1 (1785): 327–31; id. "The History of Ahmed Shah," *The Asiatick Miscellany* 1 (1785): 332–42; William Chambers, "Extracts from the Khazanah e Aamerah," *The Asiatick Miscellany* 1 (1785): 494–511; id. "A Short History of The Origin And Progress of the Marratta State, Extracted from the Khazanah e Aamerah," *The Asiatick Miscellany* 2 (1786): 86–122. See Chambers' remarks quoted in Storey, *Persian Literature*, 1:857–58. These historical extracts from Bilgrami's literary anthologies tended to skip over the poetry, however.

[48] On Hajji Imdad Allah, see Carl W. Ernst and Bruce B. Lawrence, *Sufi Martyrs of Love: Chishti Sufism in South Asia and Beyond* (New York: Palgrave Press, 2002), esp. pp. 118–21; Scott A. Kugle, "The Heart of Ritual is the Body: Anatomy of an Islamic Devotional Manual of the Nineteenth Century," *Journal of Ritual Studies* 17, no. 1 (2003): 42–60.

remarks will focus on two presentations of his life, each of which raises important criteria for the definition of the religious world of South Asian Muslims in the colonial and postcolonial eras. While one cannot necessarily take Bilgrami and Hajji Imdad Allah as typical representatives of their times, the differences between these in some ways highly comparable figures offer useful indices of major changes in outlook that have taken after the onset of British colonial rule.

To begin with, we have the hagiographic portrait of Hajji Imdad Allah by his leading disciple Ashraf ʿAli Thanvi (d. 1943), in an Urdu work entitled *Karamat-i Imdadiyya* (*The Miracles of Imdad*).[49] One of the preeminent figures of the Deoband madrasa and the author of the famous reformist manual for Muslim women, *Bihishti Zewar* (*The Heavenly Ornament*), Thanvi nevertheless composed this collection in 1317/1899 (shortly after Hajji Imdad Allah's death) as a scholarly record of the miraculous events that occurred through his master's spiritual power.[50] The title page introduces Hajji Imdad Allah as the embodiment of Sufism, "the form whose the meaning is expressed by the verses of the *Masnavi-i Maʿnavi* of Mawlana Rumi." There is an echo of Bilgrami's literary aesthetic in the Arabic ode to the master that opens up the book, though to be sure it is accompanied by an interlinear Urdu translation. And it shares the sense of prodigious narrative possibility that suffuses not only the standard Sufi hagiographies but also Bilgrami's intellectual history of Muslim scholarship. The purpose of this work, in focusing on miraculous narratives, is frankly devotional; the author proposes to fill the hearts of the saint's adherents with joy and increase their love, while at the same time augmenting the satisfaction of the common people in the perfections of the master with miracles that confirm their hearts. One such example is the following account by a disciple:

> Once this insignificant person was planning to travel from my home to the holy cities. In Bombay, I was sleeping, and in my dream I saw that the master [i.e., Hajji Imdad Allah] was present. He told me, "This time

[49] Ashraf ʿAli, *Karamat-i Imdadiyya, maʿa izafa: Zamima jadida* (Deoband: Kutub Khana Hadi, n.d.).

[50] On Thanvi (or Thanawi), see Muhammad Qasim Zaman, *Ashraf Ali Thanawi: Islam in Modern South Asia*, Makers of the Muslim World (Oxford: Oneworld, 2008); *Perfecting Women: Maulana Ashraf 'Ali Thanawi's Bihishti Zewar*, trans. Barbara Daly Metcalf (Berkeley: University of California Press, 1992).

you'll come to me in India, don't go to Mecca." I said, "Now you have come here, but I have got the fare for the ship, and every ship will go." He said, "It's not appropriate for us to go." I kept on talking, but his advice was, no—don't go this year. I opened up my eyes, and at once returned to myself, but that day was the departure of the ship. I did not comprehend the problem. The passengers boarded and the ship departed. That very day, such a storm came that the ship was damaged and the ship came back.[51]

This seems to be a typical account of the miraculous intervention of the saint to save his disciple. Yet, there is a curious rationalism in the laboriously argued answers to 10 questions about the possibility of miracles, which serve as a preface to the sequence of miracle accounts; this argumentation downplays the importance of physical miracles and draws attention instead to the spiritual miracle of fulfilling the law.[52]

Stylistically, it is surprising to see that this biography contains no chronograms whatsoever, a brusque approach in comparison to the luxuriant presentation characteristic of most Urdu lithographed books of this era. Indeed, in the temporal dimension, a new element is present when a date is unselfconsciously presented with its equivalent in the Christian calendar.[53] Nevertheless, we are not provided here with an integrated biographical account of the master, although his death is briefly described at the conclusion of the miracle stories. Instead, the presentation is fragmented and scholastic, organized like the more technical manuals of prophetic hadith sayings, grouped under the name of the transmitter; the accounts are likewise numbered in sequence, with 127 pericopes in the main body of the text. While Hajji Imdad Allah's world, like Bilgrami's, revolves around the holy cities of Arabia, the context here legitimate, legitimation, are both ok. has changed dramatically; the miracle stories of pilgrimage ships rescued from the ocean by divine and saintly intervention now incidentally feature European Christian ship captains, a sign of colonial domination that either passes without comment or else

---

[51] Ashraf `Ali, *Karamat-i Imdadiyya*, pp. 11–12.

[52] See Ernst and Lawrence, *Sufi Martyrs of Love*, pp. 120–21, for a discussion of the way Ashraf `Ali Thanvi rationalizes the religious significance of miracles through his selective interpretation of Ibn `Arabi.

[53] Ashraf `Ali, *Karamat-i Imdadiyya*, p. 40; this date citation (1306 = 1889) admittedly occurs in the supplement, which seems to have been added in 1336/1917 (p. 37).

is turned to legitimize the saint.[54] Despite the emphasis on miracles, this hagiography concentrates on the pedagogy of religious authority

A more recent Urdu work, entitled *Hajji Imdad Allah Muhajir Makki and his Successors*, portrays him in a strongly political light, in relation to the decisive crisis of the 1857 revolt against the British and the consequent exile of Hajji Imdad Allah in Arabia; this 1984 composition by Pakistani scholar Fuyuzurrahman (with a preface by Nafis al-Husayni) presents a brief biography of Hajji Imdad Allah, followed by accounts of 52 of his successors, plus another 17 more peripheral followers.[55] Written during the era of the dictatorship of General Zia, the work reflects a more confrontational view of Islamic identity clearly related to the contemporary situation of Pakistan; indeed, one may say that the emphasis on jihad in this biographical collection is very much in tune with the anti-Soviet attitude by the Pakistan government and its American patrons at the time. Neither the introduction nor the main body of this biography pays any attention to miracles at all, focusing instead exclusively on the social and political realm. The chief epithet chosen here for Hajji Imdad Allah is "the Shaykh of the Arab and the non-Arab," giving him a significance that aims to transcend any geographic limitation; the preface defines him in fact as one of the greatest saints, not only of the South Asian subcontinent but also of "the world of Islam" as a whole, so that he was the point of reference for both Muslim scholars and Sufi masters.[56] The preface is a kind of set piece for the book, describing the subject from the start in terms of a significant Sufi initiation in 1235/1819–20 at the hands of Sayyid Ahmad Shahid (1786–1831), the martyred founder of the jihad movements in British India, who was under the guidance of an important Naqshbandi reformist figure, Shah 'Abd al-'Aziz Dihlawi (1746–1824). The fact that this "initiation of blessing (*bay'at-i tabarruk*)" would have occurred when Hajji Imdad Allah, by his own account,

---

[54] Nile Green, "Saints, Rebels and Booksellers: Sufis in the Cosmopolitan Western Indian Ocean, c.1780–1920," in Kai Kresse and Edward Simpson, ed., *Struggling with History: Islam and Cosmopolitanism in the Western Indian Ocean* (London: Routledge Curzon, 2008), pp. 125–66.

[55] Hafiz Qari Fuyuzurrahman, *Hazrat Haji Imdadullah Muhajir Makki aur unke khulafa'* (Karachi : Majlis-i Nashriyat-i Islam, 1984). This author specializes in biographical works on Muslim religious scholars, especially those connected with Deoband.

[56] Other epithets given to Hajji Imdad Allah emphasize this combination of Islamic religious scholarship and mystical accomplishment. Ashraf 'Ali Thanvi referred to him as Shaykh al-'Ulama', Qutb al-'Alam (master of the scholars, pivot of the world).

was only three years old, does not lessen its importance. Just a few days later, this momentous event was followed by Sayyid Ahmad Shahid initiating Hajji Imdad Allah's future Chishti masters into the jihad movement. Hajji Imdad Allah himself was brought into the movement later on by Sayyid Nasir al-Din Dihlawi (d. 1256/1840–41), who had become the leader of the jihad movement after the founder's death. Thus, through all of his teachers, Hajji Imdad Allah was distinguished as the principal successor of Sayyid Ahmad Shahid, and therefore he and his disciples were all deeply attracted to jihad; only his father's fatal illness prevented him from sharing in his teacher's martyrdom. When the 1857 revolt against the British took place, he thus raised the standard of jihad in Thana Bhavan, but without success, so that he was forced to flee to Mecca. It is worth noting that his epithet Muhajir invokes the prophetic model of *hijra* or departure from the non-religious world in search of a divinely approved sanctuary (he had already taken the title Hajji after his first pilgrimage in 1845). He is described during his long residence in Mecca as being famed as a Sufi master and constantly visited by the Chishtis of India. It is reiterated that his service to Islam extended beyond India to the whole world, though his most eminent disciples were the founders of the Deoband movement, Muhammad Qasim Nanawtawi and Rashid Ahmad Gangohi. He and his disciples disdained sectarianism and championed Muslim unity, influencing countless followers and reviving the example of early Sufis and pious scholars.[57]

The biography proper by Fuyuzurrahman begins by identifying Hajji Imdad Allah as one of those saints who is universally recognized, describing his education in the Persian classics and his travel to Delhi to study with notable teachers, entering the Naqshbandi path, though eventually he became dedicated to the Chishti order. His participation in the 1857 revolt is described in greater detail, including his departure from India in disguise and his arrival in Mecca in 1860, where he lived a life of contentment despite all difficulties, combining the virtues of a pious warrior for the faith and the spiritual exercises of a Sufi adept. His tolerant outlook and lack of fanaticism is nevertheless stressed, along with his mastery of the *Masnavi* of Rumi, on which he indeed wrote an extensive commentary, along with a number of other titles in Urdu, mostly Sufi writings, many of them in verse. Further details of his life and writings

---

[57] Nafis al-Husayni, preface to Fuyuzurrahman, *Hazrat Haji*, pp. 6–9.

are filled out with extensive quotations from standard Arabic and Urdu biographical sources on Indian Muslim scholars (`Abd al-Hayy, Rahman `Ali) as well as the leading academic historian of the Chishti order, K. A. Nizami; the latter highlights as the major achievements of Hajji Imdad Allah not only the creation of the Deoband academy and internal reform among Muslims but also the advancement of Indian independence through the implementation of economic and military decisions. The excerpt closes with seven pages of Hajji Imdad Allah's Urdu poetry.[58]

How may we contrast Bilgrami and Hajji Imdad Allah in terms of their visions of the world? In religious terms, both were immersed in the traditions of hadith study and Sufism; although Hajji Imdad Allah was not really a specialist in the field of hadith, it certainly emerges as the main reference for his successors, as the primary focus of Deoband. There is likewise a powerful literary engagement on the part of both figures, with Persian continuing as an important medium, although the shift of literary language from Arabic to Urdu in the nineteenth century is palpable. Yet, there are significant differences. Hajji Imdad Allah was not interested in philosophy or the rational sciences, nor did he have any inclination towards the literary or religious traditions of Hindu India. Both of these shifts reflect a significant change of emphasis in the nineteenth century. There certainly was a sector of Indo-Muslim thought that continued to concentrate on philosophy, logic, and the rational sciences (epitomized by figures such as Fazl-i Haqq Khayrabadi, who was imprisoned by the British for his role in the 1857 revolt), but in this splintered intellectual environment, it was becoming increasingly difficult to bridge the gap between the intellectual and traditional Islamic sciences.[59] There are still Sufi-oriented cultural trends in South Asia that continue to embrace the poetic and musical legacies of Hindu India. But the reformist movement of Deoband to a certain extent defined itself in opposition to the rational sciences as well as in opposition to anything that could be considered similar to Hinduism. Rashid Ahmad Gangohi opposed popular practices associated with pilgrimage to Sufi shrines, despite their long acceptance in Muslim communities, precisely because they too closely resembled

---

[58] Fuyuzurrahman, *Hazrat Haji*, pp. 10–25.
[59] A. S. Bazmee Ansari, "Fadl-i Hakk," *Encyclopaedia of Islam* 2:735b.

Hindu devotional observances.[60] To be sure, one reason for the decline of philosophical studies must have been the elimination of the class of elite patrons who made possible the specialized academic study chronicled by Bilgrami in the eighteenth century. Yet British dominance surely had ideological effects as well; the crystallization of Islamic identity in opposition to the British (and to the Hindus) now trumped the intra-Islamic rivalries that had permitted Bilgrami to view the Arabs as devoid of culture and religious knowledge. Hajji Imdad Allah's exile in Mecca valorized the Arab sanctuaries as the authentic home of Islam, making India into an abode of alienation and prefiguring the concept of Pakistan as the religious realm to be reached by *hijra*.

Thus, Azad Bilgrami and Hajji Imdad Allah are separated by a gap in the pragmatics of Islamic polity. Bilgrami assumed the structures of aristocratic patronage as the basis of Muslim culture, though it must be remembered that his age, the eighteenth century, was one of extreme decentralization rather than high imperial power; in the eyes of the Europeans who viewed the subcontinent as a realm ripe for the taking, that decentralization was synonymous with civilizational decline. The conquest and overthrow of those aristocratic regimes by foreign infidels obviously caused an immense crisis for Indian Muslims. Ironically, the growth of Muslim associations in the colonial era (Deobandi, Barelwi, Ahmadi, Tablighi) created a much larger public space in India for a civil society than the charitable trusts made possible by the feudalism of the later Mughal empire. The very concept of the public was drastically redefined, as those Muslim charitable institutions were eroded by British colonial administrators and judges who, judging in the name of Islamic law but using principles of nineteenth-century England, considered the *waqf* system to be excessively oriented to private family benefit.[61] Another irony of this period was the objectification of religion as a pro-

---

[60] See my article, "An Indo-Persian Guide to Sufi Shrine Pilgrimage," in *Manifestations of Sainthood in Islam*, ed. Grace Martin Smith and Carl W. Ernst, (Istanbul: The Isis Press, 1993) pp. 43–67. It is still possible, however, for Deoband theologians to be well versed in their Rajput genealogies according to the Sanskrit epic, the *Mahabharata*; in other words, some of these Muslim reformists still identify with traditions associated with Hinduism. See Shail Mayaram, "Rethinking Meo Identity: Cultural Faultline, Syncretism, Hybridity or Liminality?", *Comparative Studies of South Asia, Africa and the Middle East* 17 (1997): 35–44 (available online at http://cssaame.dukejournals.org/content/17/2/35.full.pdf+html).
[61] Gregory C. Kozlowski, *Muslim Endowments and Society in British India* (New York: Cambridge University Press, 1985).

cess which is instrumental to other ends. This concept, accentuated by post-1857 anxiety, underlay the question posed by British colonial official W. W. Hunter in his 1871 book, *The Indian Musalmans: Are They Bound in Conscience to Rebel against the Queen*?

Clearly, the British brought a jaundiced eye to the inspection of Indian Islam. It is worth returning to the first translator of Bilgrami, William Chambers, who in 1785 provided a couple of historical extracts from Bilgrami's anthology of Persian poetry, *Khizana-i `amira* ("The Royal Treasury," composed in 1762) in an attempt to provide "real fact or... intelligence drawn from original sources" that might provide "useful knowledge" about "Eastern affairs." Chambers felt it necessary to justify the effort of translating Eastern texts despite the difficulty of the task, especially in view of the meager results that can be expected:

> But, so far as the intellectual powers are concerned, it seems vain to imagine, that nations who have ever lived under the influence of dark and confused superstitions, have constantly groaned under the yoke of lawless tyranny, and have never yet entirely emerged from a state of barbarism, could add anything considerable to the literature of Europe, furnished originally with all the lights of Grecian and Roman science, and sitting for centuries under the nurture of the mildest governments, and in the bright blaze of truth, natural and revealed; though, on the other hand, it must be allowed that they possess much, which, in its degree, deserves well to be known.[62]

Chambers went on to praise Bilgrami's narrative for its eyewitness quality and its potential to serve as a corrective in accounts of military and political events in which the French and British had been involved.[63] The European condescension toward Eastern culture and the astonishing lack of self-criticism displayed by these remarks scarcely need comment. British colonial scholarship displayed a deep ambivalence toward the civility of Persian literature, at times viewing it as superfluous to the acquisition of useful knowledge, nonetheless attracted to it; the title page of *The Asiatick Miscellany*, where Chambers's translation appeared, is adorned with an Arabic title in rhyming prose, plus the famous Persian verses from the

---

[62] William Chambers, "Extracts from the Khazanah e Aamerah," pp. 494–95.

[63] Ibid., p. 497. In this extract (pp. 500–1), Bilgrami refers once to the Christians (*Nasara*) of Pondicherry who participated in the assassination of his friend Nasir Jang; Chambers translates this term as "Europeans."

poet Sa`di that introduced his cosmopolitan ethics.[64] The study of Persian classics continued to form part of British colonial education, permitting better access to the tax and land revenue records that formed the basis of governance under the Mughals. But Macaulay's 1835 "Minute on Indian Education" established English as the new language of administration, relegating Persian, Arabic, and Sanskrit to the dusty shelves of Orientalist libraries. Indo-Muslim writers nostalgically lamented the loss of the culture of civility that had been associated with Persian literature. So one may construe the closing scene of the famous Urdu novel *Umrao Jan* ("The Courtesan of Lucknow", 1899), where the protagonist achieves her philosophical consolation by reading challenging Persian classics on ethics and philosophy (Sa`di, Tusi), pointedly excluding the courtly panegyrics of Anwari and Khaqani with their feudalistic resonance.[65]

So what have been the major changes in Indian Islam from the eighteenth to the nineteenth centuries? The question requires a much more extensive investigation than can be attempted here. Nevertheless, Azad Bilgrami and Hajji Imdad Allah furnish suggestive indices for gauging the significance of the shifts that have taken place in Muslim culture over the course of the early British regime in India. Both demonstrate distinctive characteristics of a South Asian regional identity. Yet the substantial differences between these figures cannot be fully explained except in terms of the historical changes that India experienced under the British. The regional identity of South Asian Islam was indeed reconfigured in the light of new conditions.

---

[64] The Arabic title of *The Asiatick Miscellany* was *Jawahir al-ta'alif fi nawadir al-tasanif,* "Jewels of Compositions on Rarities of Writings," which is perhaps a good equivalent of the official subtitle of the journal: "Consisting of Original Productions, Translations, Fugitive Pieces, Imitations, and Extracts from Curious Publications." The lines from Sa`di are the opening to the "Reason for the Book's Composition" in his celebrated *Bustan*: "I traveled much to the ends of the earth/spending my days with every person//I found enjoyment in every corner, gleaning fruit from every harvest" (Sa`di, *Kulliyyat*, ed. Muhammad `Ali Furughi [Tehran: Sazman-i Intisharat-i Javidan, n.d.], p. 222).
[65] Mirza Ruswa, *The Courtesan of Lucknow: Umrao Jan*, trans. Khushwant Singh and M. A. Husaini (New Delhi: Orient Paperbacks, 1961), pp. 230–31.

PART 2
Sufism, Yoga and Indian Religions

8

Sufism and Yoga according to
Muhammad Ghawth*

What has been the relationship between Sufism and yoga? The
question of yogic "influence" on Sufism has been raised from the first
Orientalist studies of Islamic mysticism because of the well-known
millennial presence of Muslims in the Indian subcontinent. Partly because
of ingrained Orientalist assumptions that Islam was legalistic and intoler-
ant, it was assumed that the mystical tendencies in the Islamic tradition
must have come from elsewhere. Thus began the quest for the "origins" of
Sufism, which were variously—and fruitlessly—sought in the doctrines
of Christian monasticism, Buddhism, shamanism, or yoga. The consensus
of scholarship now, I think, accepts Sufism as a religious phenomenon
oriented by the Qur'an and the Prophet Muhammad. Yet, one commonly
finds the assertion that Sufi practices of breathing control and meditation
somehow derive from Hindu or Buddhist yogic exercises; little proof is
ever offered for this thesis. I have spent a considerable amount of time
researching the Sufi texts that make passing reference to yoga, and it is
undeniable that certain Sufis in India were aware of yogic practices. On
a textual level, however, extended discussions of yoga are rare. Only one
work on yoga, described below, had a wide circulation in the Muslim

* This article has been developed as part of translation and study, entitled *The Pool of
Nectar: Islamic Interpretations of Yoga* (forthcoming), where the subject is discussed in
more detail. The research has been supported by a Translation Grant from the National
Endowment for the Humanities. An earlier version was presented at the American Academy
of Religion Conference in Anaheim, California, in November 1989.

world, in Arabic, Persian, Turkish, and Urdu translation. Even in this most obvious example of Muslim interest in yogic practice, however, it seems clear that yoga was integrated into the spectrum of existing Sufi practice, rather than somehow acting as a "source" for the entire Sufi tradition.

The text in question is one of the most unusual examples of cross-cultural encounter in the annals of the study of religion. The *Amrtakunda* or *Pool of Nectar* was the name of a Sanskrit or Hindi work, the original text of which is now lost. It was ostensibly translated into Arabic, according to the introduction, in 1210 in Bengal, under the title *Hawd ma' al-hayat* or *The Pool of the Water of Life*. I have prepared a critical edition and English translation of the Arabic text, which will be published with an extensive introduction dealing with the cross-cultural religious issued raised by the *Amrtakunda*.[1] For reasons too complex to discuss here, I would like to suggest that this account is fictitious and that the actual translator was a Persian scholar trained in the Illuminationist school of philosophy, probably in the fifteenth century; this unknown philosopher then went to India and encountered the teachings of hatha yoga according to the tradition of the Nath yogis (popularly called *jogis*). The anonymous translator incorporated into the introduction two symbolic narratives, one deriving ultimately from the "Hymn of the Pearl" from the gnostic *Acts of Thomas*, the other being a partial translation from a Persian treatise, *On the Reality of Love*, originally written by the Illuminationist philosopher Shihab al-Din al-Suhrawardi al-Maqtul.[2] From the dissemination of the manuscript copies of the Arabic text, it is clear that *Hawd al-hayat* was fairly well known in the Islamic world; at least 45 copies are found in libraries in European and Arab countries, the majority being in Istanbul. The content of the text was so unusual that, perhaps by default, it has been frequently assigned to the authorship of the Andalusian Sufi master Muhyi al-Din Ibn al-'Arabi; this attribution

---

[1] See *The Pool of Nectar: Islamic Interpretations of Yoga*. The Arabic text was first edited from five manuscripts by Yusuf Husain, "'*Haud al-hayat*, la version arabe de l'Amratkund," *Journal Asiatique* 213 (1928): 291–344, but unfortunately this edition contains numerous errors and omissions. My forthcoming translation is based on a superior text established by comparison of 25 of 45 extant manuscripts.

[2] Typically, the only scholar to notice these Gnostic and Illuminationist elements in the *Amrtakunda* translation was Henry Corbin, in "Pour une morphologie de la spiritualité shi'ite," *Eranos-Jahrbuch 1960*, vol. 29 (Zürich: Rhein-Verlag, 1961), esp. pp. 102–7, repeated with some variations in his *En Islam iranien, Aspects spirituels et philosophiques*, vol. 2, *Sohrawardî et les Platoniciens de Perse* (Paris: Gallimard, 1971), pp. 328–34.

is clearly erroneous.[3] The vocabulary of the text is mostly formed on the Arabic technical terminology of Hellenistic philosophy, with some Islamic overtones derived from the Qur'an and Sufism. The translator worked strenuously to render the yogic practices in a way that was understandable to a philosophically oriented reader of Arabic. Yet the *Hawd al-hayat* was only the beginning of the trajectory of the *Amrtakunda* in the Islamic world.

The Pool of the Water of Life stands out from other Arabic and Persian translations from the Sanskrit, in that it emphasized Indian spiritual practices rather than doctrines. Although al-Biruni (d. 1010) had translated Patañjali's *Yogasutra* into Arabic, he had focused on philosophical questions and omitted the topic of mantra altogether.[4] Most of the Sanskrit texts translated into Persian during the Mughal period were likewise chosen for their philosophical interest and had little relevance to religious practice. *The Pool of the Water of Life* was known to various Muslim mystics of India, some of whom had watched with interest the breathing exercises and chants of the yogis and noticed similarities with their own meditative practices.[5] Shaykh `Abd al-Quddus Gangohi (d. 1537), who was familiar with the yoga of the Naths and wrote Hindi verses on the subject, taught *The Pool* to a disciple.[6] In the sixteenth century, Muhammad Ghawth Gwaliyari (d. 1563), an Indian Sufi master of the Shattari order, translated *The Pool* from Arabic into Persian under the title *Bahr al-hayat* (*The Ocean of Life*).[7] There are at least two other less

---

[3] Osman Yahia, *Histoire et classification de l'oeuvre d'Ibn `Arabi, Étude critique*, 2 vols. (Damascus: Institut Français de Damas, 1964), 1:287–88, no. 230.

[4] Hellmut Ritter, "Al-Biruni's Übersetzung des Yoga-sutra des Patañjali," *Oriens* 9 (1956): 165–200; Bruce B. Lawrence, "The Use of Hindu Religious Texts in al-Biruni's *India* with Special Reference to Patañjali's Yoga-Sutras," in *The Scholar and the Saint: Studies in Commemoration of Abu'l Rayhan al-Biruni and Jalal al-Din al-Rumi*, ed. Peter J. Chelkowski (New York: New York University Press, 1975), pp. 29–48, esp. p. 33.

[5] E.g., Nasir al-Din Mahmud "Chiragh-i Dihli," *Khayr al-Majalis*, comp. Hamid Qalandar, ed. K. A. Nizami (Aligarh: Department of History, 1956), p. 60.

[6] For bibliographic references see S. A. A. Rizvi, "Sufis and Nâtha Yogis in Mediaeval Northern India (XII to XVI Centuries)," p. 132, quoting Rukn al-Din Quddusi, *Lata'if-i Quddusi* (Delhi: Matba`-i Mujtaba'i, 1311/ 1894), p. 41; id., *A History of Sufism in India*, vol. 1, *Early Sufism and its History in India to 1600 A.D.* (Delhi: Munshiram Manoharlal Publishers Pvt. Ltd., 1978), p. 335. Gangohi's knowledge of yoga is fully discussed by Simon Digby in "`Abd al-Quddus Gangohi (1456–1537): The Personality and Attitudes of a Medieval Indian Sufi," *Medieval India, A Miscellany* 3 (1975): 1–66.

[7] See below.

commonly known Persian translations of the Arabic text; one of these was circulated among Persian scholars of Fars in the early seventeenth century, where the Italian traveler Pietro della Valle acquired a copy in 1622. Sufis in Sind and Turkey continued to refer to *The Pool* well into the nineteenth century. The Arabic text was twice translated into Ottoman Turkish, and Muhammad Ghawth's Persian translation was itself rendered into Dakhani Urdu.[8]

Here, I would like to concentrate on the Persian translation by Muhammad Ghawth, which is of considerable importance for Sufism.[9] This Persian translation and expansion (in some copies written by Husayn Gwaliyari from the dictation of Muhammad Ghawth) was composed in the city of Broach in Gujarat, probably around 1550, in order to clarify the obscurities of the Arabic version.[10] Although Muhammad Ghawth did not have access to the Sanskrit text of the *Amrtakunda*, he had consulted extensively with contemporary yogic teachers, and his version is greatly expanded from the Arabic text. The Persian text is appropriately entitled *The Ocean of Life*, and the growth in size from a pool to an ocean parallels the expansion of the text by the addition of many new materials (e.g., the list of yogic postures in chapter four is expanded from five to 21 positions). It seems likely that he had been using the *Hawd al-hayat* as a teaching text with his disciples in the Shattari Sufi order and that his Persian translation emerged as an oral commentary on the Arabic. The teachings of the *Bahr al-hayat*, as adapted in other writings by Muhammad Ghawth, apparently occupied a significant position in the literature of the Shattari order. Some of the practices that Muhammad Ghawth incorporated into his treatise on meditation, the *Jawahir-i khamsa*, or *The Five Jewels* superficially resemble yogic exercises. The Mecca-based Shattari teacher Sibghat Allah (d. 1606) translated the latter text into Arabic as *al-Jawahir al-khams* and taught these practices to disciples from as far

---

[8] A complete description of these translations and known manuscripts are given in *The Pool of Nectar*.

[9] Here I refer to two manuscripts: Muhammad Ghawth Gwaliyari, *Bahr al-hayat*, MS 2002 Persian (Ethé), India Office Library (hereafter cited as IO); MS 6298 Persian, Ganj Bakhsh Library, Islamabad (cited as GB). More than 20 manuscripts of this text exist, along with two lithograph editions.

[10] Muhammad Ghawth, *Bahr al-hayat*, IO, pp. 2, 4.

away as North Africa and Indonesia.[11] In other words, if one wished to make a case for yogic "influence" on Sufi practice, this would seem to be the strongest possible example to make that case. There is no other known literary source on yoga so widely disseminated among Sufis.

Yet later authors in the Shattari tradition exhibited ambivalence toward the explicit description of yogic teachings in the *Bahr al-hayat*. This ambivalence towards yoga is manifest in the lengthy characterization of the *Bahr al-hayat* given by one of Muhammad Ghawth's biographers, his near-namesake Muhammad Ghawthi:

> The *Bahr al-hayat* is the translation of the ascetical work and manual of the society of Jogis [yogis] and Sannyasis, in which occur interior practices, visualization exercises, descriptions of holding the breath, and other types of meditation. . . . These two groups are the chief ascetics, recluses, and guides of the people of idolatry and infidelity. By the blessings of these very practices and repetitions of names (*adhkar*), [they have] arrived to the ladder of false spirituality (*istidraj*) and the excellent rank of visions . . . He (Muhammad Ghawth) separated all these subjects from the Sanskrit language that is the tongue of the infidels' flimsy books, dressed them in Persian, loosed the belt of infidelity from the shoulder of those concepts, and adorned them with . . . unity and *islam*, thus freeing them from the dominance of blind adherence with the overwhelming strength of true faith. The master of realization bestowed aid and assistance with Sufi repetitions of names (*adhkar*) and practices. He fashioned the Truth (*al-haqq*), which is a single casket (*huqqa*) of precious jewels, and a case for kingly rubies, from the spoils of "they are like cattle, nay, more erring" (Qur. 7.171) . . . into an ennobling crown for the Lord of "religion, for God, is *islam*" (Qur. 3.19).[12]

---

[11] See Muhammad ibn Khatir al-Din ibn Khwaja al-'Attar [Muhammad Ghawth], *al-Jawahir al-khams*, ed. Ahmad ibn al-'Abbas, 2nd ed. (Egypt: Muhammad Rif'at 'Amir, 1393/1973), pp. 3–9; Muhammad ibn 'Ali al-Sanusi, *al-Salsabil al-mu'in fi tara'iq al-arba'in*, in *al-Masa'il al-'ashar* (Cairo, n.d.), pp. 124ff.

[12] Muhammad Ghawthi, *Gulzar-i Abrar*, MS 259 Persian, Asiatic Society, Calcutta, fols. 327b–328a. Ghawthi's book is a biographical dictionary of Indian Sufis completed in 1613. The modern Urdu translation of this work considerably mutes the language of this passage, simply referring to "Hindus" instead of infidels and omitting several disparaging adjectives; cf. Muhammad Ghawthi Mandawi, *Adhkar-i Abrar, Urdu Tarjuma-i Gulzar-i Abrar*, trans. Fazl Ahmad Jewari (1326/1908; repr., Lahore: Islamic Book Foundation, 1395/1975), p. 300.

This biographer was at pains to separate the yogic practices as far as possible from their Indian origin, and he therefore argued that they had been entirely Islamized. A similar sentiment appears in a modern Urdu biography of Muhammad Ghawth, based on the work of a disciple of Muhammad Ghawth named Fazl Allah Shattari. There the text is briefly described as follows: "[On] the method of the modes and practices of the Jogi [yogi] and Sannyasi folk, in the Sanskrit language. He has translated it into the Persian language in the style of Islamic Sufism, and arranged it in the fashion of the Sufi master. This is a good book for esotericists."[13] Here too, the commentator feels the need to describe the contents of the book as having been Islamized.

Muhammad Ghawth himself saw no such ambiguity in his reworking of the yogic material. In general, he felt free to make the most remarkable equivalences between yogic terms and practices on the one hand and Sufi concepts on the other. In making these creative translations, he was following the lead of the anonymous translator of the original Arabic version. In the seventh chapter of the Arabic text, which treats the magical imagination (*wahm*), the seven Sanskrit *mantra*s or chants associated with the seven *cakra*s or spinal nerve centers are all boldly declared to be translations of the Arabic invocations of the names of God. Thus, the Sanskrit syllable *hum* is translated as "O Lord" (*ya rabb*), and *aum* is translated as "O Ancient One" (*ya qadim*). In introducing these seven great mantras, the Arabic translator remarks that "they are like the greatest names [of God] among us."[14] Muhammad Ghawth goes one better, however, providing two Arabic phrases for each Sanskrit term; he translates *hum* as *ya rabb ya hafiz*, "O Lord, O Protector," and *aum* as *ya qahir ya qadir*, "O Wrathful, O All-powerful."[15] In a discussion of breathing techniques that does not appear in the Arabic version, Muhammad Ghawth also finds equivalents for the yogic terms *hans* and

---

[13] Fazl Allah Shattari, *Manaqib-i Ghawthiyya*, Urdu trans. Muhammad Zahir al-Haqq (Agra: Abu al-Ma'ali Steam Press, 1933), p. 75. This rare lithograph has been translated from a Persian MS in the khanqah of Shaykh Wajih al-Din 'Alawi in Ahmedabad, which apparently covered the life of Muhammad Ghawth up to 941/1534–35, the remainder being added by the translator on the basis of "well-known books" (p. 80).

[14] Husain, "Amratkund," p. 330.

[15] Muhammad Ghawth, *Bahr al-hayat*, IO, pp. 91, 94; GB, pp. 82, 84.

so ham, which are pronounced during the two phases of exhalation and inhalation; the first is "an expression for the spiritual lord (*rabb ruhi*)," while the second stands for "the lord of lords (*rabb al-arbab*)."[16] There are many other examples of this kind. Semantically, such "translations" make no sense whatever; they are, rather, functional equivalents between the yogic words of power and the names of God as used by the Sufis; this is especially evident in the case of the seven great mantras, for which the Arabic equivalents are presented in a vocative form used in the Sufi *dhikr* repetitions of the names of God. Other equivalences, on the other hand, sometimes are so far-fetched as to strain credulity. For instance, the Samk'hya triad of cosmic qualities, *rajas* ("passion"), *tamas* ("darkness"), and *sattva* ("goodness"), which are here correlated with the three deities Brahma, Vishnu, and Mahesh, are bizarrely translated as "all the commands of religious law," "the blow of existence," and "equality."[17] In such a case it appears that the translator was mainly concerned to provide some kind of arbitrary equivalent from an Islamic vocabulary rather than any precise linguistic rendering. Perhaps the most remarkable equivalences made by Muhammad Ghawth involve persons, identifying primordial yogis with the prophets recognized in Islam. At one point he writes, "Their religious leader (*imam*) is Gorakh, and some say that Gorakh is an expression for Khizr (peace on our Prophet and on him)."[18] Here the archetypal yogi has been assimilated to the immortal Prophet Khizr (Arabic Khadir), who plays an important initiatic role in Sufism. There are two further identifications of this type: "That religious leader (*imam*) Chaurangi, that is, Elijah [Ilyas] (peace be upon him), and the third, 'the breath of the fish,' who is the religious leader Machindirnath [Matsyendranath, cf. Skt. *matsya*, fish], or Mina Nath, that is, Jonah [Yunus] (peace be upon him)—each one of them has attained the

---

[16] Muhammad Ghawth, *Bahr al-hayat*, ch. 4, IO, pp. 45–46; GB, p. 55; ch. 7, GB, p. 93.
[17] Muhammad Ghawth, *Bahr al-hayat*, ch. 10, GB, p. 25. Al-Biruni more accurately understood *rajas* as "exertion and fatigue," *tamas* as "languor and irresolution," and *sattva* as "rest and goodness"; cf. al-Biruni, *Alberuni's India*, trans. Edward C. Sachau (1888; repr., New Delhi: S. Chand & Co., 1964), 1:40–41. Further on these three qualities see, e.g., *The Bhagavad Gita*, trans. R. C. Zaehner (London: Oxford University Press, 1969), index, s.vv.
[18] Muhammad Ghawth, *Bahr al-hayat*, ch. 5, IO, p. 66; GB, p. 68 (omits reference to "our Prophet").

water of life."[19] Muhammad Ghawth has assimilated elements of the yogic tradition to familiar Islamic categories and persons, much as Islamic philosophers assimilated the wisdom of the Greeks and other pre-Islamic peoples to their own prophetic dispensation.

In his comparison of yogic and Islamic categories, Muhammad Ghawth not only identifies great yogis with the prophets but also implicitly puts his accounts of yogic practice on a parallel with normative religious practice in Islam. He regards the yogis' oral traditions as a parallel phenomenon to the hadith reports of the prophet Muhammad, describing them by the same Arabic term, *riwayat*, that is used for hadith transmissions. The main differences between these yogic traditions and Islamic hadith lie in their sources (Hindu deities such as Siva instead of Muhammad) and their transmitters. In the account of the "imams" of the yogis just mentioned, which is devoted to a discussion of breath control, Matsyendranath and Chaurangi are both described as presenting transmissions (*riwayat*), generally going back to Siva as an ultimate source. Muhammad Ghawth even invokes the authority of the Tantric goddess Kamak'hya Devi, who is well known in Assam and Bengal, for a technical clarification of yogic practice: "The transmitter (*rawi*) is a woman, the wife of Mahadeva [Siva], who is called Kamak'hya Devi— she says that [in the *k'hecari mudra* position] there is no need to hold the breath. . . . She is a reporter (*naqil*) from Brahma and Visnu."[20] By using terms from the normative discourse of Islamic hadith methodology, Muhammad Ghawth aims to draw the Muslim reader into the heart of the discussion of yoga by means of a format that is both familiar and authoritative.

Muhammad Ghawth frequently comments that on the practical level, the experiences of yogis and sufis are very similar. He states this emphatically with respect to the characteristic Sufi term for mystical experience, "unveiling" (*kashf*):

> Most of the "friends of God" (*awliya'-i khuda*, Sufi saints) have comprehended and explained these influences from unveiling (*kashf*), and the monks (*rahiban*) of India, who are the yogis, have unveiling that is in

---

[19] Muhammad Ghawth, *Bahr al-hayat*, ch. 5, GB, p. 68, in a marginal note marked "from another MS."
[20] Ibid., ch. 5, GB, p. 69 (following marginal corrections); IO, p. 67.

agreement with the mystical state of those who have realized the truth. Although the language differs, the explanation is the same.[21]

In a discussion of a particular repetition of a passage from the Qur'an, he states further that "Most of the sages (*hukama'*) of India have followed this practice, and have attained to their own quiddity; some Muslims have taken the same practice to completion and have reached the benefit of gnosis as is appropriate."[22] Despite the improbability of yogis devoting themselves to repeating *Surat al-Ikhlas* from the Qur'an, Muhammad Ghawth finds that the practical results of repeated chanting are very similar in both traditions, regardless of differences in semantic or religious content.

Occasionally, the Shattari master finds discrepancies between yogic teachings and standard Islamic doctrines, and these lead him to seek an explanation that will reconcile the two. In the beginning of the sixth chapter, which concerns the nature of the body, he recognizes the difference that separates the yogic and Islamic concepts of spirit and body. In an extended and revealing passage, Muhammad Ghawth sets forth the approach that he follows of seeking a kind of accord between the two positions.

> The master of the religious law (*shar'*) [i.e., the Prophet Muhammad] states that after a specific time, the entry of the spirit into the body takes place. The perfect and practiced yogis say that, without spirit, nothing abides, rather, it undergoes corruption. Especially, the point of flesh and skin does not endure a single day [without spirit]. Here lies a contradiction between the theory (*kalam*) of the yogis and the command of the religious law. A categorical reply is required, so that the decree of the religious law may accord with (*rast ayad ba*) the findings of the yogis, and so that, except for the different method (*tartib*), no doubt should attach to their words. In the end, the theory becomes a single connection (*paywand*), and each of them becomes open to advice (*pand-pazir*). With a delicate understanding one engages with the subtlety of meaning and investigates until one becomes an experiencer of truth. Then the theory (*kalam*) on both sides becomes firmly rooted in the heart and has a single substance.[23]

---

[21] Ibid., ch. 7, IO, p. 90.

[22] Ibid., ch. 3, IO, p. 31 (omitting the word "some" before "Muslims"); GB, p. 42.

[23] Muhammad Ghawth, *Bahr al-hayat*, ch. 6, IO, p. 72; GB, pp. 71–72.

The case resembles that of the early Islamic philosophers, who also had to deal with a discrepancy between the Platonic notion of the pre-existence of the soul and the prophetic emphasis on the creation of the soul by an omnipotent God. After a complicated excursus on the cosmic deployment of the spirit, Muhammad Ghawth returns to the problem of reconciling yogic and Islamic views. He concludes that while the yogic doctrine has shortcomings, their practical knowledge of the body is highly advanced and valuable for the pursuit of mystical knowledge.

> Now in the discussion of wisdom and power, plenty of difficulties have appeared. Fundamentally the words of the yogis are not correct. It is necessary to harmonize (*tatbiq dashtan*) this so that the actual condition becomes apparent, and so that their unveiling is corrected and made right. Its practice rests upon the real; its practice leads to the result of a spiritual state. The Siddha yogis say, "We are in agreement with the dervishes who realize the truth in the quiddity of spirit." Inasmuch as they speak of descent, appearance, and ascent (*tanazzul, tala 'at, taraqqi*), which rest upon the real, yet they have gone beyond the reality of recognizing the means. The yogic group has grasped the means, and they have observed and investigated it, because by the means of the body the real gnosis is discovered. . . . Therefore, the protection of the body is a duty (*fard*), because it is the means of gnosis.[24]

Again the similarity with the Islamic adaptation of Greek philosophy is striking. Just as Ibn Rushd argued that the study of philosophy is a religious duty for those who are qualified intellectuals, so Muhammad Ghawth uses a term from Islamic law, *fard*, to describe the obligatory character of the study of yoga for those who are seeking gnosis. Doctrinal differences exist but are relatively unimportant when compared with the effective realization of spiritual states for which yoga can be an effective means.

What are the practical results of Muhammad Ghawth's adoption of yogic practices into Sufi discipline? As we have seen, the equivalences that he makes between yogic and Islamic terminology, religious leaders, and spiritual experiences are functional. He acknowledges doctrinal differences but does not linger on them. As far as the direct impact on the practices of the Shattari order is concerned, the most obvious innovation

---

[24] Ibid., ch. 6, IO, pp. 76–77; GB, pp. 74–75.

is the use of chants in Hindi or Sanskrit. In speaking of the occult science called *simiya*, Muhammad Ghawth remarks that one of its bases is "the talisman [made] from the names of the most high creator; whether they are in Arabic or Hindi, the result is attained."[25] This is true whether we are concerned with the seven principal Sanskrit mantras or the Qur'anic invocations of God. Thus he further notes that

> the perfect monks and Siddha yogis have grasped these names of God most high in the Indian language, and have been occupied in reciting them. They have seen the internal result with the eye of manifestation. Having found the names in the heart, they have dived into it, and like pearl divers they have brought up the quiddity of the Essence and Attributes with praise.[26]

Thus, it will not be surprising to find that Muhammad Ghawth presents, in the ninth chapter, the "great prayer (*du'a-i kabir*)," which begins with Qur'anic invocations but shifts abruptly into a dozen lines of Sanskrit *mantra*s.[27] In his principal work on Sufi practice, *The Five Jewels*, Muhammad Ghawth also cites a *dhikr* in Hindi, which he attributes to the early Chishti Sufi master Farid al-Din Ganj-i Shakkar (d. 1265).[28]

Beyond the introduction of sacred syllables from Indian languages, which is fairly obvious, it is difficult to state precisely what has been the effect of the study of yogic practices on Sufism. In a general sense, such practices as visualization, localizing syllables in parts of the body, and repeating chants that produce occult powers, all may be considered typical of hatha yoga. Yet, these practices can also be found in many branches of Sufism unrelated to India and in the gnostic meditations of pre-Islamic traditions such as Neoplatonism. So to speak of "influences"

---

[25] Muhammad Ghawth, *Bahr al-hayat*, ch. 2, IO, p. 38; GB, p. 46.

[26] Ibid., ch. 7, GB, p. 87; IO, p. 100.

[27] Ibid., ch. 9, IO, pp. 151–52; GB, p. 13. The ninth chapter, on the subjugation of spirits, bears little resemblance to the Arabic version, which describes seven *mantra*s for control of the planetary guardians; the Persian text has an entirely different set of practices.

[28] Muhammad Ghawth, *al-Jawahir al-khams*, 2:70. The same *dhikr* was also quoted by the later Shattari author of Bihar, Imam Rajgiri (d. ca. 1718); cf. Syed Hasan Askari, "A Fifteenth Century Shuttari Sufi Saint of North Bihar," *Proceedings of the 13th Indian History Congress* (1950), p. 157; M. M. Haq, "The Shuttari Order of Sufism in India and Its Exponents in Bengal and Bihar," *Journal of the Asiatic Society of Pakistan* 16 (1971): 175 (with wide textual variations).

from one separate vessel into another, or even to raise the question in this form, is a kind of pre-judgment that does not necessarily aid in the understanding of this religious phenomenon. Muhammad Ghawth did not study yogic teachings from an academic point of view as an outside observer. His "translation" of the *Amrtakunda* text is a work framed in terms of the Islamic traditions, studded with quotations from the Qur'an and hadith. The language of "influence" does not begin to do justice to the subtlety with which he finds points of contact between the terminologies of Yoga and Sufism or to the ways in which he uses the approaches of Islamic legal discourse to categorize the study of yoga. A fuller argument regarding the wider role of yogic practice in Sufism will have to be deferred, but in the most notable case of a yogic text used by Sufis, Muhammad Ghawth's Persian translation of the *Amrtakunda*, yoga is simply a body of practices that can be successfully integrated into the overall worldview of Sufism.

9

Admiring the Works
of the Ancients
The Ellora Temples as viewed by
Indo-Muslim Authors

One of the recurrent problems in the interpretation of Indo-Muslim
identity is the attempt to ascribe a consistently Muslim attitude toward
Hindu temples. This problem arises initially with the incorporation of
building materials from Hindu temples in the construction of mosques
or other buildings commissioned by Muslim patrons. Although the
evidence for the significance of this kind of recycling is sometimes late
and retrospective, it is hard to avoid the conclusion that this phenomenon
involves the triumphal political use of trophies. Perhaps the most notable
example is the Quwwat al-Islam (or Qubbat al-Islam) mosque near the
Qutb Minar in Delhi, which contains numerous columns with partially
effaced Hindu caryatids and Jain (or Buddhist?) figures, as well as the
famous Iron Pillar.[1] This kind of triumphal reuse of temple materials and
ancient royal monuments has been seen since British times as evidence

---

[1] To this category of the trophy belongs the transport of Ashokan columns and other ancient
pillars, of which the Iron Pillar of Delhi is but one example. These trophies may be found
in royal mosques of the Sultanate period at Hisar and Jaunpur, as well as the Quwwat al-
Islam mosque of Delhi and possibly at Tughluqabad. Cf. Mehrdad Shokoohy and Natalie
H. Shokoohy, "Tughluqubad, the Earliest Surviving Town of the Delhi Sultanate," *Bulletin
of the School of Oriental and African Studies* 57 (1994): 548.

of the insatiable propensity of Muslims to destroy idols at every opportunity. Today it affords ammunition to the Hindu extremists who led the
attack on the "Baburi" mosque at Ayodhya; the supposition is that the
mosque not only rests on the site of the birthplace of Rama but also took
the place of a pre-existing temple.

There are, of course, competing theories of the exact relationship
between the Ayodhya mosque and any preceding temple. Some believe
that the mosque was built of the remains of the temple and that the construction of a mosque thus required the demolition of a temple; the reverse
of this zero-sum game is that the erection of a temple on that spot would
require the destruction of the mosque, as indeed took place in December
1992. Others like P. N. Oak assume that Muslim buildings are only
partially defaced Hindu structures so that, in theory, only a slight amount
of restoration would presumably be required to return them to their original functions, rather than full-scale destruction and reconstruction; this has
the appearance at least of a less costly program. The problem arises, however, when these modern interpretations of Muslim iconoclasm deduce
Muslim attitudes from an essential definition of Islam rather than from historical documentation of the significance that particular Muslims attached
to Hindu temples. Attempts to describe Muslims as essentially prone to
idol-smashing are confounded by the historical record, which indicates
that Muslims who wrote about "idol temples" had complex reactions
based as much on aesthetic and political considerations as on religion. The
concept of unchanging and monolithic Muslim identity accordingly needs
to undergo serious revision.

This essay is an attempt to fill out the historical dossier, by presenting
a translation and analysis of a brief text in which a Muslim author, Rafi`
al-Din Shirazi, has set forth a striking interpretation of one of the jewels
of Indian architecture, the Ellora cave temples. Shirazi viewed Ellora not
as religious architecture but as a primarily political monument, which fit
best into the category of the wonders of the world. When Shirazi's reaction to Ellora is compared with other accounts of it by Muslim authors,
with Muslim accounts of other "pagan" monuments in Egypt, and with
descriptions of Ellora by early European travelers, his aesthetic and
political reaction does not seem very unusual. This account is another
reminder that, for pre-modern Muslims, the monolithic Islam defined
by twentieth-century discourse was far from being the only or even the
primary category of judgment.

The text in question is *Tadhkirat al-muluk* (*Memorial of Kings*), a Persian history of Bijapur written by Rafi` al-Din Shirazi in 1612.[2] The author (born in Shiraz in 1540) had a long career in Bijapur government service, from the age of 30 serving Sultan `Ali `Adil Shah as a steward and scribe. In 1596, Sultan Ibrahim `Adil Shah appointed him ambassador to Ahmadnagar, and he also held posts as governor of the Bijapur fort and treasurer. Shirazi witnessed many important events over more than half a century in the Deccan, and he was also steeped in the tradition of Persian historical writing, having written abridgements of standard court chronicles such as Mir Khwand's *Rawdat al-safa`* and Khwand Amir's *Habib al-siyar*. His history is an important independent historical source comparable to the chronicle of Firishta.

In the handwritten edition of Khalidi, the outline of the text is as follows, divided into an introduction, 10 parts, and an appendix:

Introduction (1–15)

I. The Bahmani dynasty (15–35)

II–V. The `Adil Shahi dynasty (36–83)

VI. Dynasties of Gujarat, Ahmadnagar, and Golconda (84–156)

VII. Various events in the Deccan (157–96)

VIII. Ibrahim `Adil Shah, the author's patron (197–269)

IX. The Mughals (270–93)

X. The Mughals and Safavids (294–496; in some MSS this lengthy section is divided into three parts to make 12 parts in all)

Appendix. On Wonders and Rarities (497–566)

The section under discussion occurs towards the end (476–83) of the 10th part, and although its title includes the phrase "wonders and rarities," it does not fall into the appendix proper; instead, it is sandwiched between accounts of military campaigns of the Safavids and the

---

[2] I am basing this analysis on the critical edition of the text established by the late Abu Nasr Khalidi, which has been entrusted to me by his son, Omar Khalidi, to see through the press; it is to be published by the Islamic Research Foundation of the Asitan-i Quds-i Rizawi in Mashhad, Iran. For further information on this author, see my articles "Shirazi, Rafi` al-Din," in *The Encyclopaedia of Islam*, ed. H. A. R. Gibb et al., 2nd ed. (Leiden: E.J. Brill, 1960–), 9:483 (cited hence forth as EI²), and "Ebrahim Shirazi," in *Encyclopedia Iranica* (Costa Mesa, Calif.: Mazda Publishers, 1986–), 8:76.

Mughals. The appendix consists of a series of accounts of *mirabilia* of the `aja'ib` genre of wonders long established in Arabic and Persian literature.[3] Some of these wonders are related by others, although a few were seen by the author himself. These include narratives based on the Persian *Book of Kings* by Firdawsi (497–517), travelers' tales of strange islands (517–32), and accounts of the rivers and geography of India (532–43), followed by brief reports of natural wonders (544–66).

Shirazi's location of his account of Ellora in the dynastic history proper, and not in the appendix on wonders, suggests that he wished to treat it as a serious political concern, framed around a legendary Indian monarch named Parchand Rao. It thus remains separate from the superficially similar stories about fabulous islands and idol temples that occur in the appendix. Those remain comfortably in the realm of two-headed calves and other marvels, but the serious point that Shirazi wanted to make about art and royal monuments required that he situate the story of Ellora amidst similar political and military narratives. In this kind of arrangement Shirazi resembles the Egyptian chronicler of the pyramids, al-Idrisi, who kept his meticulous measurements and historical accounts of the pyramids in one chapter and saved the bizarre and the miraculous for the last chapter of his book.[4] Shirazi's chapter has, however, been circulated separately as a "Treatise on Wonders and Rarities," and in this form it would not have taken on the political coloring afforded by its contextual position in the larger history.[5] Here follows a translation of the extract:

DESCRIPTION OF THE WONDERS AND RARITIES OF THE BUILDING OF ELLORA IN DAULATABAD, WHICH PARCHAND RAO, THE EMPEROR OF INDIA, BUILT NEARLY 4,000 YEARS AGO

1. Parchand Rao was an emperor. With great majesty, he had brought under his control all the land from the border of Sind, Gujarat, the Deccan, and Telingana to the limit of Malabar, and most of the

---

[3] C. E. Dubler, "'Adja'ib," EI[2], 1:203–4.

[4] Ulrich Haarmann, "In Quest of the Spectacular: Noble and Learned Visitors to the Pyramids around 1200 A.D.," in *Islamic Studies Presented to Charles J. Adams*, ed. Wael B. Hallaq and Donald P. Little (Leiden: E. J. Brill, 1991), 65–66.

[5] Haji Muhammad Ashraf, *Catalogue of Persian Manuscripts in the Salar Jung Museum and Library*, vol. 2, *Biographies, Geography, and Travels* (Hyderabad: Salar Jung Museum and Library, 1966), 277, no. 643.

neighboring kings were his subjects. He was noble, just, and upright, and he lived in harmony with the people. The peasant and the soldier in the days of his reign were in all ways happy and free from worry. They passed all their lives in happiness, joy, contentment, and pleasure.

2. In the springtime, when the climate was perfectly mild, Parchand Rao would go on a tour of the kingdom, and he let the people partake of his magnificence. He made every effort to bring about justice and fairness. In every place that he saw abundant water, greenery, and good climate, he laid foundations for buildings, and he supplied the officials of the kingdom every resource for completing them. In this way, having traveled through the entire kingdom three times, he constructed and brought to completion lofty idol-houses (*but-khana*) outside the buildings just mentioned throughout most of his kingdom.

3. Now as for the famous Daulatabad—fine and elegant fabrics were available there, and in the neighborhoods and environs merchants brought them as gifts and donations, and they still are active and do so; wealthy merchants full of tranquility are always dwelling in that city, both Muslim and Hindu. Every year, nearly a thousand ass-loads of different kinds of silken and gold-woven fabrics are brought to its neighborhoods and environs, and general welfare prevails. The same Parchand Rao made Daulatabad his capital, and people from the four corners of the world headed in the direction of Daulatabad. Most of this multitude came to a place that was nearly five or six farsakhs away, and having built houses and gardens, they settled there; tall houses were set up with some difficulty.

4. One day in the assembly of Parchand Rao there was a discussion of the construction of buildings and abodes, and the king said, "During my reign, I have built and finished many buildings in my dominion, but these ordinary buildings do not have much permanency. I want a building that will be truly permanent so that it will be spoken of for years afterward, and there should be wonders and rarities in it so that it will endure and remain lasting for long years and uncounted centuries, and its construction will be famed and well known throughout the world."

5. Some of the architects, engineers, and stoneworkers were dedicated to the emperor and spoke his language because of the many buildings that they had made. They said, "In the region of this very city there is a mountain that is unlike any of the mountains of the world. This is because the mountains that we have seen and see today are mostly of this kind: part is bedrock, and part is soft and has cracks and fissures. In this city there is a great and lofty mountain that has absolutely no cracks, joints, fissures, or rubble. In this way, one can make a great and lofty house, which every great king can do, for lofty buildings have been repeatedly built. If one brings together all the eighteen workshops of the realm, which are famous and well-known, so that the supervisor does not need to have any other building built and he has the capacity and basis associated with that workshop and the quantity of men and animals necessary for those workshops, then they will prepare everything from stone: the assembly of the king's realm, the private palaces, the soldiers in attendance on the king—all will be carved in stone so that each will be established in the proper place. Until the dawn of the resurrection, that court, those workshops, and those people will all be preserved, each in the proper place. Such a court as this, this foundation, and this army will all be in five or six sections of stone, with the human and the other animals of proper proportions in the same form and size in which they were created, neither larger nor smaller."

6. The emperor said, "This account that you have given, if it is possible and can indeed take form, is a wonder. By all means, let them make a model from wax or chalk so that I can have a look." When the artisans, engineers, and stoneworkers heard that the emperor asked for a model, they had to come to agreement and make a completed model such as the emperor had asked for from brick, clay, and chalk. When they invited the emperor to their premises [to see the model], he became very happy, and he consented with delight.

7. Beginning from the middle of the mountain, they made a great open space in the palace, which they call the retreat (*khilwat-khana*). On all four sides of the open space, they cut open spaces (*sar-saya*, lit. "shades") in the stone, perfect in height, width, and length, with a polished and proportioned foundation. In most

places, these are carved in the fashion of great arches (*taq*) need-
ing no pillars. The carving is extremely even and polished, or
rather, is even given a luster. In some of these open spaces there
are alcoves (*bahl*, usually *bahla*, lit. "purse") with caves. Their
ability reaches such subtlety that if the master artist wished to
paint one with a brush made from a single hair, nowhere would it
be easy for him [to match their skill]. In some of the arches there
is a string of camels, and in some a stable of horses. Some are
with saddle, and some with colored blankets. There is no need to
mention the extraordinary workmanship and subtlety again. One
should compare the alcove with the palace; in each one of these
palaces, there are some human forms in the attitude of servants,
which are necessary in those palaces. One would say that all are
standing ready to serve, while some appear in such a way that one
would say they are in the act of being rejected. The remaining
animals, wild beasts and birds... are everywhere in the manner of
delivering an obligatory reply to a question. The forms of armed
and equipped soldiers, to the number of one or two hundred, are
as if ready for service, each one established in his own place. On
the courtyard in front of the palace gate, here and there, several
large and small elephants are standing in order. Around each
elephant, a few attendants stand in their regalia.

Description of the Foundation of the
Palace Fort and its Capacity

8. Four arches (*taq*) cut from stone are on one side of the courtyard,
   and within, two shorter ones are in the place of the gate.
   Symmetrical in height, breadth, and length, these four are linked
   by a single roof. Two great benches (*suffa*) are built into the great
   arches as a seat for servants, for the servants of the fort and the
   courtyard are within. Nearly five or six hundred people are sitting in their places, some standing fully armed. Outside of that,
   many weapons are carved in various places, such as swords, dag-
   gers, dirks (Hindi *katara*), spears, bows, quivers, and arrows. One
   remains in astonishment at the subtle and painstaking work. In the
   courtyard, inside the four arches, are benches, porticoes (*ayvan*),
   and rooms carved and hollowed out in the same style. On one side

are the imperial workshops, such as the armory, stable, water-works, kitchen, storehouse, and wine cellar. In every one of these palaces, there are at least fifty or sixty human forms, each one of which appears to be in the act of performing something. The skill of each workshop is cut into rock to such a degree that the human mind cannot imagine it. Everyone who goes there says that the people [in the stone reliefs] are having a party. One should spend several days at the palace if one wishes to see them all, and to understand them fully, a long lifetime would be needed. Many wild beasts and birds have also been added to these festivals to adorn the palace.

9. Proceeding behind this palace, there is a fort and some other palaces pertaining to the previously mentioned palace. Here too, a multitude of figures is made in the form of servants, done with great workmanship in a more prominent position, and the court-yard of this is greater than that in the previous palace. Some work-shops are set up in this palace, and benches, arches, and porticoes have been raised up to heaven. By way of workshops, things such as the bachelor quarters (*dar al-'azab*), goldsmith shop, fountain shop, wardrobe, treasury, and the like [have been made] with such subtlety and workmanship that a hair of a single brush could not have rendered it. The attendants of the workshops, their trade, tools, and basis of each workshop have been made to the nec-essary extent, each one being made in the performance of [the appropriate] action and each servant of these palaces has been made firm in the proper position.

A Hint of Conditions of the Court and the Arrangement of the Place of the Workmen and Attendants

10. Having made another palace with the arch and portico in per-fect proportion and having placed some smaller palaces to the sides with workmanship and beauty and the imperial throne at the front of the portico, they fixed the portrait of the emperor upon it, depicting that amount of ornament on the limbs of the emperor that is customary among the people of India, some sculpted and some in relief. Its painstaking subtlety is beyond description.

To the left and right of that throne, half-thrones have been prepared with solid foundations, and on each of these, they have sat princes and nobles of the realm. Behind the head and shoulders of the emperor are servants, friends, and relatives, each in the proper place. There are some watchmen holding swords with handkerchiefs in their hands, in the Deccan fashion. Waterbearers in their own manner and order hold vessels of water in their hands, and waiters (*shira-chi*) hold a few flagons with cups in their hands. Winebearers, by which I mean betel-leaf servers, hold trays of betel leaf in their hands with suitable accompaniments, some trays having sweet-scented things, for in each tray are cups of musk, saffron, and other items. The saucers in those trays are made in the fashion of cups, with pounded ambergris, sandalwood, and aloes, and aromatic compounds are set forth, and trays full of roses. This portico, which is subtler in arrangement than a rose, is such that the description, beauty, workmanship, and subtlety of workmanship of that assembly do not fit into the vessel of explanation.

11. In front of that portico of the court, the chief musician (*sar-i nawbatan*) and the court prefect (*shihna-i divan*) stand in the proper arrangement and position in their places. On both sides, nearly two thousand horsemen, extremely well executed, are in attendance in the proper fashion. In the courtyard of the court and the portico, across from the emperor, there are several groups of musicians, each standing with his own drum and lute; one would say that they are dancing. In the same courtyard, tumblers, jesters, wrestlers, athletes, and swordsmen exhibit their skill. One would say that each group in its particular area and assembly is right in the middle of its activity. Several famous and large elephants, which were always the apple of the emperor's alchemical eye, are in his presence, and several head of elite imperial horses, which were always present with the court drum, are present in the customary fashion.

12. So many beautiful and well-wrought things are in those buildings and courtyards that, if one wished to explain them all, he would fail to reach the goal. The listener should prepare for fatigue of the brain!

13. Outside this assembly, several other small banquet assemblies have been made and constructed, which tongue and pen are unable to explain. Three or four private palaces have been built, and in each palace are the private inhabitants, who are the women and eunuchs—more than one or two hundred. Each one is in a distinct style and position, and a detailed account of the motions and postures of those palaces would not be inappropriate; it can be generally summarized in a few words. In each of these palaces, some obscene activities—none repeated—are taking place.

14. In general, of that which is actually in existence at Ellora, not one part in a thousand has been mentioned. Few people have reached the limit of its buildings, and those who have [come] simply take in the generality of it with a glance. What is presently observable and displayed takes up nearly two farsakhs. Even further, there are places with buildings and hunting lodges, but a wall of chalk and stone has been firmly set up, so no one goes past that place. It is famous.

15. There is a smaller building like this in a village at least fifty farsakhs from Ellora. It is said that in every place, palaces, buildings, and hunting lodges have been built in the same fashion, and it is still in existence. But God knows best as to the realities of the situation.

Description of Various Matters on the Same Subject

16. There are several constructions of similar form in the neighborhood of Shiraz, and that region is called Naqsh-i Rustam and The Forty Towers (Chihil Sutun, i.e., Persepolis). In *The History of Persia*, it is well known that there were four such towers that Jamshid had made, and on top of all the towers he had made a single tall building so that these towers were pillars for that building. He spent most of his time in that building sitting on the seat of lordship and holding public audience. The people from below bowed to him and worshiped him. In that building of Ellora, most places are roofed and dark. Some places are made with illumination from windows, and most rooms have no roof

and are perfectly illuminated. Since this was three or four thousand years ago and, in that time, lifetimes were long and humans were mighty of frame and full of power and strength, such places as have been written of [above], which they made—if anyone of this age wished to make them and had a thousand people and a period of a thousand years, it is not known whether it could be carried out to completion. In fact, the intellect is astonished at that construction.

17. There was always a joke about that building which was shared between the former Burhan Nizam Shah and Shah Tahir. The Nizam Shah used to say that sodomy was brought to the Deccan during the present time by foreigners [i.e., Persians]. Shah Tahir objected that this practice is immemorial in this kingdom. Once, when they went to visit the buildings of Ellora, Shah Tahir saw a depiction of two men embracing each other. He took the hand of the Nizam Shah and brought him near that depiction, saying, "Have foreigners brought this also?" By this example, he removed the Nizam Shah's displeasure with foreigners.

Description of the Idol Temple of the Town of Lakmir

18. In the neighborhood of Bankapur is a town called Lakmir. In ancient times, it was the capital of one of the great emperors of unbelief. With the greatest architectural skill, the emperors, princes, and pillars of the realm built many idol temples in imitation of one another, extremely large and well built. Years passed, and most of the buildings fell into ruin, and only a few were still inhabited. But four hundred idol temples remained perfectly sound, having been constructed with the utmost of painstaking and elegant workmanship. At the time when we saw it, we saw many wonders and rarities, and astonishment increased upon astonishment. Out of all those, we saw one idol temple with dimensions of seventy cubits by fifty cubits. Both inside and outside of it a trough (*taghari*) had been cut in relief. Its subtlety was to the degree that in the space of a hand, in natural proportions, the forms of ten men had been made, along with the forms of ten

or fifteen animals, both beasts and birds, in such a way that the eyelashes and fingernails were visible. On the border were roses, tulips, and trees of the locality, about the size of one hand. This degree of artistry has been forgotten.

19. Imagine how much work has been done on the inside and outside of all the idol temples and how many days and how much time it took to complete them. May God the exalted and transcendent forgive the World-Protector [i.e., ʿAli ʿAdil Shah, d. 988/1580] with the light of his compassion, for after the conquest of Vijayanagar, he with his own blessed hand destroyed five or six thousand adored idols of unbelief and ruined most of the idol temples [at the battle of Talikota or Bannihatti, January 1565]. But the limited number [of buildings] on which the welfare of the time and the kingdom depended, which we know as the art of Ellora in Daulatabad, this kind of idol temple and art we have forgotten.

There are several striking aspects to this text. First of all, Shirazi makes hardly any reference to Indian religions in his description of Ellora. Second, he appreciates the monument on an aesthetic level, and he explains its origin in political terms. For him, Ellora is a royal monument that depicts the court life of an ancient king of India, making it comparable to pre-Islamic Persian monuments such as Persepolis.[6] The statue of Shiva in the Kailas temple is explained as a royal portrait. Third, and most unexpectedly, he only makes a strong bow to religion when he calls upon God to forgive his former patron, Sultan ʿAli ʿAdil Shah, for destroying the temples of Vijayanagar. This last gesture turns the stereotype of Muslim iconoclasm on its head. Shirazi acknowledges that temple destruction has taken place in military and political contexts of conquest, but he deplores it as a violation of beauty and, ultimately, as an offense against God. Although he does not mention it, the temple at Bankapur, which he also admires, was evidently the "superb temple" that ʿAli ʿAdil Shah destroyed and replaced with a mosque when he took the

---

[6] On Persepolis, see M. Streck [G. C. Miles], "Istakhr," EI², 4:219–22. It is worth noting that the author of this article attributes the defacement of human figures at Persepolis to "Muslim fanaticism," something that calls for further analysis.

city in 1575.[7] Shirazi's strong emotional and religious reaction against the destruction of temples is all the more noteworthy in view of his basically conservative Muslim attitude; his account of the religious innovations of the Mughal emperor Akbar is highly critical, closely resembling Bada'uni's negative view of Akbar rather than the universalist perspective of Abu al-Fazl.[8]

Shirazi was not the first Muslim to appreciate the importance of Ellora. The Arab scholar Mas'udi (d. 956) spent several years as ambassador to the powerful Rashtrakuta empire, under whose auspices some of the temples of Ellora were constructed; the Rashtrakutas had friendly relations with the Arabs, whom they viewed as allies against the Gurjaras of northern India.[9] In his *Meadows of Gold*, in the context of a lengthy disquisition on temples of the ancient world, Mas'udi briefly describes the temple of Ellora in the following passage, noting that in another place (unfortunately, a lost work) he has more fully discussed

> the temples (*hayakil*) in India dedicated to idols (*asnam*) in the form of Buddhas (*bidada*), which have appeared since ancient times in the land of India, and information about the great temple which is in India, known as Ellora; this is an object of pilgrimage (*yuqsadu*) from far distances in India. It has a land endowment, and around it are a thousand cells, where monks supervise the worship (*ta'zim*) of this idol in.[10]

---

[7] Mahomed Kasim Ferishta, *History of the Rise of the Mahomedan Power in India, Till the Year A.D. 1612*, trans. J. Briggs, 4 vols. (1829; repr., Lahore: Sang-e Meel, 1977), 3:84, dates this to 1573, but epigraphic evidence places this conquest in December 1575; see H. K. Sherwani and P.M. Joshi, eds., *History of Medieval Deccan, 1295–1724*, 2 vols. (Hyderabad: Government of Andhra Pradesh, 1973–74), 1:335.

[8] Iqtidar Alam Khan, "The Tazkirat ul-Muluk by Rafi'uddin Ibrahim Shirazi: As a Source on the History of Akbar's Reign," *Studies in History* 2 (1980): 41–55.

[9] André Wink, *Al-Hind: The Making of the Indo-Islamic World*, vol. 1, *Early Medieval India and the Expansion of Islam, 7th–11th Centuries* (Delhi: Oxford University Press, 1990), 303–9, esp. 305.

[10] Abu al-Hasan 'Ali ibn al-Husayn ibn 'Ali al-Mas'udi, *Muruj al-dhahab wa ma'adin al-jawahir*, ed. Muhammad Muhyi al-Din 'Abd al-Hamid, 4th ed., 4 vols. (Egypt: al-Maktaba al-Tajariyya, 1384/1964), 2:262; cf. Mas'udi, *Les Prairies d'or*, trans. Barbier de Maynard and Pavet de Courteille, ed. Charles Pellat, Collection d'Ouvrages Orientaux (Paris: Societe Asiatique, 1965), 2:547, §1424, corresponding to 4:95–96 in the nineteenth-century edition of the Arabic text by Barbier de Maynard. There are problems in the Arabic text published in Egypt; I have followed the French translators in reading *bidada* rather than *badra* (which would result in "the form of the moon" rather than "in the form of Buddhas") and Ellora (*Alura*) rather than the anomalous MS readings *al-adri*

It should be noted that in this account, Mas'udi does not distinguish between Hindu, Buddhist, or Jain temples and images; the words for "idol" in Arabic (*bidada*) and Persian (*but*) were in fact derived from Buddha (he immediately follows this reference with a vague note about the temple to the sun in Multan).[11] Indian temples are viewed here in a continuum with Roman, Egyptian, and Sabian temples, a point to which we shall return. Later references to Ellora by Muslim authors belong to the period after the Turkish conquest of the Deccan, when the temples of Ellora had ceased to function as an active religious center. According to Firishta, it was during some unofficial sightseeing at Ellora in 1307 that some Turkish soldiers stumbled across the Hindu princess Dewal Rani, whom they captured and brought to Delhi as a bride for Khidr Khan.[12] In 1318, Sultan Qutb al-Din Mubarak Shah Khalji spent a month at Ellora awaiting the return of his general, Khusraw Khan, from campaigns in Warangal.[13] A tradition related in a current gazetteer maintains that 'Ali' al-Din Hasan, founder of the Bahmani dynasty of the Deccan, visited Ellora in 1352, "taking with him those who could read the inscriptions and understand the significance of the frescoes and statuary on the walls."[14] We have seen above how the ruler of Ahmadnagar,

---

and *bilad al-ray*. Both Arabic editions are in error, however, in reading *jawarin* ("female slaves," pl. of *jariya*) in place of *jiwarun* ("resident pilgrims," pl. of *jar*, probably in this case meaning Jain monks); this led the French translators to render the last phrase as "jeunes esclaves destinées aux pèlerins qui viennent de toute l'Inde pour adorer cette idole." From what we know of Ellora under the Rashtrakutas, it would have functioned as a monastery rather than as a massive *devadasi* center.

[11] The British traveler Seely, too, was fairly vague about the relations between Hinduism and Buddhism; see J. B. Seely, *The Wonders of Ellora or the Narrative of a Journey to the Temples or Dwellings Excavated out of a Mountain of Granite at Ellora in the East Indies* (London, 1824), 197–98.

[12] Abu al-Qasim Firishta, *Gulshan-i Ibrahimi* (Lucknow: Nawal Kishor, 1281/ 1864–65), 1:117; Mahomed Kasim Ferishta, *History of the Rise of the Mahomedan Power in India*, 1:210.

[13] Banarsi Prasad Saksena, "Qutbuddin Mubarak Khalji," in *A Comprehensive History of India*, vol. 5, *The Delhi Sultanate (A.D. 1206–1526)*, ed. Mohammad Habib and Khaliq Ahmad Nizami (1970; repr., New Delhi: People's Publishing House, 1982), 436.

[14] *Aurangabad District, Maharashtra State Gazetteers*, 2nd ed. (Bombay: Gazetteers Department, Government of Maharashtra, 1977), 88. This information is apparently drawn from an important modern Urdu history of the Deccan, Muhammad 'Abd al-Jabbar Mulkapuri, *Mahbub al-watan, tazkira-i salatin-i Dakan*, vol. 1, *Dar bayan-i salatin-i Bahmaniyya* (Hyderabad: Matba'-i Fakhr-i Nizami, n.d.), 147–50, which is followed by a lengthy and enthusiastic appreciation of the Ellora caves.

Burhan Nizam Shah, and his Persian minister, Shah Tahir, used to visit Ellora for pleasure. The most surprising of all the admirers of Ellora is none other than the Mughal emperor Awrangzib, who spent years in the Deccan, first as governor under Shah Jahan and later as emperor reducing the Deccan sultanates and quashing Maratha rebels. He was buried in 1707 in the Chishti shrine complex at Khuldabad, just a few miles down the road from Ellora. In a letter, Awrangzib recorded a visit to Khuldabad, Daulatabad, and Ellora, describing the latter as "one of the wonders of the work of the true transcendent Artisan (*az `aja'ibat-i sun`-i sani`-i haqiqi subhanahu*)," in other words, a creation of God.[15] The tourist visiting Ellora today is inevitably informed that half-ruined elephants, and so on, are due to Awrangzib's fanatical destruction of idols, but there is no historical evidence to indicate that the emperor engaged in any destruction there or why he would have stopped with so much left undone. J. B. Seely, a British soldier who spent several weeks on furlough at Ellora in 1810, recorded many reports from local informants on idol smashing and cow slaughter by Awrangzib at Ellora, but he viewed them with the same skepticism that he reserved for tales of Portuguese doing the same.[16] Catherine Asher has pointed out that the reports of Awrangzib's iconoclasm in the Deccan are typically from late sources that may reflect nothing more than legends that were hung on Awrangzib; his documented acts of temple destruction were almost all associated with putting down political rebellions.[17] Ironically, some of the examples of Awrangzib's temple destruction given by these late sources are failed attempts, frustrated by snakes, scorpions, or a deity. It seems that temple destruction is viewed as an essential characteristic of Awrangzib, regardless of whether he succeeded in actually carrying it out.[18]

---

[15] Inayatullah Khan Kashmiri, *Kalimat-i-Taiyibat* (Collection of Aurangzeb's Orders), ed. and trans. S. M. Azizuddin Husain (Delhi: Idarah-i Adabiyat-i Delli, 1982), 27 (English), 13 (Persian).

[16] Seely, *The Wonders of Ellora*, 150, 165, 202, 245, 345.

[17] Catherine B. Asher, *The New Cambridge History of India*, 1:4, *Architecture of Mughal India* (Cambridge: Cambridge University Press, 1992), 254. As an example of later sources on Awrangzib's temple destruction, she notes Jadunath Sarkar, *History of Aurangzib* (Bombay: Orient Longman, 1972), 3:185 (not 285), who cites a Marathi source dated Saka 1838 (1916 C.E.).

[18] Seely's brahmin informants told him "that if Aurungzebe actually did not commit the atrocious act himself, he allowed his court" (241).

The reaction of Shirazi to the destruction of Vijayanagar's temples can be compared to that of certain Muslim writers in Egypt in the thirteenth century, who were enthusiastic admirers of the great pyramids at Giza. As Ulrich Haarmann put it, they were "deeply disturbed by the brutal demolition of intact pharaonic remains and the mutilation of pagan pictorial representations in the name of Islam, yet in reality all too often out of a very mundane greed for cheap and at the same time high-quality building materials."[19] Similarly, one may quote the physician 'Abd al-Latif, who in 1207 made the following remarks about Egyptian temples:

> It is useless to halt to describe their greatness, the excellence of their construction and the just proportion of their forms, this innumerable multitude of figures, of sculptures both recessed and in relief, and of inscriptions that they offer to the admiration of spectators, all joined to the solidity of their construction and the enormous size of the stones and materials in use.[20]

The literature of Muslim travelers in fact contains much of this kind of admiration for ancient "pagan" monuments.

The non-Islamic origin of these temples does not seem to have been a particularly big stumbling block to Muslim tourists. Some, like Shirazi, simply found religion irrelevant to their appreciation. Others were able to assimilate the non-Islamic religious traditions to acceptable categories. A number of Muslim authors interpreted the religion of the ancient Egyptians as forming part of the Sabian religion, an obscure Quranic term which permitted groups such as the Hellenistic pagans of Harran to function as "people of the book" for centuries.[21] Popular Coptic mythology combined with Hermetic lore permitted Muslims to identify the great pyramids as the tombs of Agathodaimon (Seth), Hermes (Idris), and Sab, founder of the Sabeans, or else as the constructions of the Arab ancestor Shaddad ibn 'Ad.[22]

---

[19] Haarmann, "Quest," 65. See also Haarmann, ed., *Das Pyramidenbuch des Abu Ga `far al-Idrisi (st. 649/1251)*, Beiruter Texte und Studien, 38 (Stuttgart: Franz Steiner, 1991).

[20] 'Abd al-Latif, *Relation de l'Égypte par Abd-allatiph*, trans. Silvestre de Sacy (Paris, 1810), 182, quoted in Gaston Wiet, *L'Égypte de Murtadi fils de Gaphiphe* (Paris: Librairie Orientaliste Paul Geuthner, 1953), introduction, 98.

[21] Wiet, *L'Égypte de Murtadi fils de Gaphiphe*, 60.

[22] Ibid., 2, 87–88. Further on the Arabic Hermetic histories of pre-Islamic Egypt, see Michael Cook, "Pharaonic History in Medieval Egypt," *Studia Islamica* 57 (1983): 67–104.

Further examples can be added to the dossier of Muslim tourists who wrote appreciatively of Indian temples. The Timurid ambassador `Abd al-Razzaq Samarqandi, who visited Vijayanagar at the order of Shah Rukh in 1442, reported with delight on the functioning temples he visited en route near Mangalore and Belur. He compared these temples to the paradisical garden of Iram mentioned in the Qur'an and remarked that they were covered from top to bottom "with paintings, after the manner of the Franks and the people of Khata [Cathay]."[23] Another instance is the Afghan traveler Mahmud ibn Amir Wali Balkhi, who wrote a Persian narrative of a journey from Balkh to India and Ceylon and back, completed after seven years' travel in 1631. He traveled for pleasure only, and on his return to Balkh, he was appointed to a librarian's position. He has described at length, though with some disparagement, the rituals performed at the Krishna temple constructed by Raja Man Singh near Mathura. More entertainingly, he has related his own participation in the festival at the Jagannath temple in the city of Puri, where, by his own admission, he doffed his clothes and joined the throng of pilgrims, thus participating in the dramatic rituals first hand.[24] There are undoubtedly other similar accounts.

Shirazi's aesthetic delight in Ellora places his reaction in a category separate from the moralizing reactions to vanished earthly glory, the theme of *ubi sunt qui ante nos in mundo fuere*. Shirazi would have been familiar with the great Persian poem of Khaqani (d. 1199) on the ruins of the ancient Persian palace at Ctesiphon, the famous *Tuhfat al-`iraqayn*. Unlike Khaqani and the Egyptian al-Idrisi, Shirazi does not draw an admonition (*`ibrat*) from the fall of kingly power.[25] In his view, the destruction of the temples of Vijayanagar is a cause for meditation not on the vanity of human wishes but rather on the tragedy of the loss of beauty. Shirazi's perspective contrasts with that of figures

---

[23] R. H. Major, ed., *India in the Fifteenth Century, Being a Collection of Narratives of Voyages to India...*, Works Issued by the Hakluyt Society 22 (London: Hakluyt Society, 1857), 20–21; cf. C. A. Storey, *Persian Literature: A Bio-bibliographical Survey*, 2 vols. (London: Luzac, 1927–71), 1:293–98.

[24] Mahmud ibn Amir Wali Balkhi, *Bahr al-asrar fi manaqib al-akhyar*, ed. Riazul Islam (Karachi: Institute of Central and West Asian Studies, 1980), 13–16, 32–38, of the Persian text. See Iqbal Husain, "Hindu Shrines and Practices as Described by a Central Asian Traveller in the First Half of the Seventeenth Century," in *Medieval India I: Researches in the History of India, 1200–1750*, ed. Irfan Habib (Delhi: Oxford University Press, 1992).

[25] Haarmann, "Quest," 58.

such as the Naqshbandi Sufi leader Ahmad Sirhindi, whose anti-Indian attitude led him to regard the ruins scattered over India as evidence of divine punishment for failure to pay heed to divinely inspired messengers.[26] Later, Muslim tourists at Ellora would combine moralizing reflection on the decline of ancient pagans with enjoyment of the beautiful natural and artistic setting. Here is how this kind of reflection is presented in the *Ma'athir-i `Alamgiri*, a history of Awrangzib's reign, completed in 1711:

> A short distance from here [i.e., Khuldabad] is a place named Ellora where in ages long past, sappers possessed of magical skill excavated in the defiles of the mountain spacious houses for a length of one *kos*. On all their ceilings and walls many kinds of images with lifelike forms have been carved. The top of the hill looks level, so much so that no sign of the buildings within it is apparent [from outside]. In ancient times when the sinful infidels had dominion over this country, certainly they and not demons (*jinn*) were the builders of these caves, although tradition differs on the point; it was a place of worship of the tribe of false believers. At present it is a desolation in spite of its strong foundations; it rouses the sense of warning [of doom] to those who contemplate the future [end of things]. In all seasons, and particularly in the monsoons, when this hill and the plain below resemble a garden in the luxuriance of its vegetation and the abundance of its water, people come to see the place. A waterfall a hundred yards in width tumbles down from the hill. It is a marvelous place for strolling, charming to the eye. Unless one sees it, no written description can correctly picture it. How then can my pen adorn the page of my narrative?[27]

In this passage the moralizing tone is almost a perfunctory note, inserted well in what is, for the most part, an enthusiastic report.

---

[26] Yohanan Friedmann, *Shaykh Ahmad Sirhindi: An Outline of His Thought and a Study of His Image in the Eyes of Posterity*, McGill Islamic Studies 2 (Montreal: McGill-Queen's University Press, 1971), 71.

[27] Saqi Must`ad [sicl Khan, *Ma`asir-i-`Alamgiri: A History of the Emperor Aurangzib-`Alamgir (reign 1658–1707 A.D.)*, trans. Jadu-nath Sarkar, Bibliotheca Indica 269 (Calcutta: Royal Asiatic Society of Bengal, 1947), 145 (passage dated 1094/1683); this translation is superior to that in H. M. Elliot, *The History of India as Told by Its Own Historians*, ed. John Dowson, 8 vols. (1867–77; repr., Allahabad: Kitab Mahal, n.d.), 7:189–90.

To modern Muslim scholars, Ellora provides a very different sort of lesson. Now equipped with the religious analysis that separates Hinduism, Jainism, and Buddhism, the contemporary Iranian Indologist Jalali Na'ini cites Ellora as one of a series of Indian monuments that form an outstanding ancient example of that modern religious virtue, religious tolerance.

> Apparently, prior to the edict [of Ashoka] in the Indian subcontinent, as early as the Vedic age, there was a kind of tolerance and patience between followers of various religions in terms of differing beliefs. Support for this assumption includes the hymns of the Veda and the caves of Ajanta and Ellora. In these caves the temples of three religions—Hindu, Jain, and Buddhist—are located in the bosom, the very heart of the mountains and hills of the Vindhya mountain range, about 60 miles from Aurangabad, and they can be taken as a clear sign of religious freedom and the search for peace and tranquility among the followers of the three indigenous religions of India.[28]

The vocabulary and conceptual apparatus of this remark derive from the European enlightenment rather than from medieval Islamicate culture. Nonetheless, one might characterize it as yet another Muslim reaction to Ellora, which puts the cave temples into a historical sequence constructed in terms of the relations between religions. It is also interesting to consider the estimate of Ellora by the former head of the archeological service of Hyderabad state, the well-known Muslim scholar Ghulam Yazdani:

> At Ellora the religious fervor of the followers of the Brahmanical faith has carved out in the living rock temples which might well have been considered to be the work of gods not only by the votaries of that religion but also by the most discerning critic of the period, because they are unique specimens of this kind of architecture in the world.[29]

---

[28] Muhammad Dara Shikuh, *Majma` al-bahrayn*, ed. Muhammad Rida Jalali Na'ini (Tehran: Nashr-i Nuqra, 1366/1987–88), introduction, v-vi.

[29] Ghulam Yazdani, "Fine Arts: Architecture," in *The Early History of the Deccan*, ed. Ghulam Yazdani, 2 vols. (London: Oxford University Press, 1960), 2:731.

The British, in contrast, tended to be reassured by looking at these monuments, since they saw no one in India capable of building such grandeur who thus might prove an obstacle to their plans.[30] As Seely put it, "Surely these wonderful workmen must have been of a different race to the present degenerate Hindoos, or the country and government must have been widely different from what it is at the present day."[31] We would doubtless ascribe this reaction to the colonial mentality rather than to any internal imperative derived from Christianity.

Today every Indian schoolchild is taught the names of the ancient and medieval kings of India. Harsha and Candragupta Maurya are at least as well-known as Alexander and Caesar are to western history texts. It is often forgotten that, before the nineteenth century and the prodigious antiquarian efforts of early orientalists and the Archeological Survey, these names had vanished from living memory. The rise and fall of multiple dynasties had erased the meaning of many monuments that dot the Indian landscape. Oral narratives were bound to replace lost traditions with plausible tales about the mighty men of old capable of building such wonders. We do not know what stories were told to Bijapur officials by local dwellers in the vicinity of Daulatabad about the impressive temples of Ellora, but they may well have been connected to images of the Daulatabad fort, which has notable stylistic similarities with the construction of Ellora.[32] Shirazi's political interpretation of the monument does not seem strange when compared with the explanations that were offered to Seely by his guides in 1810. Large guardian figures were still being identified with Persian terms from Indo-Muslim court life, such as *chubdar* (mace-bearer) and *pahlavan* (wrestler).[33]

It is hard to recall that, before the age of modern tourism, travelers were not likely to see evidence of what we would call a foreign culture. The first European explorers of Asia and the New World went

---

[30] Seely, *The Wonders of Ellora*, 230, quoting Lieutenant Colonel Fitzcarence.

[31] Ibid., 258.

[32] Seely (145–47) was informed that the Ellora caves were excavated by the Pandavas prior to the main action of the Mahabharata.

[33] Ibid., 139, 299. Seely also records that "two colossal figures resting on large maces" were called *dewriesdars* (172), apparently from the Hindi term *deorhi* (door) plus the Persian suffix *-dar* (holder); cf. Sarkar in *Maasir-i- `Alamgiri*, 325. Modern scholars unselfconsciously go back to the classical Sanskrit term *dwarapala* to describe the massive doorkeepers at Ellora (Surendranath Sen, ed., *Indian Travels of Thevenot and Careri*, Indian Records Series [New Delhi: National Archives of India, 1949], 320 n. 6).

equipped with fantasies like *The Travels of Sir John Mandeville*, and they saw the cannibals, Amazons, and giants that they were prepared to see. Early European engravings of Indian idols have more than a passing resemblance to Roman deities. When the Portuguese explorer Vasco da Gama and his crew arrived in India in 1498, so great was their relief in seeing buildings that were evidently not "Moorish" mosques that they accepted the Hindu temples of Calicut as Christian churches, kneeling in prayer before goddesses that they described as images of the Virgin Mary and the saints (they were evidently unconcerned by the unusually large teeth and extra arms of these images).[34] Seely notes that the first Indian soldiers sent to Egypt in British military expeditions to combat Napoleon announced in amazement that the ancient Egyptians clearly worshiped Hindu gods in their temples; this was probably the first Indian hermeneutic of pharaonic antiquities.[35] In a sense, the response of the sepoys was a repetition of the reactions of early visitors from Herodotus onwards, who described the gods of Egypt in terms of their own theologies. When Shirazi saw Ellora as analogous to Persepolis, he was only making a natural comparison from his own experience of ancient monuments. Seely did much the same when he described what he saw as Sphinxes at Ellora.[36]

Muslims were not the only ones to reinvent Ellora's significance along new lines. When the Rashtrakutas conquered the Chalukyas and took over power in the Deccan in the seventh century, in addition to adding new Hindu monuments such as the Kailas temple, they converted Buddhist viharas into Hindu temples, chiseling out many Buddha images at Ellora and covering or replacing some with images of Vishnu.[37] Architectural guidebooks unfortunately do not indicate what essential characteristic of Hinduism caused this extreme form of renovation. The Yadavas of Deogir were not a direct extension of the Rashtrakutas, and they must have formed their own interpretations of the meaning of Ellora, a monument near the center of their empire. While we can only speculate about the way the Yadavas positioned themselves in relation to Ellora, their interpretation

---

[34] K. G. Jayne, *Vasco do Gama and His Successors, 1460–1580* (London: Methuen, 1910), 55.

[35] Seely, *The Wonders of Ellora*, 156–67. It was particularly representations of the bull (i.e., Nandi) and of serpents that aroused recognition among the "Bombay Siphauees."

[36] Ibid., 156–58.

[37] Yazdani, *The Early History of the Deccan*, 2:731.

must have reflected their own self-interpretation as a successor-state to the Rashtrakutas. The founder of the Mahanabhuva sect, Cakradara, is said to have briefly established a new form of worship in Ellora that was completely unrelated to the Shaiva, Buddhist, and Jain traditions of earlier eras.[38] Ellora evidently took on a new significance among the elites of the Marathas, starting from the sixteenth century. As James Laine points out, Maloji, grandfather of the Maratha warrior Shivaji, is buried in an Islamicate tomb in the village of Ellora.[39] In the eighteenth century, Ellora evidently received further patronage from the ruling Maratha family of the Holkars, who must have interpreted the monuments in terms of their own political and religious position.[40]

European travelers such as Anquetil du Perron in 1760 and Seely in 1810 were informed by local brahmins that Buddha images in some of the caves actually represented Vishvakarma (a form of Vishnu), and Seely was given conflicting opinions about the meaning of Jain figures in a cave that the guides regarded as dedicated to Jagannath (another form of Vishnu).[41] These Hindu names for Buddhist and Jain temples are still used in current guidebooks. Anquetil was also told that a number of Ellora temples were the various tombs of Vishnu; his Brahmin informants said that other cave temples near Bombay had been built by Alexander.[42] Goddess figures at Ellora were always identified for Seely as Bhavani, following her ascendancy in modern Maratha culture. Seely occasionally caught his guides changing their identifications of images, but this he attributed to the confusion inherent in Hindu mythology rather than to any other cause.[43] Colonel Meadows Taylor, author of *Confessions of a Thug*, claimed that a Thug told him that the Ellora caves contained

---

[38] T. V. Pathy, *Elura: Art and Culture* (New Delhi: Humanities Press, 1980), 4.

[39] James Laine, "The Construction of Hindu and Muslim Identities in Maharashtra, 1600–1810," (paper presented at conference on "Indo-Muslim Identity in South Asia," Duke University, May 1995).

[40] Seely, *The Wonders of Ellora*, 152.

[41] Anquetil du Perron, *Le Zendavesta*, 3 vols. (Paris, 1771), l:ccxxxiii, cited in Jean-Luc Kieffer, *Anquetil-Duperron: L'Inde en France au XVIIIᵉ siècle* (Paris: Société d'Édition "Les Belles Lettres," 1983), 347–63 (Duperron's map of the caves, with identifications proposed by his informants, is in Bibliotheque Nationale, Nouvelles acquisitions françaises, Fonds Anquetil-Duperron, 8878); Seely, *The Wonders of Ellora*, 205ff, 238–39.

[42] Partha Mitter, *Much Maligned Monsters: History of European Reactions to Indian Art* (Oxford: Clarendon Press, 1977), 107–8.

[43] Seely, *The Wonders of Ellora*, 286.

depictions of all the methods of murder employed by the Thugs.[44] All this goes to say that Ellora, like any ancient monument, has not had a single fixed meaning over time. The precincts were constructed over centuries, with multiple religious patterns that we today distinguish by the categories of Hindu, Buddhist, and Jain. Different generations of patrons contributed their own interpretations with their commissions and constructions. Just as the monuments themselves are subject to physical modification by later visitors and patrons, so their meaning has been adjusted to the symbolic parameters of new civilizational orders.

As far as the question of Muslim iconoclasm is concerned, the evidence of Muslim travelers who visited Hindu temples does not provide justification for assuming that idol-smashing activity is easily detectable, much less the visceral instinct that it is often assumed to be. The examples cited above are not random or selective but constitute the results of a fairly extensive search for textual reactions by Muslims to Hindu temples. Why should we assume that Muslims are by nature and training iconoclastic, and when they do violence to idols or temples, why do we assume that this behavior is rooted in Islamic faith? Take the example of Babur, in an incident that took place near Gwalior in 1528. On that occasion, he recorded a bout of severe opium sickness with much vomiting. The next day, he saw some Jain statues, which he described as follows:

On the southern side is a large idol, approximately 20 yards tall. They are shown stark naked with all their private parts exposed. Around the two large reservoirs inside Urwahi have been dug twenty to twenty-five wells, from which water is drawn to irrigate the vegetation, flowers, and trees planted there. Urwahi is not a bad place. In fact, it is rather nice. Its one drawback was the idols, so I ordered them destroyed.

The following day, he visited Gwalior fort.

Riding out from this garden we made a tour of Gwalior's temples, some of which are two and three stories but are squat and in the ancient style with dadoes entirely of figures sculpted in stone. Other temples are like

---

[44] L. F. Rushbrook Williams, *A Handbook for Travellers in India, Pakistan, Bangladesh, and Sri Lanka (Ceylon)*, 22nd ed. (New York: Facts on File, 1975), 149 n. 1.

madrasas, with porches and large, tall domes and chambers like those of a madrasa. Atop the lower chambers are stone-carved idols. Having examined the edifices, we went out[45]

At that point he enjoyed an outdoor feast.

What part of Babur's behavior during these three days was Islamic? On day one, he was hung over from drug intoxication; on day two, he destroyed two naked Jain idols; and on day three, he enjoyed a pleasant excursion to Hindu temples with the governor of Gwalior fort and left the idols there intact. Why did he destroy idols on one day and enjoy them the next? His good mood on the third day may have had something to do with either his recovery from the hangover or the embassy of submission he received that morning from a major Rajput ruler. Alternatively, he may have considered it ill-mannered to destroy part of a monument he was being shown in a fort that one of his subordinates was in charge of. In any case, it is clear that it is highly problematic to predict political behavior (such as destruction of temples) from the nominal religious identity that may be ascribed to an individual or group without reference to personal, political, and historical factors.

Above all, it is noteworthy that the occasions when Muslim writers have invoked God and religion in relation to Hindu monuments have been when they have been awed by the creation of beauty. While Rafi' al-Din Shirazi, in a sense, reduced the significance of Ellora to the familiar terms of imperial monuments, he was also stirred to protest on religious grounds against the iconoclasm of his imperial patron. It does not seem accidental that at the moment of praising the extraordinary, even in what seems the stereotyped convention of the wonders of the world, the emotion of reverence should take control. It would be a shame if contemporary ideological conflicts blinded us to the perception of the profound admiration that Indian monuments like Ellora have evoked in Muslim visitors. More to the point, accounts like Shirazi's indicate that Muslims

---

[45] *The Baburnama: Memoirs of Babur, Prince and Emperor*, trans. Wheeler M. Thackston (Washington, D.C.: Freer Gallery of Art/Arthur M. Sackler Gallery, 1996),406–7; cf. Zahiru'd-Din Muhammad Babur Padshah Ghazi, *Babur-nama (Memoirs of Babur)*, trans. Annette Susannah Beveridge (1922; New Delhi: Oriental Books Reprint Corporation, 1979), 608–13. Beveridge notes that Babur's destruction amounted to cutting off the heads of the idols, which were restored with plaster by Jains in the locality.

had complex reactions to non-Muslim religious sites. Their responses could be dictated by a variety of factors, including their education and temperament, the political situation, and whether the building fell into the category of ancient wonder or living temple (Muslims seem to have enjoyed both). The popular one-dimensional portrait of Muslim iconoclasm survives as a durable stereotype because it does not acknowledge its subjects as actors in historical contexts. The iconoclasm stereotype derives not from the actual attitudes of Muslims toward temples but from a predetermined normative definition of Islam. The reasons for the appeal of such religious stereotypes, ironically, will need to be sought elsewhere.

10

The Islamization of Yoga in the *Amrtakunda* Translations*

ORIENTALIST VIEWS OF YOGA AND SUFISM

From the beginning of Orientalist studies of the Muslim world, it was axiomatic to define certain religious phenomena in terms of their origins. Because of the tendency to view all Eastern doctrines as essentially alike, Orientalist scholars of the Romantic period invariably defined Sufism as a mysticism that was Indian in origin; from the first appearance of the term in European languages, "Sufism" was characterized as essentially different from the dry Semitic religion of Islam.[1] Looking back at this early scholarship today, it is surprising that this unanimous belief in the Indian origin of Sufism was almost entirely unconnected to any historical evidence. From the days of Sir William Jones and Sir John Malcolm to relatively recent times, this opinion has had a remarkable longevity, despite the ludicrous appearance of some of these claims today. As an example one may consider the outrageous

* This article is part of my forthcoming study, *The Pool of Nectar: Muslim Interpreters of Yoga*. It is based on part of the monographic introduction to my translation of the Arabic text. An earlier version of this essay was presented at the Tantra-Muslim Esotericism-Kabbalah Conference, New York University, 5–6 April, 1998.
[1] See my *Shambhala Guide to Sufism* (Boston: Shambhala, 1997), chapter 1, for a discussion of the early Orientalist linkage of Sufism with India. Similar observations are made by Victor Pallejà de Bustinza, "Le Soufisme: les débuts de son étude en Occident," in *Horizons Maghrébins* 30: *La Walaya, Étude sur le Soufisme de l'école d'Ibn `Arabî, Hommage à Michel Chodkiewicz* (Winter, 1995): 97–107. Thanks to Zamyat Kirby for drawing the latter reference to my attention.

claim of Max Horten in a 1928 study that sought to explain Sufism as a pure expression of Vedanta: "No doubt can any longer remain that the teaching of Hallaj (d. 922) and his circle [in Baghdad] is identical with that of Samkara around 820."[2] Another pertinent example is found in an observation of William James in his 1902 Gifford Lectures, published as *The Varieties of Religious Experience*:

> In the Mohammedan world the Sufi sect and various dervish bodies are the possessors of the mystical tradition. The Sufis have existed in Persia from the earliest times, and as their pantheism is so at variance with the hot and rigid monotheism of the Arab mind, it has been suggested that Sufism must have been inoculated into Islam by Hindu influences.[3]

James' remark illustrates, innocently enough, how widely this opinion was shared at the time by the academic world in Europe and America. It is easier to see from the perspective of the later twentieth century that this opinion was conditioned by nineteenth-century racial attitudes as well as assumptions about the unchanging nature of religions.

Most specialists in Islamic studies today would find the explanation of Sufi mysticism cited by James to be quaint or objectionable, since the preponderance of evidence permits us to understand the Sufi tradition perfectly well without the slightest reference to the literary and religious traditions of India. There is really no reason to maintain, as did Eduard Sachau in 1888, that "in the Arabian Sufism the Indian Vedânta reappears."[4] The question then arises, if there is no intrinsic reference to India or Hindu texts in Sufism, what led scholars to seek such an external explanation?

Theories of cultural diffusion from a single source (like Pan-Babylonianism) had a certain logical appeal, doubtless because of their simplicity. This kind of reductionism inevitably attracted criticism. Louis Massignon's classic study of the vocabulary of Sufism contained a major section devoted to "The Role of Foreign Influences," which he rejected

---

[2] M[ax] Horten, *Indische Strömungen in der islamischen Mystik*, 2 vols., Materialien zur Kunde des Buddhismus 12–13 (Heidelberg: O. Harrassowitz, 1927–28), 2:iii.

[3] William James, *The Varieties of Religious Experience: A Study in Human Nature* (New York: New American Library, 1958), Lectures XVI–XVII, pp. 308–9.

[4] Edward C. Sachau, trans., *Alberuni's India*, 2 vols. (1888; repr., Delhi: S. Chand & Co., 1964), 1:xxxiii; cf. 1:xliii, where Sachau speaks of "the essential identity of the systems of the Greek Neo-Pythagoreans, the Hindu Vedânta philosophers, and the Sûfis of the Muslim world."

on the whole.[5] In a critical review of theories of Indian "influence" on Islamic mysticism, Moreno rightly characterized approaches like Horten's as "Indophile or Indomaniac zeal."[6] In a similar vein, Dermenghem maintained that

> The surprising thing would be if we did not find in Moslem countries something analogous to Hindu Yoga, since here are two traditions claiming the authenticity of primordial tradition. Nor is it any more surprising that, severally, these methods present a whole gamut ranging from pure intellectual contemplation to orgies of rhythm and sound. Modern Europe is almost alone in having renounced, out of bourgeois respectability and Gallican purism, the participation of body in the pursuits of the spirit. In India as in Islam, music, poetry, and the dance are spiritual exercises.[7]

He went on to observe, "This does not mean that Hindu Yoga is at the source of Moslem Sufism."[8] Thus, it has been possible for scholars such as Gardet and Eliade to entertain a comparative study of mysticism that was not historically reductive but phenomenological (and occasionally theological) in approach.[9]

But part of the genetic view of Asian religions was the habit of viewing non-Christian cultures primarily in terms of their difference from European Christianity. This was particularly prominent in the intellectual

---

[5] Louis Massignon, *Essai sur les origines du lexique technique de la mystique musulmane*, new ed. (Paris: J. Vrin, 1968), pp. 63–98, where the case of India is discussed on pp. 81–98.

[6] Martino Mario Moreno, "Mistica musulmana e mistica indiana," *Annali Lateranensi* 10 (1949): 103–219, esp. p. 198 and p. 210, where the case against influence is summarized.

[7] Emile Dermenghem, "Yoga and Sufism: Ecstasy Techniques in Islam," in *Forms and Techniques of Altruistic and Spiritual Growth*, ed. Pitirim A. Sorokin (Boston: Beacon Press, 1954), pp. 109–16, quoting p. 109.

[8] Ibid.

[9] L. Gardet, "Dhikr," EI², 2:223–27; *id.*, "Un Problème de mystique comparée: la mention du nom divin (*dhikr*) dans la mystique musulmane," *Revue Thomiste* 52 (1952): 642–79; 53 (1953): 197–216; G.-C. Anawati and Louis Gardet, *Mystique musulmane, Aspects et tendances—Expériences et techniques*, 4th ed., Études Musulmanes 8 (Paris: J. Vrin, 1986), esp. pp. 90–94, 244–45; Mircea Eliade, *Yoga, Immortality and Freedom*, trans. Willard R. Trask, 2nd ed., Bollingen Series 56 (Princeton, NJ: Princeton University Press, 1969), pp. 216–19, 408. In the end, though, Eliade could not resist the temptation of influences, which he states "were definitely exerted after the twelfth century" (p. 217). Likewise, Gardet succumbed to asserting "Indo-Iranian influence among the Mawlawiyya ('Whirling Dervishes') of Konya, and Indian through Turko-Mongol influence" for which he cites Simnani ("Dhikr," p. 224a).

climate of nineteenth-century colonialism. Theories of evolution and race were freely applied in the comparative study of religion, originally understood as a disingenuous comparison intended to reveal which religion was superior.[10] The study of religion in Christian theological faculties initially exempted Christianity from this kind of historical investigation since Christianity (in whatever form the theorist professed) was assumed to be still pure and integral, despite such arguably revolutionary events as the Protestant Reformation. If, however, other religions could be shown to be hybrids composed of various "Oriental" influences, that was a testimony to their dependent and inferior nature. In Zaehner's words, "Muslim mysticism is entirely derivative."[11] Regardless of the later progress of historical research into the relation of Christianity to the cultural and religious world into which it was born, the colonial legacy of condescension toward "Oriental religions" still lingers.

This is not to say that Sufis, particularly in India, were unaware of the ascetic and meditative practices of yogis.[12] But it is almost impossible to find any Indian textual sources on yoga that were widely known in the Muslim world. Nevertheless, in observing that the thesis of the Indian origins of Sufism was almost entirely unconnected to any historical evidence, it is important to note the single piece of evidence that forms the exception to this rule. It was Alfred von Kremer, in a wide-ranging 1873 study of Islamic civilization, who first drew attention to a short passage in a fourteenth-century Persian encyclopedia (the *Nafa'is al-funun* of Amuli) that described yogic techniques of breath control on the basis of an obviously Indian text. From this observation, which he linked with breathing practices found in Central Asian Sufi groups, von Kremer leapt to the familiar Orientalist conclusion: "We are, indeed, constrained to ascribe to Indian influences the rise of that Muslim mysticism which appears so much later and bears such a close external and

---

[10] Eric J. Sharpe ("Comparative Religion," *Encyclopedia of Religion*, 3:578–80) links the term "influence" to evolutionistic schemes that rank religions, and he optimistically considers the term to be now "seldom used."

[11] R. C. Zaehner, *Mysticism, Sacred and Profane: An Inquiry into Some Varieties of Praeternatural Experience* (London: Oxford University Press, 1961), p. 160.

[12] A survey of contacts between Sufis and yogis is provided in chapter two of *The Pool of Nectar*. See also my article "Chishti Meditation Techniques in the Later Mughal Period," in *The Heritage of Sufism*, vol. 3, *Late Classical Persianate Sufism (1501–1750): The Safavid and Mughal Period* (Oxford: Oneworld 1999), pp. 344–57.

internal resemblance to the teachings of the Vedanta school."[13] What von Kremer neglected to point out, in his enthusiasm, was that the passage on breath control occurred in the section on natural and occult sciences; the author of this encyclopedia had separately categorized Sufism as one of the Islamic sciences along with literature, law, theology, and history.[14] The connection between Indian breath control and Sufi practice was not recognized by Muslim authors, who classified the two items under different categories (this question of categorization will be raised again below). The European Orientalist assumed a genetic relationship between the two on the basis of modern prejudices extrinsic to the text. But the important thing was that von Kremer noticed a distinctively yogic text being circulated in learned Islamicate circles. This can now be identified as a version of *The Fifty Verses of Kamarupa*, which is described below.

Again, as von Kremer shows, the automatic assumption of the purely Indian origin of Sufism was axiomatic in Orientalist scholarship. In a similar case, Hartmann in 1915 noticed a report in a late Arabic text stating that one of the early founders of the Naqshbandi order in Central Asia, `Abd al-Khaliq Ghijduwani (d. 1220), was inspired by the immortal prophet Khidr to introduce the practice of breath control into Sufism. Hartmann could not resist speculating that this report concealed an Indian origin for this practice. The claim of inspiration masked the more prosaic point that Ghijduwani's native city of Bukhara was "the point of communication with Buddhist and Brahmanic Asia" and that, at this formative period in the development of the Sufi orders, they necessarily passed on the influences of their Indian environment to the rest of the Islamic world.[15] One must simply pass over with astonishment the European

---

[13] Alfred von Kremer, *Culturgeschichtliche Streifzüge auf dem Gebiete des Islams* (Leipzig: F.A. Brockhaus 1873); English trans., S. Khuda Bakhsh, *Contributions to the History of Islamic Civilization* (1904; repr., Lahore: Accurate printers, 1976), p. 119.

[14] The section on breath occurs in Shams al-Din Muhammad ibn Mahmud Amuli, *Nafa'is al-funun fi `ara'is al-`uyun*, ed. Mirza Abu al-Hasan Sha`rani (Tehran: Kitabfurusi-i Islamiya, 1379/1960), 2:360–65. The separate description on Sufism (2:2–42) leans heavily on its Islamic credentials, beginning (2:4) with emphasis on the condition of "not deviating from the rule of Islam and the path of the *shari`at*." On Amuli, see C.A. Storey, *Persian Literature: A Bio-bibliographical Survey*, vol. ii, part 3 (London: Royal Asiatic Society, 1977), pp. 355–57.

[15] Cf. Moreno, "Mistica musulmana," p. 143, citing R. Hartmann, "Zur Frage nach der Herkunft und den Anfangen des sûfitums," *Der Islam* (1915): 31–70.

parochialism that places Bukhara in the same neighborhood as India (it is roughly 1000 miles from Lahore and 2000 miles from Bengal). Here too, the argument for influence was ultimately meant to demonstrate which system is original and authentic and which is derivative. Such a tendentious motivation is also apparent in a late nineteenth-century Russian Orthodox text, which treats both yogis and Sufis as having borrowed (and bungled) the meditative techniques of the church fathers as outlined in the *Philokalia*: "It was from them [the Greek Orthodox saints] that the monks of India and Bokhara took over the 'heart method' of interior prayer, only they quite spoiled and garbled it in doing so."[16]

From the point of view of the study of religion, it is disappointing enough to see lack of historical rigor that too often accompanied Orientalist speculations about the Indian origins of Sufism. Even more problematic was the pervasive positivism and condescending Eurocentrism that increasingly replaced Romantic enthusiasm as the colonialist mentality intensified in the later nineteenth century. Von Kremer concluded his review of Islamic civilization with a heavy indictment of the errors of the Oriental:

> The more the Muslim is constrained to learn to adapt himself to the needs of the age and indeed learn them from the Europeans, whose powerful superiority he no longer fails to recognize, the more will he be induced to take the right and proper course, that of a practical life from which he has been estranged by superstitious, mystic visions and theological speculations.[17]

Here, I would like to take a different point of view, one that takes seriously the views of those who are engaged with the religious questions under discussion. If there was a text on yogic practice that was transmitted and studied in Muslim countries, how was it in fact understood? The remarks that follow are based on the study of the highly complex history of a text known by the Sanskrit title *Amrtakunda* or *The Pool of Nectar*, which survives in Arabic, Persian, Turkish, and Urdu translations in multiple recensions (see Chart 10.1). Evidence has recently come to light of a Judaeo-Arabic version produced in Yemen. This textual history indicates

---

[16] *The Way of a Pilgrim, and The Pilgrim Continues his Way*, trans. R M French (San Francisco: HarperSanFrancisco, 1991), p. 71.
[17] Von Kremer, *Contributions to the History of Islamic Civilization*, p. 123.

that the readers of this text engaged it in a process of Islamization, involving scriptural Islamic themes, philosophical vocabulary, and the terminology and concepts of Sufism. What remained was a very narrow window onto the world of Indian religions, and one that to many readers was hardly distinguishable from the standard occult and mystical practices found in Islamicate society. In short, the history of the single textual source for yogic practice in the Muslim world tells us a great deal more about its Muslim readers than it does about yoga.

THE TEXTUAL TRANSMISSION OF *THE POOL OF NECTAR*

The *Amrtakunda* or *The Pool of Nectar* (which we have come across earlier in Chapter 8 of the present volume) was the name of a Sanskrit or Hindi work, the original text of which is now lost. *The Pool of Nectar* was also connected to a work known as *Kamarupancasika* or *The Fifty Verses of Kamarupa*, which circulated in an independent Persian translation that seems to represent the earliest stage of transmission of this text by Muslim authors (see below).[18] *The Pool of Nectar* was ostensibly translated into Persian, and then Arabic, according to the introduction, in 1210 in Bengal, under the title *Hawd ma' al-hayat*, or *The Pool of the Water of Life*. The initial translation was accomplished by a Muslim scholar, Rukn al-Din al-Samarqandi, aided by a yogi who converted to Islam after losing a disputation. At an unspecified later date, the text was redacted in Arabic by an unknown author, with the aid of another yogi who converted to Islam.[19]

For reasons too complex to discuss here, and as mentioned in Chapter 8, I suggest that this account is fictitious. The earliest phase of the text (perhaps going back to the early thirteenth century) is probably represented by *The Kamarupa Seed Syllables*. This eclectic Persian text contained breath control practices relating to magic and divination, rites of the yogini temple cult associated with Kaula tantrism, and teachings of

---

[18] See Chapter 17 in this volume.

[19] The text was first edited from 5 MSS by Yusuf Husain, "*Haud al-hayat*, la version arabe de l'Amratkund," *Journal Asiatique* 213 (1928): 291–344. Unfortunately this edition contains numerous errors and omissions. My forthcoming translation is based on a superior text established by comparison of 25 MSS. I plan to publish my diplomatic edition of the Arabic text separately.

hatha yoga according to the tradition of the Nath yogis (popularly called *jogis*). All of this was placed in a context of the supremacy of the goddess Kamakhya, with frequent reference to her main temple in Assam (Kamarupa). This text was adapted by an anonymous Arabic translator, who was trained in the Illuminationist (Ishraqi) school of philosophy in Iran, probably in the fifteenth century. This anonymous Arabic translator completely rewrote the Persian text, incorporating into his introduction two symbolic narratives, one deriving ultimately from the "Hymn of the Pearl" from the Gnostic *Acts of Thomas* and the other being a partial translation from a Persian treatise, *On the Reality of Love*, originally written by the Illuminationist philosopher Shihab al-Din al-Suhrawardi al-Maqtul.[20] From the dissemination of the manuscript copies of the Arabic text, it is clear that *Hawd al-hayat* was fairly well known in the Islamic world; at least 45 copies are found in libraries in European and Arab countries, the majority being in Istanbul. None of the manuscripts is older than the late sixteenth century. The content of the text was so unusual that, almost by default, it has been frequently assigned to the authorship of the Andalusian Sufi master Muhyi al-Din Ibn al-`Arabi; this attribution is clearly erroneous, but it served to give the text a certain canonical authority, particularly in Ottoman lands.[21] The vocabulary of the text is mostly formed on the Arabic technical terminology of Hellenistic philosophy, with some Islamic overtones derived from the Qur'an and Sufism. The translator worked strenuously to render the yogic practices in a way that was understandable to a philosophically oriented reader of Arabic. The oldest recension of the Arabic version no longer exists, and the two existing later recensions show an increasing amount of Islamization of the text.

The Pool of the Water of Life stands out from other Arabic and Persian translations from the Sanskrit by emphasizing Indian spiritual practices rather than doctrines. Although al-Biruni (d. 1010) had translated Patañjali's *Yogasutra* into Arabic, he had focused on philosophical

---

[20] Typically, the only scholar to notice these Gnostic and Illuminationist elements in the *Amrtakunda* translation was Henry Corbin, in "Pour une morphologie de la spiritualité shî`ite," *Eranos-Jahrbuch 1960*, XXIX (Zürich: Rhein-Verlag 1961), esp. pp. 102–7, repeated with some variations in his *En Islam iranien, Aspects spirituels et philosophiques*, vol. 2, *Sohrawardî et les Platoniciens de Perse* (Paris: Gallimard, 1971), pp. 328–34.

[21] Osman Yahia, *Histoire et classification de l'œuvre d'Ibn `Arabi, étude critique*, 2 vols. (Damascus : Institut français de Damas, 1964), 1:287–88, no. 230.

questions and omitted the topic of mantra altogether, and his Indological works were not widely read.[22] Most of the Sanskrit texts translated into Persian during the Mughal period were likewise chosen either for political or philosophical interest and had little relevance to religious practice.[23] The Arabic text of *The Pool of the Water of Life* was known to various Muslim mystics of India, some of whom had watched with interest the breathing exercises and chants of the yogis, and noticed similarities with their own meditative practices.[24] A Chishti master, Shaykh `Abd al-Quddus Gangohi (d. 1537), who was familiar with the yoga of the Naths and wrote Hindi verses on the subject, taught *The Pool* to a disciple.[25] Shaykh Muhammad Ghawth Gwaliyari (d. 1563), an Indian Sufi master of the Shattari order, translated *The Pool* from the oldest Arabic version into Persian under the title *Bahr al-hayat* (*The Ocean of Life*).[26] Sufis from the Qadiri, Mevlevi, and Sanusi orders in Sind, Turkey, and North Africa continued to refer to *The Pool* well into the nineteenth century. The Arabic text was twice translated into Ottoman Turkish, and Muhammad Ghawth's Persian translation was itself rendered into Dakhani Urdu (see Chart 10.2). The Arabic version is still in use today; a Damascene Sufi shaykh who is an expert on the works of Ibn al-`Arabi regards it as a very important treatise.

---

[22] Hellmut Ritter, ed., "Al-Biruni's Übersetzung des Yoga-sutra des Patañjali," *Oriens* 9 (1956):165–200; Bruce B. Lawrence, "The Use of Hindu Religious Texts in al-Biruni's *India* with Special Reference to Patañjali's Yoga-Sutras," in *The Scholar and the Saint: Studies in Commemoration of Abu'l Rayhan al-Biruni and Jalal al-Din al-Rumi*, ed. Peter J. Chelkowski (New York: New York University Press, 1975), pp. 29–48, esp. p. 33. Both al-Biruni's translation of Patañjali and his description of India exist in unique manuscripts, indicating a limited circulation.

[23] See the analysis and description of Arabic and Persian translations from Indian languages in *The Pool of Nectar*.

[24] E.g., Nasir al-Din Mahmud Chiragh-i Dihli, *Khayr al-Majalis*, comp. Hamid Qalandar, ed. Khaliq Ahmad Nizami (Aligarh: Muslim University, Department of History, [1959]), p. 60; my translation is found in *Religions of India in Practice*, ed. Donald S. Lopez, Jr., Princeton Readings in Religions 1 (Princeton: Princeton University Press, 1995), p. 517.

[25] For bibliographic references see S. A. A. Rizvi, "Sufis and Nâtha Yogis in Mediaeval Northern India (XII to XVI Centuries)," p. 132, quoting Rukn al-Din's *Lata'if-i Quddusi* (Delhi: Matba`-i Mujtaba'i, 1311/ 1894), p. 41; id., *A History of Sufism in India*, vol. I, *Early Sufism and its History in India to 1600 A.D.* (Delhi: Munshiram Manoharlal Publishers Pvt. Ltd., 1978), p. 335. Gangohi's knowledge of yoga is fully discussed by Simon Digby in "`Abd Al-Quddus Gangohi (1456–1537 A.D.): The Personality and Attitudes of a Medieval Indian Sufi," *Medieval India, A Miscellany* 3 (1975): 1–66.

[26] See my "Sufism and Yoga according to Muhammad Ghawth," *Sufi* 29 (Spring 1996): 9–13, and Chapter 8 in this volume.

A document such as *The Pool of Nectar*, the only known Arabic translation of a work on hatha yoga, would seem to offer an ideal case study for determining how yoga was construed in relation to Islamic mysticism and what relation it had with Sufi practice. It is a concrete example of how a Muslim writer interpreted a characteristically Indian set of religious practices. A quick glance at the text is enough to indicate that it was definitely prepared for a Muslim readership; the text opens with an invocation of God and the Prophet Muhammad, and it is sprinkled with terms and phrases from the Islamic religious vocabulary. The translator has carefully attempted to describe practices that include Sanskrit chants or mantras, breathing techniques, postures for meditation, a version of kundalini meditation with depictions of the seven cakras or psychic centers, invocation of feminine deities, and other specific practices. My analysis of the relationship between Islamicate and Indic features of this text indicates, however, that generalities about Hinduism and Islam are relatively useless for shedding light on the significance of the text, nor does the text provide any insight into overarching questions of inter-religious exchange. Many different strands of meaning have been interwoven by the translator, who eclectically drew together practices of yoga and divination from different sources that cannot be identified with any particular surviving text on hatha yoga, providing in any case a very limited picture of hatha yoga practice.

Nevertheless, the different translations of *The Pool of Nectar* are unanimous in affirming that this is the most famous and respected scripture of India, despite the fact that no trace of it can be found today in any Indological literature. The anonymous Arabic translator concealed his identity behind a highly suspicious account of the circumstances surrounding the translation of the text, in which a leading role is played by yogis who convert to Islam and announce that their teachings are fundamentally identical with the Qur'an. The translation is prefaced with a narrative framework that adapted materials from Christian Gnosticism and Islamicate Neoplatonism, producing a complex interpretation of the religious significance and goal of yogic practice that avoids mentioning any of the principal categories of Indian metaphysics. In addition, the translator inserted into the text materials that clearly derive from standard Islamic sources. The different redactions of the Arabic text and the subsequent translations into Persian, Turkish, and Urdu contain further interpretive differences, which mostly transform Greco-Arabic philosophical concepts in the direction of Sufism. All these symbolic strategies tended to remove any sense of otherness from the yogic teachings for Muslim readers. *The Pool of Nectar* does not attempt to describe Hinduism as an autonomous religious system beyond the boundaries of Islam. In late interpretations of it, such as the description of Sufi orders by Muhammad al-Sanusi (d. 1859), yogis ended up being described as a subset of a Sufi order. In this respect, the Muslim understanding of yoga resembled the case of the enigmatic group called *Barahima* in Islamic heresiographies, whom some commentators have identified as Indian Brahmins. But a recent analysis has concluded that "there is not a single dogmatic item in the agenda of Barahima beliefs that evokes the beliefs of Hinduism. . . . the Barahima were a sect completely explicable in terms of the Islamic environment and its Judaeo-Christian heritage, and not Indians at all."[27] When translators and interpreters overuse the technique of familiarization, no trace of otherness remains, and readers see only what their training and education have prepared them to see. This over-familiarization seems to have happened with the Arabic version of *The Pool of Nectar*.

On a less sophisticated level, the Persian text of *The Fifty Verses of Kamarupa* also demonstrates an unselfconscious domestication of yogic practices in an Islamicate society. Among the breath prognostications, for instance, one learns that one should only approach "the *qadi* [Islamic judge] or the *amir* [Arabic term for ruler]" for judgment or litigation when the breath from the right nostril is favorable. Casual references mention Muslim magicians and practices that may be performed either in a Muslim or a Hindu graveyard (47b) or else in an empty temple or mosque (49b), and occasionally one is told to recite a Qur'anic passage such as the Throne Verse or to perform a certain action after evening prayer. We even hear of a Muslim from Broach who successfully summoned a yogini goddess and participated in the rites of her devotees (37a). The text is provided with an overall Islamic frame, through a standard invocation of God and praise of the Prophet at the beginning:

> Praise and adoration to that God who brought so many thousands of arts and wonders from the secrecy of non-existence into the courtyard of existence, and who adorned the sublime court with luminous bodies, who

---

[27] Norman Calder, "The Barahima: Literary Construct and Historical Reality," *BSOAS* 57 (1994): 41–50, quoting p. 46.

made the abodes of spiritual beings, and who commanded the manifestation of the sublunar world with varieties of plants and minerals, and who
made the residence and resort of animals, and who chose from all the animals humanity, creating it in the best of forms, giving the cry: "We have
created humanity in the finest of stations" (Qur. 95:4), "so bless God, the
finest of creators" (Qur. 23:14). Many blessings and countless salutations
on the pure and holy essence of the leader of the world [i.e., the Prophet
Muhammad], the best of the children of Adam, the blessings of God and
peace be upon him, and upon them all.

Likewise at the end, a quotation of a hadith saying of the Prophet and
some mystical allusions furnish a religious coloring for magical practices
(55a). These practices remain fundamentally ambiguous, however. "If
one to whom this door is opened makes the claim, he will be a prophet;
if he is good, he will be a saint; and if he is evil, he will be a magician"
(55a). As a generalization, I would like to observe that, for the average
Persian reader, the contents of *The Fifty Verses of Kamarupa* probably
fell into the category of the occult sciences, and its Indic origin would
have only enhanced its esoteric allure. The text employs standard Arabic
terms for astral magic (*tanjim*), the summoning of spirits (*ihdar*) (30b,
37b), and the subjugation (*taskhir*) of demons, fairies, and magicians.
Thus, there would be a familiar quality about the text, even when these
techniques are employed for summoning the spirits known in India as
yoginis. The chants or mantras of the yogis are repeatedly referred to
as spells (*afsun*), a Persian term of magical significance. We also read
of recognizably magical techniques such as one using a nail made from
bone (51a), which is employed nefariously with a voodoo-type doll
(51b). Another recipe uses a comb made from the right paw of a mad dog
killed with iron in rituals performed at a cremation ground (48b–49a).

ISLAMIC ELEMENTS IN THE TEXT

The Pool of Nectar contains numerous Arabic formulas and references
that locate the text in reference to standard Islamic religious themes (see
Chart 10.3). There are six clear quotations from the Qur'an in the earlier
extant Arabic recension, to which the later recension adds two more.
One *hadith* saying of the Prophet Muhammad is quoted, and another is
implicitly referred to. Terms from the vocabulary of religious practice,

particularly those relating to the names of God and prayer, are prominent. The text is, in addition, studded with pious phrases and blessings,
which occur in over half of the chapters. Cosmological terms relating
to standard Qur'anic sources appear with remarkable frequency. And
there are at least a dozen places where specific Sufi terms and themes
are invoked. All these are instances of deliberate Islamization, in which
the translator decided to use familiar terms and conventions to normalize
the foreignness of the Indian text. Three chapters (I, III, and X) contain
no Indic material whatsoever. When combined with the quotations from
Islamicate philosophical texts in the preface (see below), the net result is
that over one third of the Arabic version of *The Pool of Nectar* consists
of the translator's additions to the text.

The process of Islamization was a cumulative one. The earlier extant
version of the Arabic text (manuscript family *a*) represents a stage in this
process, which is clearly accelerated by the later version (family *b*). Not
only does family *b* add more Islamic scriptural passages and themes, it
also strips away, truncates, and distorts many Indian references. Indian
names for the planets have been garbled or omitted in both Arabic
recensions, though they are clearly preserved in the Persian translations,
perhaps because Indo-Persian scribes were familiar with the Hindi terms
(see Chart 10.4). The later recension (family *b*) omits altogether the
identification of Brahma and Vishnu with Abraham and Moses (Int.3),
the yogic term *alakh* and its translation as Allah (IV.4), the three yogis
identified with esoteric Islamic figures (V.4), the description of urethral
suction (VI.5), and most of the description of the seventh yogini (IX.9).
The manuscripts of family *b* also add further extraneous textual materials,
including an Arabic verse, inserted at the beginning of the preface, and a
treatise on the heart according to Sufi psychology, added as an appendix
after chapter X. The Islamization of the text even proceeded on the visual
level. The Arabic translation includes 14 diagrams for visualization
during meditation, of which nine relate to the cakras. A comparison of
the manuscripts indicates a subtle but unmistakable process of gramma-
tization, in which diagrams increasingly turn into Arabic letters or the
cabalistic figures common to Arabic works on occultism.

The insertion of Islamic materials into the translation of *The Pool of
Nectar* was accompanied by another technique in which Indic names and
themes were given Islamic equivalents (see Chart 10.5). The Sanskrit

term *alakh*, "the unconditioned," is translated as Allah, doubtless because of the tempting similarity of sound and their nearly identical appearance in Arabic script.[28] Brahma and Vishnu are translated as Abraham and Moses, and three legendary yogis are equated with Islamic prophets. This last identification is made in the context of a discussion of attaining complete control over the breath:

> When you have reached this station, and this condition becomes characteristic of you, closely examine three things with thought and discrimination: 1) the embryo, how it breathes while it is in the placenta, though its mother's womb does not respire; 2) the fish, how it breathes in the water, and the water does not enter it; 3) and the tree, how it attracts water in its veins and causes it to reach its heights. The embryo is Shaykh Gorakh, who is Khidr (peace be upon him), the fish is Shaykh Minanath [Matsyendranath], who is Jonah, and the tree is Shaykh Chaurangi, who is Ilyas, and they are the ones who have reached the water of life (V.4).

Several technical terms are given in their Sanskrit forms along with Arabic translations: *homa* or "sacrifice" is translated as *du`a* or "prayer," *japa* or "counted prayers" becomes `*azima* or "invocation," and the key term *yogi* (in its north Indian form *jogi*) is *murtad* or "person of discipline." *Brahmin*, the term for the priestly caste, is translated as `*alim* or "scholar." But as noted above, several of these equivalences have evaporated from the later recension of the Arabic text. The very attempt to translate an Indian name or term with an Islamic one has been abandoned in these instances. In later recensions or in quotations of the text, we find that the passage identifying the Sanskrit word *alakh* with Allah has a radically different appearance. A mid-nineteenth-century Arabic treatise on Sufi orders by the North African author Muhammad al-Sanusi (d. 1859) includes a section on the yogis (*al-jujiyya*) as a subset of the Ghawthiyya branch of the Shattariyya Sufi order; for this he clearly draws both on the writings of Muhammad Ghawth and on the Arabic text of *The Pool of Nectar*.[29] When he reaches the passage in question, he states,

---

[28] The identification of Allah with *alakh* is also found in an eighteenth-century Dakani Urdu text by a Sufi writer named Shah Turab Chishti; see his *Man samj'havan*, ed. Sayyida Ja`far, Silsila-i Matbu`at-i Abu al-Kalam Azad Oriental Research Institute 5 (Hyderabad: Abu al-Kalam Azad Oriental Research Institute, 1964), p. 1: *alak nam allah naranjan hari he*.

[29] Muhammad ibn `Ali al-Sanusi al-Khattabi al-Hasani al-Idrisi, *Al-Silsabil al-ma`in fil-tara'iq al-arba`in* (Cairo: n.p., 1989), pp. 84–87.

If one wishes to witness the hidden world, it is incumbent on him to cross his eyes over his nose, and imagine in his heart the word Allah, Allah, without moving his tongue. If he reaches the level of perfection in this practice, then magic and poison will have no influence on him, disease will not affect him, the hidden worlds will be unveiled, his prayer will be answered, and he will be famous among men for deeds of piety.

At this point it is no longer possible to see any Indian "influence" in a portrait of a practice that is indistinguishable from standard Sufi technique.

PHILOSOPHICAL FORMATIONS

It is evident that the Arabic version of *The Pool of Nectar* was composed by an Iranian philosopher familiar with the Illuminationist school because of the characteristic Illuminationist vocabulary in the treatise. The most persuasive evidence in this regard is the extensive revised Arabic version (Int.9–12) of an extract from Suhrawardi's Persian treatise *On the Reality of Love*, which is integrated with the fragmentary "Hymn of the Pearl" frame story.[30] We also find a distinctive term from Avicennan-Illuminationist psychology, "the cognizing and distinguishing rational soul for the managing of states" (Int.14), or more briefly, "the managing rational soul" (IV.1). The prominent location of this passage in the preface is clearly meant to exercise a dominant role in determining the significance of the yogic teachings of the main text. This has the distinct effect of proleptically assimilating the psychophysiology of yoga to the basic categories of Aristotelian and Avicennan psychology, even though this assimilation is not actually carried out in the text. Specifically, the text in the preface enumerates the standard Greco-Arabic list of the five internal senses, the five external senses, the seven vegetal faculties, and the two animal motor-sensory faculties, which would be familiar to any reader of later Aristotelian texts in Arabic. At the same time, the narrative suggests an overall framework for interpreting yogic practices as a means of discovering the true self through discipline of the body and mind. But there is no indication of any familiarity of philosophical anthropologies that might be found in other Sanskrit materials connected to the yogic tradition.

---

[30] These narratives are discussed in detail in *The Pool of Nectar*.

In addition to these explicit references to the Illuminationist school of philosophy, the Arabic version as a whole calls on a more diffuse kind of Arabic philosophical vocabulary, which was shared and recognized by many schools. The philosophical terms in the treatise are primarily of a cosmological significance, and they include such items as the four qualities (hot, cold, wet, dry) (VI.2–3, X.2), moderation (*al-amr al-awsat*) (IV.1, VIII.1), contraries (*diddan*) (III.4, V.2, X.2), the rational soul (*al-nafs al-natiqa*) (I.3, V.2, VI.2, X.4), the universal intellect (`aql al-kull*) (I.2, I.3), and the creator (*al-bari*) (I.2, I.3).

Intellectuals trained in the Arabic scientific curriculum would have recognized in *The Pool of Nectar* some explicit references to commonplace themes from the tenth-century encyclopedia known as *The Epistles of the Brethren of Purity*. The theme of the correspondence of the human body as microcosm and the larger cosmos as macrocosm had been well developed in Greek thought from an early period.[31] The Brethren of Purity gave an early expression to this doctrine in their encyclopedia, with strong leanings toward Pythagorean teachings. From the prominent first chapter of *The Pool of Nectar* (I.2), we can glean the following list of microcosmic-macrocosmic correspondences:

1. nostrils, eyes, ears, and mouth	seven planets
2. senses	stars
3. head	sky
4. body (*juththa*)	earth
5. bone	mountains
6. nerves	oceans
7. veins	rivers
8. hair	trees (*ashjar*)
9. skin, blood, flesh, ligaments, muscle, bone, and brain	seven climes
10. waking	day
11. sleep	night
12. happiness	spring

---

[31] On the history of this motif in the West, see George Boas, "Macrocosm and Microcosm," *Dictionary of the History of Ideas*, ed. Philip P. Wiener, 5 vols. (New York: Scribner, 1973–74), 3:126–31.

13. sadness	winter
14. hunger	summer
15. satiety	fall
16. weeping	water
17. laughing	lightning
18. heart	throne
19. brain	canopy
20. soul	universal intellect
21. intellect	creator

To this list some manuscripts from family *b* add the following items:

22. arteries	springs
23. chief limbs	mountains
24. brain	mine
25. limbs	animals

This list may be compared with a similar series of microcosmic-macrocosmic equivalences found in *The Epistles of the Brethren of Purity* (repeated or similar terms are marked in bold, with reference to the numbers in the list just given):

body (*jasad*)	**earth** (variant of no. 4)
bones	**mountains** (variant no. 5)
brain	**mines** (variant of no. 24)
belly	**ocean** (partial; no. 6)
intestines	**rivers** (partial; no. 7)
veins	streams (partial; no. 7)
flesh	dust
hair	**plants** (*nabat*) (variant of no. 8)
head to foot	civilization
back	desert
front	east
back	west
right	south

left	north
breathing	herbs
speech	thunder
cries	thunderbolts
laughing	**lightning** (variant of no. 17)
weeping	**rain** (variant of no. 16)
misery and sorrow	dark of night
sleep	death
waking	life
childhood	**spring** (partial; no. 12)
youth	**summer** (partial; no. 14)
maturity	**fall** (partial; no. 15)
old age	**winter** (partial; no. 13)[32]

The list of the Brethren of Purity continues with an additional 12 equivalences between the human condition and planetary movements, of particular relevance to astrology. The series of 25 microcosmic-macrocosmic correspondences in *The Pool of Nectar* is introduced primarily in the context of the yogic teaching regarding the sun and moon (I.1) and their association with the two opposed breaths of the right and left nostrils. As shown by the items marked in bold above, six of these correspondences are variations on correspondences given by the Brethren of Purity, and another seven give correspondences that include one of the terms in the list of the Brethren of Purity. Items 18 to 21 contain terms deriving from standard Islamicate cosmology. Manuscripts from the later recension of family *b* add four more items, one from the list of the Brethren of Purity, indicating a further stage in the domestication of the text. The Persian translation of Muhammad Ghawth (which differs widely from the Arabic text at this point) contains another four equivalences from the list of the Brethren of Purity that do not occur in any of the Arabic manuscripts of *The Pool of Nectar*, but which probably reflect the earlier Arabic recension from which his Persian translation derives.

---

[32] *Rasa'il ikhwan al-safa'*, 2:466–67.

This passage is then followed (I.3) by further reflection on the microcosm and the macrocosm, joining the language of Islamicate philosophy to citations from the Qur'an and hadith. Speculations on the microcosm and the macrocosm have certainly played an important role in Indian thought, and they are frequently found in yogic writings, but the material in this Arabic version (I.2–3) appears to be wholly unrelated to Indian sources. In Indian texts, one would normally expect specific references to correspondences between sections of the body and multiple worlds, specific geographical sites in India, etc.[33] It is hard to avoid concluding that the translator of *The Pool of Nectar*, perhaps inspired by something comparable in the yogic teaching, at this point eliminated the Indic narrative and substituted materials from exclusively Arabic sources to make the yogic teachings more comprehensible. This is not the only place in the treatise where the Brethren of Purity are invoked. A description in *The Pool of Nectar* (VI.2) regarding the prediction of the sex of the embryo in the womb, according to which direction it is facing, appears to draw directly on a passage in the writings of the Brethren of Purity.[34]

YOGIC ELEMENTS IN THE TEXT

The Arabic version of *The Pool of Nectar* contains a variety of practices. Some are not distinctively Indian or restricted to yoga but are widely found in other traditions. This is the case with the recommendation of fasting (IV.3), vegetarian diet (V.3), and sexual abstinence (VI.3, VII.11). But other practices are clearly associated with hatha yoga (see Chart 10.6). Very prominent is the description of breath control, with reference to the sun and moon breaths as associated with the left and right nostrils (I, II). The concepts of breath underlying these passages are not clearly related to standard Indian cosmologies, however.

Later Indian texts such as the *Yoga Upanisads* often employ the time unit of the *matra* to count the duration of breaths.[35] In contrast, *The Pool of Nectar* measures breaths by fingers in two passages, using a spatial

---

[33] Kalyani Mallik, *Siddha-Siddhanta-Paddhati and Other Works of the Natha Yogis* (Poona: Poona Oriental Book House, 1954), p. 39.

[34] *Rasa'il Ikhwan al-safa'*, 2:425.

[35] *Darsanopanisad* VI:3–6, in *The Yoga Upanisads*, trans. T. R. Srinivasa Ayyangar, ed. G. Srinivasa Murti (Adyar: Adyar Library, 1952), p. 137; *Yogatattvopanisad* 40–43, in *ibid.*, p. 308.

measurement rather than a temporal one. The first passage gives a list of five breaths associated with the elements, and it describes the directional orientation of four: "The breaths are five: fiery, watery, airy, earthy, and heavenly. The fiery rises up, the airy spreads out, the watery descends the extent of four fingers, the earthy descends the extent of eight fingers" (II.2). Although the number five is characteristic of Indian medical and yogic approaches to the breaths and while some of the breaths are associated with upward and downward movement, it is otherwise hard to recognize any resemblance to the Indian traditions on the breaths in this brief list.[36] The association with the elements is not found in standard Indian texts, and may be an Aristotelian touch added by the translator. The second passage details the effects of exhalation and inhalation and recommends the increase of the latter in order to prolong life:

> You will find it [breath] rising in exhalation the amount of about twelve fingers with power, and in inhalation it descends the amount of four fingers. It decreases at every breath by the power of eight fingers. So see how much it decreases every day. That is the decrease of one's life. It is appropriate that you reverse that by kindness, sympathy, and gradual approach. That is, you should inhale the breath with power and exhale it with gentleness and mildness, to the point where you inhale twelve fingers, and exhale four (V.3).

In the Persian translation of Muhammad Ghawth, this passage reads:

> Twelve fingers of breath enter, then eight fingers return, four fingers of cold wind (*sarsar*), and four of cold (*sard*). . . . When walking on foot, breath of twelve fingers enters, and two warm and two cold ones return. When exerting effort, running, or having sex, twenty-four fingers go out, and four return to place.

Oddly, the spatial measurements are missing from the account of breath in the oldest Persian translation, the portions of the *Kamarupancasika* preserved in the fourteenth-century encyclopedia of Amuli. In any case, the basic idea is apparently control of the quantity of breath in order to maximize inhalation for long life. There are occasional references to

---

[36] Kenneth G. Zysk, "The Science of Respiration and the Doctrine of the Bodily Winds in Ancient India," *Journal of the American Oriental Society* 113 (1993): 198–213.

the finger as a spatial measure of length related to breath control in the *Yoga Upanisads*, but these do not correspond with the life preservation technique mentioned here.[37]

Physiological techniques mentioned in the text include the purification of body by postures recognizable as yogic asanas (IV.4–8). The Arabic text acknowledges the traditional number of 84 postures but describes only five (although the Persian translation of Muhammad Ghawth, relying on an earlier version of the Arabic, describes 21 postures). These are difficult to match with the descriptions of asanas in standard hatha yoga texts, but from the descriptions, we may recognize the Virasana, Kukkutasana, and Uttana Kurmasana among these five. The Arabic text emphasizes the physical and psychic health benefits of these postures. It is notable that the yogic word *alakh* is repeated in each position; this reinforces the association with the Nath or Kanphata yogis, for whom this is a characteristic utterance. Among these physiological techniques appears to be a version of the *khecari mudra*, described as staring at the tip of the nose and drinking the "nectar" of saliva (II.5, II.7). Unlike standard hatha yoga accounts of this practice, this description emphasizes the crossing of the eyes (vividly illustrated in some manuscripts) as the chief element, which permits the retention of semen during sexual intercourse; the swallowing of nectar is also modestly credited with curing sores and headache.[38] Another yogic technique that occurs here is a variation of the *vajroli mudra*, which makes possible return of the semen by urethral suction (VI.5). Curiously, the discussion of retention of semen is embedded in a lengthy section on procreation and embryology according to Galenic medical principles, leading to the equivalent of the philosophical proverb, "Every animal is sad after sex" (VI.4).

Visualization is another prominent feature of *The Pool of Nectar*, particularly in the lengthy chapter VII on the magical imagination (*wahm*), treated as a generic term for mental and magical powers. Normal Islamic discourse gives *wahm* the pejorative meaning of "illusion" or "prejudice," and *wahm* also has various technical meanings

---

[37] In the *Trisikhibrahmanopanisad*, 53–55 (*The Yoga Upanisads*, p. 100), the vital breath is described as being 12 "digit-lengths" longer than the body, which is 96 "digit-lengths," evidently meaning a unit the size of the fingertip. The recommendation in this case, however, is to shorten the air to the length of the body in order to know Brahman.

[38] Cf. Eliade, *Yoga*, pp. 247–48, for accounts of the *khecari mudra* which describe the swallowing of nectar as responsible for the retention of semen.

in Aristotelian philosophy as the "estimative faculty" (Lat. *aestimatio*, Gk. *sunesis, phronesis*) and "compositive imagination" (Gk. *phantasia logistike*). But *wahm* in the sense of "magical imagination" seems to presuppose a correspondence with some unstated Indic term, possibly *dharana* or *kalpana*. It is defined in *The Fifty Verses of Kamarupa* as "the knowledge of breaths" (16a), and in the translator's introduction, magical imagination is also linked with the term "discipline" (*riyadat*), which is the standard Arabic-Persian translation for yoga. I am open to suggestions about other interpretations of this term. At any rate, this practice takes the form of the visualization in sequence of seven locations corresponding to the standard yogic cakras, from the seat to the crown of the head. Each cakra is described in terms of a color and a diagram, but instead of being linked to Hindu gods and letters of the Devanagri alphabet, the cakras are connected with the planets. While some of the *bija-mantra*s contain phonemes recognizable to Indologists, others are beyond retrieval, doubtless due to the difficulties of preserving the chants in Arabic script (see Chart 10.4). The demythologization of the cakras, and their planetary placement, has the effect of likening the cakra meditation and the implicit upward movement of the kundalini to the ascension of the soul through the planetary spheres, a major theme in Islamic, Iranian, and Jewish traditions.

The seven Sanskrit mantras or chants associated with the seven cakras are all boldly declared to be translations of the Arabic invocations of the names of God. Thus, the Sanskrit syllable *hum* is translated as "O Lord" (*ya rabb*), and *aum* is translated as "O Ancient One" (*ya qadim*). In introducing these seven great mantras, the Arabic translator remarks that "they are like the greatest names [of God] among us." Muhammad Ghawth goes one better, however, in his Persian translation, providing two Arabic phrases for each Sanskrit term; he translates *hum* as *ya rabb ya hafiz*, "O Lord, O Protector," and *aum* as *ya qahir ya qadir*, "O Wrathful, O All-powerful."[39] In a discussion of breathing techniques that does not appear in the Arabic version, Muhammad Ghawth also finds equivalents for the yogic terms *hams* and *so ham*, which are pronounced during the two phases of exhalation and inhalation; the first is "an expression for the spiritual lord (*rabb ruhi*)," while the second stands for "the lord of

---

[39] *Bahr al-hayat*, India Office Library MS, pp. 91, 94; Ganj Bakhsh MS, pp. 82, 84.

lords (*rabb al-arbab*)."[40] There are many other examples of this kind. Semantically, such "translations" make no sense whatever; they are, rather, functional equivalents between the yogic words of power and the names of God as used by the Sufis; this is especially evident in the case of the seven great mantras, for which the Arabic equivalents are presented in a vocative form used in the Sufi *dhikr* repetitions of the names of God.

Chapter IX of *The Pool of Nectar* amplifies on the cakra meditations in Chapter VII with elaborate instructions for summoning seven female deities or "spiritual beings" (Ar. *ruhaniyyat*) who are evidently the chief yoginis (there are a total of 64 of these entities). These seven are usually called Mother Goddesses in yogic circles.[41] In this text, however, they are assimilated to the seven planets, as in Chapter VII. Here as well, it seems that the planetary organization is a deliberate attempt by the translator to familiarize the subject, in this case by likening the summoning of Indian goddesses to well-known Middle Eastern occult practices involving planetary spirits. The phrase "subjugation of spirits" (*taskhir al-arwah*) in the title of Chapter IX is the normal Arabic name for this kind of occultism. The yoginis are summoned with incense and mandalas. Instructions here call on the practitioner to act like a son and a brother with the goddesses, in order to obtain the numerous favors they can bestow. Lengthy Sanskrit mantras addressed to these beings must be repeated thousands of times (see Chart 10.7).

The worship of the female deities known as yoginis seems to have been at its height in India from the ninth to the twelfth centuries, but it continued in various places until at least the eighteenth century. Vidya Dehejia has described at length the open-air yogini temples found at remote sites where these deities were honored.[42] While the description of the yoginis in *The Pool of Nectar* is brief, *The Fifty Verses of Kamarupa* describes them at length as the key to knowledge of all things. At the beginning of the section on breath, we are told,

---

[40] *Bahr al-hayat*, ch. 4, India Office Library MS, pp. 45–46; Ganj Bakhsh MS, p. 55; ch. 7, Ganj Bakhsh MS, p. 93.

[41] W. W. Karambelkar, "Matsyendranatha and his Yogini Cult," *Indian Historical Quarterly* 31 (1955): 367.

[42] Vidya Dehejia, *Yogini Cult and Temples: A Tantric Tradition* (New Delhi: National Museum; Sole distributors, Publications Division, 1986).

So say those sixty-four women, "By the command of God (who is great and majestic), who one day gave us this science, we shall not speak of this science. By the God by whose command the 18,000 worlds exist, this is an oath, that this is the science of magical imagination, for whatever is in the earth and heaven is in the grasp of the children of Adam. We tell everything, for everything that goes on in all the world is all known and made clear by the science of magical imagination" (16a).

Furthermore, they say,

> By the command of God most high, and the masterful teaching they have taught us, between the moon and the sun one can know whatever goes on in all the world. We teach a science of who comes, and from where, and what he asks. Also know that this science lengthens life and makes one near immortal (17a).

The knowledge that the yoginis confer makes poison harmless, cures the sick, removes desire, and enables one to control all persons and things in the world. These "spiritual beings" are invulnerable to injury by sword or fire; their hair and nails cannot be cut; they hear from a distance and travel anywhere in an instant (23b). Each of the 64 yoginis has a particular spot in India, and they go to delightful places to enjoy themselves at feasts, dressed in gold and jewels, wearing crowns and wreaths, revered by the *devs*; they will never die, grow old, or get sick before the day of judgment, but all appear to be 20 years of age (30b–31a). These beings are in fact the principal objects of worship among the Hindus, who carve idols of them. "Just as we have prophets, saints, and miracle workers, so the Hindus have faith in them" (31a). Many of their names are given, though the Persian script leaves many ambiguities: Tutla, Karkala, Tara, Chalab, Kamak, Kalika, Diba, Darbu (31b), Antarakati (44b, 46b), Chitraki (56a), Ganga Mati (45a), Sri Manohar (45a), Katiri (30a), Parvati (49b), Suramati (44b), Susandari (44b), Talu (30a). Of course, as Vidya Dehejia has pointed out, no two lists of names of yoginis are the same. Sometimes adepts may have sexual relations with the yoginis (39a), but at other times they regard them as sister and mother (46b). "She is the yogini and you are the yogi" (48a). Benefits of association with them include money (44b) and food (48b).

As a comprehensive description of Indian religious practices, a narrative limited to Kamakhya and the yoginis might seem a bit eccentric. Brahmins are mentioned, but only as occasional sources of information about *The Fifty Verses of Kamarupa* and its interpretation. This is clearly a narrow sample, but what is it based on? In terms of the categories that are available today, we could probably say that this text reflects practices of the yogini temple cult that are associated with Kaula tantrism.[43] There is also some connection with the Nath or Kanphata yogis, as indeed Matsyendranath is usually considered the introducer of the yogini cult among the Kaulas, and the name of Gorakhnath is invoked once (51a) in the text.[44] Beyond that general indication, we find multiple strands of Hindu tradition popping up in an incidental fashion. This text assumes a system of nine cakras rather than the seven cakras current in most Nath yoga writings (19b, 20a, 25a). Meditative exercises are given that concentrate on raising the Sakti from the navel up the spinal column (17b, 18a, 28a). A standard list of supernormal powers (*siddhis*) is provided (54a).[45] Occasional mantras appear to contain the phrase "Krsna avatar" (48b, 53a). We are told of the temple of Mahakala in Ujjain where many siddhas or magicians are said to live (24b, 37a). The story of Siva (Mahadev) and the churning of the ocean is told at length (31b–32b). While long accounts are given of the temple of the goddess Kamakhya, nothing is said about the animal sacrifices associated with that site today. The basic teachings of *The Fifty Verses of Kamarupa*, however, are the use of breath for divination and the summoning of yoginis to obtain various goals; hatha yoga meditation is certainly linked to these practices.

The representation of yogic practices in *The Pool of Nectar* and *The Fifty Verses of Kamarupa* was highly selective, to say the least. In one sense, this is not surprising, if these texts are the result of the adventitious contact of one or two enterprising Muslim scholars with a mixture of esoteric Indian teachings. It includes unusual practices not attested elsewhere, such as a combined visualization of all seven cakras into a composite diagram (VII.14, VIII.5). Among the benefits of the practices mentioned in *The Pool of Nectar* are familiar yogic powers (*siddhis*), such as taking on an animal form or another human body, whether living or dead (*parakaya-pravesa*) (VII.12–15). At the same time, there are

---

[43] Ibid., pp. 30, 36.
[44] Ibid., pp. 74–75.
[45] See Eliade, *Yoga*, p. 88, n.

non-yogic powers, such as the prediction of the time of death by visual meditation, a practice common in early tantric works on sorcery (*kriya tantra*) that predate hatha yoga (VIII.1–5). There are also sexual practices that use breathing techniques derived from early Indian magical and divinatory texts (II.4). There are two different accounts of the breaths that are pretty much incompatible (five breaths in II.2; three breaths in V.3). The Arabic version of *The Pool of Nectar* has an otherwise unattested selection of five asana postures, while the Persian translation of Muhammad Ghawth provides 21, the names of which do not overlap with any known work on hatha yoga.[46] It is difficult to identify the *bija-mantras* in Chapter VII, though here, as with the longer mantras of Chapter IX, the problem may lie in part in the inherent difficulty of representing Sanskrit (especially short vowels) in Arabic script. In any case, despite the translators' claims regarding the scriptural authority of their texts, the representation of yogic practices that they provided was arbitrary and selective, and it was heavily colored both in context and in interpretation by a strongly established set of Islamic conventions.

TRANSLATION AS HERMENEUTICS

What is the function of a translation such as *The Pool of Nectar*? The account of the origin of the text domesticates it in an Islamic context through the conversion of yogis to Islam. The two frame stories invoke particular interpretive approaches linked to the gnostic myth of the soul and the Illuminationist allegory of the senses and psychic faculties. The actual mechanism of translation is applied unevenly throughout the text. Sometimes purely Islamic terms and symbols are unselfconsciously placed in the text as adequate descriptions of Indian originals. This has the result that many of the original Indian terms and symbols can only be recovered by the use of resources of modern Indology outside of this text. The Islamizing tendency is most evident in the later stages of manuscript production; there, the most common recension of the Arabic dispenses with most of the Indian elements of the text. Sanskrit originals are also dropped when techniques are being introduced that would be new to Arabic readers,

---

[46] Several manuscripts of the Persian translation contain miniature illustrations of the 21 asanas. One of these MSS is in the Chester Beatty Library in Dublin, another is in the Salar Jung Library in Hyderabad, a third is in the private collection of Simon Digby, and the fourth has recently been acquired by the University of North Carolina at Chapel Hill.

particularly in the sections on chanting, visualization, and postures. In an intermediate stage of translation, Indic names and terms are retained alongside their Islamic "translations." Yet, there is a certain residue that remains untranslatable, particularly in the Sanskrit mantras that are transmitted in Arabic script. In short, *The Pool of Nectar* exhibits conflicting tendencies in its modes of translation, which are never fully resolved.

In approaching his task, the Arabic translator seems only to have felt the limitations imposed by the audience's unfamiliarity with technical terminology; he was not limited by social and religious constraints. A glance at the Indian names and terms that are transmitted in the text along with their Arabic translations (Chart 10.3) shows that major theological translations relating to God and the prophets are entertained without hesitation. It must be repeated, however, that some of the Indic terms can only be recovered with difficulty through recourse to modern Indological sources. Given the almost exclusively extra-Indian distribution of manuscripts (only one of 45 is found in India), it is hard to believe that any readers of the Arabic text would have been in a position to recognize that the text contained Sanskrit terms.

In other cases, the translator evidently felt that it was pointless to retain the Indian originals for a cluster of other important terms. "Mantra" is almost certainly the term underlying the Arabic term *dhikr* or "recollection," referring to the seven powerful "words" or "names" in chapter VII, which consist of seed-syllables like *aum*. "Yantra" is probably the Indic original translated as *shakl* or "diagram." Curiously, the term "yoga" is only mentioned by implication once in the text, in the title to chapter IV on yogic postures; there it is represented by the Arabic term *riyada* or "exercise," which is from the same root as found in the Arabic word (*murtad*) used as a translation of "yogi." The unstated Indian term with the most theological baggage is probably *yogini*, "female yogi," which in the text refers to semi-divine beings rather than humans. The translator renders this as *ruhaniyya* or "spiritual being," which might seem equivocally to conceal polytheistic goddesses behind an innocuous looking front. Still, it is worth noting that earlier Arabic translators of Greek authors such as Plotinus used the same Arabic term *ruhaniyya* to translate the Greek term *theos* or "god."[47]

---

[47] 'Abd al-Rahman Badawi, *Aflutin 'inda al-'Arab [Plotinus Among the Arabs]*, 2nd ed. (Kuwait: Wakalat al-Matbuat, 1977), index, p. 248.

Jan Assmann has proposed a model of translation with respect to the Hellenistic age that is suggestive for the Islamicate translations of Indic texts.[48] The complete and selfconscious translations of divinities from one culture to another was a common feature of ancient near eastern societies. The best known such case was Herodotus' translation of the Egyptian gods into familiar Greek ones: Amun was Zeus, Re was Helios, etc. Where there is easy translation from one pantheon to another, Assmann argues, conversion is not an issue. As long as there is the possibility of translation there is no need of conversion. If all religions basically worship the same gods there is no need to give up one religion and to enter another one. This possibility only occurs if there is one religion claiming knowledge of a superior truth. It is precisely this claim that excludes translatability. If one religion is wrong and the other is right, there can be no question of translating the gods of the one into those of the other. Obviously they are about different gods.[49] It is only when one insists on the untranslatability of key religious figures that "the cosmotheistic link between god and world, and god and gods, is categorically broken." Thus, Jewish and Christian views of the incomparability of God precluded identification with the interchangeable "pagan" deities of the Hellenistic world. Following an idea put forward by G. W. Bowersock, Assmann maintains that the Greek culture of Hellenism was a vehicle through which many non-Greek cultures forcefully expressed their own distinctiveness. From the Jewish or Christian perspective, however, differences between Hellenistic religions were so trifling as to be meaningless. Hellenism, by furnishing an overarching system of equivalences, created a cosmopolitan consciousness of a fairly unified pagan world.

A number of the features described by Assman in the Hellenistic case have parallels in the Islamicate cultures where *The Pool of Nectar* was produced and read. As with the Hellenistic age, the Arabic culture of the high caliphate and the Persianate culture of the middle periods of Islamic history were characterized by the creation of vast ecumenic imperial structures, in which minorities of many kinds expressed

---

[48] Jan Assmann, "Translating Gods: Religion as a Factor of Cultural (Un)Translatability," in *The Translatability of Cultures: Figurations of the Space Between*, ed. Sanford Budick and Wolfgang Iser (Stanford: Stanford University Press, 1996), pp. 25–36. Assmann unfortunately includes in his model an account of "syncretistic translation" that is far from clear.
[49] Ibid., p. 31.

themselves through the dominant language.[50] The ethnic identities of non-Arab peoples found expression through the Arabic language in the Shu'ubiyya movement, and non-Muslims made use of Persian for both religious and historical purposes. In Islamicate societies, the legal authority of the Islamic religion continually existed in tension with universalizing tendencies of Hellenistic origin embodied in the philosophical tradition. As a consequence, there were always significant aspects of the Islamicate cosmos that were not exclusively Islamic; this is the justification for Hodgson's term "Islamicate." Indeed, from the perspective of the most thoroughgoing exponents of philosophy (e.g., Ibn Sina), all religions (including Islam) were special modifications of the universal truths of philosophy, intended for mass consumption. The standard minimalist concept of Islam current in the mass media today identifies it with authoritarianism, legalism, and violent iconoclasm. The Muslim equivalents of Tertullian would doubtless be horrified by the contents of *The Pool of Nectar* and would reject out of hand any consideration of murmuring Sanskrit mantras to feminine deities. Yet, the sophisticated Neoplatonism of the Muslim Illuminationists (like that of, say, the Christian Platonist Marsilio Ficino in Renaissance Italy) permitted the translation and assimilation of "pagan" themes, deities, and practices, without a sense of radical difference.[51] Still, the text makes a kind of concession to the absolute demands of Islamic religious authority, by making sure that the bearers of foreign knowledge (the yogis) become converted Muslims, and even authorities on Islamic law.

In a way, the fortunes of *The Pool of Nectar* resemble the important texts that Robert E. Buswell has called Chinese Buddhist apocrypha. These were often original texts composed in China but presented as translations of important and authentic Buddhist scriptures from India. "Such texts were sometimes written in association with a revelatory experience, but often were intentionally forged using false ascriptions as a literary device both to enhance their authority as well as to strengthen

---

[50] See Eric Voegelin, *Order and History*, vol. 4, *The Ecumenic Age* (Baton Rouge: Louisiana State University Press, 1974).

[51] The Persian scholar Mulla Zayn al-Din of Lar, from whom Pietro della Valle obtained a manuscript of *The Fifty Verses of Kamarupa* in 1622, belonged to a sect "which attributed intelligences to the sun, moon and stars, and venerated them as angels of a superior order who would intercede with God and seek his protection" (J. D. Gurney, "Pietro della Valle: The Limits of Perception," *BSOAS* 49 [1986]: 113).

their chances of being accepted as canonical."[52] They took a strategy of making Buddhism intelligible by explaining it in terms that would be familiar to Chinese readers, even to the extent of creating new scriptures out of whole cloth. The analogy with *The Pool of Nectar* is not exact; there was some kind of textual basis for the translations of *The Pool of Nectar*, even if it may have been primarily an esoteric teaching restricted to oral transmission. But the Arabic translator clearly wanted to establish the canonical authority of his work, and part of his technique consisted of adding enough of the familiar Islamicate structures of authority to convince his readers to pay attention. He opened his translation with the following sentence: "Now in the land of India there is a respected book, known to its religious scholars (*'ulama'*) and philosophers (*hukama'*), called *Amrtakunda*, that is, *The Pool of the Water of Life* (Int.2)." The primary task was to draw attention to the book's credentials. The Chinese Buddhist apocrypha sometimes adopted another technique found in *The Pool of Nectar*, i.e., overcoming the distance between Buddhism and Chinese thought by declaring that Lao Tzu and Confucius were theophanies of Buddhas and bodhisattvas.[53] This is precisely the hermeneutic of equivalence adopted by the translator of *The Pool of Nectar*, when he has the yogi announce that Brahma and Vishnu are Abraham and Moses or when he identifies major yogis with Islamic prophets. In each case, this approach permits the use of a dominant discourse (Chinese or Islamicate) to render the foreign Indian teachings.

A similar translation strategy can be seen in the remarks of the earlier Persian translator of the related *The Fifty Verses of Kamarupa* :

> Thus says the translator of the book: In India I saw many books with complete information about every science. Most of their books are in verse, because they memorize verse better, and one's nature inclines to it more. I found a book which they call *Kamarupancasika*, which is one of their choicest books; they have great faith in this. It contains two types of science.
>
> One is the science of magical imagination (*wahm*) and discipline (*riyadat*); they have no kind of science that is greater or more powerful than this. On the basis of this science they affirm things that intellect does not accept, but

---

[52] Robert E. Buswell, Jr., "Introduction: Prolegomenon to the Study of Buddhist Apocryphal Scriptures," in *Chinese Buddhist Apocrypha* (Honolulu: University of Hawaii Press, 1990). Thanks to Charles Orzech of UNC-Greensboro for drawing this reference to my attention.
[53] Ibid., p. 10.

they believe in it, and among them it is customary. For each of these things they adduce and show a thousand proofs and demonstrations. Regarding the subject of this science, this is a summary, which they have affirmed.

The other is a science that they call *s[v]aroda* [i.e., divination]. Their scholars and sages observe their breath; if their breath goes well, they perform their tasks, but if the breath goes ill, they do no work, but strenuously avoid it. They have taken this subject to the height of perfection. The common people of India know nothing of this, and they are not privy to this secret, nor do they know anything. They call this the science of [reading] thought (Arabic *damir*) (fols. 2a–2b).

As with the Arabic version of *The Pool of Nectar*, here we are confronted with a powerful book, alleged to be of the highest authority in India, though in the same breath we are told that it is secret and known only to a few. The Persian translator frequently returns to both the themes of the book's scriptural authority and its hidden esoteric character. Thus, in another passage he writes,

This book is known throughout India, and among the Hindus no book is nobler than this. Whoever learns this book and knows its explanation is counted as a great scholar and wise man. They serve him, and whoever is occupied with the theory and practice of this they call a jogi and respect him greatly. They serve him just like we respect the saints and the masters of struggle and discipline (15b).

The translator speaks of information gathered from Brahmin informants, regarding practices such as employing the "greatest name" of God (40b) and summoning the goddess Lakshmi for sexual relations (43b), and he testifies to his own success in employing these techniques. In addition, on several occasions the translator cites another text, which he calls "the thirty-two verses of Kamak Dev," which may have been a separately circulating text with similar contents.[54] He frequently emphasizes the verse character of the original, and several Hindi *doha* verses are quoted

---

[54] In one place (26a) the translator says, "Know that thirty-two verses in the Indian language have been transmitted from the sayings of Kamak. Now Kamak chose a certain kind from those, and added something else to it, and this poem is called *Kamak baray tajanka* (?)." Elsewhere he adds, "This is all a commentary on the thirty-two verses, which someone has written in the Indian language, in which many practices are mentioned, and in which are strange and wonderful sciences which all the practitioners of imagination (*wahm*) and magicians are agreed upon and pleased with" (29a). Once (15b) he says, "Now they put this book into 85 verses, and versified it in the Indian language."

in Persian script (26b, 27a, 29a). The translator stresses the difficulty of the task of translation. "Then I rendered it from the Indian language to the Persian language, taking many pains, and it was read to a group of brahmins and scholars, and it was compared, corrected, and clarified (16a)." Despite this advertisement of scholarly authority, which makes suspicious use of the terminology of Arabic literary production, on other occasions the translator confesses that the material he is dealing with is more than obscure. After giving a lengthy Hindi passage in Arabic script, he remarks, "I presented these verses to a group of the scholars of India, brahmins, and jogis, and they could not explain it, but were incapable of understanding it, for the words are strange and difficult" (27a). Thus, it is not clear to what extent this represents a single text or a selection from yogic verses available from oral sources but represented as scripture.

A comparable case of translation and scriptural authority can be found in the sixth-century Persian physician Burzoy, who traveled to India in search of wonderful plants that can restore the dead to life. He eventually learned from Indian sages that the miraculous plant was really an allegory for wisdom. He returned to Persia with a strongly ascetic inclination and an aversion to religious dogma, bringing with him a selection of Indian literature (Pancatantra, Hitopadesa) that he translated into Middle Persian. This was later translated into Arabic by Ibn al-Muqaffa` under the title *Kalila wa Dimna*, eventually becoming one of the greatest popular trans-missions of literature prior to the invention of print.[55] It is striking to see how the Arabic version of this text preserves the strategies of treating this book of wisdom as divinely inspired and a source of great benefit: "The cause of the copying of this book and its transmission from the land of India to the kingdom of Persia was an inspiration from God Most High, by which he inspired Chosroes Anushirvan [the Persian king]."[56] Or again:

> Regarding his desire for knowledge and devotion to it, he heard of one of the books of the philosophers of India, among their kings and scholars, rare and highly prized by them. It was the root of all their culture and the head of all their knowledge, the guide to every benefit and the key to the search for the hereafter and the work of salvation.[57]

---

[55] François de Blois, *Burzoy's Voyage to India and the Origin of the Book of Kalilah wa Dimnah*, Prize Publication Fund 23 (London: Royal Asiatic Society, 1990).

[56] Ibid., p. 90, col. a, lines 39–41.

[57] Ibid., p. 91, col. b, lines 61–63.

This highly charged religious language, and the frequent reference to the philosophers and sages of India in other passages, became a well-known literary pattern in Islamicate literature (including the account of Burzoy in the Persian *Book of Kings* by Firdawsi); this popular book was several times translated into Persian and many other languages. This is the same language and the same geographic trajectory employed by the Arabic translator of *The Pool of Nectar*, when he announced that "in the land of India there is a respected book, known to its religious scholars (`ulama'*) and philosophers." The fame of *Kalila wa Dimna* in Arabic would have made the theme of the mysterious book from India a familiar echo.

Looking over the many different versions and recensions of the *Amrtakunda* translations produces a peculiar esthetic effect, character-ized by sensations of erasure and overwriting. There is a palimpsest effect when one can see the earliest versions and chart the changes that have taken place in later ones, many of them by whitewashing and then writing over their predecessors. This experience would not have been available to readers of the separate versions of this text, but remains a luxury only accessible today through retrospective scholarly researches. The Islamizing tendency is the most notable overall effect in the transmission of the text, and it clearly becomes stronger in the later versions.

Early Orientalist theories of the Indian origins of Sufism have never been supported by documentation, although that lack of historical evidence hardly seems to have troubled the most ardent upholders of this view. This single historical document on hatha yoga, through its multiple translations, has indeed furnished a channel for certain Indian practices into the Islamic world. But the net result has been that the popularization of this text has been achieved primarily by adding Islamic terms, names, and even whole chunks of texts to make the text more accessible; it has even been ascribed to the authorship of one of the great Sufi theorists, Ibn al-`Arabi. Although it may have appeared that one irreducibly foreign element remained in the text, i.e., the Sanskrit mantras in Chapter IX, even these could be assimilated to the category of non-Arabic divine names or placed alongside occult talismans alleged to be in Hebrew, Syriac, or Chaldean. Thus when Mevlevi dervishes copied out the Ottoman Turkish version of this text a hundred years ago, they thought of it as a familiar genre of Sufi text with some interesting occult applications; they did not have the slightest notion that they were chanting garbled Sanskrit mantras addressed to Hindu goddesses. That conclusion would be left to foreign scholars, who alone had the resources and the motivation to re-Indianize the text. Influence is in the eye of the beholder.

CHART 10.1

Manuscript symbols for the translation of *The Pool of Nectar*

I. Arabic

The edition of Yusuf Husain: A
Family *a*, the earlier and fuller existing recension: B–J (9 MSS).
Family *b*, the later, revised recension: K–Y (15 MSS).
Fragments Z^1–Z^2, based on *a*, containing only the beginning of the "Hymn of the Soul" passage.
Other known manuscripts not used in this study: MSS AA–UU.
Total: 49 copies.

II. Persian (Per^1 and Per^2 are based on a lost recension of Arabic predating both *a* and *b*, while Per^3 is the source of the Arabic text).

Per^1, the translation of Muhammad Ghawth: Per^{1}A–Per^{1}W (21 MSS, plus two lithographed editions).
Per^2, the translation of Muhammad ibn `Abd al-Razzaq: Per^{2}A–Per^{2}C (3 MSS, each a separate recension).
Per^3, *The Kamarupa Seed Syllabus* (anonymous), incorporating *The 32 [or 84] Verses of Kamakhya* (2 complete MSS, plus one abridgement).
Total: 29 copies.

III. Turkish

Tur^1, based on family *a*: Tur^{1}A–Tur^{1}D (3 MSS, plus the printed version).
Tur^2, based on family *b*, translated by Salah al-Din: Tur^{2}A–Tur^{2}D (4 MSS).
Total: 8 copies.

IV. Urdu: Only one copy (Urd), based on Per^1.

CHART 10.2

Putative literary transmission of *The Pool of Nectar*

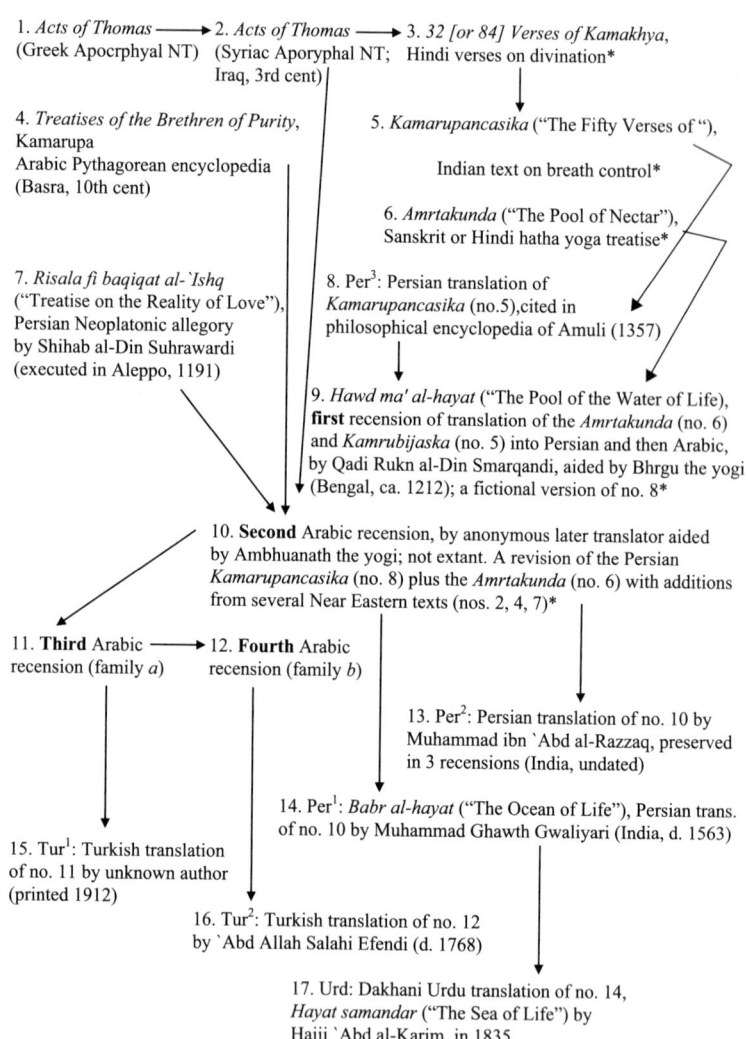

1. *Acts of Thomas* ———▶ 2. *Acts of Thomas* ———▶ 3. *32 [or 84] Verses of Kamakhya,*
(Greek Apocrphyal NT) (Syriac Aporyphal NT; Hindi verses on divination*
Iraq, 3rd cent)

4. *Treatises of the Brethren of Purity,*   5. *Kamarupancasika* ("The Fifty Verses of "),
Kamarupa
Arabic Pythagorean encyclopedia   Indian text on breath control*
(Basra, 10th cent)

6. *Amrtakunda* ("The Pool of Nectar"),
Sanskrit or Hindi hatha yoga treatise*

7. *Risala fi baqiqat al-`Ishq*   8. Per³: Persian translation of
("Treatise on the Reality of Love"),   *Kamarupancasika* (no.5),cited in
Persian Neoplatonic allegory   philosophical encyclopedia of Amuli (1357)
by Shihab al-Din Suhrawardi
(executed in Aleppo, 1191)

9. *Hawd ma' al-hayat* ("The Pool of the Water of Life),
first recension of translation of the *Amrtakunda* (no. 6)
and *Kamrubijaska* (no. 5) into Persian and then Arabic,
by Qadi Rukn al-Din Smarqandi, aided by Bhrgu the yogi
(Bengal, ca. 1212); a fictional version of no. 8*

10. **Second** Arabic recension, by anonymous later translator aided
by Ambhuanath the yogi; not extant. A revision of the Persian
Kamarupancasika (no. 8) plus the *Amrtakunda* (no. 6) with additions
from several Near Eastern texts (nos. 2, 4, 7)*

11. **Third** Arabic ———▶ 12. **Fourth** Arabic
recension (family *a*)   recension (family *b*)

13. Per²: Persian translation of no. 10 by
Muhammad ibn `Abd al-Razzaq, preserved
in 3 recensions (India, undated)

14. Per¹: *Babr al-hayat* ("The Ocean of Life"), Persian trans.
of no. 10 by Muhammad Ghawth Gwaliyari (India, d. 1563)

15. Tur¹: Turkish translation
of no. 11 by unknown author
(printed 1912)

16. Tur²: Turkish translation of no. 12
by `Abd Allah Salahi Efendi (d. 1768)

17. Urd: Dakhani Urdu translation of no. 14,
Hayat samandar ("The Sea of Life") by
Hajji `Abd al-Karim, in 1835

CHART 10.3

Islamicate elements in the Arabic translations of *The Pool of Nectar**

Qur'anic References

The spirit "is from the command of my Lord" (17:85)	Int. 3
"a single soul" (4:1, etc.)	I.3
"lotus tree of the boundary" (53:14)	III.1
"farthest mosque" (17:1)	III.1
"companions of the right hand" (56:27, etc.)	III.3
"companions of the left hand" (56:41)	III.3
"right-hand valley" (28:30)	III.4
God "does what he wants" (3:40)	IV.8 (*b*)
God "orders what he wishes" (5:1)	IV.8 (*b*)

Sayings of the Prophet Muhammad (hadith)

"He who knows himself knows his lord"	
"Hearts are between two finders of the Merciful one" III.1–2	I.3

Islamic law and theology

obligatory (*mafruda*)	IV.3
Greatest Name of God	IV.4(*b*), VII.2
names of God	VII.1
prayer (*du`a*)	IX.10
invocation (`*azima*)	IX.10

Pious Phrases

praise of God and the Prophet	Int. 1, X.11
God's mercy upon him	Int. 4
the weakest of the servants of God most high	Int. 5

---

* References are to chapter and section of the text. References followed by (*b*) indicate manuscripts from the last recension of the Arabic text and are only found in the later recension.

God willing	Int. 6, VII.12
the creator (may his majesty be exalted)	I.2
the creator (there is no god but he)	I.2
God, who is great and mighty	II.5, IV.4
blessings of God on saints and prophets	III.4
blessings of God on Sufis	III.4(*b*)
God knows best	IV.9(*b*), VII.15(*b*), VIII.5(*b*)
by the command of God	VI.1
taking refuge with God from the accursed Satan	III.3, VI.4(*b*)
knowledge of power from God	VII.6

Islamic cosmological terms

throne	I.2
canopy	I.2
jinn	IV.7, VII.6–8, VII.11
angel	Int. 10.4, III.3, IV.6, VII.6, VII.11
devil	Int. 10, III.2–3
spirit	I.3, IV.8, VI.3, VI.5, VII.11, IX.1, IX.9, X.4
hidden world	Int. 3, II.5, IV.5, V.4, VII.3, VII.6, VII.14
water of life	Int.14, II.7, V.4, VI.5

Philosophical terms and concepts†

contraries (*diddan*)	III.4, V.2, X.2
creator (*bari*)	I.2, I.3
four qualities (hot, cold, wet, dry)	VI.2–3, X.2
four humors	VI.1, VI.3

---

† It should be added that excerpts from two philosophical texts are contained in the Arabic *Pool of Nectar*, a fragmentary Arabic version of the Gnostic Hymn of the Soul (Int.7–8, 13–14; X.11) and an Arabic translation of the central section of Shrawardi's Persian allegory, *On the Reality of Love* (Int.9–12). There are also quotations from the Arabic *Epistles of the Brethren of Purity* (I.2, VI.2)

five elements	II.2, VI.1
moderation (*al-amr al-awsat*)	IV.1, VIII.1
rational soul (*al-nafs al-natiqa*)	Int.13, I.3, IV.1, V.2, VI.2, X.4
universal intellect (*'aql al-kull*)	I.2, I.3
omne animalis post coitum triste	VI.4

Sufi terms

gnosis of reality (*ma'rifat al-haqiqa*)	Int. 5
disciple (*murid*)	Int. 6, III.4
annihilated (*mumahhaq*)	Int. 8
spiritual state (*hal*)	II.5, IV.8(*b*)
constellations of the heart	III.1
unveiling (*mukashafa*)	III.4
discipline (*riyada*)	III.4
striving (*mujahada*)	III.4
station (*maqam*)	III.4, IV.8
little food, little speech, little sleep	IV.4
path (*tariq*)	IV.8(*b*)
"taste" or experience (*dhawq*)	V.4
recollection or chant (*dhikr*)	V.4, VII.2
meditative practice (*ishtighal*)	IX.2

CHART 10.4

Planets, cakras, mantras, dhikrs, and yoginis in *The Pool of Nectar*

Chapter VII			Chapter IX				
Planet	Name	Cakra	Mantra	Dhikr	Name	Yogini	
1. Saturn	*Sanicar**/**Zuhal**	seat	*hum*+	**ya rabb**	**Zuhal**	*Kali*	
2. Mars	*Mangal*/ **Mirrikh**	genitals	*aum*+	**ya qadir**	**Mirrikh**	*Tira*	
3. Jupiter	*Brhaspali**/ **Mushtari**	navel	*hrim*+	**ya khaliq**	**Mushtari**	*Kalkala*	
4. Sun	*Bhanu**/**Shams**	heart	*brinsrin*	**ya karim**	**Shams**	*Badamta*	
5. Venus	*Sukr*/**Zahra**	throat	*bray*	**ya musakhkhir**	*Sukr*	*Saras[w]ati*	
6. Mercury	*Budh**/ **Utarid**	eyebrows	*yum*	**ya `alim**	**`Utrarid**	*Nari*	
7. Moon	*Candra*/**Qamar**	brain	*hansamansa*	**ya muhyi**	*Candra*	*Tuqla*	

NB: The spelling of Indic names and terms in Arabic script offered formidable difficulties to copyists, and as a result, frequently they are corrupted or omitted from manuscripts. Indic terms are in *italics* while Arabic terms are in **bold**. Common Hindi planet names marked with an asterisk (*) have been restored from the Persian translations, and mantras marked with a plus sign (+) are reconstructed according to Sanskrit parallels.

Although the planets in Ch. VII are given both Indian and Arab names (the former sometimes garbled), in Ch. IX, two planets (Venus and the moon) are given Indian names while the other five planets have just Arabic names; presumably this is due to the inconsistency of copyists. The names of the yogini goddesses in Ch. IX are mostly unrecognizable, except for Kali and Saraswati.

CHART 10.5

Indian names and terms in *The Pool of Nectar* with Arabic translations
(terms in brackets are speculative reconstructions)

Sanskrit	Arabic
braham	`alim (Int. 2): "scholar"
yogi	**murtad** (Int. 2): "ascetic, person of discipline"
Brahma & Visnu	**Ibrahim & Musa** (Int. 3): Abraham and Moses
alakh: unconditioned	**Allah** (II.5): God
[*yoga*]	**riyada** (IV, title): "exercise, discipline"
Gorakh (yogi)	**Khidr** (V.4): deathless prophet
Matsyendra (yogi)	**Yunus** (V.4): Jonah
Chaurangi (yogi)	**Ilyas** (V.4): Elijah
[*mantra*]	**dhikr** (V.4): "recollection, chant"
[*yantra*]	**shakl**, pl. **ashkal** (VII.1–15) : "diagram"
[*mantra*]	**al-ism al-a `zam** (VII.2): "the Greatest Name" of God
mandala	**mandala** (IX.2): "magic circle"
homa: oblation, sacrifice	**du`a** (IX.10): "prayer"
japa: counted prayer	`**azima** (IX.10): "invocation"

CHART 10.6

Yogic elements in the Arabic translation of *The Pool of Nectar*

sun and moon breaths	I.1–2, II.1
five breaths	II.2
prognostication by breath	I.3–4
sex practices from divinatory and magical texts	II.4
retention of semen	II.5, VI.5
khecari mudri, drinking nectar	II.5
prevention of disease	II.6–8
asana postures	IV.2–9
eighty-four siddhas	IV.2
kundalini (?)	V.1
three breaths	V.2
measuring breath, breath control	V.3–4
celibacy	VI.3–4, VII.13
vajroli mudra, urethral suction	VI.5
mantras	VII.1–9
seven cakras	VII.2–9
occult powers (*siddhis*)	VII.10–15
predicting time of death (pre-hatha yoga kriya tantra)	VIII.2–5
yoginis	IX.1–10
mandala	IX.2
homa	IX.10
japa	IX.10

CHART 10.7
Sample variations in Arabic transcription of
mantras in *The Pool of Nectar*

The following mantras, transliterated in Arabic script, occur in Chapter
IX, "On the Knowledge of the Subjugation of Spirits," where they
invoke seven chief yogini goddesses who are assimilated to the seven
planets. Notable variations occur in all MSS. Some Indic terms can
be distinguished, including standard seed syllables (*aum*, *hum*), the
concluding phrase *bodhi svaha*, and references to divinities, demons,
and spirits (*devata*, *devi*, *rakshasa*, *bhut pret*).

1. Saturn
   Husain: **malka tuni sandar sandar varbha rabi wakna mas daja-
   raha rabi aum kalfar yadin fum but svaha**
   Paris: **awwam kalka wamui nam nam but svaha**
   Paris marg.: **dalalasakak adiri sidi sil wadihawas raktabas san-
   haha uli aum kalfa didas**

2. Mars
   Husain: **trira devi tazkar mari bhuskafa sakfihar fi deva devata
   nari humum trira devi tarkar nari nam nam but svaha**
   Paris: **hum trira deva tarkaz marani bhusankah safkaharni devad
   devatha arni hum trira devi nam nam but svaha**

3. Jupiter
   Husain: **aum rhin kal kala dev `ind munh nam ham but svaha
   bwani kahir kahran hum rhin**
   Paris: **aum rhin kalka devi nam nam but svaha**

4. Sun
   Husain: **narayan bawayn aum tashrin hum badamiya devi nam
   nam but svaha**
   Paris: **aum hasrin brin hum badmah evi mark lujani hans kuni
   tasrin brin**

5. Venus

   Husain: **aum aum sarasati devi aum nam nam but svaha**

   Paris: **aum a iyi sarasati devi aum nam nam thumm but svaha**

6. Mercury

   Husain: **aum yum tari hu tala devi ithna rabi des des tara fi makash bhut pret tarani adam hum tara devi adam nam nam but svaha**

   Paris: **aum yum tara devi mara tanari das des marani rak`hes bhut pret aum baram nara devi aum nam tam but svaha**

7. Moon

   Husain: **aum tum tawa natari des des tara fi rak`hash bhut pret tawani adam yum adu adi adam nam nam svaha aum huwayna tutla devi nam nam svaha**

   Paris: **aum hansa tutla devi nam nam but svaha**

Sources: Yusuf Husain, "*Haud al-hayat*, la version arabe de l'Amratkuud," *Journal Asiatique* 213 (1928), pp. 291–344; and MS Paris, Bibliothéque Nationale, Ar. 1699.

11

Muslim Studies of Hinduism? A Reconsideration of Persian and Arabic Translations from Sanskrit

What have been the historical relationships between the Islamic and Hindu religious traditions? Variations on this question inevitably come to mind in any attempt to assess the significance of the past dozen centuries of South Asian civilization, during which time significant Muslim populations have played important roles, interacting with Indian religions and cultures from a variety of perspectives. Although frequently this kind of question is posed in terms of assumptions about the immutable essences of Islam and Hinduism, I would like to argue that this kind of approach is fundamentally misleading, for several reasons. First, this approach is ahistorical in regarding religions as unchanging, and it fails to account for the varied and complex encounters, relationships, and interpretations that took place between many individual Muslims and Hindus. Second, it assumes that there is a single clear concept of what a Hindu is, although this notion is increasingly coming into question; considerable evidence has accumulated to indicate that external concepts of religion, first from post-Mongol Islamicate culture, and eventually from European Christianity in the colonial period, were brought to bear on a multitude of Indian religious traditions to create a single concept of Hinduism. Third, there is a significant difference between medieval

Islamicate and modern European approaches to Indian religion and culture. It is the thesis of this essay that, although many Muslims over the centuries engaged in detailed study of particular aspects of Indian culture, which may appear in a modern perspective as religious, there was for the most part no compelling interest among Muslims in constructing a concept of a single Indian religion, which would correspond to the modern concept of Hinduism. While this thesis could be tested in many different contexts, the translations from Sanskrit into Arabic and Persian offer a particularly promising ground for examining Muslim approaches to Indian culture.

The cultural movement between the Indic and Islamicate civilizations has spanned well over a millennium. The translation movement between the Indian and Islamic cultures is still rarely studied, though as a cross-cultural event the movement from Sanskrit into Arabic and Persian is comparable in magnitude and duration to the other great enterprises of cross-cultural translation (Greek philosophy into Arabic and Latin, Buddhism from Sanskrit into Chinese and Tibetan). The following sketch is offered to suggest new lines of interpretation, to clarify the significance of this translation movement. The impetus for establishing this taxonomy is a larger study in which I analyze the translations of a text on hatha yoga, *The Pool of Nectar*, into Arabic, Persian, Turkish, and Urdu.[1] I should emphasize that the classification outlined here is still tentative, especially since the bulk of the Persian translations from Sanskrit still remain in unedited manuscripts. In most cases, little progress has been made since the work of turn-of-the century manuscript cataloguers.[2] This

---

[1] This study, entitled *The Pool of Nectar: Muslim Interpreters of Yoga*, is in preparation and should go to press soon. My critical edition of the Arabic text, together with the principal Persian translation, will be published separately.

[2] For surveys, see Hermann Ethé, "Neupersische Litteratur," part d) "Übersetzungen aus dem Sanskrit," in *Grundriss der iranischen Philologie*, ed. Wilh. Geiger and Ernst Kuhn (Strassburg: Verlag von Karl J. Trübner, 1896–1904), 2:352–55; A. B. M. Habibullah, "Medieval Indo-Persian Literature relating to Hindu Science and Philosophy, 1000–1800 A.D.," *Indian Historical Quarterly* 1 (1938): 167–81; M. A. Rahim, "Akbar and Translation Works," *Journal of the Asiatic Society of Pakistan* 10 (1965): 101–19; N. S. Gorekar, "Persian Language and Sanskritic Lore," *Indica* 2 (1965): 107–19; Muhammad Bashir Husayn, "Mughliyya dawr mēñ Sanskrit awr ʿarabī kē fārsī tarājim," in *Tārīkh-i adabiyyāt-i Musulmānān-i Pākistān u Hind*, ed. Maqbul Beg Badakhsani, vol. 4, part 2, *Fārsī adab (1526–1707)* (Lahore: Punjab University, 1971), pp. 774–804; Muhammad Akram Shah, "Dastānēñ," in ibid., pp. 866–73; N. S. Shukla, "Persian Translations of Sanskrit Works," *Indological Studies* 3 (1974): 175–91; Fathullah Mujtabai, "Persian

large field of research is therefore basically unexplored, and it is to be hoped that this study will encourage more work along similar lines.

As a first analytical approach to the subject, I suggest that among the translations from Indian languages into Arabic into Persian, four main categories of texts stand out as having special importance: 1) early Arabic and Persian translations on practical arts and sciences; 2) Persian translations of epics from the time of Akbar, having primarily political significance; 3) Persian translations of mostly metaphysical and mystical texts from the time of Dara Shikuh; and 4) Persian translations of works on Hindu ritual and law commissioned by British colonial officials. To this list one may also add original Persian works on Indian religions by Hindus as well as recent Indological studies by Iranian scholars. As this division suggests, attitudes toward Indian religion as reflected in these translations tended to be defined by the particular political and intellectual interests of the translators, rather than by any internally generated sense of the coherence of Indian religious traditions. I would argue that it is only in the fourth phase, in the British colonial period, that Persian and Arabic translations from Indian languages were viewed as representing Hindu religion as it is understood today.

PRACTICAL ARTS AND SCIENCES

The initial interest of the early Arabic translators from Sanskrit was primarily in scientific works on mathematics, medicine, toxicology, astronomy, and alchemy; a number of works of this kind were translated

---

Translations of Hindu Religious Literature," in *Yādnāma-i Ankitīl Dūparūn/Anquetil Duperron Bicentenary Memorial Volume*, ed. Farhang Mihr (Tehran: Nashriya-i Anjuman-i Farhang-i Īrān-i Bāstān, 1351/1973), pp. 13–24, with Persian translation in Persian section, "Tarjuma-hā-yi fārsī-i āṣār-i dīnī-i Hindūvān," pp. 76–106; id., "Persian Hindu Writings: Their Scope and Relevance," in his *Aspects of Hindu Muslim Cultural Relations* (New Delhi: National Book Bureau, 1978), pp. 60–91; Shriram Sharma, *A Descriptive Bibliography of Sanskrit Works in Persian*, ed. Muhammad Ahmad (Hyderabad: Abul Kalam Azad Oriental Research Institute, 1982). The most important catalogues include Hermann Ethé, *Catalogue of Persian Manuscripts in the India Office Library* (1903; repr., London: India Office Library & Records, 1980), and Charles Rieu, *Catalogue of the Persian Manuscripts in the British Museum*, 3 vols. (1879–83; repr., London: The Trustees of the British Museum, 1966). Many important items are also listed in D. N. Marshall, *Mughals in India, a Bibliographical Survey*, vol. 1, *Manuscripts* (Bombay: Asia Publishing House, 1967). I have not seen Muhammad Riza' Jalali Nā'ini, *Tarjuma-hā-yi fārsī az kutub-i sānskrīt* (Delhi, 1973).

during the heyday of the `Abbasid caliphate in the ninth and tenth centuries, apparently by Indians residing in Baghdad, though few of these survive.[3] A well-known result of this scientific exchange was the transmission of Indian numerals and the zero notation, later known in Europe as Arabic numbers. The same practical emphasis was also characteristic of some of the early translations from Sanskrit into Persian commissioned by the Turkish sultans of Delhi. As an example, when Sultan Firuz ibn Tuqhluq besieged the hill fortress of Nagarkot (Kangra) in 1365, his army plundered nearby temples and acquired a library of 1,300 Sanskrit books. Out of this booty, only a single work, "a book on natural philosophy and auguries and omens," was translated into Persian by a court poet, under the title *Dalā'il-i Fīrūz Shāhī* (*The Demonstrations of King Firuz*); from the description it seems that this work contained elements of astronomy and divination. Although this particular treatise seems not to have survived, a historian of the Mughal period who saw it commented that it was a useful work, "containing various philosophical facts both of science and practice."[4] Bada'uni, who perused the same work in Lahore in 1591, found it "moderately good, neither free from beauties nor defects," and he commented that a number of works had been translated from Sanskrit during the time of Firuz, mostly on "profitless" subjects such as music and dance.[5] In all these instances, there seems to be little interest in the religions of India, at least in comparison with the practical sciences. The story of Sultan Firuz indicates that, despite the possibility of access to a full range of Sanskrit texts, the specific interests of potential patrons of translation remained quite limited in terms of subject-matter.[6]

---

[3] See *The Fihrist of al-Nadīm: A Tenth-Century Survey of Muslim Culture*, ed. and trans. Bayard Dodge, 2 vols. (New York: Columbia University Press, 1970), 2:589–90 (Arabic translators from Sanskrit), 645 (astronomical and medical texts), 736 (occultism), 826–36 (fragmentary survey of Indian religions). A list of all known titles and manuscripts of Indian texts translated into Arabic is found in Fuat Sezgin, *Geschichte des arabischen Schrifttums* (Leiden: E. J. Brill, 1969–), 3:187–202 (medicine); 4:118–19 (alchemy); 5:191–202 (mathematics); 6:116–21 (astronomy); 7:89–97 (astrology).

[4] Nizamuddin Ahmad, *The Ṭabaqāt-i-Akbarī*, trans. B. De, Bibliotheca Indica 300 (1911; repr., Calcutta: The Asiatic Society, 1973), 1:249.

[5] `Abdu-'l-Qādir ibn-i-Mulūkshāh al-Badāonī, *Muntakhabu-'t-tawārīkh*, trans. George S. A. Ranking, Bibliotheca Indica 97 (Calcutta: The Asiatic Society of Bengal, 1898), 1:332.

[6] On the basis of Jain records, Mahdi Husain has suggested that Jain scholars writing in Sanskrit were the "philosophers" with whom Sultan Muhammad ibn Tughluq (d. 1351) associated. If correct, this would still indicate a fairly specialized interest in a minority

This practical trend in Muslim attitudes toward Indian thought seems to have been the rule, though there were some exceptions. Stories of Buddhist origin, particularly the cycle later known in Europe as Barlaam and Ioasaphath, were related by Muslim authors such as the tenth-century Brethren of Purity (Ikhwan al-Ṣafa'), who employed these stories particularly for moralizing purposes.[7] The only early Muslim scholar to show sustained interest in Indian religious and philosophical texts was the great scientist and philosopher al-Biruni. He translated a number of Sanskrit works into Arabic (including selections from Patañjali's *Yogasūtras* and the *Bhagavad Gītā*) in connection with his encyclopedic treatise on India.[8] Although the authors of Arabic books on sects and heresies, such as al-Shahrastani (d. 1153), generally devoted a section or a few pages to the religions of India, no other Arabic writer followed in al-Biruni's footsteps as a specialist on Indian religion and philosophy.[9] Wilhelm Halbfass has attempted an assessment of al-Biruni's contribution, praising him for his fair and objective approach to India:

A clear awareness of his *own* religious horizon as a particular context of thought led him to perceive the "otherness" of the Indian religious philosophical context and horizon with remarkable clarity . . . Unlike

tradition that is not today considered part of the "Hindu" fold. See his *Tughluq Dynasty* (Calcutta: Thacker Spink & Co. Pvt. Ltd., 1963), pp. 315–39.
[7] Ian Richard Netton, *Muslim Neoplatonists: An Introduction to the Thought of the Brethren of Purity (Ikhwān al-Ṣafā')* (London: George Allen & Unwin, 1982), pp. 89–94.
[8] Eduard Sachau, trans., *Alberuni's India* (1888; repr., Delhi: S. Chand & Co., 1964); Hellmut Ritter, "Al-Birūni's Übersetzung des Yoga-sūtra des Patañjali," *Oriens* 9 (1956): 165–200; Bruce B. Lawrence, "The Use of Hindu Religious Texts in al-Birūni's *India* with Special Reference to Patanjali's Yoga-Sutras," in *The Scholar and the Saint: Studies in Commemoration of Abu'l Rayhan al-Bīrūnī and Jalal al-Din al-Rūmī,* ed. Peter J. Chelkowski (New York: New York University Press, 1975), pp. 29–48; Shlomo Pines and Tuvia Gelblum, "Al-Birūni's Arabic Version of Patañjali's *Yogasūtra*: A Translation of his First Chapter and a Comparison with Related Sanskrit Texts," *BSOAS* 29 (1966): 302–25; id., "Al-Birūni's Arabic Version of Patañjali's *Yogasūtra*: A Translation of the Second Chapter and a Comparison with Related Texts," *BSOAS* 40 (1977): 522–49; id., "Al-Birūni's Arabic Version of Patañjali's *Yogasūtra*: A Translation of the Third Chapter and a Comparison with Related Texts," *BSOAS* 46 (1983): 258–304.
[9] Bruce B. Lawrence, *Shahrastānī on the Indian Religions* (The Hague: Mouton, 1976); idem, "al-Birūni and Islamic Mysticism," in *Al-Bīrūnī Commemorative Volume*, ed. Hakim Mohammed Said (Karachi: Hamdard Academy, 1979), p. 372; id., "Birūni, Abū Rayḥān. viii. Indology," *Encyclopaedia Iranica* (1990), 4:285–87.

Megasthenes, Biruni did not "translate" the names of foreign deities, nor did he incorporate them into his own pantheon, and of course he did not possess the amorphous "openness" of syncretism and the search for "common denominators." That is why he could comprehend and appreciate the other, the foreign as such, thematizing and explicating in an essentially new manner the problems of intercultural understanding and the challenge of "objectivity" when shifting from one tradition to another, from one context to another.[10]

Halbfass's admiration for the scholarly achievement of al-Biruni is certainly justified, but these remarks call for some qualification. First of all, as stated earlier, al-Biruni's perception of the "otherness" of Indian thought was not just hermeneutical clarity with regard to a pre-existing division; it was effectively the invention of the concept of a unitary Hindu religion and philosophy. Furthermore, Halbfass's praise of al-Biruni's bold proclamation of "otherness" obscures the fact that he had to engage in a remarkably complex interpretation of his sources with many "Islamizing" touches. His translation of Patañjali's *Yogasūtras* was based on a combination of the original text with a commentary that is still not identified, all rephrased by al-Biruni into a question-and-answer format. Like the translators of polytheistic Greek texts into Arabic, al-Biruni rendered the Sanskrit "gods" (*deva*) with the Arabic terms for "angels" (*malā'ikah*) or "spiritual beings" (*rūḥāniyyāt*), surely a theological shift amounting to "translation." He was, moreover, convinced on a deep level that Sanskrit texts were saturated with recognizable philosophical doctrines of reincarnation and union with God, which required comparative treatment: "For this reason their [the Indians'] talk, when it is heard, has a flavour composed of the beliefs (`aqā'id) of the ancient Greeks, of the Christian sects, and of the Sufi leaders."[11] Consequently, al-Biruni made deliberate and selective use of terms derived from Greek philosophy, heresiography, and Sufism to render the Sanskrit technical terms of yoga. But, al-Biruni's rationalistic approach to Indian religions remained isolated and almost forgotten, while his Arabic version of Patañjali was

---

[10] Wilhelm Halbfass, *India and Europe: An Essay in Understanding* (Albany: State University of New York Press, 1988), pp. 26–27.
[11] Ritter, "Al-Birūni's Übersetzung," p. 167; Pines and Gelblum, "Al-Birūni's Arabic Version," pp. 309–10.

described by at least one reader as incomprehensible.[12] There is some superficial reference to al-Biruni's work on India and the Patañjali translation in the *Bayān al-adyān* or *The Explanation of Religions* of Abu al-Ma'ali, written in Ghazna in 1092.[13] It appears, however, that the principal readers of al-Biruni's work on India were interested mainly from a historical and administrative point of view; the world-historian and Mongol minister Rashid al-Din (d. 1318) drew extensively on al-Biruni's geographical information, while the Mughal wazir Abu al-Fazl 'Allami (d. 1602) apparently had al-Biruni's work in mind when he compiled a detailed but uncritical survey of Indian thought in his Persian gazetteer of Akbar's Indian empire.[14] Today, both al-Biruni's work on India and his translation of Patañjali exist in unique manuscripts, suggesting an extremely limited circulation. I would like to suggest that al-Biruni's concept of a unified Indian religion, as a polar opposite to Islam, lay forgotten until it was resurrected in an even more radical form by European scholarship a century ago; the growth of the Muslim concept of Hindu religion took place largely without reference to al-Biruni. Since Sachau's edition (1886) and translation (1888) of al-Biruni's work on India was undertaken at the suggestion of the board of the Oriental Translation Fund and was entirely subsidized by Her Majesty's India Office, it is tempting to locate this work's historical importance primarily within the larger political concerns of colonial Orientalism.[15] Al-Biruni's rationalistic and reifying approach to religion, which had practically no impact on medieval Islamic thought, is much more palatable to the modern taste, and this explains his popularity today.

---

[12] Pines and Gelblum, "Al-Birūni's Arabic Version," p. 302, n. 1, quoting the incomprehension of Ibrahim ibn Muhammad al-Ghazanfar al-Tibrizi; Fathullah Mujtabai, "Al Biruni and India: The First Attempt to Understand," in his *Aspects of Hindu Muslim Cultural Relations*, p. 51, n. 52, cites reactions to the Patañjali translation by Persian authors Abu al-Ma'ali in his *Bayān al-adyān* and Mir Findiriski in his translation of the *Yoga vāsiṣṭa*.

[13] Abu al-Ma'ali Muhammad al-Husayni al-'Alawi, *Bayān al-adyān dar sharḥ-i adyān wa maẕāhib-i jāhilī wa islāmī*, ed. 'Abbas Iqbal Ashtiyani, Muhammad Taqi Danish Puzhuh, and Sayyid Muhammad Dabir Siyaqi (Tehran: Rawzanah, 1376/1998), pp. 23–24, 98; H. Massé, trans., "L'Exposé des religions," *Revue de l'Histoire des Religions* 94 (1926): 17–75; A. Christensen, "Remarques critiques sur le *Kitāb bayāni-l-adyān* d'Abū'l-Ma'āli," *Le Monde Oriental* 5–6 (1911–12), pp. 205–16; Lawrence, *Shahrastānī*, pp. 89–90.

[14] Halbfass, *India and Europe*, pp. 29–30 (Rashid al-Din), 32–33 (Abu al-Fazl); Abū 'l-Fazl 'Allāmi, *The Ā'īn-i Akbarī*, trans. H.S. Jarrett, ed. Jadunath Sarkar, 2nd ed. (1948; repr., New Delhi: Oriental Books Reprint Corporation, 1978), 3:vii–lx, 141–358.

[15] Sachau, *Alberuni's India*, Preface, p. l.

HISTORICAL AND POLITICAL TEXTS

The second large category of translations from Sanskrit consists of the mostly epic texts rendered into Persian during the time of Akbar. This phase of translation was dominated by historical and political considerations. Most modern discussions of the Mughal period, which speak confidently about translation of Sanskrit *religious* texts into Persian, fail to notice any ambiguity in the phrase "religious text." Today, with a comfortably solid notion of Hindu religious texts in place in the curriculum, we have no hesitation in treating epic works like the *Mahābhārata* and the *Rāmāyāna* as religious. Nonetheless, the prominent courtly and martial features of these texts furnish the occasion for questioning the assumption that the Mughals viewed their contents as religious. As we have seen, the early translations from Sanskrit into Arabic and Persian focused primarily on practical arts and sciences. Patrons of Persian learning in the later Indo-Muslim courts were also interested in translations on practical subjects, such as erotics, mathematics, astronomy, medicine, farriery, and, in particular, music.[16] Rarely, we hear of pre-Mughal translations of epic texts from Sanskrit into Persian. As early as the eleventh century C.E., a partial Persian translation of an old recension of the *Mahābhārata* was achieved, and in the fourteenth century C.E., the *Bhagavāta Purāna* was translated.[17] The ruler of Kashmir, Zayn al-`Abidin (d. 1470), had the *Mahābhārata* translated into Persian, along with the Sanskrit metrical history of Kashmir, *Rājatarangiṇī*; he was, moreover, a patron of Sanskrit literature, and he commissioned the Sanskrit historian Srivara to translate Jami's romantic Persian epic on

---

[16] See, for instance, works on erotics and farriery translated from Sanskrit to Persian and dedicated to `Abd Allah Qutbshah of Golconda (d. 1672) and Muzaffar Shah II of Gujarat (d. 1526), listed by Marshall, *Mughals in India*, p. 227, no. 792; p. 548, no. 621A. On Indian music see the numerous translations listed by Ethé, *Catalogue of Persian Manuscripts*, nos. 2008–33, and in particular Husaini, *Indo-Persian Literature*, pp. 227–47, for a detailed description of the *Lahjat-i Sikandar Shāhī*. For further examples of translations on practical subjects see also C. A. Storey, *Persian Literature: A Bio-bibliographical Survey* (London: Luzac & Company, Ltd., 1972), 2:4–5, 17, 26 (mathematics); 38, 93 (astronomy); 231, 253–54, 266 (medicine); 394–96 (farriery); 412–22 (music); 439, no. 13 (alchemy).

[17] On the early *Mahābhārata* version, see J. T. Reinaud, *Fragments arabes et persans inédits relatifs a l'Inde, anterieurement au XIe siècle* (1845; repr., Amsterdam: Oriental Press, 1976), pp. 17–29. The *Bhagavāta Purāna* translation is described by J. Aumer, *Die persischen Handschriften der K. Hof- und Staatsbibliothek in München* (Munich, 1866), cited by Ethé, *Catalogue of Persian Manuscripts*, no. 1952, col. 1091.

Joseph and Zulaykha into Sanskrit.[18] But, the remarkably high number of translations of the epics commissioned by the Mughal emperors suggest that they have a special importance connected with the political posture of that dynasty. In this connection it should be recalled that collections of Sanskrit narrative literature, principally the *Pañcatantra* and the *Hitopadeśa*, had been translated into middle Persian during the Sasanian period; when stories from this tradition were later put into Arabic by Ibn al-Muqaffa' (d. 759) under the title *Kalīla wa Dimna*, they were valued in Arabic literature primarily for their political significance.[19]

The political context for the Mughal interest in Sanskrit lies in the imperial program devised by Akbar and followed in varying degrees by his successors. Although earlier writers on the Mughals have treated this interest primarily as an indication of liberal personal religious inclinations on the part of Akbar, this romantic conception should yield to a more realistic analysis of policy aspects.[20] It is highly anachronistic to read an Enlightenment virtue of "tolerance" into the religious politics of the Mughal era. The original precedent for Akbar's policies of patronage of multiple religions is probably best sought in the Mongol era, when the prudent insurance policy of the "pagan" Mongols gave generous treatment to Buddhists, Christians, Taoists, and Muslims. Akbar's family conceived of their regime as a continuation of the neo-Mongol empire of Timur (Tamerlane); like Timur, Akbar was furnished with a genealogy that included Chingiz Khan, but in his case, it was extended to include the Mongol sun-goddess Alanquwa. The symbolism of world-domination inherent in the Mongol political tradition was given an ingenious philosophical and mystical twist in the writings of Akbar's minister Abu al-Fazl, who interpreted Akbar's role in terms of the Neoplatonic metaphysics of Ishraqi Illuminationism and the Sufi doctrine of the Perfect Man. This metaphysical apparatus was invoked not merely for its own

---

[18] Syeda Bilqis Fatema Husaini, *A Critical Study of Indo-Persian Literature during Sayyid and Lodi Period, 1414–1526 A.D.* (Delhi: M. S. Publication, 1988), pp. 15, 85; Richard Schmidt, *Das Kathakautukam des Çrivara verglichen mit Dschami's Jusuf und Zuleikha* (Kiel : C.F. Haeseler, 1893); id., *Srivara's Kathakautukam, die geschichte von Joseph in Persisch-Indischem Gewande, Sanskrit und Deutsch* (Kiel : C.F. Haeseler, 1898).

[19] Walter Harding Maurer, "Pañcatantra," *Encyclopedia of Religion* (1987), 9:161–64.

[20] See most recently John F. Richards, *The Mughal Empire*, vol. I.5 of *The New Cambridge History of India* (Cambridge: Cambridge University Press, 1993), pp. 36–40, 44–47.

philosophical consistency but essentially to undergird the authority of Akbar in an eclectic fashion.[21]

While coinage with Sanskrit formulas and patronage of different religious institutions (including "Hindu" ones) was a feature of most Indo-Muslim regimes, what distinguished the Mughals under Akbar was their attempt to re-focus all religious enthusiasm of whatever background onto the person of the emperor.[22] Akbar's sponsorship of the translation of Sanskrit works was part of the overall literary phase of his reign, which included the regular reading aloud of works from the canon of Persian court literature, history, and Sufism. He assigned to the task a number of courtiers who were scholars of Persian but presumably ignorant of Sanskrit; they were assisted, however, by Sanskrit pandits so that, from a literary point of view, the translation process probably involved a considerable amount of oral explication in vernacular Hindi prior to the composition of the Persian "translation." Some translators, like Bada'uni, assisted in this project much against their own inclinations. The extent of the sustained translation enterprise can be judged from the numerous manuscript copies, some lavishly illustrated, and the repeated revisions and new translations (in both poetry and prose) of particularly valued texts.[23] In political terms, the inclusion and translation of Sanskrit works was designed to reduce intellectual provincialism and linguistic divisiveness within the empire.[24] Sanskrit and Hindi romances, such as the story of Nala and Damayanti, seem to have been integrated into a literary continuum along with Near Eastern fables like the story of Majnun and Layla or the tales of Amir Hamza. Abu al-Fazl appears to regard the epic *Mahābhārata* and *Ramāyāna* primarily as histories of ancient India

---

[21] See the stimulating essay of Peter Hardy, "Abul Fazl's Portrait of the Perfect Padshah: A Political Philosophy for Mughal India—or a Personal Puff for a Pal?", in *Islam in India, Studies and Commentaries*, vol. 2, *Religion and Religious Education*, ed. Christian W. Troll (New Delhi: Vikas Publishing House Pvt. Ltd., 1985), pp. 114–37.

[22] For coinage with Sanskrit and patronage of non-Muslim religious institutions, see my *Eternal Garden: Mysticism, History, and Politics at a South Asian Sufi Center*, SUNY Series in Muslim Spirituality in South Asia (Albany: State University of New York Press, 1992), pp. 47–53. On Akbar as the center of all religions, see Harbans Mukhia, *Historians and Historiography During the Reign of Akbar* (New Delhi: Vikas Publishing House Pvt. Ltd., 1976), p. 70.

[23] John Seyller, *Workshop and Patron in Mughal India: The Freer Ramayana and other Illustrated Manuscripts of `Abd al-Rahim* (Zurich: Artibus Asiae, 1999).

[24] Khaliq Ahmad Nizami, *Akbar & Religion* (Delhi: Idarah-i-Adabiyat-i Delli, 1989), pp. 180–81.

with biographical and philosophical overtones. This even holds true of Puranic extensions of the epic, such as the *Harīvamsa*, which Abu al-Fazl describes only as a biography of Krishna. Akbar himself entitled the Persian translation of the *Mahābhārata* as the *Razmnāmah* or *The Book of War*, underlining its character as a martial epic.

Abu al-Fazl's complicated vision of the purpose of the *Mahābhārata* translation is worth examining in detail. On the one hand, he observes that the epic does contain remarkable philosophical and cosmological perspectives of great complexity. Abu al-Fazl notes that at least 13 different Indian schools of thought are mentioned in the text.[25] On the other hand, he points out that a quarter of its 100,000 verses are devoted to the martial epic of the war between the Kauravas and the Pandavas, making it a vade mecum for the conduct of war and battle, and much of the remainder is "advice, sermons, stories, and explanations of past romance and battle *(bazm o razm)*."[26] In one long passage in his introduction to the Persian translation of the Mahabharata, Abu al-Fazl recounts a series of justifications for the translation project, all couched as an expansion of his encomium to his patron Akbar, who is eulogized in the most hyperbolic of terms. Abu al-Fazl outlines five major objectives: reducing sectarian fighting among both Muslims and Hindus; eroding the authority of all religious specialists over the masses; deflating Hindu bigotry towards Muslims by revealing questionable Hindu doctrines; curing Muslim provincialism by exposing Muslims to cosmologies much vaster than official sacred history, and providing access to a major history of the past for the edification and guidance of rulers (the traditional ethical justification for history). This passage is translated here in full:

(1) In a smuch as the fine method of physicians of the body in physical remedies is always such [as the body], the pleasing disposition of the physicians of the soul will be according to a higher method. So why should this not be the noble nature of the chief healer of chronic illnesses of the soul [i.e., Akbar]? When with

---

[25] Abu al-Fazl, in Muhammad Riza Jalali Na'ini and Narayan Shankar Shukla, ed., *Mahābhārat, buzurgtarīn manẓūma-i kuhna-i mawjūd-i jahān*, Persian trans. from Sanskrit by Mīr Ghīyās al-Dīn `Alī Qazwini Naqib Khan et al., Hindshināsi 15–18, 4 vols. (Tehran: Kitābfurūshi Ṭuḥūri, 1358–59/1979–81), 1:xx.

[26] Ibid., 1:xl–xli.

his perfect comprehension he found that the squabbling of sects of the Muslim community (*millat-i Muḥammadī*) and the quarreling of the Hindus increased, and their refutation of each other grew beyond bounds, his subtle mind resolved that the famous books of each group should be translated into diverse tongues. Thus both factions, by the blessing of the holy words of the revered perfect one of the age [again, Akbar], holding back from excessive fault-finding and perversity, should become seekers of God. Having become aware of each other's virtues and vices, they should make laudable efforts to rectify their own states.

(2) Likewise, in every group there are some who account themselves religious authorities, on the basis of extreme, frivolous, and ignorant theories that have been advanced. They have made representations that are far from the royal road of firm wisdom, with frauds and deceptions that are memorable for the masses. These unfortunate deceivers, whether from ignorance or irreligiousness, confirm themselves in a different style in accordance with their selfish and lustful goals, having concealed the books of the ancients, the advice of the righteous, the sayings of the wise, and the weighty deeds of predecessors. Whenever the books of both factions are translated with a clear expression, understandable to the masses yet pleasing to the elite, the tabula rasa of the masses attains reality, and is rescued from the idiocies of fools pretending to be wise, thus reaching the goal of reality.

Therefore, the sublime decree went forth concerning the book of the *Mahābhārata*, written by masters of genius, containing most of the principles and applications of the beliefs of the Brahmins of India, than which there is no book more famous, greater, or more detailed among this group. The wise of both factions and the linguists of both groups, by way of friendship and agreement, should sit down in one place, and should translate it into a popular expression, with the knowledge of judicious experts and just officials.

(3) Likewise, the irreligious partisans and credulous leaders of India have a belief in their own religion that goes beyond all measure, and whether from lack of discrimination or ingrained injustice, they consider the embellishments of their beliefs to be free from

error, taking the path of blind imitation. Having made certain representations to the artless masses, they are prevented from realizing their goals and become rooted in false beliefs. They regard the group of those who are connected to the religion of Muḥammad (*dīn-i Aḥmadī*) as utterly foolish, and they refute this group ceaselessly, although they are unaware of its noble goals and special sciences.

Therefore, the subtle intellect [of Akbar] desired that the book of the *Mahābhārata*, which contains the jewels of the goals of this group, should be translated with a clear expression, so that deniers should restrain their denial and refrain from intemperance, and so that the artless believers, having become somewhat embarrassed by their beliefs, should become seekers of God.

(4) Likewise, the common people among the Muslims, who have not read well the pages of scriptures and religious books, and who have not opened the admonition-seeing eye to the diverse histories of the age belonging to the Chinese, the Indians, etc., and who have not even read the words of the great ones of their own religion, such as Imam Ja`far Sadiq, Ibn `Arabi, and others, believe that the beginning of humanity was some seven thousand years ago. They consider the scientific realities and intellectual subtleties that are famous and well-known among the peoples of the world as the products of the thinking of the men of the past seven thousand years. Therefore the beneficent mind (of Akbar) decided that this book, which contains the explanation of the antiquity of the universe and its beings, and is even totally occupied with the eternity of the world and its inhabitants, should be translated into a quickly understood language, so that this group favored by divine mercy should become somewhat informed and retreat from this distasteful belief [in the recent creation of the world]. It will become clear that these subtle sciences and subtle understandings have no obvious end, and these precious jewels of wisdom have no beginning.

(5) Likewise, the minds of most people, especially the great kings, love to listen to histories, for the wisdom that is contained in the divine makes the science of history attractive to their hearts, for it supplies admonition for the wise. Taking counsel from the past and

counting it as bounty for the present time, they may expend their precious hours in that which is pleasing to God. Therefore kings are most in need of listening to the tales of their predecessors. Thus the wisdom-nourishing mind [of Akbar] had complete oversight on the translation of this book, which contains illustrious examples of this science. For this reason a group was gathered together of wise men who know languages, distinguished for broad wisdom and wide reading, far from partisanship and contentiousness and close to justice and equity, and they translated the aforementioned book with deliberation and penetration, with clear expressions and familiar terms. Different groups of people love to take copies to different corners of the world.[27]

Abu al-Fazl was interested in the philosophical and religious content of the epic, from the perspective of an enlightened intellectual whose cosmopolitan vision had moved him out of a strictly defined Islamic theological perspective. But, I think it is fair to say that this intellectual project was thoroughly subordinated to the political aim of making Akbar's authority supreme over all possible rivals in India, including all religious authorities. The translation of the Sanskrit epics was not an academic enterprise comparable to the modern study of religion; it was instead part of an imperial effort to bring both Indic and Persianate culture into the service of Akbar.

The historiographical continuity between Sanskrit and Persian literary traditions can be glimpsed further in the case of Tahir Muḥammad Sabzawari, an official in the employ of Akbar, who, in 1011/1602–3, made abridged prose translations of the *Bhāgavata Purāna*, the *Mahābhārata*, and its appendix the *Harīvamsa*.[28] Four years later, when he wrote a world history in Persian called *Rawżat al-ṭāhirīn* or *The Garden of the Pure*, one of the five sections contained Indian historical

---

[27] Ibid., xviii–xx. In translating the third sentence of this passage, I have emended the printed text to read *juḥūd-i hunūd* ("the quarreling of the Hindus") instead of *juḥūd u hunūd*. Also, in the first sentence of the second paragraph under point (3), I read *ra`s* instead of *raghs* (meaning *ra`s wa samīn*, i.e., jewels).

[28] Ethé, *Catalogue of Persian Manuscripts*, no. 1955.

traditions culled from the *Mahābhārata* and other Sanskrit epics.[29] The only translated text that Abu al-Fazl specifically refers to as scriptural or religious is an incomplete version of the *Atharva Veda*, "which, according to the Hindus, is one of the four divine books."[30] No copy of this survives, however. Another popular Sanskrit text, the *Singhāsan Battīsī* or *Thirty-Two Tales of the Throne*, concerned the fortunes of the ancient Indian king Vikramaditya; one of the Persian translations of this work presented to Akbar was entitled *Shāhnāmah* or *The Book of Kings*, the very same as the title of Firdawsi's epic on Persian kingship.[31] The evidence suggests that one of Akbar's purposes was the absorption of Indian traditions of kingship into a form that he could take advantage of. One of the likely political fruits of the translation project was the rumor, noticed by the European traveler Oranus, that Akbar was the 10th incarnation of Vishnu.[32] Another piece of symbolic fallout was the custom of weighing the emperor in gold, which, as Abu al-Fazl noted, was a custom that Indian tradition associated with both beatitude and universal monarchy.[33] Perhaps most importantly, Akbar's project succeeded in permitting the interweaving of two historical narratives. Many Persian world histories and histories of Mughal India continued to portray a single line of political authority drawn exclusively through Muslim rulers, back through the sultans of Delhi to their Central Asian and Iranian predecessors. But a significant number of Indo-Persian dynastic histories would place the later Mughals in a series of "the kings of India" beginning with Yudhishthira and the heroes of the *Mahābhārata*.[34] In the same vein, Firishta (d. ca. 1633) prefaces his famous history of Indo-Muslim dynasties with an account of Indian epic history drawn from the *Mahābhārata* that is completely interwoven with the heroic cycles of the

---

[29] Marshall, *Mughals in India*, no. 1768.
[30] Abu al-Fazl, *The Āʾīn-i Akbarī*, 3:110–12. This translation, entitled *Atharban* in Persian, was entrusted to Badaʾuni, but he abandoned it after failing to find a competent pandit.
[31] Marshall, *Mughals in India*, no. 384.
[32] J. Talboys, ed., *Early Travels in India (16th & 17th Centuries)* (1864; repr., Delhi: Deep Publications, 1974), p. 78.
[33] Abu al-Fazl, *The Āʾīn-i Akbarī*, 3:307. For the practice of weighing the emperor, see Mubarak Ali, *The Court of the Great Mughuls, Based On Persian Sources* (Lahore: Book Traders, 1986), pp. 51–53.
[34] Storey, *Persian Literature*, 1:133 ff (general histories), 1:442 ff. (histories of India).

Persian *Book of Kings*.[35] Eventually, as a result of this process, the Ranas of Udaipur and the Sisodia Rajputs, noble Hindu houses in Mughal service, adopted genealogies traced to Persian kings.[36]

METAPHYSICAL AND MYSTICAL TEXTS

After the political phase of translation we can distinguish a third group of Persian translations from the Sanskrit, in this case focusing on works that may be called metaphysical or mystical. This type of translation typically mediated Vedantic philosophical and mystical texts through a loose oral commentary provided by Indian pandits; this was rephrased in the Sufi technical vocabulary, presenting the texts as a kind of gnosis (Persian *ma'rifat*) and frequently amplifying their contents by the insertion of Persian mystical verses. Many Sanskrit works were translated by members of the circle of Akbar's great-grandson Dara Shikuh (d. 1659). Banwali Das, also known as Wali Ram (d. 1667–68), an accomplished poet and historian in Dara Shikuh's service, produced a Persian translation of *Prabhodacandrodaya*, a Vedantic theological allegory in dramatic form composed by Krishna Das for the eleventh-century Chandella king Kirtivarman. This translation was entitled *Gulzār-i ḥāl yā ṭulū'-i qamar-i ma'rifat*, meaning *The Rose-garden of Ecstasy, or the Rising of the Moon of Gnosis*; Banwali Das regarded the text as a veritable "bouquet of reality and gnosis." In describing the genesis of the original text, Banwali Das related it to classical Indian metaphysical works, calling the latter "books of Sufism and unity (*taṣawwuf wa tawḥīd*)" and "texts of Sufism."[37] It is also likely that Banwali Das had a hand in a translation of the shorter version of the *Yoga Vāsiṣṭha*, a treatise on Vedantic metaphysics that employs narrative to explore the nature of illusion and reality; this was commissioned by Dara Shikuh

---

[35] Mahomed Kasim Ferishta, *History of the Rise of the Mahomedan Power in India, Till the Year A.D. 1612*, trans. J. Briggs, 4 vols. (1829; repr., Lahore: Sang-e Meel Publications, 1977), 1:xlv–lxiii.

[36] James Tod, *Annals and Antiquities of Rajast'han, or The Central and Western Rajpoots of India*, 2 vols. (1829–32; repr., London: George Routledge & Sons Limited, 1914), 1:192.

[37] *Gulzār-i ḥāl yā ṭulū'-i qamar-i ma'rifat/Prabodhachandrodaya*, Persian trans. from Sanskrit by Banwali Das, ed. Tara Chand and Amir Hasan 'Abidi (Aligarh: Aligarh Muslim University, 1967), pp. 6–7.

because of his dissatisfaction with earlier versions.[38] Another scholar in the service of Dara Shikuh, Chandarbhan Barahman (d. 1657–58), translated a Vedantic work of Śankara, the *Ātma-vilāsa*, under the title *Nāzuk khayālāt* or *Subtle Imaginings*.[39] Both of these Hindu *munshī*s (or scribes) were intensively involved in the Persianate culture of the Mughal court, and both wrote Persian poetry in the Sufi mystical style; Banwali Das even took instruction from Dara Shikuh's Sufi master Mulla Shah, and in his translation work from Sanskrit, he was forced to rely on the oral Hindi commentary of a well-known pandit. There were other contemporary students of Indian mysticism outside the circle of Dara Shikuh, such as ʿAbd al-Rahman Chishti (d. 1683), who produced a Sufi interpretation of the *Bhagavad Gītā* in a text called *Mirʾāt al-ḥaqāʾiq* or *The Mirror of Realities*.[40]

In addition to translations, one may include in the metaphysical category several original Persian treatises by Muslim authors from different historical periods, who explored questions raised by Vedantic texts and related them to Islamicate philosophical and mystical themes. An early example of this kind of text is Fayzi's *Shāriq al-maʿrifa* or *The Illuminator of Gnosis*, which dealt with topics taken from the *Yoga Vāsiṣṭha* and the *Bhāgavata Purāna*; as the title suggests, this study was carried out in terms of categories derived from the Ishraqi or Illuminationist philosophy of Suhrawardi.[41] Another transitional text was an early version of the *Yoga Vāsiṣṭha* translated by Nizam al-Din Panipati at the request of Prince Salim (later Jahangir) in 1597. This

---

[38] Storey, *Persian Literature*, 1:450–52. See *Jūg bashist/Yogavāsiṣṭha*, Persian trans. from Sanskrit by Banwali Das, ed. Tara Chand and Amir Hasan ʿAbidi (Aligarh: Aligarh Muslim University, 1967). See also Swami Venkatesananda, trans., *The Concise Yoga Vāsiṣṭha* (Albany, NY: State University of New York Press, 1984); Wendy Doniger O'Flaherty, *Dreams, Illusion and Other Realities* (Chicago: University of Chicago Press, 1984); and my review of the latter in *Journal of Asian and African Studies* 20 (1985): 252–54.

[39] Storey, *Persian Literature*, 1:570–72; this was printed at Lahore in 1901. See also Sharif Husain Qasemi, "Čandra Bhān Barahman," *Encyclopaedia Iranica* (1990), 4:755–56. Another unidentified work on Hinduism by Chandarban, in question and answer form, is found in Berlin. See Wilhelm Pertsch, *Die Handschriften-Verzeichnisse der Königlichen Bibliothek zu Berlin*, IV, *Perischen Handschriften* (Berlin: Buchdr. der Koünigl. Akademie der Wissenschaften, 1888), no. 1081/2.

[40] Roderic Vassie, "ʿAbd al-Rahman Chishti & the Bhagavadgita: 'Unity of Religion' Theory in Practice," in *The Legacy of Mediaeval Persian Sufism*, ed. Leonard Lewisohn (London: Khaniqahi Nimatullahi, 1992), pp. 367–78.

[41] Ethé, *Catalogue of Persian Manuscripts*, no. 1975.

translation, which Dara Shikuh considered unreliable, was conceived as part of the encyclopedic collection of edifying literature initiated by Akbar, and this particular work was regarded by Salim as falling into the same category with Sufi writings. Prince Salim remarked,

> When expert Arabic linguists, specialists in the different sciences, connoisseurs of the arts of poetry and prose, historians, and Indian pundits entered the noble presence in the style of his imperial majesty, . . . the *Ma̲s̲navī* of Mawlana Rumi, the *Z̤afarnāmah* [a history of Tamerlane], the memoirs of Babur, other written histories, and collections of stories were read out in turn. Stories containing morals and advice were conveyed to the august hearing. In these days, it is commanded that the book *Yogavāsiṣṭha*, which contains Sufism (*taṣawwuf*) and provides commentary on realities, diverse morals, and remarkable advice, and which is one of the famous books of the Brahmins of India, should be translated from the Sanskrit language to Persian.[42]

The translator, however, felt that the Brahmins were closer to the ancient philosophers (i.e., the Greeks), and in any case, he proclaimed his intention to gloss over any contradictions, which must be purely verbal.

Dara Shikuh himself supervised the Persian translation of 50 of the most important Indian scriptures, the Upanishads, under the title *Sirr-i Akbar* or *The Greatest Mystery*.[43] He is also credited with a translation of the *Bhagavad Gītā* entitled *Āb-i zindagī* or *The Water of Life*, and a version of the Vedas.[44] Another Sanskrit work translated for Dara is the *Aṣṭavakragītā*, a dialogue on liberation.[45] What is most distinctive about Dara Shikuh's approach to Indian texts is that he treats them as

---

[42] *Jūg bashisht*, p. xxx.

[43] Erhard Böbel-Gross, *Sirr-i akbar, Die Persische Upanishad Übersetzung des Mogulprinzen Dārā Shikūhs* (Marburg, 1962); a Hindi translation from the Persian is available under the title *Sirre akabara*, ed. Salama Mahaphuza (New Delhi: : Meharacanda Lachamanadasa Pablikesansa, 1988).

[44] The ascription of this *Gītā* version to Dara Shukuh is described as doubtful by Storey, *Persian Literature*, 1:996, n. 1. On the Veda translation, see the description of an autograph MS, Brij Mohan Birla Research Centre, Ujjain (connected with Vikram University, Ujjain), cited in *Motilal Banarsidass Newsletter* (August 1983), p. 9.

[45] Berlin MS 1077/3. Another copy is described by Nazir Ahmad, "Notes on Important Arabic and Persian MSS, found in Various Libraries in India—II," *Journal of the Asiatic Society of Bengal* 14 (1918): cxcvix-ccclvi, esp. p. ccxxix, no. 24, dated 1676.

scripture, in the same category as the Psalms of David, the Gospel, and the Qur'an.[46] Sufis such as Mirza Mazhar Jan-i Janan (d. 1781) also made this theological concession, but typically with the stipulation that such ancient scriptures had been abrogated by the most recent revelation, the Qur'an.[47] Dara Shikuh viewed the Upanishads as hermeneutically continuous with the Qur'an, providing an extended exposition of the divine unity that was only briefly indicated in the Arabic scripture. Among Dara Shikuh's original contributions was a comparative study in Persian of the vocabulary of Hindu and Islamic esotericism, entitled *Majma` al-baḥrayn* or *The Meeting-place of the Two Oceans*.[48] It is interesting to note that this Persian work has been translated into Arabic, Urdu, and Sanskrit.[49] The *Majma` al-baḥrayn* has unfortunately been subjected to superficial interpretations deriving from the inadequate edition and English translation of the text made by Mahfuz-ul-Haq in 1929; luckily, this has been superseded by a superior critical edition published by the Iranian scholar Jalali Na'ini in 1956, which was revised again in 1987.[50] Just to give one example of the problems in the first edition, Mahfuz-ul-Haq translated the title as *The Mingling of the Two Oceans*,

---

[46] Mir Findariski (d. 1640), who produced a translation of the *Yogavāsiṣṭha*, showed a similar attitude in these verses: "These words are just like water to the world, pure and enlightening like the Qur'an. / When you have passed through the Qur'an and Prophetic sayings, no one [else] has this way of speaking" (*Jūg bashisht*, p. xxxi).

[47] Yohanan Friedmann, "Medieval Muslim Views of Indian Religions," *Journal of the American Oriental Society* 95 (1975): 214–21.

[48] See the studies of Jean Filliozat, "Sur les Contreparties indiennes du soufisme," *Journal Astiatique* 268 (1980): 259 73, and Daryush Shayegan, *Les Relations de l'Hindouisme et du Soufisme d'après le Majma` al-Bahrayn de Dârâ Shokûh*, Collection Philosophia Perennis (Paris: Éditions de la Différence, 1979); id., "Muḥammad Dārā Shukūh, Bunyānguẕār-i `irfān-i taṭbiqi," *Īrān Nāmah* 1, no. 2 (1990).

[49] The Arabic version of *Majma` al-baḥrayn* by Muhammad Salih ibn Ahmad al-Misri, completed before 1771, is found in the Buhar collection (National Library, Calcutta), MS 133 Arabic. The Urdu translation by Gokul Prasad, entitled *Nūr-i `ayn* or *Light of the Eye*, was lithographed at Lucknow in 1872. For the Sanskrit version, see Roma Chaudhuri, *A Critical Study of Dārā Shikūh's Samudra-sangama*, 2 vols., Prācyavāni-mandira Comparative Religion and Philosophy Series 2 (Calcutta: Prācyavāni-mandira, 1954).

[50] *Majma`-ul-baḥrain or The Mingling of the Two Oceans*, ed. M. Mahfuz-ul-Haq, Biblioteca Indica 246 (Calcutta: Asiatic Society of Bengal, 1929); *Muntakhabāt-i āṣār-i Muḥammad ibn Shāhjahān Qādirī Dārā Shukūh*, ed. Muhammad Riza Jalali Na'ini (Tehran: Kitābfurūshī Iqbāl, 1335/1956); *Majma` al-baḥrayn*, ed. Muhammad Riza Jalali Na'ini (Tehran: Nashr-i Nuqrah, 1366/1987 88).

intending it as a heavy-handed metaphor for the literal syncretism, or mixing together, of two religions (Hinduism and Islam) conceived as oceans. He evidently was unaware, or considered it unimportant, that the phrase "the meeting-place of the two oceans" is Qur'anic (18:60). In the Qur'an, this phrase refers to the place where Moses found the water of eternal life and the mysterious servant of God usually identified as Khizr.[51] The allusion to the contrast between the legalistic prophet Moses and the esoteric gnostic Khizr forms the basis for Dara Shikuh's description of the importance of this text.

Dara Shikuh states that after having immersed himself in the truths of Sufi doctrine, he desired to comprehend the doctrines of the Indian monotheists (*muwaḥḥidān*) and realizers of truth (*muḥaqqiqān*).

> Since [this book] is the meeting place of the realities and gnostic truths of two groups that know God (*ḥaqq-shinās*), it is known as *The Meeting-place of the Two Oceans*. . . . I have written this investigation in accordance with my own mystical unveiling and experience (*kashf u zawq*), for the sake of my own family, and I have nothing to do with the common people of either community.[52]

This focus on esoteric truth and the caustic disregard for external religion that was so characteristic of Dara Shikuh is described in a distorted fashion by Mahfuz-ul-Haq as "an attempt to reconcile Hinduism and Islam."[53] This simplistic terminology suggests again that Hinduism and Islam are monolithic and unchanging hostile essences that need to be pacified. Dara Shikuh's interest was in a particular kind of mystical and esoteric knowledge that was shared, in his view, by a small elite within both communities; this he had observed in conversations with Sufis and with accomplished Indian mystics such as Baba La'l Das. The Hindu and Muslim masses, however, were utterly ignorant of this gnosis. Dara Shikuh implicitly accepted the politicized terminology that equated the Hindu with unbelief or infidelity (*kufr*), even as he questioned, from a

---

[51] A. J. Wensinck, "al-Khaḍir," *Shorter Encyclopaedia of Islam*, p. 232b.

[52] *Majmaʿ al-baḥrayn*, ed. Jalali Na'ini, p. 2; cf. Mahfuz-ul-Haq, ed., *Majmaʿ-ul-bahrain*, p. 38.

[53] Mahfuz-ul-Haq, ed., *Majmaʿ-ul-bahrain*, Introduction, p. 27; the phrase is repeated by Storey, *Persian Literature*, 1:994.

Sufi perspective, the opposition between infidelity and Islam.[54] His focus on esoteric doctrine from a Sufi perspective made his approach to Indian religion highly selective.

ANGLO-PERSIAN TEXTS

The last major category of Persian translations from Sanskrit and other Indian languages consists of an extensive series of works commissioned by British colonial officials in India, but it may also be expanded to include other Persian translations utilized by Europeans for the study of Hindu law, religion, and cosmology. This phase may be known for convenience as Anglo-Persian literature. Here, at last we have a series of texts that deal tentatively with "Hindu" or (as it was then known) "Gentoo" religion, from the perspective of religion as understood in Christian Europe. Warren Hastings commissioned a Persian translation of a Sanskrit compendium on Hindu law for the use of East India Company officials, and in 1776, Nathaniel Halhed (d. 1830) produced an English version of this under the title *A Code of Gentoo Laws*, one of the first translations of a Hindu text available in Europe.[55] A Persian paraphrase of the laws of Manu was prepared for Sir William Jones, and the manuscript contains English and Devanagari marginalia as well as a piece of doggerel Persian verse by Jones using the pen-name

---

[54] In the opening lines of *Majma' al-bahrayn* (p. 1), Dara Shikuh quotes a version of a famous verse by the poet Sana'i (d. 1131), "Infidelity and religion (*kufr wa dīn*) are both following in your path, crying, `He alone, he has no partner!`" This verse is a quotation from the beginning of the Sana'i's classic Sufi epic *Ḥadīqat al-ḥaqīqat*. In its original context, it is an illustration of the Sufi concept of mystical infidelity as non-duality (see my *Words of Ecstasy in Sufism*, SUNY Series in Islam [Albany: State University of New York Press, 1985], pp. 63–96). In Dara Shikuh's version, however, the verse reads, "Infidelity and *islām*," giving it a political character implying Hindu and Islamic communities or doctrines. In this he followed the same wording (and implications) as Abu al-Fazl, who is said to have engraved this verse on a temple used by Indian "monotheists" (*muwaḥḥidun*) in Kashmir (Abu'l Fazl, *Ā'īn*, 1:liv–lvi). Ironically, this verse as quoted here by Dara Shikuh was seized upon by Awrangzib as evidence of his brother's apostasy from Islam, despite its classical origins in the Sufi tradition (see Anees Jahan Syed, *Aurangzeb in Muntakhab-al lubab* [Bombay: Somaiya Publications Pvt. Ltd, 1977], p. 77).

[55] Rosanne Rocher, *Orientalism, Poetry, and the Millennium: The Checkered Life of Nathaniel Brassey Halhed, 1751–1830* (Delhi: Motilal Banarsidass, 1983), pp. 48–72.

"Yunus."[56] Hastings commissioned in 1784 the composition of a Sanskrit text on chronology and cosmology, *Purānārtha Prakāśa*, from which a Persian translation was prepared in 1786 by Zurawar Singh, also on the instructions of Hastings; this, in turn, was put into English by Halhed.[57] Another untitled work on cosmogony, mythology, and history compiled from Sanskrit sources was commissioned by Hastings and composed by one Karparam, of whom Halhed writes that he was "a Moonshy [i.e, *munshī* or scribe] in the Persian Translator's office at Calcutta. He was well versed in Hindoo learning, and his knowledge of the Persian and Arabic, added to Sanscrit and Bengalee, gave advantage over most of the Pandeets."[58] Sir John Murray in 1796 commissioned an unknown author to compose a Persian work entitled *Zakhīrat al-fu'ād* or *The Treasury of the Heart* as a work on Hindu religious duties based on "the Śastra, the purana, the pandits, and the Veda reciters (*bēd-khwānān*)." While this contained information from both scriptural and oral sources on festivals, cosmogony, and castes, it also provided a guide to the tilak marks worn by various religious groups on the forehead, with illustrations.[59]

Regional and sectarian emphases accompanied the encyclopedic tendency in the study of Hinduism through Persian. Some Persian translations were produced for Jonathan Duncan by Anandaghana "Khwush," who rendered several puranic texts on sacred Hindu places of pilgrimage. His lengthy *Baḥr al-najāt* or *The Sea of Salvation* (completed 1794) was taken from the *Kāśī-khandā* section of the *Skanda purāna*, describing the mythic features of Benares, and his Persian *Gayā mahātmya* (1791)

---

[56] Pertsch, *Die Handschriften-Verzeichnisse*, no. 1082. Since this curious Persian verse by Jones (in the meter of the *Shāhnāmah*) may not have been noticed by his biographers, it may be worth translating, as follows: "Act thus with goodness and justice, Yunus, with compassion for creatures and fear of God, / so that after your death, all humanity, in Indian and China, will bless you. / Your companions will lament over your bier, the Musulman wailing with lacerated breast, / the Brahman reciting the Veda over it, and the Sufi scattering wine over it."

[57] Ethé, *Catalogue of Persian Manuscripts*, no. 2003; Rieu, *Catalogue of the Persian Manuscripts*, 1:63–64 (the Sanskrit text is Or. 1124, the Persian trans. is Add. 5655, and the English version is Add. 5657, fols. 163–94). A similar work composed by Kanchari Singh in 1782 is found in Berlin (Pertsch, *Die Handschriften-Verzeichnisse*, no. 1083).

[58] Rieu, *Catalogue of the Persian Manuscripts*, 1:63 (Add. 5654).

[59] Pertsch, *Die Handschriften-Verzeichnisse*, no. 1076; cf. Rieu, *Catalogue of the Persian Manuscripts*, 2:792b/ii. On Murray (d. 1822), who commissioned a number of Persian treatises, see Storey, *Persian Literature*, 1:1145, n. 1; ibid., 2:375 (works on agriculture).

concerned the virtues and rituals of Gaya in Bihar.[60] The transitional role of Anandaghana is reflected by a collection of Persian Sufi poems that he completed at the same time (1794) on the model of Rumi's *Maṣnavī*, extolling among other things the virtues of Benares and the thought of Dara Shikuh.[61] A number of works on Burmese Buddhism were trans-lated into Persian after 1779 from the Mugh language at the instance of Sir John Murray and others; these included Jataka stories as well as works on law, cosmology, and medicine.[62] Some Sanskrit Jain works in Devanagari script, accompanied by commentaries in Persian, were pre-pared for the French adventurer General Claude Martin in 1796. Andrew Sterling between 1812 and 1821 commissioned an accountant at the Jagannath temple to write Persian translations of Orissi writings about the temple and on local history.[63] Works of a proto-anthropological cast were also produced, prefiguring the later census categories. Among these was *Riyāẓ al-maẕāhib* or *The Garden of Religions*, which was composed by a Brahmin named Mathuranath at the request of John Glyn in 1812 and dedicated to the Governor-General of India, Lord Moira; this was a description of Hindu castes and sects, as well as religious orders and non-Vedic groups such as Jains and Sikhs, and it was found very useful by the early Indologist H. H. Wilson.[64] A similar work on castes and men-dicant orders was compiled by Col. John Skinner in 1825 from Sanskrit sources that he had translated to Persian. This curious manuscript, enti-tled *Tashrīḥ al-aqwām* or *The Description of Peoples*, contained over one hundred illustrations by native artists.[65]

---

[60] Ethé, *Catalogue of Persian Manuscripts*, nos. 1959, 1962.

[61] Ethé, *Catalogue of Persian Manuscripts*, nos. 1725, 2905.

[62] Pertsch, *Die Handschriften-Verzeichnisse*, no. 1089 (Jātaka), 1090–91 (law), 1093 (cos-mology), 1094–95 (medicine).

[63] Pertsch, *Die Handschriften-Verzeichnisse*, 1078/3–4.

[64] Rieu, *Catalogue of the Persian Manuscripts*, 1:64 (Add. 24,035); Sayyid ʿAbd Allah, *Adabiyyāt-i fārsī mēñ Hindū'ūñ kā ḥiṣṣa*, Silsila-i Maṭbūʿāt-i Anjuman-i Taraqqi-i Urdū (Hind) 187 (Delhi: Anjuman-i Taraqqi-i Urdū [Hind], 1942), p. 215, no. 5. This Urdu study is now available in a Persian translation by Muhammad Aslam Khan, *Adabiyyāt-i fārsī dar miyān-i Hindūvān* (Tehran: Bunyād-i Mawqūfāt-i Duktur Maḥmūd Afshār, 1371/1992).

[65] Rieu, *Catalogue of the Persian Manuscripts*, 1:65–67 (Add. 27,255); Nora M. Titley, *Miniatures from Persian Manuscripts: A Catalogue and Subject Index of Paintings from Persia, India and Turkey in the British Library and the British Museum* (London, 1977), no. 372. See further on Skinner and Company art Mildred Archer and Toby Falk, *India Revealed: The Art and Adventures of James and William Fraser 1801–35* (London: Cassell, 1989), index, s.n. Skinner.

In addition to the commissioned works, a number of manuscripts of Persian translations of Sanskrit texts such as the *Mahābhārata* bear the marginal comments of the English officials who owned them. Among such works in the India Office Library, there are quite a few bearing the comments of Richard Johnson, who acquired several of these copies in 1778, and there are even a couple of manuscripts annotated by Sir Charles Wilkins (d. 1826), England's first notable Sanskritist after Sir William Jones. Halhed's collection of a dozen annotated Persian translations of Sanskrit texts, some accompanied by his own English summaries and translations, forms the core of the British Library's collection of this branch of literature.

This body of translations commissioned by the British is sufficiently large to be indicative of a separate trend and approach to the study of Indian religion, for the special purpose of familiarizing British colonial administrators with the religion of their Hindu subjects. This had a practical purpose beyond the concerns of pure historical scholarship. Witness the project that Sir William Jones took up for the East India Company: the compilation of a digest of Hindu law from Sanskrit texts for the express purpose of serving as a reliable legal source for personal law in the British-run court system. Not only the Persian translations from the Sanskrit commissioned by the British, but also previous Mughal-era translations (whether belonging to the political or metaphysical categories described above), were all subsumed into a single vision of the religion of the Hindus, from the perspective of the British administrators who used Persian as the language of governance in India. It is often forgotten that Persian, the language of administration and government revenue records in the Mughal empire, continued to be the medium of government in the British East India Company until the 1830s, and in some regions, as late as the 1860s. It should not be surprising, then, that figures such as Hastings regarded Persian translations as a perfectly adequate basis for establishing their knowledge of Hindu religion; they evidently considered it to be a medium transparent enough for their purposes. Nonetheless, the interest of the British administrators in discovering the textual basis for personal law for Hindus eventually led them to take extraordinary steps to set up a dyadic opposition between Hinduism and Islam.[66]

---

[66] Rosane Rocher, "British Orientalism in the Eighteenth Century: The Dialectics of Knowledge and Government," in *Orientalism and the Postcolonial Predicament: Perspectives on South Asia*, ed. Carol A. Breckenridge and Peter van der Veer (Philadelphia: University of Pennsylvania Press, 1993), pp. 215–49.

Until the formation of a solid European tradition of Sanskrit scholarship, the earlier Orientalists continued to rely on these Persian translations as the best available guides to Hindu philosophy and religion. The Upanishads were initially introduced to Europeans through several versions of Dara Shikuh's Persian translation: first, the partial English translation of Halhed in 1782; next, Anquetil Duperron's Latin version in 1801, which had a significant impact on European thinkers such as Schopenhauer; and then a German translation from Duperron's Latin, completed by Franz Mischel in 1882.[67] European scholars drew upon Abu al-Fazl's account of Indian philosophy for some of their earliest descriptions of this subject.[68] The Sanskrit collection of stories about King Vikramaditya, *Singhāsan Battīsī*, was also made known initially through a French version of a Mughal-era Persian translation in 1817.[69] As late as 1831, a partial English version of the *Mahābhārata* was made available via the Persian translation sponsored by Akbar.[70]

This period when Persian was the primary mode of access to Hindu religious thought has been largely forgotten in European scholarship. The next generation of Sanskritists after Sir William Jones, particularly British officials such as Sir Charles Wilkins and H. H. Wilson, were usually still familiar with Persian because of their administrative involvement. Increasingly, however, Sanskrit became a subject unto itself, achieving a high level of academic prestige, particularly in the German universities. As scholars began to have full and independent access to Sanskrit literature, they soon cast aside the earlier interpretations gained via the medium of Persian. I would suggest that the mode of scholarship that came to dominate the European study of Sanskrit, especially outside of British circles, selfconsciously tried to stand apart from the naive practicality of Halhed and Hastings. Following the model of the

---

[67] On Duperron's translation, entitled *Oupnek'at, id est secretum tegendum*, see Annemarie Schimmel, *Mystical Dimensions of Islam* (Chapel Hill, NC: University of North Carolina Press, 1975), p. 361; Bikrama Jit Hasrat, *Dara ShikohShikoh, Life and Works*, 2nd ed. (New Delhi: Munshiram Manoharlal, 1982), pp. 255–58.

[68] J. G. Schweighaeuser, "Sur les sects philosophiques de l'Inde," *Archives literaires de l'Europe* 16 (1807): 193–206.

[69] M. Lescallier, trans., *Vikramacaritra: Le Trone enchanté*, 2 vols. (New York: J. Desnoues, 1817).

[70] David Price, *The last days of Krishna and the sons of Pandu from the concluding section of the Mahābhārata translated from the Persian version made by Naqıb Khan, in the time of the Emperor Akbar, published together with miscellaneous translation* (London: Oriental Translation Fund, 1831).

Greek and Latin classics, Sanskrit became a classical study; applying the methods of textual criticism developed by Renaissance scholars, Sanskritists began to look for the original textual archetypes, the *Ur*-text uncorrupted by medieval intrusions. The Persian translations were seen as inaccurate, biased, and faulty guides, an embarrassment to the serious study of true Hinduism. They are now mentioned only as curiosities or passed over in silence. They are no longer relevant to the modern study of classical Hinduism, which has been defined precisely as the original Indian religion as distinct from the foreign influence of Islam. We can see this attitude at work already in Sir William Jones:

> My experience justifies me in pronouncing that the Mughals have no idea of accurate translation, and give that name to a mixture of gloss and text with a flimsy paraphrase of both; that they are wholly unable, yet always pretend, to write Sanskrit words in Arabic letters; . . . from the just severity of this censure I except neither Abul Fazl nor his brother Faizi.[71]

This classicist approach unfortunately has the side effect of relegating to insignificance the participation of Hindus in Persianate and Islamicate culture, together with any effect that this may have had in the development and reinterpretation of Hindu religious thought.[72] While the period of British sponsorship of Persian translations from Sanskrit was brief, perhaps three quarters of a century, it represents a decisive step in the transition toward the eventual establishment of Islam and Hinduism as separate fields of study.

There are a number of other literary phenomena besides the translations from Sanskrit that challenge the standard notion of fixed boundaries between Hinduism and Islam. Little work has been done, for instance, to study the direct patronage of Sanskrit literature by Muslim

---

[71] Sir William Jones, *Works* (London, 1794), 1:422, quoted by Habibullah, "Medieval Indo-Persian Literature," p. 167.

[72] The detailed study of European Indology by Raymond Schwab, *The Oriental Renaissance: Europe's Rediscovery of India and the East, 1680–1880*, trans. Gene Patterson-Black and Victor Reinking (New York: Columbia University Press, 1984), does not address the significance of the Persian translations at all but stresses in a classicist manner the importance of access to original Sanskrit texts.

rulers.[73] While most Sanskrit works dedicated to sultans were belletristic court poetry, some Hindu and Jain officials in the employ of Muslim rulers wrote Sanskrit religious and legal treatises in which they mention their sovereigns.[74] A few Sanskrit works can be found that attempt to construct a relationship between Islam and ancient Hindu scriptures. As an example, a short Sanskrit text called the *Alla [Allāh] Upanishad* was apparently composed by one of Akbar's courtiers, in order to identify the Muslim deity with the gods of the Vedas, assisted by a combination of the Muslim call to prayer and tantric seed syllables. As late as the nineteenth century, many pandits considered this text a reliable, if obscure, formulation of Vedanta (the curious political context of this work is indicated by its substitution of "Muhammad Akbar," i.e., the emperor Akbar, for the Prophet Muhammad). Indian scholars trained in the classical style of Orientalist scholarship apparently succeeded in eliminating this work from the canon of Hindu scripture. R. Mitra, in 1871, trenchantly dismissed this work as "apocryphal," "the gross religious imposition" of a "Muhammadan forger" who was betrayed by incorrect Sanskrit grammar and stylistic inconsistencies.[75] I would suggest, to the contrary, that such "apocryphal" works could provide an important source for understanding the way that Hindus understood Islamic theology and ritual in certain political contexts. Another important area for contact between Hindu and Muslim culture is the participation of Muslim authors in

---

[73] M. M. Patkar, "Mughal Patronage of Sanskrit Learning," *Poona Orientalist* 3 (1938): 164–75; C. H. Chakravarty, "Muhammadans as Patrons of Sanskrit Learning," *Sāhitya Parishad Patrika* 44, no. 1; S. Sulaiman Nadwi, "Literary Progress of the Hindus under Muslim Rule," *Islamic Culture* 12 (1938): 424–33, 13; (1939): 401–26; D. C. Bhattacharyya, "Sanskrit Scholar of Akbar's Time," *Indian Historical Quarterly* 13 (1937): 31–36; Jatindra Bimal Chaudhuri, *Muslim Patronage to Sanskritic Learning*, part 1 (1942; repr., Delhi: Idarah-i Adabiyat-i Delli, 1981); S. A. I. Tirmizi, "Sanskrit Chronicler of the Reign of Mahmud Begarah," in *Some Aspects of Medieval Gujarat* (Delhi: Munshiram Manoharlal, 1968), pp. 45–54.

[74] Upendra Nath Day, *Medieval Malwa, A Political and Cultural History, 1401–1562* (Delhi: Munshi Ram Manohar Lal, 1965), pp. 367–70, 422–28, 437–39; M. R. Ranbaore, "Hindu Law in Medieval Deccan," in *History of Medieval Deccan (1295–1724)*, ed. H. K. Sherwani and P. M. Joshi, 2 vols. (Hyderabad: The Government of Andhra Pradesh, 1973–74), 2:529; V. W. Paranjpe Shastri, "Language and Literature—Sanskrit," in ibid., 2:128–29.

[75] Bábu Rájendralála Mitra, "The Alla Upanishad, a spurious chapter of the Atherva Veda—text, translation, and notes," *Journal of the Asiatic Society of Bengal* 40 (1871): 170–76.

indigenous Indian literary genres in modern Indian languages. This often resulted in the use of Hindu themes and structures in surprising ways, as in *Padmāvati*, an Eastern Hindi (Awadhi) adaptation of Rajput epic as mystical yogic allegory, written by a Sufi author, Muhammad Ja'isi; here the unexpected shift is that the Turks are the villains of the piece.[76] Since this category of literary creation covers a large number of unedited texts in a variety of Indian languages, I will only allude to it here in passing as an important topic for research.[77] I am ignoring for the purposes of this discussion the extensive participation by Hindu authors in secular Persian literature, in which they played important roles in the composition of court histories, literary anthologies, and poetry. A sociological study of the effects of Persianate culture on the Kayasths and other groups who served Mughal and other Indo-Muslim bureaucracies would be of considerable interest. Another important topic crying out for treatment is the description of Indian religions by Zoroastrian authors in the Dasatiri literature, especially the important seventeenth-century survey of religions called *Dabistān-i maẕāhib*.[78]

Of particular significance for the study of religion is a series of original Persian writings on Indian religion written by Hindus, including doctrinal summaries of "classical" Hindu teachings as well as biographies of figures of the medieval bhakti movements. The eighteenth century seems to have been a particularly rich time for the production of these Hindu Persian works.[79] As an example, one may consider *Makhzan al-ʻirfān* or *The Treasury of Gnosis* by Rup Narayan, written in 1717 in Lahore as a guide to the holy places of Braj.[80] A survey of Hindu creeds, festivals, rituals,

---

[76] Shantanu Phukan, "Through a Persian Prism: Hindi and Padmavat in the Mughal Imagination," (PhD diss., University of Chicago, 1999).

[77] For a brief survey, see Ronald Stuart McGregor, *Hindi Literature from its Beginnings to the Nineteenth Century*, A History of Indian Literature VIII/6 (Wiesbaden: Otto Harrassowitz, 1984), pp. 23–24, 26–28, 63–73, 150–54; S. M. Pandey, "Kutuban's *Miragāvatī*: its content and interpretation," in *Devotional literature in South Asia: Current research, 1985–1988*, ed. R. S. McGregor (Cambridge: Cambridge University Press, 1992), pp. 179–89.

[78] See most recently M. Athar Ali, "Pursuing an Elusive Seeker of Universal Truth – the Identity and Environment of the Author of the *Dabistan-i Mazahib*," JRAS, Series 3, 9.3 (1999), pp. 365–73.

[79] There is considerable information on this topic in ʻAbd Allah, *Adabiyyāt-i fārsī*. See also Ahmad Munzavi, *Fihrist-i mushtarak-i nuskha-hā-yi khaṭṭī-i fārsī-i Pākistān* (Islamabad: Markaz-i Taḥqiqāt-i Fārsi-i Irān u Pākistān, 1363/1405/1985), 4:2135–200, for a comprehensive list of titles and manuscripts of Persian works on Hinduism, both translations and original works.

[80] Rieu, *Catalogue of the Persian Manuscripts*, 1:62 (Egerton 1027), copied in 1766.

and ascetic practices, *Haft tamāshā* or *The Seven Displays*, was written in 1813 by a Hindu convert to Islam known by the pen-name Qatil, at the request of a learned Shiʻi scholar of Lucknow.[81] One of the last notable examples of original theological reflection by a Hindu in this medium was Raja Ram Mohan Roy (d. 1833), in his *Tuḥfat al-muwaḥḥidīn* or *The Gift of the Monotheists*, written in Persian with an Arabic preface.[82] While some of these texts were written as straightforward expositions of Hindu doctrines or rituals, others engaged more directly with Islamic religious thought, and in the nineteenth century, they even began to take on the form of apologias for Hinduism against the stereotyped criticisms found in Muslim polemical literature. To this category belong two Persian works composed by Andarman around 1866, *Tuḥfat al-islām* or *The Gift of Islam*, and *Pādāsh-i islām* or *The Revenge of Islam*, both written in defense of Hindu religion.[83] Also worthy of interest is *Madīnat al-taḥqīq* or *The City of Demonstration*, written by Karparam in Samvat 1932/1875 as a refutation of a Persian work that attacked Hinduism.[84] One even finds a work called *Taḥqīq al-tanāsukh* or *The Demonstration of Reincarnation* by Anantram, son of Karparam (possibly identical with the Karparam just mentioned), composed in 1875 clearly as a defense of that doctrine commonly associated with Hinduism.[85] One suspects that these works emerged from the climate of religious disputation that resulted from the attacks of Christian missionaries upon Islam, Hinduism, and Sikhism. The fact that they were written in Persian at such a late date may be explained by the continued administrative use of Persian in the Punjab through the 1860s. Even the least self-conscious of these productions necessarily engaged in a complex cross-cultural hermeneutic by the very choice of

---

[81] Rieu, *Catalogue of the Persian Manuscripts*, 1:64 (Or. 476), copied 1850.

[82] Abid Ullah Ghazi, "Raja Rammohun Roy (1772–1833): encounter with Islam and Christianity, the articulation of Hindu self-consciousness," (PhD diss., Harvard University, 1975), pp. 95–98.

[83] ʻAbd Allah, *Adabiyyāt-i fārsī*, p. 216, no. 10, both found in the Lahore Public Library.

[84] Ibid., p. 216, no. 11, where the offensive treatise is identified as *Tuḥfat al-Hind*. This seems unlikely, since that work is primarily an account of Indian arts and culture that is not in any way critical; see Mirza Khan ibn Fakhr al-Din Muhammad, *Tuḥfat al-Hind*, ed. Nur al-Hasan Ansari, Zabān u Adabiyyat-i Fārsi 39 (Tehran: Bunyād-i Farhang-i Īrān, 1354/1975). Perhaps what is meant is the similarly entitled *Ḥujjat al-Hind* of ʻAli Mihrabi, which consists of a polemical dialogue between two birds on the merits of Hindu mythology and Islam. The dating of the text by the Indian Vikrama or Samvat era, rather than the Islamic calendar, is a telling index of the polemical character of this work.

[85] ʻAbd Allah, *Adabiyyāt-i fārsī*, p. 216, no. 12, found in Punjab University Library, Lahore.

the Persian words used to render technical terms from the vocabulary of Hindu religious texts. This neglected field of literature would seem to be especially promising for the study of the concrete relationships that individual Hindu authors worked out to position themselves in relation to the dominant Indo-Muslim court culture.

Finally, it should not be forgotten that the tradition of Persian Sanskritic learning established by Akbar and Dara Shikuh still continues today among a small circle of Iranian scholars. Daryush Shayagan, in addition to his French study of Dara Shikuh, has also written a large survey in Persian on *The Religions and Philosophical Schools of India*.[86] The prolific Muhammad Riza Jalali Na'ini has, in collaboration with Indian scholars, produced an impressive series of text editions of Persian translations from Sanskrit, including works by Dara Shikuh as well as a critical edition of the *Mahābhārata* translation sponsored by Akbar.[87] He has in addition authored an original Persian translation of the *Rig-veda*, a study of the Sikh religion, an analysis of Hindu mysticism, a comparative study of language and religion among the ancient Aryans, a reconsideration of the treatment of Indian religions in Shahrastani's Arabic theological survey, and an edition of Dara Shikuh's Persian translation of the *Bhagavad Gita*.[88] To this should be added two Sanskrit-Persian lexicons, co-authored by Jalali Na'ini and Indian scholar N. S. Shukla.[89] Fathullah

---

[86] Daryush Shayagan, *Adyān wa maktab-hā-yi falsafī-yi Hind*, 2 vols. (Tehran: Dānishgāh-i Tihrān, 1967).

[87] Besides the previously mentioned editions of Dara Shukuh's *Majma' al-baḥrayn* and the *Mahābhārata*, see Dara Shukuh, trans., *Ūpānīshād (Sirr-i akbar)*, ed. Tara Chand and Muḥammad Riza Jalali Na'ini, 3rd ed., 2 vols. (1963; repr., Tehran: Intishārāt-i 'Ilmi, 1368/1989).

[88] Muhammad Riza' Jalali Na'ini, *Guzīda-i sarūd-hā-yi rīg vedā* (Tehran: Chāp-i Tābān, 1348/1969); id., *Ṭarīqa-i Gurū Nānak va paydāyī-i āyīn-i Sik* (Tehran: Chāp-i Tābān, 1349/1970); id., *Ādāb-i ṭarīqat va khudāyābī dar 'irfān-i hindū* (Tehran: Chāp-i Tābān, 1347/1968); id., *Khwīshāvandī-i zabān va maẕhab-i qadīm-i dū qawm-i āryā-yi Īrān wa Hind* (Benares University, 1971); Shahrastāni, *Ārā-yi Hind (bakhshī az kitāb al-milal wal-niḥal*, new ed. Muṣṭafā Khāliqdād 'Abbāsi, ed. Muhammad Riza' Jalali Na'ini (Tehran: Chāp-i Tābān, 1349/1970); Dara Shikuh, trans., *Bhagavad Gītā*, ed. Muhammad Riza' Jalali Na'ini (n.p., 1957).

[89] Muhammad Riza' Jalali Na'ini and N. S. Shukla, *Lughāt-i sānskrīt maẕkūr dar kitāb mā lil-Hind-i 'Allāma Bīrūnī* (Tehran: Chāpkhāna-i Khurrami, 1353/1975); id., *Farhang-i fārsī prakāsh (farhang-i sānskrīt bi-fārsī)* (n.p., 1354/1976); id., *Farhang-i Sanskrīt-Fārsī* (Tehran : Pizhūhishgāh-i 'Ulūm-i Insānī wa Muṭāla'at-i Farhangī, 1996). Cf. also Chittenjoor Kunhan Raja, *Persian-Sanskrit grammar*, (New Delhi: Indian Council for Cultural Relations, 1953), and Muhammad 'Ali Hasani Da'i al-Islami, *Khwudāmūz-i zabān-i Sanskrīt [Teach Yourself Sanskrit]*, 2nd ed. (Tehran : Shirkat-i Danish, 1982).

Mujtabai wrote a Harvard dissertation on the Persian translation of the *Yoga Vāsiṣṭha* by Mir Findiriski.[90] Outside the circle of scholarly Iranian Indologists, the prominent Iranian philosopher Jalal al-Din Ashtiyani has engaged with Indian religions in a series of critical volumes on comparative religion based largely on European scholarship.[91] Nur al-Din Chahardihi, an indefatigable researcher on the topic of Islamic esotericism, has also turned his attention to Indian traditions. In addition to writing his own study of yoga (which he practices), he has also reprinted a treatise on yoga and divination called *Muḥīṭ-i ma'rifat* (*The Ocean of Gnosis*) of Satidasa son of Ram Bha'i "'Arif," written in 1753–54 and published in Lucknow in 1860. This work, containing 16 chapters on metaphysics, yoga, and divination, is based on the Hindi (Bhak'ha) work *Svarodaya* of Charana Dasa, pupil of Sukhadevji, and the translation contains a considerable amount of sophisticated Persian verse.[92] Modern Persian translations of literary works by Kalidasa and Tagore have also been published in Iran and Afghanistan.[93] In Iran, it seems, there remains a keen interest in Indian religion and thought, partially prompted by a sense of the proximity of ancient Indian and Iranian cultures, but which may be expected to continue and resurface in the future.

To sum up, then, the translations from Sanskrit into Arabic and Persian fall into four classes: practical arts and sciences, political works (based on epics), metaphysical and mystical treatises, and works on Hindu religion and law commissioned by the British. The first three categories, which characterize the translations done for Muslim patrons, have little to do with the modern concept of religion. It is only when the lens of the modern European notion of religion is applied that one can view

---

[90] Fathullah Mujtabai, "Muntakhab-i Jug-basasht or, Selections from the Yoga-vasistha," (PhD diss., Harvard University, 1976).

[91] Muhandis Jalal al-Din Ashtiyani, *Idiāl-i bashar; tajziya wa taḥlīl-i afkār-i 'irfān-i būdīsm wa jaynīsm, maẓāhib-i hindī*, Majmū'a- i 'irfān 5 (*The Ideals of Humanity: Analysis of the Mystical Thought of the Indian Religions of Buddhism and Jainism*, The Mysticism Collection 5) (Tehran: Chāpkhāna Ḥaydari, 1377/1999).

[92] Carandas Sukhadevji, *Svarodaya*, Persian trans. from Hindi by Satidasa son of Ram Bha'i "'Arif," *Muḥīṭ-i ma'rifat* (Lucknow, 1860); reprint ed. Nur al-Din Chahardihi, *Asrār-i panhānī-i maktab-i yūg* (*Hidden Secrets of Yoga Teaching*) (Tehran: Nashr-i Pārsā, 1369/1991).

[93] Kalidasa, *Śakuntala*, Persian trans. by Hadi Hasan, *Shakuntala yā khatīm-i mafqūd* (Tehran, 1956), also trans. 'Ali Asghar Hikmat (Delhi: Chapkhanah-i "Q", 1957); Rabrindranath Tagore, *Gitanjali*, Persian trans. by Ravan Farhadi, *Surūd-i nayāyish* (Kabul, 1975).

pre-modern Muslims as having had a clear notion of Hinduism. What are the implications of this conclusion? I would suggest that this points to the need further to complicate our picture of Hindu-Muslim interaction, not to derive it from predetermined concepts of the essential characteristics of a religion. If we wish to take account of historical change within religious traditions and to understand the diversity within the traditions that, for convenience, we treat as unitary, then it is important to pay close attention to the historical and political concerns that inform any individual act of inter-religious interpretation. To understand a multi-century process of inter-civilizational interpretation, such as the Arabic and Persian translations from Sanskrit, it is necessary to take seriously the hermeneutical structures and categories that guided the efforts of those interpreters. Above all, it is important to try, as much as possible, to avoid reading anachronistic concepts into pre-modern materials. Only then can we fully appreciate the rich density and texture of the complex religious patterns that are woven into the life of South Asian culture.

12

Situating Sufism and Yoga

"The natives of all unknown countries are commonly called Indians"

—Maximilian of Transylvania, De molucco (1523)

ORIENTALISM AND ESSENTIALISM IN
THE STUDY OF RELIGION

Since the Protestant Reformation, the dominant concept of religions has been one of essences unconditioned by history.[1] The nature of religious traditions can best be understood, from this perspective, by analyzing religions into their original components. Scholars have used various metaphors to describe how one religion "borrows" doctrines or practices from another, which is consequently the "source" by which it is thus "influenced." By a mechanical and ahistorical conception of a religion as a pure and unchanging essence, variations from what was perceived to be the norm (or from the definition of a religion as defined by scholars) could be easily explained as the result of importing a foreign doctrine or practice. This terminology, which is highly abstract and metaphorical, is rarely questioned in the intellectual history approach to religious studies, even though it tends to make religions rather than people into agents. How often have we read that a particular school or thinker "was influenced" by so-and-so? Even those who reject a particular case of alleged influence unconsciously accept it as a category of analysis.

---

[1] See my *Following Muhammad: Rethinking Islam in the Contemporary World* (Chapel Hill, NC: University of North Carolina Press, 2003; New Delhi: Yoda Press, 2005), chapter 2, for a discussion of modern concepts of religion.

Once influence has been established, it is felt, one has said something of immense significance; the phenomenon has been explained—or rather, explained away. There is in addition an implicit evaluation in this kind of language. "Sources" are "original" while those "influenced" by them are "derivative." This kind of analysis contains so many problematic and subjective assumptions that it is hard to see how it helps clarify anything. I would like to argue that what the Germans call *Quellenforschung* ("search for origins") often misses the point by excluding or minimizing the significance of an author's reinterpretation of sources. As Wendy Doniger observes with respect to the study of myth, "The problem of diffusion is more basic than the mechanical complexities or political agendas of this sort of tale-tracking. For on the one hand, diffusion still fails to account for the particular genius of each telling."[2] In the comparative study of religion, this approach also perpetuates an implicitly Protestant concept of religions as ideologies competing for world domination, and any evidence of dependence on foreign influences is a sure sign of weakness. This model is fine if one is engaging in missionary activity, but for an analytical appreciation of the nature of religion, it has serious flaws.

One of the chief examples of this search for sources and influences in religious studies was the study of early Christianity and its relationship to the religions of late antiquity. Early scholars in this field liked to talk about "Oriental-Gnostic" influences on Christianity, deriving from India. Such borrowing sometimes was said to have been carried out by the elite or, alternatively, by the superstitious masses; though the favorite explanation was deliberate borrowing from paganism by priests, who were keen to aggrandize their power by this deception. As Jonathan Z. Smith has pointed out, Protestant anti-Catholic polemics are the key to understanding this jaundiced view of early Christianity.[3]

The language of "influence" becomes especially suspect when we consider its history. The term is originally astrological, denoting the ethereal emanations of the stars that control terrestrial events; subsequently it came to mean "the inflowing . . . or infusion (into a person or thing) of any kind of divine, spiritual, moral, immaterial, or secret

---

[2] Wendy Doniger, *The Implied Spider: Politics and Theology in Myth* (New York: Columbia University Fresco and 1998), p. 141.

[3] Jonathan Z. Smith, *Drudgery Divine: On the Comparison of Early Christianities and the Religions of Late Antiquity* (Chicago: The University of Chicago Press, 1990), pp. 21–22, 34.

power or principle." One can also see this archaic notion at work in the term *influenza*, based on the notion that this viral disease was caused by the influence of maleficent stars. Most recently, influence means, more abstractly, the exertion of power by one person or thing over another, in a manner that is only perceptible by its effects.[4] In the history of ideas, influence therefore signifies the "authority of prestige over the ideas or over the will of another."[5] Since the Enlightenment, it is above all in intellectual history that the term "influence" has come to function as a major category of analysis. The task of the historian of ideas was seen as simplifying complicated philosophical systems into their basic components, much like a chemist reducing compounds to elements. In the quest for these basic factors, in the phrase of Arthur Lovejoy, the history of ideas "is especially interested in the processes by which influences pass over from one province to another."[6] If it is correct to trace this enterprise to astrology, then the historian of ideas would resemble a latter-day astrologer, charting the influences of the stars of our intellectual cosmos. This chemist, or perhaps better, alchemist, reduces the intellectual compounds of history to their essential elements, and in the process may attain the philosopher's stone of academic immortality. This kind of detective work can be seen as the principal thrill of the hunt in scholarship. "Spotting certain thematic likenesses or disclosing related verb patterns between as well as within texts seems to inaugurate the excitement fueling the critical act."[7] Unfortunately, the connections discerned by the history of ideas may exist only in the mind of the theorist. As Jonathan Z. Smith observes, "Similarity and difference are not 'given.' They are the result of mental operations."[8] The mechanical character of the influence metaphor obscures the role of selection and intentionality that takes place in any thinker's evaluation of previous formulations, and it privileges the superior position of the analyst who triumphantly announces the detection of decisive influence of one thinker upon another. If we

---

[4] *Oxford English Dictionary*, s.v. "influence."

[5] André Lalande, *Vocabulaire technique et critique de la philosophie*, 5th ed. (Paris: Presses Universitaires de France, 1947), p. 498, which also stresses the astrological origin.

[6] Arthur O. Lovejoy, *The Great Chain of Being: A Study of the History of an Idea* (1936; repr., Cambridge, MA: Harvard University Press, 1976), p. 16.

[7] Louis A. Renza, "Influence," in *Critical Terms for Literary Study*, ed. Frank Lentricchia and Thomas McLaughlin (Chicago: The University of Chicago Press, 1990), p. 187.

[8] Smith, *Drudgery Divine*, p. 51.

wish, in contrast, to understand how complex intercultural exchanges take place, it will be necessary to re-examine the freight of meaning carried by this kind of metaphorical language, which all too often substitutes for analysis. We need a wider range of categories that take account of acts of interpretation, appropriation, and resistance.

Another example of a problematic metaphor is the vaguely disapproving term "syncretism," which by its neo-Greek etymology metaphorically suggests either pouring two different liquids together or allying two independent forces. The term was originally introduced during the Protestant Reformation as a derogatory description of misguided attempts to reunite Catholics and Protestants. The underlying assumption was that these two religions were irrevocably separate; those who attempted to rejoin them were attempting to combine two alien substances or powers. Subsequently the term was used to refer to philosophical and religious positions that identified various deities of the ancient world as being simply different aspects of the same god or goddess. By the nineteenth century, syncretism was a familiar term in religious studies, usually applied disparagingly to non-Christian contexts.[9] I would like to suggest that the concept of syncretism is problematic in the study of religion because of the underlying assumptions that either of its etymologies conveys. If religions are treated either as homogeneous substances or autonomous individuals, this vastly oversimplifies the question. Any one-sided characterization of the "essence" of such a religion makes historical change, complexity, or diversity into a deviation from the norm. Syncretism, by proposing that religions can be mixed, also assumes that religions exist in a pure unadulterated state. Where shall we find this historically untouched religion? Is there any religious tradition untouched by other religious cultures? Has any religion sprung into existence fully formed, without reference to any previously existing religion? If pure and irreducible religions cannot be found, a logical problem follows; syncretism becomes a meaningless term if everything is syncretistic.[10]

---

[9] *Encyclopaedia of Religion and Ethics* (Edinburgh: T. & T. Clark; New York: C. Scribner's Sons, 1908–26), "Syncretism," an article that is sensitive to the polemical historical origins of the term. Oddly, the 1987 *Encyclopedia of Religion* more or less accepted syncretism as a legitimate category and offered no critical analysis of the concept.

[10] See Robert D. Baird, *Category Formation and the History of Religions*, 2nd ed., Religion and Reason 1 (Berlin: Mouton de Gruyter, 1991), pp. 142–52; Tony K. Stewart and Carl W. Ernst, "Syncretism," *South Asian Folklore: An Encyclopedia*, ed. Peter J. Claus and Margaret A. Mills (New York: Garland Publishing, Inc., 2003).

The term "religion" itself lends itself to equivocation as well. We use the term equally to describe the interior consciousness of a single believer, the religious community as a corporate entity, and the vast historical complex of tradition as it has accumulated over the course of centuries. If this ambiguity is not clarified, then misconceptions easily occur. If the discussion concerns an author normally assigned to one religious tradition, who nonetheless deals with concepts or texts customarily associated with another religion, is this an inter-religious exercise? Does the author necessarily have a consciousness of overstepping a boundary? If one applies a fixed abstract notion of religion to this kind of analysis, the result can be a mechanical history of ideas with a bias toward doctrine as the essence of religion.

To speculate briefly on the reasons for the powerful urge to find unity or genetic relationship in diverse religious phenomena, one may point to the disorientation of Christian Europe by the colonial encounter with other civilizations. The dislocation of the Christian version of sacred history was perhaps inevitable, once the ancient and independent civilizations of China and India were clearly in view. Likewise, the authority ascribed to tradition underwent severe questioning after the discovery of the New World, unaccounted for in the works of the ancients revered throughout Europe.[11] Another major factor in the need to define religious genealogies was the anxiety over the very existence of Judaism and Islam, which has continued to be a defining factor in European modernity. Yet, the impulse to give history a single line of meaning, as an alternative to sheer arbitrariness, still expressed itself, not in theology but in various scientific theories of cultural diffusion. These ranged from Abel-Remusat's 1824 essay explaining the historical relation between Greek and Chinese thought (based on a comparison of Lao-Tzu and Heraclitus) to the excesses of the Pan-Babylonian school at the turn of the century, which sought to derive all forms of religion from Babylonia via a process of cultural diffusion. As philosopher of history Eric Voegelin observed,

A *horror*, not *vacui* but *pleni*, seems at work, a shudder at the richness of the spirit as it reveals itself all over the earth in a multitude of hierophanies, a monomaniacal desire to force the operations of the spirit in history on the one line that will unequivocally lead into the speculator's present.

---

[11] Donald. E. Pease, "Author," in *Critical Terms for Literary Study*, pp. 105–20.

No independent lines must be left dangling that conceivably could lead into somebody else's present and future.[12]

Similarity between two formulations could be explained as the result of historical dependency. Thus, we can explain the farfetched but self-assured Romantic pronouncements about the essential identity of all Oriental (i.e., non-European) religions in their Indian core. The rough edges of particularity, smoothed out by reducing formulations to a doctrinal core, could be safely disregarded as accidental. The real meaning of religious phenomena was to be found in the exercise of theoretical imagination through comparison and detection of sources.

Another factor in the quest for influences is reflexive and contrary to the first, viewing non-Christian cultures primarily in terms of their difference from European Christianity. This was particularly prominent in the intellectual climate of nineteenth-century colonialism. Theories of evolution and race were freely applied in the comparative study of religion, originally understood as a disingenuous comparison intended to reveal which religion was superior.[13] The study of religion in Christian theological faculties initially exempted Christianity from this kind of historical investigation, since Christianity (in whatever form the theorist professed) was assumed to be still pure and integral, despite such events as the Protestant Reformation. More than other literary texts, the Christian scriptures were accorded the authority of tradition in a way that defined authenticity both through the witness of history and the sanction of divine truth. If, however, other religions could be shown to be hybrids composed of various "Oriental" influences, that was a testimony to their dependent and inferior nature. Despite the later progress of historical research into the relation of Christianity to the cultural and religious world into which it was born, the colonial legacy of ambivalence toward "Oriental religions" still lingers. In addition, it is also important to recognize the extent to which Romantic concepts of the "mystic East" were

---

[12] Eric Voegelin, *Order and History*, vol. 4, *The Ecumenic Age* (Baton Rouge, LA: Louisiana State University Press, 1974), p. 3.

[13] Eric Sharpe ("Comparative Religion," *Encyclopedia of Religion*, 3:578–80) links the term "influence" to evolutionistic schemes that rank religions, and he optimistically considers the term to be now "seldom used."

a screen for debates about religion in the European Christian context.[14] Problematic issues coded under the names of mysticism and pantheism could be projected in this way onto a foreign Oriental screen.

The problem with the comparative approach to religion just mentioned is its irrelevance and lack of significance with reference to the religious phenomena that are being described. The magisterial comparison by the scholar detecting "influences" previously unsuspected by anyone else exhibits a disconnection from historical tradition that can border on solipsism. Some scholars, secure in their conviction as to the essential nature of "classical" Islam, still have contempt for any attempt to discover what later Muslims have thought about their predecessors and how their religious interpretations have evolved over time. I would like instead to turn attention to the internal dynamic of the evolving tradition insofar as it is available to us in individual examples provided by history, and its self-interpretation. We need to understand the origins of religious traditions as formulated by participants as well as the factual beginnings noted by academic observers.[15] As a gesture to indicate the dethronement of the magisterial observer, I wish to be explicit about abandoning the project of comparative religion, insofar as it entails essentialist assumptions about religion.[16]

Recent critical scholarship on the concept of religion has stressed the provisional and heuristic nature of religious categories, proposing in place of the essentialist model a polythetic analysis of religion. This is analogous to a model already familiar in zoology and anthropology, in which "it was no longer true that what was known of one member of a class was thereby known of the other members ... classes of creatures were grouped by what were in fact family resemblances."[17] This means that multiple and even conflicting authoritative positions can be included under the rubric of a single religious category; definitions of religions

---

[14] Richard King, *Orientalism and Religion: Postcolonial Theory, India and 'The Mystic East'* (London: Routledge, 1999), pp. 33, 97, 118–45.

[15] For Marc Bloch's distinction between origins and beginnings as applied to the study of religion, see Carl W. Ernst and Bruce B. Lawrence, *Sufi Martyrs of Love: Chishti Sufism in South Asia and Beyond* (New York: Palgrave Press, 2002), pp. 48–49.

[16] Ironically, the book in which I argue against an essentialist interpretation of Islam, *Following Muhammad*, is catalogued by the U.S. Library of Congress categories under "Islam—Essence and Character."

[17] Rodney Needham, "Polythetic Classification: Convergence and Consequences," *Man* 10 (1975), pp. 349–69, quoting pp 350, 352. See also Doniger, *The Implied Spider*, p. 143–45.

based on unvarying sets of characteristics are no longer acceptable since they implicitly entail endorsement of one authoritative position rather than another. It is especially noteworthy to see the flexibility of analytic categories in recent scientific thought, since the phrase "comparative religion" was clearly based upon the earlier notion of "comparative zoology," so that it evidently perpetuates an outmoded notion of unvarying genus and species in the definition of religions. Recent helpful approaches include Talal Asad's notion of religion as a discursive tradition, in which one can recognize the persistence of authority without adopting the Protestant concept of religion as belief.[18] Avoiding essentialism means striking a practical balance between similarity and difference, and it makes simple comparison a problematic enterprise, by abandoning a number of *a priori* prejudices about religion that are no longer justifiable. While there is in fact a strong emerging argument for non-essentialist interpretations of religion among academics, essentialism still dominates in ideological, media-driven, and mass marketing concepts of religion, as we shall see below.

> *"This is the practice of the Jogis; this is not an activity of the community of Muhammad. Nevertheless, it is correct."*
>
> —*Muhammad Muhyi al-Din, ca. 1748*

SUFI INTERPRETERS OF YOGIC PRACTICES

The foregoing remarks on the study of religion expand on a problem that has dogged the modern study of religion since its inception. As I have argued elsewhere, since the beginning of Orientalist scholarship over two centuries ago, it was an unquestioned assumption that Sufism was somehow derived from Hinduism, so it was not really Islamic at all.[19] This conceit has endured through the nineteenth century until recent

---

[18] Talal Asad, *Genealogies of Religion: Discipline and Reasons of Power in Christianity and Islam* (Baltimore: Johns Hopkins UP, 1993).

[19] For a general review of early scholarship on Sufism, see Carl W. Ernst, *The Shambhala Guide to Sufism* (Boston: Shambhala Publications, 1997), chapter 1. I have presented a more detailed series of remarks on the theory of the Indian origins of Sufism in "The Islamization of Yoga in the Amrtakunda Translations," *Journal of the Royal Asiatic Society*, Series 3, 13, no. 2 (2003): 199–226, and Chapter in this volume.

times. In Zaehner's words, "Muslim mysticism is entirely derivative."[20] Orientalists and romantics alike agreed that mysticism must always and inevitably derive from India. The lack of historical evidence for this assumption demands that one seek elsewhere for an explanation of what one scholar has called "Indomaniac zeal."[21] In part, no doubt, there was some attraction in the elegance and simplicity found in theories of cultural diffusion from a single source. One typical example of the romantic Orientalist interpretation of Sufism was E. H. Palmer's 1867 translation of an important thirteenth-century Persian text by `Aziz al-Din Nasafi, which Palmer entitled *Oriental Mysticism*. "Steering a mid course between the pantheism of India on the one hand and the deism of the Coran on the other, the Sufis' cult is the religion of beauty .... Sufiism is really the development of the Primaeval Religion of the Aryan race."[22] Arguments used to support this contention wavered between focusing on yogic practice and the philosophical doctrines of Vedanta as the essence of Indian mysticism.

Let me make it clear that I have no interest in upholding the purity of Islamic mysticism from pollution by foreign sources. That would simply be a reversal of the comparativist project of Orientalism. As J. Z. Smith points out,

> It is as if the only choices the comparativist has are to assert either identity or uniqueness, and that the only possibilities for utilizing comparisons are to make assertions regarding dependence. In such an enterprise, it would appear, dissimilarity is assumed to be the norm; similarities are to be explained either as the result of the 'psychic unity' of humankind, or the result of 'borrowing.'[23]

If we are to avoid these essentialist dichotomies, the polythetic approach to religion is extremely helpful. No longer is it necessary to attack or

---

[20] R. C. Zaehner, *Mysticism Sacred and Profane: An Inquiry into some Varieties of Praeternatural Experience* (New York: Oxford University Press, 1961), p. 160.

[21] Martino Mario Moreno, "Mistica musulmana e mistica indiana," *Annali Lateranensi* X (1949), pp. 103–219, citing p. 198.

[22] E. H. Palmer, *Oriental Mysticism: A Treatise on Sufiistic and Unitarian Theosophy of the Persians* (1867; repr., London: Frank Cass & Co. Ltd, 1969), pp. x–xi. Palmer dedicated this treatise to Napoleon III, whom he described as a great patron of "European Orientalism."

[23] Smith, *Drudgery Divine*, p. 47.

defend arguments of influence or authenticity since it is now possible to acknowledge freely that numerous examples of hybrid and multiplex symbols, practices, and doctrines can be at work in any particular religious milieu. Nevertheless, it is still worthwhile to dissect essentialist and Orientalist interpretations of religion, particularly when they take the form of what literary critics call "strong misreadings," in which a theorist triumphantly proposes a revolutionary explanation based on newly detected alleged sources and origins.

What, then, is the data regarding the relationship between Sufism and yoga, apart from *a priori* assumptions about Oriental mysticism? In an earlier chapter, I have traced the history of the single text, *The Pool of Nectar*, which, in multiple versions and translations, made available to Muslim readers certain practices associated with the Nath jogis and the teachings known as hatha yoga (in standard North Indian pronunciation, yogis are called jogis).[24] These practices include divination by control of breath through the left and right nostrils, summoning female spirits that can be identified as yoginis, and performing meditations on the cakra centers accompanied by recitation of Sanskrit mantras. All this material was increasingly Islamized over time, in a series of translations into Arabic, Persian, Ottoman Turkish, and Urdu. This remarkable text, and a number of other examples that I will mention, make it abundantly clear that in certain Sufi circles there was an awareness and use of particular practices that can be considered yogic (although the question of defining yoga and the perspective from which it may be identified still needs to be clarified). Contrary to Orientalist expectations, however, Sufi engagement with yoga was not to be found at the historical beginnings of the Sufi tradition, and it was most highly developed, unsurprisingly, in India.[25] Moreover, the knowledge of yoga among Indian Sufis gradually became more detailed over time. The most exact accounts of hatha yoga in Sufi texts, using technical terms in Hindi, occur in writings from as late as the nineteenth century, although these texts typically juxtapose yoga materials alongside Sufi practices without any real attempt at integration

---

[24] Ernst, "Islamization of Yoga."
[25] To gauge the relative importance of these yoga practices for Sufism considered broadly, I would point to a recent encyclopedia article on Sufism (5000 words), in which I devoted two sentences to yoga; see "Tasawwuf," in *Encyclopedia of Islam and the Muslim World*, ed. Richard Martin (New York: Macmillan Reference U.S.A., 2003), 2:684–690.

or synthesis. The Sufi interest in hatha yoga was very practical and did not (with certain notable exceptions) engage with philosophical texts of Vedanta or other Sanskritic schools of thought.[26]

The foregoing brief summary of the *Pool of Nectar* translations has just introduced a number of technical terms that will remain methodologically problematic if we do not pause for some basic attempts at historical and descriptive definition. What do we mean by Sufism and yoga? "Sufism" is by its nature an outsider's term, belonging to the Enlightenment catalog of ideologies and creeds identified as "isms." As such, it inevitably stands in tension with the insider vocabulary of spiritual vocations and ethical ideals of the Sufi tradition.[27] Historically, what we call Sufism may be considered a typical and prominent trend in most Muslim societies, gradually crystallizing as a selfconscious movement in the ninth and tenth centuries. Despite the strong emphasis upon the Qur'an and the Prophet Muhammad in Sufi thought and practice, Sufism has been disassociated from Islam in both Orientalist scholarship and modern Muslim reformist polemics for the past 200 years so that now it is a highly contested subject. Sufism can refer to a wide range of phenomena, including scriptural interpretation, meditative practices, master-disciple relationships, corporate institutions, aesthetic and ritual gestures, doctrines, and literary texts. As a generic descriptive term, however, Sufism is deceptive. There is no Sufism in general. All that we describe as Sufism is firmly rooted in particular local contexts, often anchored to the very tangible tombs of deceased saints, and it is deployed in relation to lineages and personalities with a distinctively local sacrality. Individual Sufi groups or traditions in one place may be completely oblivious of what Sufis do or say in other regions.

"Yoga" is a term that may be even harder to define. Georg Feuerstein maintains that "Yoga is like an ancient river with countless rapids, eddies, loops, tributaries, and backwaters, extending over a vast, colorful terrain of many different habitats."[28] Some regard it mainly as a philosophy linked to important Sanskrit texts, particularly Patañjali's *Yoga*

---

[26] For the larger context of this translation movement, see Carl W. Ernst, "Muslim Studies of Hinduism? A Reconsideration of Persian and Arabic Translations from Sanskrit," *Iranian Studies* 36 (2003), pp. 173–95.

[27] See Ernst, *Shambhala Guide to Sufism*, chapter 1.

[28] Georg Feuerstein, *Yoga: The Technology of Ecstasy* (Los Angeles: Jeremy P. Tarcher, Inc., 1989).

Sutras. For others, yoga signifies primarily meditative ascetic practices frequently associated with the god Shiva in Hindu teachings, though yoga is also widespread in Buddhist and Jain contexts. The yogic material that the Sufis mostly encountered was a highly specialized tradition called hatha yoga (literally, "the yoga of force"), associated with charismatic figures of the tenth to twelfth centuries, especially Matsyendranath and Gorakhnath. The lineage that preserves the hatha yoga teachings is known collectively as the Nath *siddhas* (adepts) or Kanphata ("split-ear") jogis, due to the distinctive wooden inserts and large rings they put in their ears during initiation.[29] The early Nath jogis were associated with the erotic practices of Kaula Tantrism, and prominent in their pantheon are the feminine deities known as yoginis or female yogis. Hatha yoga has a much more complicated psycho-physical set of techniques than the classical yoga of Patañjali, and it is presented with a minimum of metaphysical explanation. Special practices include manipulation of subtle physiology including psychic centers called cakras, retention of semen, pronunciation of syllabic chants or mantras with occult efficacy, and the summoning of deities. Despite their ascetic emphasis on sexual restraint, the Kanphata jogis have become over the past millennium a recognizable hereditary caste.[30]

Yet in the attempt to provide even such brief descriptions of both Sufism and yoga, we are faced with an especially challenging problem arising from the gap between scholarly analyses of the history of religions and the way in which these traditions are appropriated in the global marketplace of contemporary thought, especially under the rubric of New Age spirituality. Although the scholarly Orientalist argument about Sufism and yoga addressed issues of authenticity and dependence related to anxieties about Islam and the relegation of mysticism to India, the attraction of both Sufism and yoga today rests primarily on the extent to which both traditions can be seen as transcending any religious definition. The accelerating distrust of authority that still marks the legacy of the

---

[29] David Gordon White, *The Alchemical Body: Siddha Traditions in Medieval India* (Chicago: The University of Chicago Press, 1996); George Weston Briggs, *Gorakhnath and the Kanphata Yogis* (1938; repr., Delhi: Motilal Banarsidass, 1980), pp. 179–250; Shashibhusan Das Gupta, *Obscure Religious Cults*, 3rd ed. (Calcutta: Firma KLM Private Limited, 1976), pp. 191–210, 392–98; Feuerstein, *Yoga*, pp. 277–302.

[30] Daniel Gold and Ann Grodzins Gold, "The Fate of the Householder Nath," *History of Religions* 24 (1984): 113–32.

Enlightenment values experience over doctrine and authenticity over institutional approval.[31] The most popular forms of Sufism in Europe and America are those that minimize or ignore any form of Islamic identity. Rumi is the bestselling poet in America precisely because he is seen as going beyond all religions.

With yoga the definitional problem in relation to religion is even more severe. Yoga is often seen as the very basis of all spirituality or, alternatively, as a physical technique for stress reduction that can be embraced by anyone regardless of religious affiliation. According to some estimates, over five million Americans practise yoga, and in most cases, they do so in settings (physical education, YMCA classes) that downplay or ignore any connection whatever with Hindu religious traditions. A quick survey of recent library acquisitions on the topic of yoga yields a series of titles that emphasize its universal accessibility: *Yoga for Americans*; *Yoga for All*; and, inevitably, *The Complete Idiot's Guide to Yoga*. Glossy magazines on yoga are available at supermarket counters, and newspapers describe the yoga fashion accessories available for "today's yoginis."[32] So when we use the term yoga now, it carries multiple burdens—the sublime philosophy of transcendence associated with Patañjali, the intricate and esoteric psycho-physical system of the Nath jogis, and also the mass marketing category of yoga as the generic basis of mysticism in all religions. Modern scholarship is not immune from these grandiose concepts of yoga.[33]

When one turns to the historical context for the encounter of Sufism and yoga, it is a curious coincidence that the arrival of Sufis in India took place not long after the Nath or Kanphata jogis became organized, that is, by the beginning of the thirteenth century. While ascetic orders certainly had existed in India for many centuries, the Naths appear to have had a remarkable success at this particular time. The Nath jogis did not observe the purity restrictions of Brahminical ritual society and were free

---

[31] "The modern age conflates authoritarianism with authority, hence tends to suspect the latter (and its poetic representatives) as in fact embodying the former. Only when the notion of authority becomes a pejorative social term can anxiety concerning it spread to other areas like literature and criticism" (Renza, "Influence," p. 197).

[32] Sara Steffens, "Yoga Baring: Find your Inner Fashionista with Exercise Gear," *Raleigh News & Observer*, March 15, 2004.

[33] Frits Staal, *Exploring Mysticism: A Methodological Essay* (Berkeley: University of California Press, 1975).

to drop in for meals at Sufi hospices, which in turn were open to any and all visitors. While hardly representative of "Hindu" culture as a whole, the jogis were perhaps the only Indian religious group with whom Sufis had much in common. This was also an encounter between two movements that shared overlapping interests in psycho-physical techniques of meditation, and which competed to some extent for popular recognition as wonder-workers, healers, and possessors of sanctity. [34] Moreover, in a country where cremation was the preferred funeral method, both groups practised burial; Sufi tombs, to the untutored eye, must have fit the model of the lingam shrines or *samadhis* set up over jogis, who were customarily buried in the lotus position.[35] The similarity between jogis and Sufis extended to the point that the heads of Nath jogi establishments became known by the Persian term *pir*, the common designation for a Sufi master. While it is sometimes suggested that this name was adopted defensively to deter Muslim rulers from wiping the jogis out,[36] from the historical evidence it seems clear that many Muslim rulers were quite familiar with the characteristic specialities of jogis, and it is striking that the Mughals in particular became patrons of jogi establishments.[37] Acculturation by the jogis to selected Islamicate norms seems a more likely reason than the presumption of religious persecution for the jogis' adoption of such a title.[38]

The theoretical problem with the Orientalist influence model is that, even in cases where Sufis clearly recognize a particular technique (such as breath control) as being associated with Indian yogis, this does not explain the significance of the practice as adapted by Sufis. Recently, Jürgen Paul returned to the influence model to inquire into the case of

[34] For a stimulating sociological comparison of Hindu and Islamic asceticism, see Marc Gaborieau, "Incomparables ou vrais jumeaux? Les renonçants dans l'hindousime et dans l'islam," *Annales: Histoire, Sciences Sociales* 57 (2002): 71–92.

[35] Briggs, *Gorakhnath and the Kanphata Yogis*, pp. 39–40; Mircea Eliade, *Yoga: Immortality and Freedom*, trans. Willard Trask (Princeton, NJ: Princeton University Press, 1989), pp. 422–23.

[36] G. S. Ghurye, *Indian Sadhus* (Bombay: Popular Prakashan, 1964), p. 139, argues protective dissimulation from the proximity of Jogi shrines and pilgrimage sites to Muslim population centers and the alleged conversion of two shrines at Gorakhpur into mosques by `Ala' al-Din Khalji (d. 1316) and Awrangzeb (d. 1707).

[37] B. N. Goswamy and J. S. Grewal, *The Mughals and the Jogis of Jakhbar, Some Madad-i-Ma`ash and Other Documents* (Simla: Indian Institute of Advanced Study, 1967).

[38] On Sufi terms in yogi centers, see Véronique Bouillier, *Ascètes et rois: Un monastère de Kanphata Yogis au Népal* (Paris: CNRS Editions, 1997), pp. 91–93.

Naqshbandi Sufis in Central Asia. Using what he calls a phenomenological comparison, he proposed a concept of Indian influence based on deliberate study, consideration, and adoption of religious practices such as vegetarianism, celibacy, and breath control. There seems to have been a clear awareness among these Naqshbandis that breath control, a central technique at least since the time of Baha' al-Din Naqshband (d. 1390), was also common among Indian yogis. Paul therefore concludes that these Central Asian Sufis were "inspired by non-Muslim Indian mystical techniques."[39] Yet, the significance of this breath control technique would seem to be affected by the fact that, among these Naqshbandis, breath control invariably was used to accompany *dhikr* recitation formulas in order to make this meditation continuous, with a focus on such typically Islamic chants such as *la ilaha illa allah* (there is no god but God). In other words, if breath control was used to enhance the effect of Islamic meditation formulas, to what extent can it be considered "inspired by non-Muslim Indian mystical techniques"?

Another example raises questions about the influence model, in this case concerning a major systematization of Sufi psycho-physical meditative practice. `Ala' al-Dawla Simnani (d. 1336) was one of the chief figures in the Kubrawi Sufi order in Central Asia, whose vast literary output was matched by his extensive activities in training disciples. Heir to an already highly developed system of meditation established by his teacher Nur al-Din Isfarayini (d. 1317) and others, Simnani incorporated earlier practices and articulated a spiritual method of considerable complexity, based on interior visualization of seven subtle centers (*latifa*, pl. *lata'if*) within the body, each associated with a particular prophet and a color.[40] The system of seven subtle centers developed by Simnani underwent further evolution in India in the Naqshbandi order, from the fifteenth

---

[39] Jürgen Paul, "Influences indiennes sur la *naqshbandiyya* d'Asie centrale?", *Cahiers d'Asie Centrale* 1–2 (1996) : 203-217. In a similar vein, William S. Haas observed that the *dhikr* technique of the Algerian Rahmaniyya order "has as its centre a thoroughly elaborated technique of breathing, obviously of Indian origin," and so he speculated that the nineteenth-century founder of the order must have gone to India; see "The Zikr of the Rahmanija-Order in Algeria: A Psycho-physiological Analysis," *Moslem World* 33 (1943), pp. 16–28, citing p. 18.

[40] Henry Corbin, *En Islam iranien: Aspects spirituels et philosophiques*, vol. 3, *Les Fidèles d'amour, Shî`isme et soufisme*, Bibliothèque des Idées (Paris: Gallimard, 1972), pp. 275–355; Nuruddin Abdurrahmân i Isfarâyinî, *Le Révélateur des mystères: Kâshif al-Asrâr*, ed. and trans. Hermann Landolt (Paris: Verdier, 1986), "Étude Preliminaire," pp. 38–49.

through the late nineteenth century, resulting in a new assignment of six subtle centers to particular parts of the body. A typical version of the Naqshbandi subtle centers puts the heart (*qalb*) two fingers below the left breast, the spirit (*ruh*) two fingers below the right breast, the soul (*nafs*) beneath the navel, the conscience (*sirr*) in the middle of the breast, the mystery (*khafi*) above the eyebrows, and the arcanum (*akhfa*) at the top of the brain.[41]

One could argue that the Naqshbandi-Kubrawi system has a certain similarity with the yogic concept of seven cakras or subtle nerve centers located along the region of the spine, although some of the Sufi centers are clearly unconnected with the spinal region. Both systems include visualization of appropriate colors and sometimes images in particular bodily locations so that one might assume either that the Sufi practices were based on earlier unspecified Indian yoga techniques or that figures like Simnani would have been interested in contemporary yogis. From his biography, however, it appears that Simnani, much against his inclination, was forced to engage in disputations with Buddhist monks at the court of the Mongol ruler Arghun; in these debates, Simnani showed considerable theological hostility to the Buddhists. Although they were probably from Mahayana schools with highly developed yogic techniques of their own, Simnani showed no interest in discussing meditation practices with them.[42]

Recent research has shown that there was considerable practical variation among Sufis in the number of subtle centers, the colors assigned to each subtle center, and even their physical locations in the body. Arthur Buehler has described the adjustable Naqshbandi system of subtle centers as "a heuristic device for the disciple to develop a subtle body or a subtle field with which to travel in non-material realms."[43] Similar variations occur within hatha yoga practices.[44] Despite their

---

[41] Muhammad Dhawqi Shah, *Sirr-i dilbaran* (4th printing, Karachi: Mahfil-i Dhawqiyya, 1405/1985), pp. 298–99.

[42] Jamal J. Elias, *The Throne Carrier of God: The Life and Thought of `Ala' ad-dawla as-Simnani* (Albany: State University of New York Press, 1995), pp. 18, 26; for Simnani's concept of subtle substances or centers, see pp. 79–99.

[43] Arthur Frank Buehler, *Sufi Heirs of the Prophet: The Indian Naqshbandiyya and the Rise of the Mediating Sufi Shaykh*, Studies in Comparative Religion (Charleston, SC: University of South Carolina Press, 1998), p. 112; cf. pp. 103–16 for a full account of the *latifa* system.

[44] Agehananda Bharati, *The Tantric Tradition* (Garden City, N.Y.: Anchor Books, 1970).

comparability, however, the Sufi techniques do not seem to have any intrinsic relation with the psycho-physiology of yoga, and they rarely make reference to the characteristic yogic descriptions of subtle nerves (*nadis*), the breaths, the sun and moon symbolism, or the *kundalini*. In addition, Sufi texts contain a multi-level prophetology and mystical Qur'anic exegesis tied to each of the seven subtle centers so that distinctive Islamic symbolisms are embedded in the system. As will be indicated below, some Naqshbandi Sufis like Ahmad Sirhindi showed explicit hostility toward the practices of jogis and Brahmins. Major manuals of Sufi contemplative practice from remoter areas, such as *Miftah al-falah* or *The Key to Salvation*, by the Egyptian Sufi master Ibn 'Ata' Allah of Alexandria (d. 1309), make no reference to any identifiable Indian yoga technique.[45] Judgments about sources and influences of such practices necessarily ignore the significance accorded them in Sufi interpretations. Enamul Haq, who argued for the yogic origin of the Naqshbandi subtle centers, was forced to explain away the differences by begging the question, calling the Sufi system "quite imperfect and immature . . . due to the ignorance of anatomical knowledge of the Sufis who were far inferior to the Indian Yogins with respect to the scientific knowledge of human body."[46]

This being said, it is striking to see a very late Urdu text that makes explicit comparison between the Naqshbandi system of subtle centers and the yogic cakras. After giving a lengthy description of a six-center version of the Naqshbandi method, Ghawth 'Ali Shah Qalandar Qadiri (d. 1880) remarked in conversation that "These six subtle centers are also in the Sannyasi teaching, the six lotuses (*k'hat kanwal*) or six cakras, according to the *Yoga sastra*." He then enumerated these six lotuses according to a complex yogic scheme that includes a different number of petals for each lotus, which are ordered according to the Sanskrit alphabet; these are depicted in a diagram included in the published version of his discourses, in the form of a long-stemmed plant with groups of petals

---

[45] Ibn 'Ata' Allah al-Sikandari, *Miftah al-falah wa misbah al-arwah* (Egypt: Matba'at Mustafa al-Babi al-Halabi wa Awladuh, 1381/1961); Ibn 'Ata' Allah, *The Key to Salvation & the Lamp of Souls*, trans. Mary Ann Koury Danner (Cambridge, UK: The Islamic Texts Society, 1996).

[46] Muhammad Enamul Haq, *A History of Sufi-ism in Bengal*, Asiatic Society of Bangladesh Publication 30 (Dacca: Asiatic Society of Bangladesh, 1975), p. 139. This study based on a 1937 dissertation, relies to a considerable extent on older Orientalist literature.

bunched together at the level of each lotus. In the upper right corner of the diagram, there is also a drawing of a throne-like platform, with a marginal note on the diagram reading, "Here the student must visualize his guru or *pir* sitting on the throne, [thinking that] 'From the treasury of hidden emanation, an ocean of light has poured over my heart.'" In the brief comment that follows this diagram, Ghawth ʾAli Shah remarked,

> The method of this practice is that through visualization one should trans-
> fer each [Sanskrit] letter from the petal to the inside of the stem. Having
> imagined the stem as a single great river, after reaching the *brahmanda*
> [the cakra at the crown of the skull], one transfers [the letter] above. When
> all the letters are collected above, then in due order the subtle centers
> become active, and the entire body becomes luminous.[47]

This account shows a remarkably detailed knowledge of yoga, gained probably through contact with nineteenth-century jogis, rather than from the vaguely titled book mentioned in this passage (when the transcriber of these discourses inserted the description of the lotuses and their petals, he introduced it only as coming from "a certain sage" [*kisi gyani*]). Although Ghawth ʾAli Shah juxtaposes the Naqshbandi subtle centers and the yogic cakras as similar, this late comparison does not attempt to bridge the conceptual and technical gap between the two meditative systems. This kind of comparison is more a testimony to the author's willingness to bring in the evidence of Indian sages as external confirmation of doctrines and practices based on traditional Islamic sources.[48]

In recent times, Naqshbandi Sufi leaders in northern India have taken significant steps to spread their teachings among Hindu disciples, including a number of Hindu masters who explain the Naqshbandi cosmology with terms from classical hatha yoga. These Naqshbandi branches (centered particularly on Kanpur) constitute what is in effect a new Sufi-based school

---

[47] Gul Hasan Qadiri, *Tadhkira-i ghawthiyya* (Delhi: Matbaʿ-i Faruqi, 1298/1881), pp. 148–50. This section is omitted from the English translation of this text, Gul Hasan, *Solomon's Ring: The Life and Teachings of a Sufi Master*, trans. Hasan Askari (London: Altamira Press, 1998), but see pp. 185–93 for "Encounters with Hindu Sages."

[48] See the brief section entitled "Conversation with Mahapurusa Sannyasi Mata," ibid., pp. 139–44 (trans. Askari, pp. 155–60), which acts as a Hindu supplement to four lengthy chapters on the divine unity based on the Qur'an, hadith, and Sufi authorities (pp. 22–139). Other passing references to yogic practices discussed by Ghawth ʾAli Shah are found on pp. 52 (a mantra with translation), 332 (Hindi verses ascribed to Amir Khusraw on the anahita or unstruck sound).

of yoga, known as Ananda-yoga. Particularly important practices of these groups include silent recitation of the name Allah to awaken the cakras. The overall doctrine of the identity of the microcosm and the macrocosm, common to both Islamicate and Indic traditions, permits a wide-ranging series of analogies between Sufi notions of subtle centers with yogic cakras.[49] This recent development, which inverts the Orientalist view of the relation between Sufism and yoga, is a striking indication of the way in which the history of religion can defy the expectations of essentialism.

Keeping in mind these cautions about the comparative approach, we can briefly survey here some important examples of how Sufis appropriated or interpreted yogic practices, with attention to the most important text, *The Pool of Nectar*. The earliest sources, from the fourteenth century, depict Sufis with a range of reactions to the teaching and practices of the jogis, ranging from skeptical criticism to frank admiration. On the critical side, Sharaf al-Din Maneri (d. 1381), for instance, felt that contemporary jogis did not understand the full meaning of the sayings they had inherited.[50] The Chishti saint Burhan al-Din Gharib (d. 1337) believed that a certain yogi of his acquaintance used fraudulent alchemical techniques and supplemented these with drugs and the assistance of spirits.[51] Some Sufis criticized yogic practices such as meditation and ascetic exercises, on the grounds that in themselves they were devoid of spiritual grace; following the prescribed Islamic religious duties was much more beneficial. Such was the position, not surprisingly, of the doctrinally emphatic Naqshbandi Sufi, Shaykh Ahmad Sirhindi (d. 1624), who regarded jogis, Brahmins, and other non-Muslim ascetics (such as Plato and other ancient Greek philosophers) as irremediably misguided.[52] Likewise, a Sufi teacher in India

---

[49] Thomas Dähnhardt, "La scienza sufica dei centri sottili presso una scuola contemporanea di *yoga*," *Asiatica Venetiana* 2 (1997): 19–29; id., *Change and Continuity in Indian Sufism: A Naqshbandi Mujaddidi Branch in the Hindu Environment* (New Delhi: D.K. Printworld, 2002).

[50] Simon Digby, "Encounters with Jogis in Indian Sufi Hagiography," (unpublished paper presented at the Seminar on Aspects of Religion in South Asia, University of London, January 1970), p. 6.

[51] Carl W. Ernst, *Eternal Garden: Mysticism, History, and Politics at a South Asian Sufi Center*, SUNY Series in Muslim Spirituality in South Asia (New York: State University of New York Press, 1992), p. 328, n. 361.

[52] Ahmad Sirhindi, *Maktubat i imam i rabbani*, 2 vols. (1392/1972; repri., Istanbul: Isik Kitâbevi, 1977), 1:130 (letter 52); 1:366 (letter 221); 1:394 (letter 237); 1:666 (letter 313); 2:157 (letter 55).

named Muhammad Muhyi al-Din displayed considerable ambivalence when a disciple questioned him in 1748 about the divination techniques for estimating the end of one's life, as explained in an early version of *The Pool of Nectar* known as the *Kamrubijaksa*. "This is the practice of the Jogis," he replied; "this is not an activity of the community of Muhammad. Nevertheless, it is correct."[53]

All the same, considerable evidence shows that Sufis commented with interest on particular yogic techniques and concepts, and many of them seem also to have been familiar with versions of *The Pool of Nectar*. The Chishti master Nizam al-Din Awliya' (d. 1325) found one yogi's concept of bodily control impressive, and he was also intrigued by yogic accounts of the effect of different days of the month on the conception of children (until his master indicated to him that he would live a celibate life). His disciple Nasir al-Din Chiragh-i Dihli (d. 1356) commented in passing on the yogic practice of breath control in comparison to that practised by Sufis:

> The essence of this matter is restraint of breath, that is, the Sufi ought to hold his breath during meditation. As long as he holds his breath, his interior is concentrated, and when he releases his breath, the interior is distracted, and it destroys his momentary state. . . . Therefore the Sufi is he whose breath is counted. The adept is the master of breath; this has but a single meaning. The accomplished jogis, who are called *siddha* in the Indian language, breathe counted breaths.[54]

Nasir al-Din's disciple Muhammad al-Husayni Gisu Daraz (d. 1422) felt that breath control was essential for Sufi disciples. In a manual of discipline composed in 1404, he remarked,

> Following the habit of stopping the breath, as is done among the jogis, is necessary for the disciple, but not everyone can do it to the extent that those people can. Those who follow this habit must completely abstain from association with women. Diminution of intake of food and drink permits

---

[53] *Kamrubijaksa*, Pakistan National Museum, Karachi, MS 1957-1060/18-1, fol. 2b (marginal comment).

[54] Nasir al-Din Mahmud Chiragh-i Dihli, *Khayr al-majalis*, comp. Hamid* Qalandar, ed. Khaliq Ahmad Nizami, Publication of the Department of History, Muslim University 5, Studies in Indo-Muslim Mysticism 1 (Aligarh: Muslim University, Department of History, n.d. [1959]), pp. 59-60 (session 12).

the performance of required and supererogatory prayers in the case of one of fixed abode, and the traveler retains mobility. One should avoid idle talk. If control becomes habitual, many thoughts can be banished; thought is natural to the carnal soul.[55]

Nonetheless, Gisu Daraz was extremely careful to limit the extent to which yogic practice was acceptable. "Except for breath control, which is the specialty and support of the jogis, it is necessary for the disciple to avoid all their other kinds of practices. These two points which I have written respecting the jogis are also incumbent on [advanced] Sufis."[56]

Another Chishti, Ashraf Jahangir Simnani (d. 1425), is credited by his biographer with a victory over a yogi, and he was also familiar with mantras of the Naths used for purposes of curing snakebite and similar purposes, which he regarded as magical charms (*afsun*).[57] The later Chishti master 'Abd al-Quddus Gangohi (d. 1537) was probably more familiar with the yoga of the Naths than anyone else in that order. He wrote Hindi verses on the subject under the pen-name "Alakhdas" or "Servant of the Absolute." It is in connection with 'Abd al-Quddus that we find the earliest external reference to the Arabic version of *The Pool of Nectar*, which he is said to have taught to a disciple, Sulayman Mandawi, in the late fifteenth century, in exchange for instruction in Qur'anic recitation.[58] He also composed a treatise called *Rushd nama* or *The Book of Guidance* with

---

[55] Gisu Daraz, *Khatima-i adab al-muridin al-ma'ruf bi-khatima,* Urdu trans. Mu'in al-Din Darda'i (Karachi: Nafis Academy, 1976), p. 158, no. 168.

[56] Ibid., p. 171, no. 205.

[57] Ashraf Jahangir Simnani, *Lata'if-i ashrafi,* comp. Nizam Gharib Yamani, 2 vols. (Delhi: Nusrat al-Matabi', 1295/1878), 2:396.

[58] Simon Digby, "'Abd Al-Quddus Gangohi (1456-1537 A.D.): The Personality and Attitudes of a Medieval Indian Sufi," *Medieval India, A Miscellany* III (1975): 1–66, citing p. 36, equivalent to Rukn al-Din Quddusi, *Lata'if-i Quddusi* (Delhi: Matba'-i Mujtaba'i, 1311/1894), p. 41, anecdote 5. From this source it is known that 'Abd al-Quddus composed a *Risala-i qudsi*, possibly in answer to Mandawi's questions on the yogic text and a manuscript of this text is preserved in Lahore; cf. Muhammad Bashir Husayn, *Fihrist-i makhtutat-i Sherani* (Lahore: Danishgah-i Panjab, 1969), 2:224, no. 1236. On examination, however, the manuscript (22 fols.) turns out to be a conventional Sufi treatise with no reference to yogic practices. On Sulayman Mandawi (d. 945/1538–9, reportedly aged over 150), whose Quranic recitation was inspired by the Prophet and 'Ali during his 50 years of austerities in Mecca, see Muhammad Ghawthi Mandawi, *Adhkar-i abrar, Urdu tarjuma-i gulzar-i abrar,* trans. Fadl Ahmad Jewari (1326/1908; repr., Lahore: Islamic Book Foundation, 1395/1975), pp. 243–44.

considerable yogic content.[59] Later masters of the Chishti order such as Nizam al-Din Awrangabadi (d. 1729) and Hajji Imdad Allah (d. 1899) continued to include descriptions of yogic mantras in Hindi alongside Arabic *dhikr* formulas, together with explicit accounts of yogic postures (although the latter account tends to be much abbreviated). In this way Nizam al-Din Awrangabadi gave a brief account of yogic mantras in his lengthy survey of Sufi meditative practices, *Nizam al-qulub* or *The Order of Hearts*:

> Recollection (*dhikr*) in the Hindi language. Towards the sky [say] "*tuñ*," and towards oneself [say] "*huñ*," though some also [say] "*huñ*" towards the heart. Or one says to the right, "*uhi hi*," and to the left, "*wuhi hi*." Or one says to the right, "*inhañ tuñ*," to the left, "*inhañ tuñ*," towards the direction of prayer (*qibla*), "*inhañ tuñ*," towards heaven, "*uhañ tuñ*." In the heart one strikes "*inhañ tuñ*," though some say towards the ground, "*inhañ tuñ*," towards heaven, "*uhañ tuñ*," and in the direction of the heart, "*inhañ tuñ*."

> Another recollection (*dhikr*) in the Hindi language. One sits cross-legged just like the position of the jogis. One turns the head and eye toward heaven and recites this recollection one thousand times, or recites it even more. In the end a world favors one's wishes. One says this very word: "*uhi uhi*." But one of the eighty-four postures (Hindi *baithak*) has been selected as having the benefit and special quality of all the postures, and it is as follows. One sits cross-legged and brings up both feet, placing the sole of the left foot beneath the genitals, and holding the right foot near it. Then one looks at the stomach and brings the breath up and collects it at the navel, and takes it toward the back. One closes the mouth and holds the tongue firmly on the palate. Then one practices magical imagination (*wahm*), that is, one internally thinks, "*uhi hi*," and one remains hungry and without sleep. If he remains three days together without food or sleep, and remains occupied with this practice, he attains an unconsciousness that produces in him the unveiling of hidden things. He then returns to consciousness or becomes enraptured and intoxicated (*majdhub u mad'hush*).[60]

[59] For bibliographic references see S. A. A. Rizvi, "Sufis and Nâtha Yogis in Mediaeval Northern India (XII to XVI Centuries)," *Journal of the Oriental Society of Australia* 7 (1970): 119–33, citing p. 132, quoting Rukn al-Din's *Lata'if-i Quddusi*, p. 41; idem, *A History of Sufism in India*, vol. 1, *Early Sufism and its History in India to 1600 A.D.* (Delhi: Munshiram Manoharlal Publishers Pvt. Ltd., 1978), p. 335; S. C. R. Weightman, "The Text of *Alakh Bani*," in *Devotional literature in South Asia: Current research, 1985–1988*, ed. R. S. McGregor (Cambridge: Cambridge University Press, 1992), pp. 171–78. Gangohi's knowledge of yoga is discussed at length by Simon Digby in "'Abd Al-Quddus."
[60] Nizam al-Din Awrangabadi, *Nizam al-qulub* (Delhi: Matba`-i Mujtaba'i, 1309/1891–92), p. 32. This text is discussed in detail in Ernst and Lawrence, *Sufi Martyrs of Love*, chapter 2.

This account of yogic mantras from the fifteenth chapter of this survey of *dhikr* techniques resembles the Hindi chant of Farid al-Din Ganj-i Shakkar, the only Hindi chant that Muhammad Ghawth (discussed below) included in his Arabic meditation manual, *The Five Jewels*.[61] Although it is said that Nizam al-Din Awrangabadi had contact with living yogis, he generally prefers to cite yogic practice via Sufi authorities and texts deriving from different Sufi orders.[62]

Along with the Chishtis, it is probably the Shattari Sufis who most integrated yoga into their practice without any hesitation, giving particular emphasis to the mantra.[63] Though the historical origins of this Sufi order are obscure, it seems that it was introduced to India by ʿAbd Allah Shattari (d. 1485), the first Sufi to use that name. The same order is known as the ʿIshqiyya or Bistamiyya in Iran and Central Asia. The latter name points to the association of the Shattaris with the Iranian Sufi Abu Yazid al-Bistami, one of the most powerful early representatives of the ecstatic form of Sufism. There are, on the other hand, traditions that link the Shattaris with the Qadiri order, which trace its origin to the master of sober Sufism, Junayd of Baghdad (d. 910). The characteristic meditative practice of repetition of the Qurʾanic names of God (*dhikr*, plural *adhkar*) formed a prominent part of ʿAbd Allah Shattari's teaching, though only fragments of his written work have

---

[61] I have heard oral commentaries on these Hindi mantras, suggesting a simple mystical interpretation: "*uhañ tuñ*" resembles modern Hindi for "you are there," while "*inhañ tuñ*" sounds like "you are here," so the chant would underscore the presence of God everywhere. Thanks to the late Prof. M. R. Tarafdar for this suggestion.

[62] K. A. Nizami, *Tarikh-i mashayikh-i Chisht* (Delhi: Idarah-i Adabiyyat-i Delli, 1985), 5:174–75; cf. Digby, "ʿAbd al-Quddus," p. 51. In the *Kashkul-i Kalimi* (Delhi: Matbaʿ-i Mujabaʿi, n.d.), Shah Kalim Allah (p.30) describes the single most efficacious postures of yoga according Shaykh Bahaʾ al-Din Qadiri (Shattari?), and he explains the yogi "unstruck sound" (pp. 40–41) with reference to the comments of Miyan Mir of Lahore (Qadiri) and Shaykh Yahya Madani (Chishti).

[63] See Khaliq Ahmed Nizami, "The Shattari Saints and Their Attitude towards the State," *Medieval India Quarterly* 3 (1950): 56–70; Syed Hasan Askari, "A Fifteenth Century Shuttari Sufi Saint of North Bihar," *Proceedings of the 13th Indian History Congress* (1950): 148–57; M. M. Haq, "The Shuttari Order of Sufism in India and Its Exponents in Bengal and Bihar," *Journal of the Asiatic Society of Pakistan* 16 (1971): 167–75; Athar Abbas Rizvi, *A History of Sufism in India* (Delhi: Munshiram Manoharlal Publishers Pvt. Ltd., 1983), 2:151–73.

survived.[64] Certainly in the work of Shaykh Baha' al-Din Shattari (d. 1515) there is evidence of an interest in Indian spiritual practices; his work *Risala-i Shattariyya* or *The Shattari Treatise* contains repetitions of divine names in Hindi, alongside the divine names in Arabic and Persian. The fourth and last chapter is entitled, "On various Arabic, Persian, and Hindi *adhkar*, with attention to certain methods (*suluk*) of the jogis and their *adhkar*, which they recite with magical imagination (*wahm*), the sentences that they recite in meditation, and other incantations (*da`awat*) related to them."[65] Thus, by the beginning of the tenth/sixteenth century, a member of the Shattari order was able to produce a systematic account of yogic mantras and visualization practices, assimilated and even incorporated into the conceptual structure of Sufi tradition.[66]

But, it is particularly with Muhammad Ghawth Gwaliyari (d. 1563), one of the most influential Shattari masters, that yoga became a significant element in the repertoire of Sufi practice. Muhammad Ghawth was notable both for his spiritual teachings and for his political influence with the first Mughal emperors. His spiritual career began with a 13-year period of meditation in the hills around the fort of Chunar in eastern Uttar Pradesh, where he came into contact with jogis who

---

[64] `Abd al-Haqq Muhaddith Dihlawi al-Bukhari, *Akhbar al-akhyar fi asrar al-abrar*, ed. Muhammad `Abd al-Ahad (Delhi: Matba`-i Mujtaba'i, 1332/1913–14), p. 176. Two manuscripts reportedly containing works by `Abd Allah Shattari are *Risala-i `Abd Allah Shattari*, MS Khudabakhsh Library, Patna; and *Tawba wa dhikr*, an anonymous treatise containing sayings of Hallaj and `Abd Allah Shattari, MS Karachi, National Museum 1965-210-21, cit. Ahmad Munzawi, *Fihrist-i Mushtarak-i Nuskha-ha-yi Khatti-i Farsi-i Pakistan* (Islamabad: Markazi-i Tahqiqat-i Farsi-i Iran wa Pakistan, 1363/1405/1984), 3:1365, no. 2447.

[65] Baha' al-Din ibn Ibrahim al-Ansari Shattari, *Risala-i Shattariyya*, MS 297/61 no. 318, Osmania University, Hyderabad, available as microfilm 1018, Middle East collection, University of Chicago, fols. 2a–3a. Unfortunately this copy lacks the fourth chapter. The use of the term imagination (*wahm*) is characteristic of *The Pool of Nectar* (ch. VII).

[66] See Hermann Ethé, Catalogue of Persian Manuscripts in the India Office Library (1903; repr., London: India Office Library & Records, 1980), no. 1913, col. 1060; numerous other copies are found in libraries in India and Pakistan. See also the undated work by Ishaq (a disciple of one `Abd al-Rahman Shattari), titled *Ma`rifat-i anfas*, MS 873(i) Persian (suppl. cat. I), Asiatic Society, Calcutta, which Dara N. Marshall described as "a Persian version of a Hindu tract on metaphysics"; *Mughals in India, A Bibliography* (Bombay: Asia Publishing House, 1967), p. 207, no. 728. From the title, *The Knowledge of Breaths*, it appears to deal with breath control.

were probably visiting the jogi shrine located in the fort.[67] Muhammad Ghawth completed a Persian translation and expansion of *The Pool of Nectar* in Gujarat, probably around 1550, partly out of dissatisfaction with an existing Persian translation and partly in order to clarify the obscurities of the Arabic version.[68] One of the apparently insoluble problems in the study of Indian mantras was the inappropriateness of the Arabic alphabet for precise transliteration of Hindi or Sanskrit terms, a problem complained about by a number of readers. This is an especially acute problem, because as everyone knows, charms and spells must be pronounced exactly right in order to retain their efficacy. Although Muhammad Ghawth did not have access to any Sanskrit text of *The Pool of Nectar*, he incorporated his knowledge of contemporary hatha yoga. His version is greatly expanded from the existing Arabic text, with considerable differences based in part upon his access to an earlier recension of the Arabic version that no longer survives. It seems likely that he had been using *The Pool of Nectar* as a teaching text with his disciples in the Shattari Sufi order and that his Persian translation emerged as an oral commentary on the Arabic. The teachings of *The Pool of Nectar*, as adapted by Muhammad Ghawth, apparently occupied a significant position in the literature of the Shattari order. Most of the material on cakras in chapter VII may be found in a manual of Shattari teachings written by Muhammad Rida Shattari of Lahore (d. 1706), *Adab-i muridi* or *The Manners of Discipleship*.[69]

In this connection it is necessary to mention Muhammad Ghawth's popular mystical treatise, *Jawahir-i khamsa* or *The Five Jewels*, first composed in the shaykh's youth and later revised in 1549.[70] The Mecca-based Shattari teacher Sibghat Allah (d. 1606) later translated this text into Arabic, and under his successors, these practices were taught to disciples from as far away as North Africa and Indonesia; through these Shattari channels, North African authors such as al-Sanusi learned of jogis in the guise of a Sufi order called al-Jukiyya, with their own distinctive *dhikr*

---

[67] Briggs, *Gorakhnath and the Kanphata Yogis*, p. 82.

[68] Carl W. Ernst, "Sufism and Yoga according to Muhammad Ghawth," *Sufi* 29 (Spring 1996): 9–13.

[69] Muhammad Riza Shattari Qadiri Lahuri, *Adab-i muridi*, MS 5319 `irfan, Ganj Bakhsh, Islamabad (Munzawi, *Fihrist-i Mushtarak-i*, 3:1218, no. 2149), pp. 31–32, 62–78.

[70] Muhammad Ghawthi Mandawi, *Gulzar-i abrar* (MS 259 Persian, Asiatic Society), fol. 326a.

formulas.[71] *The Five Jewels* deserves comment here, because, despite the assertions of certain nineteenth-century Orientalists, it in fact contains hardly anything that might be considered Indian in content. Nevertheless, Hughes' popular *Dictionary of Islam* (first published in 1885, and still in print) described it as follows: "This book is largely made up of Hindu customs which, in India, have become part of Muhammadanism," without explaining what that could mean.[72] In reality, the text consists almost entirely of prayers in Arabic, together with instructions on how they can be used as charms to gain particular results, or else recited as *dhikr* recitations in familiar Sufi style. The first section (or "jewel") explains how one may deepen one's devotional life through the Islamic ritual prayer. The second section concerns prayer using the divine names, while the third describes the use of the divine names as "invocations (*da`wat*)" to obtain specific goals (this is the longest section of the book). The fourth section deals with the specific techniques of the Shattari order, and the fifth is devoted to the way to see God. The text contains a single *dhikr* formula in Hindi, attributed, not to any yogi, but to the early Chishti Sufi master Farid al-Din Ganj-i Shakkar (d. 1265).[73] For the Shattari Sufis' understanding of the practices of yoga, the Persian translation of *The Pool of Nectar* is the primary source, rather than *The Five Jewels*. Its continued popularity is attested both by a large number of manuscripts and a nineteenth-century Urdu translation by a Qadiri Sufi in southern India.

Further citations from *The Pool of Nectar* can be found up through the nineteenth century. Because of the wide circulation of the Arabic version of *The Pool of Nectar* in Ottoman lands, Turkish Sufis there cited its

---

[71] See Muhammad ibn Khatir al-Din ibn Khwaja al-`Attar [Muhammad Ghawth], *al-Jawahir al-Khams*, Arabic trans. from Persian by Sibghat Allah, ed. Ahmad ibn al-`Abbas, 2nd ed. (Egypt: Muhammad Rif`at `Amir, 1393/1973), pp. 3–9; Muhammad ibn `Ali al-Sanusi, *al-Salsabil al-mu`in fil-tara'iq al-arba`in*, in *al-Masa'il al-`ashar* (Cairo, n.d.), pp. 124ff.

[72] Thomas Patrick Hughes, *A Dictionary of Islam* (1885; repr., Delhi: Oriental Publishers, 1973), s.v. "Da`wah," pp. 72–78. Cf. also Ja`far Sharif, *Islam in India or the Qanun-i-Islam, the Customs of the Musalmans of India*, trans. G. A. Herklots, ed. William Crooke (1921; repr., Oriental Books Reprint Corporation, 1972), pp. 219–31, for examples of practices taken from *The Five Jewels*. Marc Gaborieau has discussed these practices in detail in "L'Ésotérisme musulman dans le sous-continent indo-pakistanais: un point de vue ethnologique," *Bulletin d'Études Orientales* 14 (1993) : 191–210.

[73] Muhammad Ghawth, *al-Jawahir al-khams*, 2:70. The same *dhikr* was also quoted by the later Shattari author of Bihar, Imam Rajgiri (d. ca. 1718); cf. Askari, "A Fifteenth Century Shuttari Sufi Saint," p. 157; Haq, "The Shuttari Order," p. 175 (with wide textual variations).

practices as part of the continuum of Sufi experience, many of the manuscripts being attributed to the great Andalusian Sufi master Ibn `Arabi (d. 1240); we shall return to this pseudonymous attribution below. The popularity of the text led to its being translated twice into Ottoman Turkish during the eighteenth century, and one of these translations was printed in Istanbul in 1910; the text was particularly popular among Sufis of the Mevlevi order. One Ottoman testimony to this text was provided by a certain Muhammad al-Misri, who, in a Turkish catechism on Sufism in question-and-answer form, cited the importance of breath control by quoting from *The Pool of Nectar*; the passage in question (I.2) describes how control of the "sun" and "moon" breaths in the right and left nostrils can make one impervious to heat and cold.[74] Sir Richard Burton also encountered a reference to the teachings of *The Pool of Nectar* in Sind in the early nineteenth century in an unnamed writing by a Sufi named Mahmud of Karya (evidently Mahmud Nizamani of Kara, d. 1818). Burton cited an unspecified treatise on Sufism by Mahmud which referred to the frame story at the beginning of *The Pool of Nectar* (Int.2-4), in which a Hindu sage from Kamru came to Lakhnauti and converted to Islam after losing a disputation with Qadi Rukn al-Din Samarqandi, and "from a Hindoo work, the Amirat Kandha [i.e., *Amritakunda* or *Pool of Nectar*], composed a treatise in Arabic and named it Hauz el Hayat [*Pool of Life*]."[75] Burton took this story as a sign of the "popular belief" as to the Indian origin of Sufism, a subject on which he (unlike Sir William Jones and many others) declined to take a position. Although these fragmentary references testify to the wide diffusion of *The Pool of Nectar*, they also indicate that it was

---

[74] John P. Brown, "On the Tesavuf, or Spiritual Life of the Soffees, Translated from the Turkish of Mohemmed Missiree," *Journal of the American Oriental Society* 8 (1856): 95–104, quoting the *Hawd al-hayat* on pp. 99–100; reprinted in id., *The Dervishes; or, Oriental Spiritualism* (London: Trübner and Co., 1868), pp. 359–70, quoting the *Hawd al-hayat* on p. 365; also reprinted in Hughes, *A Dictionary of Islam*, s.v. "Sufi," pp. 615a–617b, where the quotation from *Hawd al-hayat* occurs on p. 616a. It is not clear which author or text was translated here by Brown; a manuscript of a Turkish catechism by Niyazi Muhammad Misri (d. 1697), similarly entitled *As'ila wa ajwiba-i mutasavvifana* (Reşit 353, fols. 25–32, Suleimaniye Library, Istanbul), does not contain this passage.
[75] Richard F. Burton, *Sindh* (1851; repr., Lahore: Khan Publications, 1971), pp. 199, 405. Unfortunately, in the absence of the text of Nizamani it is difficult to know which version of the text he had in mind. Several Persian works by Mahmud Nizamani of Kara, including two collections of the discourses (*malfuzat*) of his master Pir Muhammad Rashid (d. 1827) are listed by Munzawi, *Fihrist-i Mushtarak-i*, 3:1383, no. 2481; 3:1548, no. 2840, 3.1840, no. 3416.

used very selectively. A similar instance arises in the case of the fifteenth-century Yemeni Jewish scholar Alu'el, who cited the yogic teachings on the positive and negative qualities of right- and left-hand breaths from *The Pool of Nectar* in his exegesis of a Biblical text (Genesis 13:9).[76] In such a case, the ultimately Indian material was only of significance insofar as it contributes to the main point the author is making.

While the scope of this essay is limited primarily to Arabic, Persian, and Urdu sources, it should nevertheless be pointed out that a more extensive engagement with yogic tradition took place among Indian Sufis through regional Indic languages, especially on the frontiers of Bengal and the Punjab. It may be that the process of translation into literary Persian and Arabic imposed certain limits on the transmission of Indian religious concepts, whether because of the highly developed cosmological and psychological vocabulary tied to Islamic and Hellenistic sources or because of the specific teaching requirements of Sufi orders. Literary composition in local languages may have been less prone to this difficulty. The sixteenth-century eastern Hindi romance *Padmavat* by Muhammad Ja'isi, a Chishti Sufi, contains a far more extensive picture of yogic physiology and practice than *The Pool of Nectar.*[77] The same is true of a host of Bengali Muslim authors who explored the themes of yogic physiology and cosmology with considerable technical skill. Here, we find full details of the cakras, the nerves, drinking nectar, and other yogic themes, together with more extensive metaphysical concepts, combined with certain Islamic identifications. A work suggestively called the *Yoga-Qalandar* identifies the cakras with Sufi mystical stations and substitutes angels for Hindu deities in the cakras. There is even a biography of Gorakhnath called *Goraksa-vijaya* written by a Muslim author named Fayd Allah.[78] In the Indus region, while this level of immersion

---

[76] Y. Tzvi Langermann, *Yemenite Midrash: Philosophical Commentaries on the Torah*, Sacred Literature Series (San Francisco: HarperSanFrancisco, 1996), pp. 276–77.

[77] White, *Alchemical Body*, pp. 260–62.

[78] For suggestive reviews of this literature, see Momtazur Rahman Tarafdar, *Husain Shahi Bengal 1494–1538 A.D., A Socio-Political Study*, Asiatic Socity of Pakistan Publication 16 (Dacca: Asiatic Society, 1965), pp. 198–225; id., "Influence of the Natha cult on the growth of Sufism in Bengal," in *Shi`a Islam, Sects and Sufism: Historical Dimensions, Religious Practice and Methodological Considerations*, ed. Frederick De Jong (Utrecht: Publications of the M. Th. Houtsma Stichting, 1992), pp. 97–104; Enamul Haq, *Sufi-ism in Bengal*, pp. 368–422; David Cashin, *The Ocean of Love: Middle Bengali Sufi Literature and the Fakirs of Bengal* (Stockholm: Association of Oriental Studies, Stockholm University, 1995).

in yogic concepts did not occur, the yogi became a popular figure in poetry written in Punjabi and Sindi. The writings of the great Sindh poet and Sufi `Abd al-Latif B'hita'i (d. 1752) furnish a very positive evaluation of jogis. He himself had worn the ochre robe and wandered like a Hindu sannyasin, visiting the major jogi places of pilgrimage in the Indus region while traveling with jogis for a space of three years. One of his cycles of poetry, the "Sur Ramkali," is dedicated to the praise of the ideal jogis.[79] Bullhe Shah (d. 1758), a Punjabi Sufi poet, used folklore motifs that portray the archetypal yogi as the mystical beloved.[80] It has been suggested that he was familiar with the Persian translation of *The Pool of Nectar* through his master Shah `Inayat Qadiri (d. 1735), author of the *Dastur al-`amal* or *The Handbook of Practice*, a work that discusses yogic teachings.[81] Much remains to be done in the evaluation of the significance of yogic themes in these literatures.

****

"Baba Ratan the Hajji, that is, Gorakhnath, having been the nurse of the Prophet [Muhammad], and having nourished the revered Messenger, taught the Prophet the path of yoga."

—*Dabistan*

COMPETING RHETORICAL STRATEGIES OF SUFIS AND JOGIS

Much of the historical evidence for the interaction of jogis and Sufis appears to lie in Sufi hagiographical texts, and this material is definitely written from a Sufi point of view. The first attempt to analyze and classify accounts of jogis in Sufi literature was made by Simon Digby in an

---

[79] Motilal Jotwani, *Shah Abdul Latif: His Life and Work* (Delhi: University of Delhi, 1975), pp. 29, 33–34, 126, 140–41.

[80] Denis Matringe, "Krsnaite and Nath elements in the poetry of the eighteenth-century Panjabi Sufi Bullhe Sah," in *Devotional literature in South Asia: Current research, 1985–1988*, ed. R. S. McGregor (Cambridge: Cambridge University Press, 1992), pp. 190–206; J. R. Puri and T. R. Shangari, *Bulleh Shah, the Love-intoxicated Iconoclast* (New Delhi: Radha Soami Satsang Beas, 1986), pp. 117–18, 169–70; Lajwanti Rama Krishna, *Pañjabi Sufi Poets A.D. 1460-1900* (New Delhi: Ashajanak Publications, 1973), pp. 71–74.

[81] Maqbul Beg Badakhshani, "Adabi manzar," in *Tarikh-i adabiyat-i Musalmanan-i Pakistan o Hind*, ed. Sayyid Fayyaz Mahmud (Lahore: Punjab University, 1971), 4:129; cf. Rama Krishna, *Pañjabi Sufi Poets*, pp. 65–66, where Shah `Inayat's commentary on the *Jawahir-i khamsa* of Muhammad Ghawth is also cited.

oft-cited unpublished paper.[82] Digby classifies these stories into several categories, most of which involve the conversion of the yogis to Islam: 1) spontaneous conversion of the yogis in the presence of Sufis; 2) magical contests between yogis and Sufis, in which the yogi is vanquished and converts to Islam; 3) magical contests leading to conversion of the yogi, in which a contested sacred site is yielded to the Sufi; 4) a Sufi's refusal of gifts from a yogi; and 5) casual reference to the lore and practices of the yogis. In these stories it is clear that one of the key issues is the rivalry between Sufis and jogis in terms of miraculous powers. The Sufi sources generally maintain that even when jogis perform what appear to be miracles, these must be considered in a different light than actual miracles performed by Sufi saints, who are inspired by God. Following an old distinction, Sufi writers often classify the powers of these non-Muslim charismatic figures as false miracles (*istidraj*) of Satanic inspiration, as contrasted with the genuine miracles (*karamat*) that God permits saints to perform. From the perspective of this study, it is remarkable that only one of the five categories of stories concerns the interest of Sufis in yogic techniques and practices; the first four categories all have to do with establishing the religious and thaumaturgical superiority of the Sufis over the jogis.

As Digby points out, the numerous hagiographic accounts of encounters between Sufis and jogis (or other Hindu figures) almost always depict the yogi acknowledging the superior spiritual power of the Sufi.[83] There is necessarily a theological element of triumph in this kind of narrative. This is evident in a story told by Nizam al-Din Awliya' (d. 1325), describing a yogi who challenged a Sufi to a levitation contest. While the yogi could rise vertically in the air, with God's help the Sufi was able to fly first in the direction of Mecca, then to the north and south, before returning to accept the submission of the yogi; the flight in the direction of Mecca surely indicates the religious

---

[82] Digby, "Encounters with Jogis." See also Simon Digby, *Wonder-Tales of South Asia* (Jersey: Orient Monographs, 2000), pp. 140–220, "The Tale of Gorakh Nath"; pp. 221–33, "Medieval Sufi Tales of Yogis."

[83] Similar stories from the Deccan are related by Richard M. Eaton, *Sufis of Bijapur 1300-1700; Social Roles of Sufis in Medieval India* (Princeton, NJ: Princeton University Press, 1977), pp. 53–54, 110–11, 132–33.

character of the victory.[84] While this basic pattern emerged in texts of the fourteenth century, the most grandiose versions derive from the later Mughal period, as in an extravagant hagiography called *Siyar al-aqtab* or *Lives of the World-Axes*, completed by Ilah-diya Chishti in 1647. In the biographical account of Mu'in al-Din Chishti, his arrival in India is described as the result of a divine command issued to him by God from the Ka'ba in Mecca. He consequently arrived in Ajmer, with orders to unleash holy war on the infidel king, and he immediately threatened to destroy the idol temples there. He conspicuously slaughtered and ate a cow, arousing the wrath of the local populace, but they were unable to harm him. Such was his power that the deity (*dev*) worshipped in the local temple converted to Islam and became his disciple. Then the yogi Ajaypal arrived with 1,500 followers, but his numerous magical assaults on the Sufi were all rendered ineffective by the saint's power. In what becomes a typical episode in this kind of story, the yogi then took to the air and flew away on his deerskin, but the Sufi sent his shoes up in the air to beat the yogi into humble submission, and so the yogi returned and converted to Islam, becoming a disciple of Mu'in al-Din and at the same time gaining the boon of immortality. The story then continues with the refusal of the Raja of Ajmer to convert to Islam, leading Mu'in al-Din to proclaim the forthcoming victory of Sultan Shihab al-Din and the establishment of the Delhi Sultanate.[85] The story contains several elements missing in earlier Sufi biographies of Mu'in al-Din, particularly the emphasis on conversion to Islam and strident imperialism, so that it crosses the line between hagiography and royal historiography The story's triumphalism thus has a strong political dimension as well as a theological one.[86] These stories of one-upmanship over jogis were not limited to Sufis, however. To this class of triumphal encounters belongs the important biography of the Sikh founder-figure, Guru Nanak, who is

---

[84] Nizam al-Din Awliya' Bada'oni, *Fawa'id al-fu'ad*, comp. Hasan 'Ala Sijzi, ed. Muhammad Latif Malik (Lahore: Malik Siraj al-Din and Sons, 1386/1966), p. 84; trans. Bruce B. Lawrence, *Nizam Ad-Din: Morals for the Heart* (New York: Pauist Press, 1992); cf. Digby, "Encounters," p. 12.

[85] Ilah-diya Chishti, *Siyar al-aqtab*, pp. 124–33, trans. Simon Digby, *The Shrine and Cult of Mu'in al-Din Chishti of Ajmer*, by P. M. Currie, Oxford University South Asian Studies Series (Delhi: Oxford University Press, 1992), pp. 72–81.

[86] Ernst, *Eternal Garden*, pp. 90–91.

depicted as confounding the Nath siddhas of his day with his profound teachings on the nature of the "true jogi."[87] A similar appeal to the ideal of the "true jogi" occurs in an Isma`ili hymn, in which the Isma`ili imam establishes his superiority to the Nath jogi Kanipha.[88]

The triumphal rhetoric of the tales of Sufis humbling jogis is matched by an unusual literary phenomenon, in which extensive expositions of yogic teachings occur in pseudonymous texts that are ascribed to well-known Sufis. Most of the Arabic manuscripts of *The Pool of Nectar* in Istanbul libraries are attributed to the authorship of the great Andalusian Sufi master, Ibn `Arabi. The founder of the Indian Chishtiyya, Mu`in al-Din Chishti, is likewise said to be the author of an extremely popular work on yoga that is found under several different titles, most commonly called *Wujudiyya* (*The Treatise on Existence*). This treats the subtle nerves and breath control, using the standard Hindi terms of yogic physiology; at the same time, the yogic material is followed by meditations on the Arabic names of God, but the Sufi and yogic materials remain separate, without any attempt to integrate them.[89] Another such work is the *Risala-i haft nam* (*Treatise on the Seven Names*), also called *Haft ahbab* (*The Seven Friends*), a composite work attributed to the early Sufi Hamid al-Din Nagawri (d. 1295) and others, sometimes classified as a work on alchemy. Each of the seven chapters is separately entitled with a phrase containing the number seven. The second chapter, by Gyan Nath the Jogi alias "Felicitous" (Persian *sa`adatmand*), is entitled in Hindi as

---

[87] Max Arthur Macauliffe, "Life of Guru Nanak: Chapter XIII," in *The Sikh Religion*, Vol. 1 (Oxford: Oxford University Press, 1909), http://www.sacred-texts.com/skh/tsr1/tsr116. htm; W. H. McLeod, *Guru Nanak and the Sikh Religion* (Oxford: Clarendon Press, 1968), p. 141.

[88] Dominique-Sila Khan, "Conversation between Guru Hasan Kabiruddin and Jogi Kahipha: Tantra Revisited by the Isma`ili Preachers," in *Tantra in Practice*, ed. David Gordon White, Princeton Readings in Religions (Princeton, NJ: Princeton University Press, 2000), pp. 285–95.

[89] I have consulted copies of this and another Persian text on yoga ascribed to Mu`in al-Din Chishti, kindly provided by Pir Zia Inayat Khan from his personal collection, both entitled *Risala-i wujudiyya*. Munzavi (*Fihrist-i Mushtarak-i*, 3:2101–3, no. 3820) lists ten MSS of this title in Pakistan, the earliest dated 1084/1673–74; see also Muhammad Bashir Husayn, *Fihrist-i makhtutat-i Shafi` (ba-farsi o urdu o panjabi) dar kitabkhana-i Professor Doctor Mawlawi Muhammad Shafi`*, ed. Ahmad Rabbani (Lahore: Danishgah-i Panjab, 1392 q./1351 sh./1972), pp. 261–62, no. 305. A text with the same title in Calcutta (Ivanow, ASB Curzon 460/5) is attributed to Farid al-Din Ganj-i Shakkar.

Sat sagar (*The Seven Oceans*) and is written in Hindi with a Persian translation. The third chapter, *The Seven Stars*, is credited to Sulayman Mandawi (d. 1538–39), a prominent Muslim scholar who had studied the Arabic version of the *The Pool of Nectar* with `Abd al-Quddus Gangohi, but the remaining authors are obscure.[90] These yogic texts appropriated by Sufi tradition form a literary equivalent to the submission of jogis to Sufis (like that of Ajaypal to Mu`in al-Din Chishti) in the later hagiographic legends.[91]

The process of inter-religious appropriation was not entirely one-sided, however. Jogis and other ascetics on the fringes of society appear to have been open to friendly exchanges with Muslims from an early date. The Persian merchant and traveler Buzurg ibn Shahriyar, writing around 953, commented that the Kapalika ascetics of Ceylon "take kindly to Musulmans and show them much sympathy."[92] The Tibetan Buddhist historian Taranath, writing in the thirteenth century, was critical of the Nath jogis for following Shiva rather than the Buddha, and what was more, "They used to say that they were not even opposed to the Turuskas (Turks)."[93] The jogis went on to mythologize their encounter with Sufism and with the Indo-Muslim culture represented by Turkish and Mughal emperors. A mural on a Nath jogi temple in Nepal displays the submissive visit of the Ghurid sultans in the twelfth century.[94] Legends about the humiliation of hostile Muslims, the efforts of Muslim rulers to become disciples of jogis, and the reconstruction of jogi temples after their destruction by Muslims (especially by the late

---

[90] Muhammad Bashir Husayn, *Fihrist-i makhtutat-i Sherani* (Lahore: Danishgah-i Panjab, 1969), 3:566; Munzavi, *Fihrist-i Mushtarak-i*, 3:842, citing also Charles Rieu, *Catalogue of the Persian Manuscripts in the British Museum*, 3 vols. (1879–83; repr., London: The Trustees of the British Museum, 1966) 2:486. Other MSS are cited by C. A. Storey, *Persian Literature: A Bio-bibliographical* Survey (London: Luzac & Company, Ltd., 1972), 2:438, no. 3.

[91] On the general problem of pseudonymous authorship in Sufi texts, see my "On Losing One's Head: Radical Hallajian motifs in works attributed to 'Attar," in *Farid al-Din `Attar and the Persian Sufi Tradition*, ed. Leonard Lewisohn (London: I. B. Tauris, forthcoming).

[92] Buzurg ibn Shahriyar, *The Book of the Marvels of India*, French trans. L. Marcel Devic [1883–86], English trans. Peter Quennell (New York: The Dial Press, 1929), p. 132.

[93] *Taranatha's History of Buddhism in India*, trans. Lama Chimpa and Alaka Chattopadhyaya (Simla: Indian Institute of Advanced Study, 1970), p. 320.

[94] Bouillier, *Ascètes et rois*, pp. 68–75 (this mural is reproduced in color in the unnumbered plate on the second-to-last page before p. 129).

Mughal emperor Awrangzeb, d. 1707) are common.[95] These triumphal stories should probably be seen as part of a tradition of rhetorical inversion of Mughal authority rather than as historical evidence of temple destruction, to judge from the legendary proliferation of such stories about Awrangzeb.[96]

From their conversations with Sufis over the years, the jogis also undoubtedly picked up a fair amount of information about the Sufi orders and their Islamic origins. They had a special interest in a relatively late figure known as Abu al-Rida Ratan, or simply Baba Ratan, who was buried in the Punjabi village of Bhatinda in 1243. He is well known throughout the Islamic lands as one who claimed Methuselah-like longevity; according to his own account, he had been born over 600 years previously in India, had heard rumors of the appearance of the Prophet Muhammad in Arabia, and had gone to meet him in person and became his follower. Thus, he was able at this late date to relate hadith reports from the Prophet with no intermediary. Although challenged by some Islamic scholars, his authenticity was accepted by others, such as the famous Ibn Hajar al-`Asqalani, and he was adopted as patron saint of the gardeners' guild in Istanbul.[97] Jogis of a later date confidently told the Zoroastrian author of the *Dabistan* that Baba Ratan had in fact been Gorakhnath and that he had initiated the Prophet into the practices of hatha yoga; this was one of the main reasons for the successful spread of Islam. Here is the full account of the jogis' philosophy of religious history, according to the *Dabistan*:

---

[95] Bouillier, *Ascètes et rois*, pp. 116–18; Briggs, *Gorakhnath and the Kanphata Yogis*, pp. 70 (Awrangzeb as rejected disciple of Gorakhnath), 92, 94–95, 105, 144 (Akbar as initiate). See also the account of a Nath yogi's relationship with Shah `Alam II (d. 1809), translated by David Gordon White, "The Wonders of Sri Mastnath," in *The Religions of India in Practice*, pp. 399–411.

[96] Carl W. Ernst, "Admiring the Works of the Ancients: The Ellora Temples as viewed by Indo-Muslim Authors," in *Beyond Turk and Hindu: Rethinking Religious Identities in Islamicate South Asia*, ed. David Gilmartin and Bruce B. Lawrence (Gainesville, FL: University Press Florida, 2000), pp. 198–220.

[97] J. Horovitz, "Baba Ratan, the Saint of Bhatinda," *Journal of the Punjab Historical Society* 2 (1913-14): 97–117; `Abd al-Hayy ibn Fakhr al-Din al-Hasani, *Nuzhat al-khawatir wa bahjat al-masami` wa al-nawazir*, 2nd ed. (Hyderabad: Da'irat al-Ma`arif al-`Uthmaniyya, 1386/1966–), 1:112–18. Manuscripts of a collection of Persian translations of his hadith transmission are noticed by Munzawi, *Fihrist-i Mushtarak-i*, 3:1544, no. 2838.

The Jogis are a famous group in India. "Yoga" in Sanskrit means "to unite" (Persian *payvastan*), and these people take themselves to have attained God. They call God *alak* (Hindi *alakh*, "pure"), and in their belief the chosen one of God, rather his Essence, is Gorakhnath. Likewise, Machhindernath and Cauranginath are among the Siddha saints, that is, perfect ones. According to them, Brahma and Vishnu and Mahesh are [merely] angels, but they [the jogis] are students and disciples of Gorakhnath, just as today some of them claim to be connected to each of these. This group consists of twelve *panth*s . . . [the author enumerates these]. *Panth* is what they call a sect (*firqa*). It is their claim that the masters of all religions, communities, and teachings coming from the prophets and saints are students of Gorakhnath; whatever they have attained is attained from him. The belief of this group is that Muhammad (peace be upon him) was trained by a student of Gorakhnath, but from fear of the Muslims they cannot say it. Rather they say this, that Baba Ratan the Hajji, that is, Gorakhnath, having been the nurse of the Prophet, and having nourished the revered Messenger, taught the Prophet the path of yoga. When among Muslims, they are scrupulous about fasting and ritual prayer, but when with Hindus, they practice the religion of this group. None of the forbidden things is prohibited in their sect, whether they eat pork according to the custom of Hindus and Christians, or beef according to the religion of Muslims and others. . . . In the belief of this group, even if every path proceeds from Gorakhnath, and every sect may be connected to Gorakh, still in their view they have travelled the path that is connected to one of the twelve orders of yoga.[98]

The Nath Jogi tradition of incorporating Islamic prophets into its own narrative is still alive today. A recent visitor to the central Nath temple at Gorakhpur gives the following surprising account:

I visited the Gorakhnath Mandir with my wife in February 1998. There we saw, among other things, a hall adorned with ... statues of the masters claimed by the Nath lineage. Statues were of Muhammad, as well as of Abraham (and Jesus, etc.). Below was a small board explaining that

---

[98] Mobad Shah [Muhsin Fani, attr.], *Dabistan al-madhahib* (Bombay, 1262/1846), pp. 149–50. Instead of "Baba Ratan," the lithograph text erroneously reads "Baba Rin," a mistake caused by misplacing two dots. This error is repeated, moreover, both in the recent Tehran edition and in the highly inaccurate 1843 translation of Shea and Troyer; cf. *The Dabistán or School of Manners*, trans. David Shea and Anthony Troyer, reprint ed, abridged by A. V. Williams Jackson (Washington: M. Walter Dunne, 1901), pp. 239–40.

Muhammad was in fact a Nath yogi, and that the Mecca was in fact a Shaiva center, known in some Purânas as Makeshvar.[99]

This particular incorporation of Muhammad into Hindu tradition has not been publicized, however. Jogis had made a further observation to their Zoroastrian interlocutor, which they normally refrained from making to their Muslim acquaintances: the spiritual power of mosques could be easily explained by the striking resemblance of the *mihrab* (prayer-niche) and the minaret towers to the *yoni* (vulva) and *lingam* (phallus) of Shaivite worship, for which reason the prayer-niche and minaret were always found together.[100] The jogis reasoned that these prominent architectural features were responsible for the spread of Islam. The various accounts of jogis and saints who had miraculous experiences at Mecca without becoming Muslims, including the famous story of Guru Nanak, founder of the Sikhs, evidently belong in this category of Indian mythologies, which relativized the sacred sources of Islam and subordinated them to Indian figures and categories.[101] Ratan Nath is, in any case, a name firmly ensconced in yogic tradition, and in Indian stories unrelated to the long-lived hadith scholar, he figures as a Nath in the third generation after Gorakhnath.[102]

The relationship between Islam and yoga is further complicated by the participation of Muslims in the Nath Jogi tradition. Out of the 13 principal Nath sub-orders described by Briggs, one, the Rawal or Nagnath order, located in the Punjab, consists of Muslims despite being originally derived from Shiva. Two of the six minor sub-orders, the Handi Pharang and the Jafir Pirs, are also Muslim in composition, as their names suggest; although they are Kanphatas and undergo the customary initiations, the Hindu jogis do not eat with them.[103] The 1891 Indian census, which listed all jogis under the category of "miscellaneous and disreputable vagrants," gave figures indicating that over 17 per cent of jogis were Muslims, even though by 1921 the proportion of

---

[99] Letter of David DuBois, 4 June 2003.
[100] *Dabistan.*, p. 157; trans. Shea and Troyer, p. 251.
[101] Ibid., p. 147 (Akamnath); trans. Shea and Troyer, p. 235.
[102] Briggs, *Gorakhnath and the Kanphata Yogis*, p. 92.
[103] Ibid., pp. 66, 71.

Muslims had fallen to less than 5 per cent.[104] It is difficult to interpret these figures without more knowledge of the social context, but they are still an interesting index of continuing existence of Muslim jogis in recent times; it is impossible to tell whether they were originally jogis who became Islamized or Muslims who were drawn into the ranks of the jogi orders.

Beyond the ranks of the jogis themselves, Muslims also formed relationships with jogi shrines, both as pilgrims and as administrators. Ratan Nath's disciple, known as Kaya Nath or Qa'im al-Din, has both Muslim and Hindu followers who have built for him separately a samadhi and a tomb, and one can find numerous examples of this kind of dual religious shrine for jogis in the Punjab and in the Deccan.[105] The important jogi shrines of Hinglaj (now in the province of Baluchistan in Pakistan) and Amarnath (in the Indian Himalayas) have for centuries been in the custody of Muslims, who regulate the pilgrimage rites in those places. In the case of Amarnath, the famous ice *lingam* in the cave there was apparently discovered several centuries ago by local Muslim shepherds, who announced this prodigy to their Hindu acquaintances. The shepherds' descendants to this day preside over the annual pilgrimage and take a good percentage of the revenue, though their position has recently been threatened by the attempts of Kashmiri militant groups to harass the pilgrims.[106] At Hinglaj, the story is told that at one time a Muslim woman in charge of the shrine required pilgrims to become Muslims in order to perform the rituals. Consequently, on their return to India proper, at a site near Karachi, the pilgrims would receive a brand mark of Shiva, to indicate that they were remade Hindus; we are not told how they dealt with circumcision.[107] These examples, which fall outside the elite circles of the Sufi orders, illustrate the difficulty of drawing firm lines separating Muslim and Hindu identities in the yogic tradition. In institutional terms, dual-use shrines exhibit a profound ambiguity that allows different groups to claim ownership without any sense of contradiction.

---

[104] Ibid., pp. 4–6, with 1891 figures of 214,546 yogis in all India and 38,137 Muslim jogis in the Punjab, and 1921 figures of 629,978 Hindu yogis and 31,158 Muslim yogis.

[105] Ibid., p. 66; J. J. Roy Burman, *Hindu-Muslim Syncretic Shrines and Communities* (New Delhi : Mittal Publications, 2002).

[106] Saba Naqvi Bhaumik, "Journey's End," *Indian Express*, 7 August 1994.

[107] Briggs, *Gorakhnath and the Kanphata Yogis*, pp. 106–7, 109–10.

The ambiguous relationship between Sufism and yoga may finally be summarized in the striking identification of the founder-figures of the Nath tradition and the esoteric initiators of Islamic lore, which is announced for the first time in *The Pool of Nectar*.

> When you have reached this station, and this condition becomes characteristic of you, closely examine three things with thought and discrimination: 1) The embryo, how it breathes while it is in the placenta, though its mother's womb does not respire; 2) the fish, how it breathes in the water, and the water does not enter it; 3) and the tree, how it attracts water in its veins and causes it to reach its heights. The embryo is Shaykh Gorakh, who is Khidr (peace be upon him), the fish is Shaykh Minanath [Matsyendranath], who is Jonah, and the tree is Shaykh Caurangi, who is Ilyas, and they are the ones who have reached the water of life (V.4).

The precise significance of this identification is elusive and problematic. The first case recalls ancient Indian associations of the embryo's breath as dispensing with inhalation and exhalation, a goal of yogic breathing exercise.[108] The comparison with Khidr rests loosely on his association with water. In the second case, the fish clearly explains the association of Matsyendra ("lord of the fish") with the Prophet Jonah, who spent three days in the belly of a fish. The third case is more obscure. Caurangi Nath figures alongside Gorakh in the Marathi tradition as a disciple of Matsyendra Nath, and his name comes up in various lists of *Siddhas*.[109] Ilyas (Elijah) is one of the figures in Islamic lore who was granted immunity from death, and he is often pictured as flying in heaven like a bird and sitting in a tree. Tibetan tradition preserves traditions relating to Caurangi in the biographical literature devoted to the 84 *siddhas*. There Caurangi is described as a prince falsely accused of improper advances by his stepmother; as a punishment, he suffered dismemberment and was left under a tree in the forest but was subsequently saved and initiated into yoga by Matsyendra with the assistance of Gorakh.[110] The parallel here probably rests loosely on the tree as the witness to the miraculous

---

[108] Eliade, *Yoga: Immortality and Freedom*, pp. 110, 395, 419; cf. also the Chinese concept of embryonic breathing, ibid., pp. 59–62.

[109] Das Gupta, *Obscure Religious Cults*, pp. 203, 208; cf. p. 200 for an etymology.

[110] Keith Dowman, trans., *Masters of Mahamudra: Songs and Histories of the Eighty-Four Buddhist Siddhas*, SUNY Series in Buddhist Studies (Albany: State University of New York Press, 1985), pp. 81–90.

restoration of Caurangi's limbs and as the paradisical site of Elijah's deathless abode. In any case, the three identifications revolve around the practice of breath control, expressed through these allegories. Thus, breath control and meditative practice is the underlying theme of the comparison between the Sufi and yogic traditions.

The rhetorical effect of identifying Islamic prophets with Hindu jogis is one of appropriation, but such a radical claim could amount to making the claimed tradition dependent and inauthentic. Discomfort seems to have arisen in several quarters. A Muslim objection appeared in a polemical text of uncertain date entitled *Hujjat al-Hind* or *The Proof of India*, which takes the form of a Muslim critique of Hinduism in story form. One of the criticisms of the text is directed against the Nath jogis, as follows:

> Yet they have no proof which they can show or establish, except idle tales and verses (*caupad*) which the Jogis have ascribed to them [the *Naths*]. They also say, 'We talk of Gorakh and you of the Prophet Khidr; we talk of Cauranga and you of Ilyas; we of Macchendar and you of the Prophet Yunus [Jonah].' This also is false: nay, it is unbelief (*kufr*).[111]

The comparison is briefer than what occurs in *The Pool of Nectar*, omitting the references to breath control and meditation, but the figures are the same. It is possible that this identification, like the mythology of Ratan Nath, originated among the jogis as a way of constructing their relationship to Islam through narrative. On the other hand, the comparison may have originated with the translator of *The Pool of Nectar*, in precisely the reverse manner. There is no way to decide this issue at present, but the inevitable triumphalism of the comparison was evidently seen as problematic, not only by Muslims but also by Hindus.

A similar reference to *The Pool of Nectar* occurs in the *Dabistan-i madhahib* or *The Academy of Religions*, to which brief reference has already been made. The *Dabistan* was written in Persian in seventeenth-century India by Mobad Shah, a Zoroastrian author belonging to the school of Adhar Kayvan. This text is a highly complex philosophical and

---

[111] Mihrabi, *Hujjat al-Hind*, trans. Digby, "Encounters," p. 4. Digby dates this text to around 1400 and locates it in the Deccan, but Munzavi (*Fihrist-i Mushtarak-i*, 2:952–54, no. 1613; 2:1086, no. 1852) dates this to the period of Shahjahan, although the oldest of the nine MSS he describes (no. 4642, in a Peshawar library) is dated to the ninth/fifteenth century Marshall gives two dates: "not later than 1084/1673" (no. 221) and 1055/1645 (no. 1809).

mystical treatise, in which Sufism, Ishraqi Illuminationism, and strands of Indian religious thought and practice (including yoga) form the basis for an original mystical reinterpretation of Zoroastrian tradition; the work contains, for instance, extensive descriptions of Zoroastrian techniques corresponding to yogic meditations. The *Dabistan* was highly regarded as an authoritative work on comparative religion during the early period of Orientalism, by Sir William Jones for instance, but critical nineteenth- and twentieth-century scholars rejected it, seeing its creative approach to religious history as nothing but a fraud. Modern Iranian scholars espe- cially have been particularly harsh in their criticism of this work. Much of the fanciful vocabulary that this text attributed to ancient Iranian sages was incorporated into the standard early dictionaries of Persian, an event that current philologians regard as an embarrassment.[112] In any case, the author of the *Dabistan* remarks as follows concerning *The Pool of Nectar*:

> I saw the *Amritakunda*; it was also translated into Persian, and entitled *Hawd al-hayat* (*The Pool of Life*). There it is said, "Gorakhnath is an expression for Khidr, and Machhinder [Matsyendra] for Yunus [Jonah]." This opinion in the *Amritakunda* is baseless; as often as they speak of Gorakhnath, so frequently the name of Alakh or Brahma appears, which is correct.[113]

The quotation from *The Pool of Nectar* (corresponding to V.4 of the Arabic text) follows the Persian translation of Muhammad Ghawth, but it is abbreviated to omit the reference to Caurangi and Ilyas. Evidently the author of the *Dabistan* felt that the identification of archetypal jogis with figures from Islamic sacred history was mistaken, since contempo- rary yogic tradition viewed Gorakhnath as a manifestation of divinity,

---

[112] See H. Corbin, "Adar Kayvan," *Encyclopedia Iranica*, 3:183–87, along with the edi- tor's critical addendum directly refuting Corbin; cf. also Fath-Allah Mojtaba'i, "Dabestan-e Madaheb," ibid., 6:532–34, where the evidence for authorship is discussed as well. A bril- liant new interpretation of the Dabistan and the Zoroastrian historiography of the Adhar Kayvan movement is provided by Mohamed Tavakoli-Targhi, "Contested Memories: Narrative Structures and Allegorical Meanings of Iran's Pre-Islamic History," *Iranian Studies* 29 (1996): 149–75.

[113] *Dabistan*, p. 153; Mobad Shah [Kaykhusraw Isfandiyar, attr.], *Dabistan-i madhahib*, ed. Rahim Riza-zada Malik, Adabiyyat-i Dasatiri 1, 2 vols. (Tehran: Kitabkhana-i Tahuri, 1362/1983), 1:162 (where Alakh is misspelled as *lak*). The English translation of Shea and Troyer is hopelessly incorrect at this point.

better referred to either as *alakh* or the god Brahma. Either the author of the *Dabistan* or his jogi informants rejected the identification of the Sufi and yogic traditions as ultimately implausible because the Islamic prophet alleged as the equivalent of Gorakh was not his equal in spiritual power; this contemptuous dismissal raises the rhetorical stakes by declaring that Gorakh is divine and no mere prophet. So, while breath control was admittedly the most likely point of contact between these two groups, the construction of competing rhetorical narratives was part of a contest for supremacy rather than an explanation of an acknowledged common origin.

> *"When among Muslims, they [the Nath jogis] are scrupulous about*
> *fasting and ritual prayer, but when with Hindus, they practice the*
> *religion of this group."*
>
> —*Dabistan*

CONCLUSION

How can we meaningfully situate Sufism and yoga, in light of the preceding discussion? Let us sum up the evidence. Indian Sufis and Nath jogis regarded each other as distinguishable groups, with overlapping interests in psycho-physical discipline and with often competing roles as spiritual leaders. While some yogic practices were, to a certain extent, compatible with Sufi disciplines, it is historically impossible to derive one entire system from the other. Different Indian Sufi groups, particularly the Chishti and Shattari orders, incorporated certain yogic practices into their repertory of techniques, but this addition did not fundamentally alter the character of existing Sufi practices; Hindi mantras, for instance, were infrequent in Sufi texts and clearly subordinate to Arabic formulas of Qur'anic origin. *The Pool of Nectar* was probably the most important single literary source for the diffusion of knowledge about yoga through Islamicate languages. Sufis and jogis alike both felt the need periodically to take account of the other group, and this acknowledgement took the form of competing narratives, including conversion stories, liminal figures like Baba Ratan the hadith scholar, pseudonymous Sufi authorship of yogic texts, and the identification of primordial jogis with the esoteric prophets of Islam. The repeated insistence on the identification of Sufi and yogic themes reveals a stubborn sense of difference.

All these observations suggest that we must find a way to describe this sense of difference without essentialism. If it is true that Sufis assimilated and adapted certain yogic practices, to what extent did Sufis show resistance to incorporating yoga into their own worldview? I would suggest that we can answer this question best by dividing the material into three separate categories: yogic practices, jogis as individuals belonging to an identifiable group, and the abstract notion of yoga as a religious doctrine. With regard both to yogic practices and jogis as individuals, there is a variable spectrum among Sufis, ranging from complete appropriation of certain yogic material (breath control, chants, meditation techniques, jogis, and even goddesses) to wary approval and even complete rejection; it is not possible to reduce this range of reactions to a single formula. A critical issue for assessing this process of assimilation is the character of the strategies of translation that Sufis adopted to present the Indic data in Islamicate garb. Our most notable text, *The Pool of Nectar*, presents a number of identifications between Islamic and Indic personalities; in addition to the identification of the three jogis with Islamic prophets, we are also told that Brahma is Abraham, and Moses is Vishnu. A brahmin is equivalent to a Muslim scholar (`alim`), and a jogi is an ascetic (*murtad*). Equivalents are also provided for a couple of minor practices; the Hindi term *japa* or counted prayer is equivalent to `azima` or invocation, and *homa* or sacrifice is equivalent to *du`a* or prayer.[114]

Yet, some extremely important yogic terms are entirely missing from this account. Nowhere in all this Sufi literature, as far as I can determine, is the term yoga ever mentioned.[115] Likewise, the extremely important technical terms *mantra*, *yantra* (diagram), and *cakra* are never spelled out, although they are described at length and in detail with numerous examples. All these critical terms for yogic practice are completely subordinated to Islamicate categories and represented by Arabic terms; mantra is replaced by *dhikr*, yantra by *shakl* (shape), cakra by *mawda`*

---

[114] See Ernst, "Islamization," chart 10.5, for these translations, and Chapter 10 in the present volume.

[115] Shah Kalim Allah in passing refers to the postures of yoga (*baihak-i jog*) and also mentions "the endless sound (*sawt-I sarmadi*),…which in youga (*jog*) they call anahid [*anahita*]" (*Kashkul-i Kalimi*, pp. 30, 39). But these mentions of yoga (*jog*) are extremely rare.

(place), and yoga itself by *riyada* (asceticism). Only with the benefit of Indological resources, which were unavailable to pre-modern readers of *The Pool of Nectar* and kindred texts, can we plausibly restore the Indic originals. While there seems to be a clear recognition among Sufis of the existence of the Nath Jogis as a sociological group and of their practices as distinctive, the discursive tradition of Sufi teaching was powerful enough to make the independent existence of something called yoga completely irrelevant precisely because yogic practices could be assimilated into a Sufi perspective without much effort. In short, there is no Sufi concept of yoga as a completely separate system. It would probably be safe to say that there was likewise no hatha yoga concept of Sufism as a separate entity. The highly abstract language of essentialism contributes nothing to our understanding of this phenomenon of historical difference.

The old Orientalist debate about yoga as the source of Sufism was based on a "strong misreading," denying the apparent significance of a tradition by triumphant announcement of origins and influences detected only by modern scholars. Anxieties about textual authority and about the very existence of Islam continue to fuel such grandiose projects, as one can see in the recent attempt of "Christoph Luxenburg" (a pseudonym) to unveil the Qur'an as a text, not written in Arabic, but in Syriac, in this way proposing that the entire Islamic tradition is based on a faulty reading of a Christian lectionary. Luxenburg's announcement that the "white-eyed" virgins of the Qur'an are in reality white raisins was considered important enough to be featured on the front page of the *New York Times*, which does not often happen with large German tomes on Semitic philology.[116] Meanwhile, the New Age essentialism views Sufism and yoga as forms of spirituality that contest for the position of the mysticism that is most authentic because it is least authoritative. Despite their appeals to the history of religions, neither of these approaches is particularly historical. Against such strong misreadings, and their quest to find the essential origins of religion either

---

[116] *New York Times* (2 March 2002). Luxenburg's book was also the subject of an article in *Newsweek* (25 July 2003), which was banned in Pakistan. For a critical review of Luxenburg's book, see François de Blois in *Journal of Qur'anic Studies* 5 (2003): 92–97. For the importance of the debunking of the Qur'an as a theme in recent Euro-American culture, see Ernst, *Following Muhammad* chapter 3.

in debunked sacred texts or in a bland universalism, we can offer alternate forms of interpretation. Wendy Doniger favors a more provisional form of categorization:

> An appropriate metaphor, I think, for the network of diffused narratives with no common origin is not the family tree that folklorists used to favor, but rather a banyan tree, which must have an original root but sends down so many subsequent roots from its branches (other variants) that one can no longer tell which was the original. The pattern of banyan roots is rather like a Venn diagram of family resemblances, or the web of an invisible spider.[117]

In this sense, polythetic approaches to categorizing religious traditions offer a flexibility and an attention to historical difference that is not held hostage to the all-or-nothing comparativist constructions of source and influence. Abandoning essentialism, and getting rid of binary formulations, is an important part of the project of anthropologizing and provincializing Europe, particularly in terms of decentering and relativizing Protestant concepts of religion.[118] For religious studies scholars, an important task for the future will be to explain these non-essentialist interpretations of religion in a way that can be relevant to the broader public spheres beyond the academy.

---

[117] Doniger, *The Implied Spider*, p. 139. For a Venn diagram-style description of Chishti Sufism, see *Sufi Martyrs of Love*, pp. 2–4.

[118] King, *Orientalism and Religion*, pp. 187–89, 209.

13

Two Versions of a Persian Text on Yoga and Cosmology: Attributed to Shaykh Mu`in al-Din Chishti*

As we have seen in previous chapters, one of the most intriguing aspects of the development of Sufism in South Asia has been the interaction of Sufis with the spiritual traditions of India, especially yoga. Much has been written on this theme, though frequently in a speculative manner.[1] It is therefore important to look for concrete examples of Sufi appropriation of yogic materials that can serve as the basis for an accurate historical reconstruction of the way in which these traditions were engaged. An excellent example for case study is a short Persian text on yoga and meditation that is attributed to the famous founder of the Indian Chishti Sufi order, Shaykh Mu`in al-Din Chishti (d. 1236). A number of different versions of this treatise are found in manuscripts held in different libraries, often with different titles, though there is a

---

* Although I generally prefer to avoid using diacriticals, in order to avoid confusion with technical terms in this essay I use the transliteration system of Persian from the *International Journal of Middle East Studies*. For Indic retroflex consonants, I use an apostrophe. Proper names and book titles are left without diacritical marks.

[1] For an overview of the issues surrounding the relationship of Sufism and yoga, see Carl Ernst "Situating Sufism and Yoga," *Journal of the Royal Asiatic Society*, Series 3, 15, no. 1 (2005): 15–43; and id., "The Islamization of Yoga in the *Amrtakunda* Translations," *Journal of the Royal Asiatic Society*, Series 3, 13, no. 2 (2003): 199–226.

fair amount of overlap in the contents. Most commonly, it is called the "Treatise on the Human Body" (*Risala-i Wujudiyya*); although Sufi metaphysicians and Islamicate philosophers generally interpret the key term in the title (*wujūd*) as the abstract concept of existence, it also has an archaic meaning of "body," and it is systematically treated in that way in these texts, as we shall see. It is also entitled the "Treatise on the Nature of Yoga" (*Risala-i Sarmaya-i Jog*), using the North Indian pronunciation in Persian script (thus we see *jōg* for the Sanskrit term yoga, and *jōgi* for yogi), and there are other variant titles for what appears to be substantially the same text.[2]

While it is attractive to consider that the founder of the Indian Chishti order may have written this work on yoga and cosmology, this attribution is in all likelihood fictional. Legend is replete with accounts of Mu'in al-Din Chishti engaging in thaumaturgic contests with the jogi Ajaipal, but these stories are clearly part of the hagiographic tradition, in which Sufis inevitably were victorious over the jogis. As is well known, the successors of Mu'in al-Din, notably Shaykh Nasir al-Din Mahmud Chiragh-i Dihli (d. 1356), were quite certain that he never wrote anything at all.[3] The manuscripts of this text are all late; none is older than the late seventeenth century. The two manuscripts I have used for this translation (one entitled *Treatise on the Human Body* and the other called *Treatise on the Nature of Yoga*) belong to the library collection of Pir Zia Inayat-Khan, and both appear to be quite recent copies, written on modern paper, though they are undated. Since there are significant differences between the two copies, I have translated them side-by-side to facilitate comparison.

---

[2] MSS include 6314 Ganj Bakhsh, Islamabad, entitled simply "Treatise of Mu'in al-Din Chishti," cited by Ghulam-'Ali Arya, *Tariqa-i Chishtiyya dar Hind wa Pakistan* (Tehran: Kitabfurushi-i Zavvar, 1365/1987), p. 100. Other examples include the "Treatise on Horizons and Souls" (*Risala-i afaq wa anfus*), 1754 India Office Library, London, fols. 272–4; and the "Treatise on Wayfaring, on the Status of the Human Veins" (*Risala dar suluk dar sha'n-i rag-ha-yi adami*), MS 152 Pir Muhammadshah Dargah, Ahmedabad, fols. 1–15. The latter two citations I owe to Dr. Scott Kugle. There are at least nine other MSS in libraries in Pakistan, of which the two oldest are dated 1084/1673; for details, see Ahmad Munzavi, *Fihrist-i mushtarak-i nuskha-ha-yi khatti-i farsi-i Pakistan* (Islamabad: Markaz-i Tahqiqat-i Farsi-i Iran u Pakistan, 1363/1405/1985), 3:2101–3, no. 3820.

[3] See Carl W. Ernst and Bruce B. Lawrence, *Sufi Martyrs of Love: Chishti Sufism in South Asia and Beyond* (New York: Palgrave Press, 2002).

Why should such a collection of teachings with Indic psycho-physical practices be attributed to Mu'in al-Din Chishti? In one sense, this pseudo-epigraphic attribution is an indication of the seriousness with which Indian Sufis approached the practices of yoga. In other words, these teachings were important enough that they should have been part of the teaching of the greatest Sufi master in the Chishti tradition. This attribution is paralleled by the phenomenon we see in the circulation of the most important Arabic work on hatha yoga, *The Pool of Nectar*, which in many manuscripts is attributed to the great Andalusian Sufi master Shaykh Muhyi al-Din Ibn 'Arabi (d. 1240).[4] From a strictly historical perspective, neither attribution can really be sustained, but it is striking to see that people felt that this should have been the case.

The text is divided into three short chapters (the numbered paragraphs are my own addition). Chapter 1 begins abruptly, omitting the customary praise of God and the Prophet Muhammad, and it consists of an account of the subtle physiology of hatha yoga, with emphasis on the three veins that parallel the spinal column.[5] It relates in detail an esoteric system of breath control related to a complicated cosmology, which assumes the concept of the human body as the microcosm related to the larger universe as macrocosm. Many details are obscure and demand more explanation than the text provides, which presumably would be available from oral commentary by a master. Most of this chapter is clearly Indic in origin.

Chapter 2 carries on with a number of similar themes, especially the microcosm-macrocosm analogy, but it is predominantly Islamicate in substance, with frequent quotations from the Qur'an (passages in Arabic are printed in bold). The cosmological analogies are drawn mainly from Arabic sources such as the *Epistles* of the Pure Brethren, which in turn draw on Pythagorean antecedents; many of these analogies are also found in the preface to *The Pool of Nectar*. There are a few significant touches from the classical Sufi tradition, such as the four types of soul in 2.1 (also listed in Diagram 13.1).

---

[4] See Ernst, "Islamization of Yoga."

[5] For detailed accounts of these yogic teachings, see Mircea Eliade, *Yoga, Immortality and Freedom*, trans. Willard R. Trask, 2nd ed., Bollingen Series 56 (New Jersey: Princeton University Press, 1969); David Gordon White, *The Alchemical Body: Siddha Traditions in Medieval India* (Chicago: The University of Chicago Press, 1996); George Weston Briggs, *Gorakhnath and the Kanphata Yogis* (1938; repr., Delhi: Motilal Banarsidass, 1980).

Chapter 3 has an interestingly composite structure, in which the metaphysical levels and archangels of Islamicate cosmology are linked to the breaths of yogic practice (3.1–6). In the *Treatise on the Nature of Yoga*, these are accompanied by what are now unintelligible mantras; unfortunately, the inability of the Persian script to represent short vowels inevitably resulted in chaos whenever it was used for the transcription of Sanskritic phrases. Nevertheless, the text asserts that the realization of these levels is closely related to the supreme spiritual states associated with the Prophet Muhammad. Indeed, the text goes on to link these states with knowledge revealed during the Ascension of Muhammad to heaven; moreover, it maintains that this knowledge was then conferred on Mu`in al-Din Chishti, either spontaneously by the Prophet Muhammad or through the agency of Mu`in al-Din's master, Shaykh `Uthman Harwani (3:7–8). In other words, the principal teachings of this text are alleged to be the essential import of what the Prophet Muhammad received during his most sublime spiritual experience. At this point, Mu`in al-Din is warned not to transmit this esoteric teaching to just anybody, but the restrictions are generous enough to include sincere followers of the Chishti order in later generations (3.9). The text concludes with reflections on the two supreme stations known as Sultan Nasir and Sultan Mahmud, followed by additional comments on the subtle nerves of yogic teaching, the visualization of Muhammad, and the 99 names of God (3.10–11). Both manuscripts feature meditative diagrams of nested squares to illustrate the cosmological doctrines.

A detailed comparison of the two versions reveals considerable differences in portraying what is undoubtedly the same core teaching. The Sanskrit terms for yogic concepts such as the nerves are spelled with many variations, indicating the likely oral nature of this transmission (e.g., the central vein called *sukhumnā* uses the Hindi pronunciation of the Sanskrit *suṣumṇā*, while the parallel veins, known as *idā* and *pingalā* in Sanskrit, are here made into a rhyming pair, either *hingarā* and *pingalā*, or else *ingalā* and *pingalā*). Some of the Indic terms are no longer recognizable (to this reader, at least), and these are marked with question marks. The variations between the texts are not limited to spelling; in a number of places, there appear to be obvious mistakes in counting, and in the recording of ordinary Persian words; I have attempted to account for these discrepancies in the notes and in parenthetic remarks. The general impression is of texts that are basically transcriptions of oral teachings given at different times and places, by disciples who may have had a more or less sure grasp of the contents.

The overall significance of these writings is difficult to gauge. Today, the presence of Indic spiritual teachings in Sufism can be a source of discomfort to Sufi orders who find their Islamic credentials questioned by fundamentalists. Likewise, the emphasis on purifying Hinduism from foreign accretions would make the Islamic references in these texts awkward for modern Vedantic schools of yoga. Yet, these composite teachings clearly point to a concept of the world in which not only the fixed religious boundaries of today, but also the rigid separation of soul from matter, were not even conceivable.[6] In that sense, these Sufi apocryphal texts on yoga, despite their inconsistencies and their sometimes formidable esotericism, may still have much to teach us.

Treatise on the Nature of Yoga	*Treatise on the Human Body*
Chapter 1	**Chapter 1**
1.1 Know that in the human being the first thing that appeared was the vein called *sukhumnā* [Sanskrit *suṣumā*]. Then came *ingalā* and *pingalā*. From these three, the nine *nāt'ak* (?) became manifest, and from the nine *nāt'ak*, the 360 veins and the 16 digits (*kalā*) came into existence. But the goal of those is the three veins, and their principle is one, which is called *sukhumnā*.	He clarified that first is the vein *sukhumnā* [*suṣumā*]. Then there were the nine *ranātak* (?), the 316 60 [i.e., the 360]. Then there were the 360 and 16,000. But the goal of those is the three, and their principle is one, which is our *sukhumnā*.

---

[6] For an illuminating commentary on the role of yogic anatomy in Sufism, see Scott Kugle, *Sufis and Saints' Bodies: Mysticism, Corporality, and Sacred Power in Islam*, Islamic Civilization and Muslim Networks Series (Chapel Hill, NC: University of North Carolina Press, forthcoming), Chapter 7.

1.2 Know that the top of the *sukhumnā* vein is in the navel, and its root is in the middle of the *darzālat* (?). This vein draws breath from the navel, and that breath reaches the station of the navel by the path of the *darzālat*. From there it rises upward. The *ingalā* and *pingalā* are the veins of the left and right of the *sukhumnā*. Whenever the seeker draws breath from the navel, it is through the *sukhumnā*. Then it comes to the heart. From that place, it divides in three parts, and going between flesh, skins, and arteries, it enters into the brain. Then, going out between the two eyebrows, it picks up. When the seeker wishes to hold his breath, and to become aware of its substance, he closes the nine doorways (i.e., the nine orifices of the body), and he eats mild and scanty food, so that during a 40-day retreat, a knot [*bandh*] appears, beneath the breast; in the second retreat, it is at the waist; and in the third retreat, the knot appears above. When these three knots are firmly established, the breath being in the midst of the knot, it happens three times.

By way of knowing the veins which are in the existence of human beings, the principle is from the navel, and the root of the *sukhumnā* is open in the middle which is the *izālat* (?). And the *hingarā* and *pingalā* which are there are to the left and right of the *sukhumnā*. Then, the seeker draws breath from the navel until it comes from the heart, having gone through the *sukhumnā*, to the heart. Then, above the heart there are three parts, and going between flesh, vein, and skin, it comes to the head. It circles three times, then, either going out between the eyebrows it goes out, comes to its place, and there turns around three times and stays. This is because of the following. When the seeker closes and locks the nine doorways, if he is able to eat little and lightly, during a 40-day retreat a knot appears and nine fingers of breath come out. Each finger's length is 250 years of life. Then, until the second 40-day retreat, if he practises asceticism until the second knot occurs, then until the third 40-day retreat, if he performs asceticism, the planetary guardians will become guides for them. Their principle has five aspects: earth, water, wind, fire, and perfect light. But four of these are dominant.

Diagram 13.1

From *Treatise on Existence*

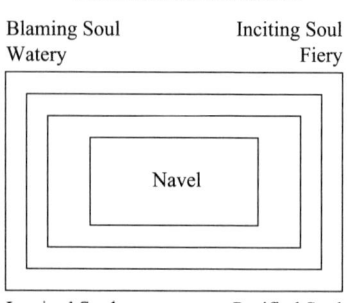

Blaming Soul   Inciting Soul
Watery   Fiery

Navel

Inspired Soul   Pacified Soul
Earthy   Airy

Diagram 13.2

From *Treatise on the Nature of Yoga*

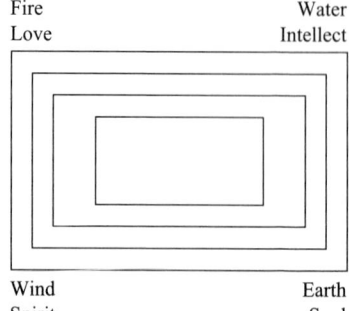

Fire   Water
Love   Intellect

Wind   Earth
Spirit   Soul

1.3 Then he goes by the way of the breath from the mother's womb. There are six doorways there, within the folds of the navel, in the midst of the knot of the throne, which has three doorways on the right side and three doorways on the left side. Having opened these six doorways, he enters the window of the loins (or lumbar window). There he travels through 28 stations; in each station is a governor. He knows them, for their principle is from five things, and in each one of them a single attribute is dominated, and four attributes [are dominant?]. From those five people, 28 people appear. Five are of earth, and their color is yellow. Five are from water, and their color is white. Eight of them are from air, and their color is green. Five are from fire, and their color is red. Five are from light, and the color of that is black.

Every one of these is dominated by them. They have a master who flows and returns to that work, saying, "also they give information about themselves and about their reality." They are of five kinds. One is watery; seven people appear,[7] with these characteristics: five are of earth, whose color is yellow; five are of water, whose color is red; eight are from air, whose color is green; five are of fire, whose color is black; five are of light, whose color is white.

1.4 These 28 stations are the circle of substances, the 28 elements (or explanations), and the 28 stations of the left. Those 28 stations have three knots and three whirlpools; there, the breath becomes three lotuses (*bāraj*).

There are 28 circles which are the stations of the moon, and there are 28 stations, and there are 28 stations on the left. In these 28 stations, there are 3 knots, for here the breath goes around three times.

1.5 At that time, this sign appears: at the time of inhaling breath, after reaching this degree, in a week he takes in five [breaths] from the stomach, and the stomach becomes right. The proof of it is that he consumes [burns] whatever he eats. If he does not eat something, he has no need of food. A mighty power appears in him, and the stomach being right, it [the breath] goes between the flesh, skin, and blood. In every inhalation of breath, three times amidst them at that time, the flesh and blood decrease. The sign of that is that whatever is hidden is unveiled to him.

Then this sign appears: the seeker who inhales the breath, the gut has five *barā* (?). The gut becomes right; then after it becomes right, it is the gut. However much he eats, he consumes. And if he does not eat, he does not desire it. Much power appears in him. Then the gut becomes right and the breath is between the flesh, skin, blood, and vein, for a week. Between the flesh and skin every time he inhales, three times the breath comes. Then blood and flesh decrease. This sign becomes evident, that whatever is a hidden secret becomes manifest and unveiling is clear.[8] By the command of God Most High, the work of the seeker is complete, **and God knows best what is right.**

---

[7] This version here appears to be confused, and should probably read with the other version, "and from those five people, 28 people appear."

[8] Reading *sirr* (secret) instead of *sīr* (full; milk); the word *tīr* (arrow) after *kashf* (unveiling) is inexplicable.

Chapter 2	Chapter 2
2.1 When God (glory be to Him) wished to make Himself manifest, and to see Himself, He created four things from the four elements, and four breaths. The first is the light that He separated from His pure essence. It became established in four degrees, in this likeness: the divine realm (*lāhūt*), the realm of potency (*jabarūt*), the angelic realm (*malakūt*), and the human realm (*nāsūt*), just like fire, air, water, and earth. In these four pillars are the four natures, the four proximate angels, and the very four friends of our revered Prophet (God bless him and his family and grant him peace)—may God be pleased with them. And from the very four souls—inciting (*ammāra*), blaming (*lawwāma*), inspired (*mulhama*), and pacified (*muṭma'inna*)—it is just as it is given in the division of the four elements: air is related to the spirit, water is related to the intellect, fire is related to love, and earth is related to the soul. Even so, the inciting soul is related to fire, the blaming soul is related to water, the inspired soul is related to air, and the pacified soul is related to earth (refer to Diagram 13.1).	The Revered Master Mu`in al-Din Hasan Sanjari[9] (may God sanctified his conscience) was there. My dear! God Most High from nonexistence made Adam and from the five (i.e., four) elements created the four existences, and the four souls became evident. At first the Real Most High wished that which He made to become a light separate from Himself. It became evident through the four levels from the substance of longing for the Essence (which is splendid and sublime), in this likeness that He made separate from Himself. Water, fire, earth, and air He calls these very four pillars, and these very four angels and four natures, the proximate one to that Revered One, and these very four friends of the cave[10] of the revered Prophet (may God bless him and his family and grant him peace). This direction is in this likeness, and again these four souls became evident. First is the inciting soul, second the blaming soul, third the pacified soul, and fourth the inspired soul, just as it is given in the division of the four elements. Wind is related to the Holy Spirit, water is related to the intellect, fire is related to love, and earth is related to the soul. Likewise, the inciting soul is related to fire, the pacified soul is related to earth, and the inspired soul is related to water (refer to Diagram 13.2).

---

[9] This common spelling of one of the names of Mu`in al-Din Chishti is based on an old misreading of Sijzi as Sanjari.

[10] "Friend of the cave" (yār-i ghār), here applied to all of the first four caliphs (called "the four friends" in the parallel text), is an epithet normally reserved for Abu Bakr, who sheltered with the Prophet Muhammad in a cave as they departed Mecca for Medina.

2.2 Know that the Real Most High has created with his power everything in the
world, and he has also created in the
human being, just as in the word of the
Most High: **"We shall show them our
signs on the horizons"** (Qur. 51:21)
**"and in your souls; do you not then
have insight?"** (Qur. 41:53).[11] God Most
High has created 12 zodiacal signs in
heaven and has also created them in the
human being.

Also, God Most High has created
in the horizons with signs, which is
established by reason of this verse
of the Qur'an. The noble verse: **"We
shall show them our signs on the
horizons"** (Qur. 51:21) **"and in
your souls; do you not then have
insight?"** (Qur. 41:53). And another
example, God Most High as created 12
zodiacal signs in heaven, and has also
created their likes in the human being.

2.3 First, the head is Aries, Taurus is the
shoulders, Gemini the hands, Cancer
the arm, Leo the breast, Virgo the belly,
Libra the navel, Scorpio the genitals,
Sagittarius the thigh, Capricorn the leg,
Aquarius the shank, and Pisces the sole
of the foot.

First, the head is Aries, Taurus is the
shoulders, Gemini the hands, Cancer
the arm, Leo the breast and the heart,
Virgo the belly, Libra the navel,
Scorpio the pudenda, Sagittarius the
thighs, Capricorn the leg, Aquarius the
shank, and Pisces the sole of the foot.

2.4 And the seven planets that wander
through these 12 zodiacal signs correspond as follows: the sun is the heart,
Jupiter the liver, the moon the lungs
(*shush*), Mercury the kidney (*gurda*),
Saturn the spleen (*supurz*), Mars the
brain, and Venus (*zuhra*) the gall bladder
(*zahra*).

Also, the seven stars that wander
throughout these 12 zodiacal signs
are also created in the human being,
that is: the sun is the heart; Jupiter the
liver; the moon, sun, and Mars are
the gall bladder (*talkha*); Venus is the
kidney; Saturn is the spleen (Hindi
tillī); and Mercury is the brain.

2.5 And God (glory be to Him who is Most
High) created 360 days, and the existence
of the year came about from the total of
those. The zodiacal signs of the heavens
cover 360 degrees, and on the face of
the earth there are 360 mountains and
360 great rivers. In the human being 360
individual bones stand in the place of
mountains, and 360 veins in the place of
the rivers. 360 pieces of flesh are in place
of the 360 degrees of the zodiac, and 360
pieces of skin in place of the days.

Also, God Most High created in the
year degrees, and likewise there are
360 in the human being, and they
became evident in the number of
bones. The 360 pieces of bone are
like mountains. Also, these are like
the 360 pieces of flesh. The 360 veins
are like rivers, and the 360 rivers are
created in different regions.

---

[11] The juxtaposition of these two verses from the Qur'an is evidently due to the similarity
of the phrase at the beginning of the second citation to the phrase that continues the first
citation: "We shall show them our signs on the horizons and in their souls" (Qur. 51:21)

2.6   The belly of a man is like the sea, and the hair is like trees, and in the forest and meadow there are biting worms and the like; and genital worms are in that position. The face is like a building and dwelling place. The back is like a desert and wasteland. In the world there are four seasons, and in the human such as these exist: childhood is spring, youth is summer, maturity is a fall, and old age is the rainy season.

The belly is like the sea, and hairs are like trees . . . The face[12] is like buildings [and] dwellings. The back is like a desert. Also, the four seasons— spring is like childhood, summer like youth, fall like maturity, and winter like old age.

2.7   Corresponding to thunder is the human voice, lightning to laughter, and rain to tears. Know that the ear drinks water from the bladder, and its water becomes clear from bitterness. The eye drinks water from the liver, and because of that, its water is difficult. The nose drinks water from the lungs, and therefore its water is dirty. The tongue drinks water from the heart, and its water is sweet. Intellect is in the brain, modesty (*ḥayā'*) in the eye, understanding is in the ear, knowledge in the breast, and thought is in the heart (*qalb*).

Also, the voice is just like thunder, and laughter[13] just like lightning, and weeping of the eye just like rain. For other stations are in existence. First is the tongue, then the nose, then the ear, then the eye. Also the ear drinks water from the bladder and that water is bitter. The nose drinks water from the lungs, and that water is dirty. The tongue drinks water from the heart, and that water is sweet. Also intellect [is in] the brain, the forehead (*jabīn*) is in the eye, understanding is in the ear, knowledge is in the breast, and thought in the bodily frame (*qālib*).

2.8   The Revered Creator created seven heavens, as in his divine saying, **"We arranged one level upon another"** (Qur. 84:19). First is the heaven of Saturn, second the heaven of Jupiter, third heaven of Mars, fourth heaven of the sun, fifth the heaven of Venus, sixth the heaven of Mercury, seventh the heaven of the moon. And these are the five veils in the human being. Four proofs have become evident by this reality: fire, air, water, and earth. The essence of the heavens is the elements of the earth, the essence of the earth is plants, and the essence of plants is animals, and the essence of animals is the human, and the essence of the human is the Real **from every perspective.** Brother seeker! One should know and be familiar with these four breaths, and one should also know their quantity. What is the quantity of these four breaths, and what power do they have?

Also, the Creator of the world created the seven levels of heaven. First is the heaven of Saturn and, second the heaven of Jupiter, third heaven of Mars, fourth the heaven of the sun, fifth the heaven of Venus, sixth the heaven of Mercury, and seventh the heaven of the moon. The station of Sultan Mahmud is upon it and air is dominant. In this way[14] it is said that the seeker should know these four breaths, for what quantity of power do these four breaths have? One should know the demonstration and one should gaze there. It has been said, so one should realize this point in the presence of the master.

---

[12] The manuscript reads *dar vay*, which should be emended to rūy as the other version has it.
[13] The text reads either khastan (injure) or jastan (jump), apparently a mistake for the well-established equivalency of laughter (Persian khandan) with lightning (Amrtakunda 1.2).
[14] Several garbled and unrecognizable words follow, in the place corresponding to an Arabic phrase in the other version.

	Chapter 3, The Science of the Point
3.1 From this, by way of demonstrating the meaning of knowledge, a subtle point is reached, demonstrating this very subtle point. In each principle there is a word, and in each word there is a station.	For it is said that one should demonstrate that every principle has a word; one that exists, each one is the principle of a word: the stations of humanity, the angelic realm, the realm of might, and divinity.[15]
Verse:	Verse:
Divinity is fivefold, my son. The angelic realm is the branch of that tree. The realm of might is the leaf, behold it. The realm of humanity in the world is just like fruit.	The trees are five, my son. The angelic realm is the branch of that tree. The realm of might is the leaf, behold it. The realm of humanity of all the world is like fruit.
In the place of divinity is the tongue, the station of the Holy Spirit. Gabriel knows it. The place of Gabriel is **"the praised station"** (Qur. 17:79). Gabriel is earthy, and the "praised station" is also earthy, its color is yellow, and its taste is thick. But it draws the breath 12 fingers out from the body. In the Indian language, they call this *mangalī mandala vartākamal lahndar* (?).	Again, even in the place of divinity is another station of the realm of might, which is the tongue, and that is the station of the Holy Spirit. Gabriel knows it. The place of Gabriel is **"the praised station"** (Qur. 17:79); the praised station is earthy, its color is yellow, and its taste has subtleties. But it tries to breathe out 12 fingers from this.
3.2 In the place of the angelic realm is the nose, and its station is the navel; Israfil knows it. Israfil is airy, and his color is green, and his taste is sour. But it draws the breath eight fingers out of the body, and in the Indian language they call this *barkamal lūlī* (?).	Another station is in the three navels (?), and it is the nose. Israfil knows it. Israfil is also airy, and his color is green, and his taste is sour. [It draws] out eight fingers from the body.

Diagram 13.3
From *Treatise on the Nature of Yoga*

Fire   Water
Azra'il   Michael

Wind   Earth
Israfil   Gabriel

---

[15] The word "eight" (*hasht*) appears here without any apparent significance, and it does not fit metrically into the following verse.

3.3   In the place of the realm of might is the eye, and its station is the top of the head. Michael knows it, and Michael is watery, and the station of the top [of the head] is also watery. Its color is white, and its form is like the form of the new moon, and its taste is sweet. But it draws the breath 16 fingers out of the body, and in the Indian language they call this *shatadhal kamal barawwan hathil* (?).

The existence of the station of the angelic realm is the eye. Michael knows it, and Michael is watery and the station of the top [of the head] is also watery. Its color is white, and its form is like the new moon, and its taste is sweet. And this goes 16 fingers of breath outside.

3.4   In the place of humanity is the ear, and ʿAzraʾil knows it. ʿAzraʾil is fiery, and the station of the ear is also fiery, and its color is red. Its taste is bitter. But it draws the breath four fingers out of the body, and in the Indian language they call this *madkamal amal* (?).

Another station, divinity, is the ear. ʿAzraʾil knows it. ʿAzraʾil is fiery, and the station of the ear is all fire, its color is red, and its form is (?). Its scent and flavor are bitter. From this it goes out four fingers of breath (refer to Diagram 13.3).

3.5   That is the station of Sultan Nasir; that is **"the praised station"** (Qur. 17:79), the light of Majesty, the light of Beauty, the light of Muhammad, and the light of Ahmad. And these are the four bodies: the subtle body, the gross body, the body of eternality (*baqaʾ*), and the body of annihilation (*fanaʾ*). These are the four spirits: the lowly spirit, the lofty spirit, the Holy Spirit, and the angelic (*malakī*) spirit.

That is the station of Sultan Mahmuda and Sultan Nasira, the lights of Majesty, the light of beauty, the light of the One, the light of Muhammad, and the light of Mahmud. These are the four bodies: the subtle body, the gross body, the body of annihilation, and the body of eternality. And these are the four spirits: first the lowly spirit, second the lofty spirit, third the Holy Spirit, fourth the heavenly spirit. **"Truly God encompasses everything"** (Qur. 4:108).[16]

3.6   Then, from the demonstration of the quantity of these four breaths, when one draws them all in as a single breath, in a particular fashion from one place of the breath to another, as is written above, one practices until that air (*bād*) of "the praised station" and Sultan Nasir becomes dominant. As long as the seeker does not traverse these four breaths, **"annihilation in the master"** (*fanāʾ fi al-shaykh*) does not take place, and there is no **"eternality with God"** (*baqāʾ billāh*).

One learns the practice of these four breaths by heart from the master. When one draws in[17] these four breaths all at once in a particular fashion, one holds the breath from one place to another, and thus it is written in Chapter 1, and even so it is explained, until with that breath with "the praised station," Sultan Mahmud,[18] and Sultan Nasir become dominant. In this way, the seeker should traverse all four paths at once, all four; that station then becomes available until **"annihilation in the master and eternality with God"** occur.

---

[16] The quotation from the Qurʾan is inexact but parallels both 4:108 and 41:54.
[17] Reading *bi-kashad* (draws in) as in the other version, instead of *yikshahr* (a single town).
[18] Several words appear with no apparent meaning (*yād wa wa yād*), possibly reflecting the shape of the word "air," *bād*.

3.7 One should know these four breaths and perform the action. These four airs in the human being have an emperor, but they are in the following of a single person, and this is the light of Muhammad, which rides all the four elements. The light of Muhammad is the light of the One (*aḥad*). The seeker should [know] that just as the One was, even so it is again, and that the being of the light of Muhammad is in acquisition from this. Wayfarers on this path are given no access to the Ascension without this acquisition. For it is not possible, because the planetary governors become dominant, not allowing anyone to enter as long as it is not the request of the Real (glory be to Him who is exalted).

Then one should know these four breaths and contemplate them. These four that exist from the human being each have an emperor, but they are a single person through following speech; that is, the points on which they rest are the light of Muhammad. It has come to be just as it was, and even so it is again, and this is the acquisition of the light of Muhammad, which the advanced masters, who were both scholar and practitioner, will become.

3.8 Know that this is the acquisition of the Revered Prophet (May God bless his family and grant him peace), which Gabriel had taught. And that time when my master and savior, Lord `Uthman Harwani (May God sanctify his conscience) had bestowed grace and kindness upon this beggar (i.e., Mu`in al-Din Chishti), he took my spirit to the presence of that Revered One (May God bless him and his family and grant him peace). He said, "Lord! This is a child who is worthy of succession." The Revered messenger of God (May God bless him and his family and grant him peace) gave me this much knowledge and this divine acquisition, saying, "Mu`in al-Din! God Most High taught this acquisition to Gabriel (peace be upon him), and Gabriel taught it to me. The time when God Most High wished to manifest his prophecy, he separated me from that place, and I became united with this acquisition. The day when this practice was completed was the very time when the Ascension became my destiny. Then prophecy became manifest. Mu`in al-Din! I bestow this very acquisition upon you!"

Then he gave them guidance, that is, it is the acquisition of the Ascension, but it is possible that one should know that in this matter the Prophet provided information to be about the foregoing, and bestowed this acquisition. He said, "Mu`in al-Din!" God Most High had taught this acquisition to Gabriel. At the time when the Real Most High was manifesting his Messenger, that which God had done was also united with this acquisition. That day when the practice was completed became the very occasion of the Ascension. So the origins were manifest to our Messenger, and he said, "Mu`in al-Din! I also bestowed this acquisition upon you." The time when the acquisition was obtained was the very time when the Ascension became my destiny, because that is to write, **"humanity is My secret."**

3.9 I came to this side (i.e., the world) and became occupied with this acquisition. At the time when this practice was completed I reached the height; at that moment this beggar experienced the Ascension, but permission was not given to write about the secret. Again I presented my case to the Revered One with a thousand entreaties and laments, and permission was granted, on the condition that he stated: "Do not speak[19] of this to every seeker and disciple, except to someone who is a sincere seeker and has more or less learned the knowledge so that this secret should not go from house to house." Brother! This acquisition is something to be realized. First, one goes before the master; when the master knows[20] that the realizations have clearly taken place for the seeker, then he authorizes this acquisition.

Since there was no permission [to reveal] this secret and these words were hidden, again I requested with a thousand entreaties and laments. I obtained permission from the Revered One, on this condition: "Do not ever tell this secret to every seeker, every friend, every poor man, and every master, except if it is a sincere seeker and a sincere friend, who has more or less learned the knowledge of unity. Holding these words, tell him, but otherwise these words should not go from house to house." Brother! This is the acquisition of the saints and the ascetics. If they experience realization by this path, then they are the perfect master, and so these realizations become evident for this seeker.

3.10 He says that spirits have two forms: one lofty and the other lowly. He adds two forms to all four forms, and again, these two forms both have a station: one is Sultan Mahmud and the other is Sultan Nasir. He is a single traveler in two forms, and the other is the stationary one. The seeker should know and become familiar with the form of the traveler and know his color, as is said above, so the seeker does not make a mistake. Most of this form of the traveler reaches the form of the stationary one, and that form of the stationary one attains witnessing of the Real, and here he attains the reality of the 99 Names.

Then, he tells of this acquisition, that spirits have two forms: one lofty and the other lowly. Know that he adds these four forms in the midst of two forms. One should know that these two forms have two stations: one is Sultan Nasir and the other is Sultan Mahmud. The other two forms that exist—one is the traveler and the other is stationary. Thus the seeker should know and be familiar with the form of the traveler. And that which he knows, just as is said above, is so that the seeker may not experience opposition. If this form of the traveler attains the form of a stationary one, he also attains the witnessing of the Real; from here, which was reality, he becomes familiar with the name of God Most High

---

[19] The text reads "speak," which is clearly an error for "do not speak."
[20] Reading *bi-dā nad ki* for *bi-dān ki* ("know that").

3.11 The master tells the seeker to direct his gaze down to the nose, in the *barra* (?) of the nose. This is from the point of view that these two eyes which they call sun and moon, which are related to both chief veins which in the Indian language are called *ingalā* and *pingalā*, both of which are related to the *sukhumnā* vein, which is the vein of life—they hold these two, the sun and moon, in the middle of the *sukhumnā* vein. They efface their own image, in the form that we displayed; in this form, visualization is added, in the form of the master, which shows the outer view. For which master is commanding to gaze above the nose? In the midst of the nose is the station of the angelic realm, and the form of the place is displayed in a thousand ways, external and internal. But every form that he displays expresses the fact that the form of the master is visualized in the glance. He does not pass by that visualization until the visualization of the form of the master is added in the form of Muhammad and he attains the visualization of Muhammad. The visualization of Muhammad attains the visualization of God. Then the reality of the 99 names becomes manifest, and those 99 names are effaced in a single name. The one that exists, that is "A" (*alif*), and it became the inhalation of "He" (*huwa*), and the station of M (*mīm*), and from M is N (*nūn*). Farewell.

So that both eyes, which they call sun and moon, both of which are connected to the chief veins, which in the Indian language they call *mangalā* and *pingalā*—both veins are connected to the soul, and the vein of life in the Indian language is called *sukhumnā*. The two are called sun and moon, and in the midst of the *sukhumnā* rests a color that has no form. And the form that we displayed, this form is understood by the form[21] in the form of the master, which is displayed in the outer view. Which is the time when the master says [gaze] "at the nose"? Because the nose is the station of the angelic realm, and it displays the form of the Angels in a thousand ways, external and internal. But that form which he displays[22] expresses the fact that it is the form of the master himself. This form is by the form of the master, and the form of the master is by the form of Muhammad. This form that is attained after this reaches the form by the form of the visualization of Muhammad, and the visualization of Muhammad is by the forms of Unity. By the reality of the 99 names,[23] the Creator Most High became manifest. And so it was that the one name Mahmud became effaced, and the one name that is, that was "A" (*alif*), and it became the inhalation of "He" (*huwa*), and "He" made M (*mīm*) by his own station, and from M **"N (*nūn*) and the pen"** (Qur. 68:1) is illuminated. **The goal is the goal**, and this is it. It is finished and complete.

---

[21] The text has the ungrammatical feminine plural *surāt* (forms).

[22] The text adds here an unintelligible word, *makish*

[23] The text by shifting a dot mistakenly gives "was" (*būd*) instead of "ninety" (*nuvud*).

14

Fragmentary Versions of the Apocryphal "Hymn of the Pearl" in Arabic, Turkish, Persian, and Urdu*

INTRODUCTION

Of all the religious literature of the ancient world, there are a number of texts that continue to attract interest in many unexpected quarters. One of these is the "Hymn of the Pearl" or "Hymn of the Soul" from the apocryphal *Acts of Thomas*, which, despite the rarity of its survival in a single Syriac manuscript and a unique Greek version, since its rediscovery in the nineteenth century still casts a spell over many readers. Interpretations of this text vary widely, ranging from the view that it represents the core spiritual teachings of Eastern Christianity to the notion that it is primarily a Manichean treatise about the descent of the soul into the body.[1]

* Research for this article was supported by the National Endowment for the Humanities and the American Research Institute in Turkey. I also gratefully acknowledge the assistance of Dr Canguzel Zulfikar, who at my request kindly established the text and translation of the Ottoman Turkish version of the "Hymn of the Pearl." All other translations are mine.

The editorial board is grateful to Dr Eyal Gineo for his assistance with the Turkish segment of this article.

[1] See Bentley Layton, *The Gnostic Scriptures: a Translation with Annotations and Introductions* (Garden City, NJ: Doubleday, 1987), pp. 366–375; Paul-Hubert Poirier, *L'Hymne de la perle des Actes de Thomas: introduction, texte, traduction, commentaire,*

It is striking to notice some of the contemporary uses to which the "Hymn of the Pearl" has been put. It was cited by William Butler Yeats in his poem "A Vision," and a collection of poems by Polish author Czeslaw Milosz bears its title. The text has been the subject of recent workshops on spiritual development offered by the Gnostic Society of Los Angeles, the New Veda Ashram of Queensland, Australia, and by a leader of an Iranian Sufi order in Europe, and it has also been investigated as a model for psychological processes.[2] The celebrated passage about the garment of the soul that occurs in the "Hymn of the Pearl" has been considered as evidence supporting the identification of the Shroud of Turin as the garment used to wrap the body of Jesus Christ, and the Hymn has also been seen as a parallel to an important Mormon liturgical text.[3] Artists and musicians have been fascinated with the text, which has been re-created as a deluxe "artist's book," as the inspiration for avant-garde classical music, and as a song text in cabaret and jazz fusion

---

Homo Religiosus 8 (Louvain-la-Neuve: P. Pierier, 1981); Hans Jonas, *The Gnostic Religion: The Message of the Alien God and the Beginnings of Christianity*, 2nd ed. (Boston, Beacon Press, 1963); Davidson, *The Robe of Glory: An Ancient Parable of the Soul* (Shaftesbury, Dorset & Rockport, MA: Element Books, 1992); Patrick J. Hartin. "The Search for the True Self in the Gospel of Thomas, the Book of Thomas and the Hymn of the Pearl," *Hervormde teologiese studies* 55 (1999): 1001–21; Jacques Méhard, *Le Chant de la Perle: poème gnostique*, Collection Gnostica (Paris: Cariscript, 1991); Johan Ferreira, *The Hymn of the Pearl* (Sydney: St. Pauls Publications, 2002); A. F. J. Klein, *The Acts of Thomas: Introduction, Text, and Commentary*, 2nd ed, Supplements to Novum Testamentum 108 (Leiden: Brill, 2003).

[2] These examples include an online version of William Wright's 1871 translation with a 75-minute audio commentary by Dr Stephen Hoeller of the Gnostic Society of Los Angeles (http://www.gnosis.org/library/hymnpearl.htm); a workshop by Les Dyer of the New Veda Ashram in Queensland, Australia (http://www.lesdyer.com/); the International Workshop on Spiritual Evolution offered by Dr. Seyed Mostafa Azmayesh, London, August 2003 (http://icchome.org/events/london_082903.pdf). See also D. D'Rozario, "Hymn of the Pearl: A Psychological Analysis of the Process of Migration," *Australian Journal of Psychology* 55 (2003): S177–S181.

[3] Albert R. Dreisbach, *Thomas & the Hymn of the Pearl* (Atlanta: The Atlanta International Center for the Continuing Study of the Shroud of Turin, Inc., 2000), http://www.shroud.com/pdfs/dreisbc2.pdf; J. W. Welch and J. V. Garrison, "The 'Hymn of the Pearl': An Analysis of an Early Christian Poem in Latter-Day Saints (Mormon) Hymnody: An Ancient Counterpart to 'O My Father.'" *Brigham Young University Studies* 36 (1997): 127–38.

performances.[4] It has even been depicted in an illustrated children's book published by a press devoted to the works of G. I. Gurdjieff.[5]

With a text capable of eliciting so many responses from different readers, it would not be surprising to learn that the "Hymn of the Pearl" also found attentive audiences in the languages of Asia, although, up to now, there has not been any evidence for the text circulating in those milieus.[6] I offer below brief and fragmentary versions of the Hymn into Arabic, Turkish, Persian, and Urdu, accompanied by English translations of each version (refer to Tables 14A.2–5). These different versions have all been extracted from a remarkably eclectic source, the multiple translations of a work on hatha yoga known as the *Amrtakunda* or *The Pool of Nectar*[7], which has been discussed at length in previous chapters of the present volume.

What was the "Hymn of the Pearl" doing in Islamicate versions of a work on yoga, and how was it understood by readers? In an effort to supply an interpretive framework for readers of *The Pool of Nectar*, the anonymous Arabic translator inserted two symbolic narratives into the

---

[4] See the "Unique Artist's Book," hand painted and lettered by Douglas Shafer, offered for sale by Priscilla Juvelis Rare Books for $6500 (http://juvelisbooks.com/catalog27-51%20 and%20above.html); "Éclats de perle" (2002), by Canadian composer Gilles Gobeil, on *Métamorphoses 2002 — 2e concours biennal de composition acousmatique* (http://www.electrocd.com/cat.e/mr_2002.pis.html); the New World Performance Lab's "Stairway to Paradise: a Cabaret Soul Journey," a 2004 musical and dramatic production in Cleveland, Ohio, featuring Megan Elk singing popular American songs juxtaposed to the ancient tale "The Hymn of the Pearl" (http://www.buchtelite.com/2004/1019/arts_01.shtml); and the performance of the Los Angeles jazz fusion group Beth the Sybil, using the text of "The Hymn of the Pearl" as translated by Willis Barnstone, trans., The Other *Bible*, (New York: Harper Collins, 1984), pp. 309–13, (http://beththesybil.com/reviews/reviews.html; email from Beth the Sybil dated August 1, 2005).

[5] Nonny Hogrogian, *The Pearl: Hymn of the Robe of Glory* (Aurora, OR: Two Rivers Press, 1979).

[6] The ever elusive Idries Shah maintained that a version of the "Hymn of the Pearl" appeared as a Sufi teaching story entitled "The King's Son," which he attributed to Amir Sultan of Bukhara, who taught in Istanbul and died in Bursa in 1429; see his *Tales of the Dervishes* (New York: Dutton, 1970), pp. 217–18. As usual, Shah provided no source for his version of the story. Kruse, who sees the "Hymn of the Pearl" as an Eastern Christian variation on the "prodigal son" theme of the New Testament, argues for its influence on the Lotus Sutra of Mahayana Buddhism, in "The Return of the Prodigal," *Orientalia*, n.s., 47 (1978): 163–214.

[7] See Carl W. Ernst, "The Islamization of Yoga in the Amrtakunda Translations," *Journal of the Royal Asiatic Society*, Series 3, 13, no. 2 (2003): 199–226, and Chapter in the present volume.

introduction as a frame story for the text. The first of these two stories (numbered in my unpublished edition and translation of *The Pool of Nectar* as Int.7–8, Int.13–14, X.11) is, as I will argue, a fragmentary version of the "Hymn of the Pearl." The second story (Int.9–12), drawn from a Persian narrative written by the Illuminationist philosopher Suhrawardi (d. 1191), is a philosophical allegory about the psycho-physical faculties, inserted in the middle of the first story.[8] It is possible that the translator chose these tales to replace a Hindu frame story featuring the deities Shiva and Parvati or the yogi Gorakhnath, as is common in hatha yoga texts, but that cannot be determined since there is no trace of the original *Amrtakunda* surviving independently in any Indic language. In any case, these two intertwined tales were evidently designed to provide interpretative avenues to the yoga text, suggesting how the Arabic translator wished the reader to come to grips with these Indian practices.

The original "Hymn of the Soul" or "Hymn of the Pearl" is a brief and charming story, set in Parthian Iran, allegorically depicting the journey of the soul from its transcendent home to the exile of the material world. To summarize the story very briefly, a prince of the East is sent by his royal parents into Egypt to rescue the pearl of knowledge from the great dragon that guards it. While in Egypt, the prince eats of the local food and forgets his identity, but he is awakened by a message sent to him in the form of a bird. He subsequently returns to his homeland, where he is united with his heavenly self in the form of a jeweled garment. Despite its fame in recent times, the "Hymn" occurs as an interpolation in only two manuscripts of the *Acts of Thomas*, part of the apocryphal New Testament; the Syriac version is in verse (in a unique manuscript from Baghdad dated to 936), and the Greek is in prose (in a single eleventh-century manuscript). It has been suggested that the "Hymn" was composed in Gnostic, possibly Manichean, circles, and that it was subsequently adopted by Christians in the Mesopotamian city of Edessa in the early third century. According to that scenario, it was then introduced into the Syriac *Acts*

---

[8] This extract is the sixth chapter of Suhrawardi's *Treatise on the Reality of Love* (*Risala fi haqiqat al-'ishq*), found in Shihab al-Din Yahya Suhrawardi, *Oeuvres philosophiques et mystiques de Shihabbaddin Yahya Sohrawardi*, ed. Henry Corbin, Opera metaphysica et mystica 2 (Tehran: Institut Franco-Iranien, 1954) 3:273–81; W. M. Thackston, Jr., trans, *The Mystical & Visionary Treatises of Shihabuddin Yahya Suhrawardi* (London: Octagon, 1982), pp. 62–75, esp. pp. 66–69.

of Thomas, where it is described as a hymn sung by the Apostle Thomas during his imprisonment in India.

THE DIFFERENT ISLAMICATE VERSIONS OF THE "HYMN OF THE PEARL"

The primary version of the "Hymn of the Pearl" known in Islamicate circles is in the introduction to the anonymous Arabic text known variously as *The Mirror of Meanings on the Understanding of the Microcosm*, *The Pool of the Water of Life*, or *Do-it-yourself Medicine*. Composed probably in the fifteenth century by an Iranian author steeped in the Illuminationist school of philosophy, it drew on accounts of yogic breath control, divination, and summoning of Hindu Goddesses, contained in 10 chapters that follow the introduction. The conclusion of the "Hymn" is, however, postponed to the closing lines of the tenth and final chapter of the yogic text (X.11). Exactly how the "Hymn of the Pearl" may have been transmitted into Arabic is still unclear, although it is conceivable that Syrian Christian intellectuals communicated the story to Muslim philosophers in some of the eclectic salons of later `Abbasid Baghdad. The Arabic version exists in two recensions, one of which (*a*) preserves the Indic material fairly well, while the other (*b*) drops several Indic references and introduces a significant number of Islamizing touches.[9] The majority of these manuscripts are in the libraries of Istanbul, with a few others scattered among libraries in Arab and European countries; this distribution is clearly due to the fact that the Arabic *Pool of the Water of Life* was commonly (though erroneously) attributed to the patron saint of the Ottoman Empire, the Andalusian Sufi master Muhyi al-Din ibn `Arabi (d. 1240).

A separately circulating version of the Arabic "Hymn" narrative indicates that, outside Sufi circles, Muslim philosophers viewed this story as equivalent to the symbolic tales of Ibn Sina (Avicenna).[10] Corbin was the first to point out that the initial frame story in *The Pool of Nectar* (Int.7–8, 13–14) is strongly suggestive of the "Hymn of the Pearl"; he

---

[9] For further details, see Chapter 10 in this volume.
[10] For these stories, see Henry Corbin, *Avicenna and the Visionary Recital*, trans. Willard R. Trask (Irving, TX: Spring Publications, 1980), passim.

initially made this suggestion with reference to two Arabic manuscripts attributed to Ibn Sina (Z^1, Z^2).[11] These two manuscripts, based on recension *a*, contain the main portion of the fragmentary "Hymn" narrative from *The Pool of Nectar*, but without the Suhrawardian tale. Later on, Corbin became acquainted with the Arabic edition of the *Amrtakunda* published by Yusuf Husain, and he then realized that this was the source of the tale found in the two Ibn Sina manuscripts.[12] In both of these Ibn Sina manuscripts, the "Hymn" story occurs as the second of three narratives that form an appendix to a commentary on Ibn Sina's famous poem on the soul. The first of the three stories is the allegorical *Treatise of the Bird* by al-Ghazali, and the third is a commentary on the Prophetic saying, "People are asleep, and when they die they awake."[13] Both manuscripts lack the concluding paragraph of the frame story (X.11), so it appears that the compiler of these Ibn Sina manuscripts had no access to the full version of the story other than via the introduction to the Arabic *Pool of Nectar*, or else it was not realized that the conclusion was to be found at the end of the yogic text. The interpretive context suggests that readers of this Arabic version of the "Hymn" belonged to the mystically inclined philosophical milieu characteristic of later Avicennism and Illuminationism.

Directly dependent on the two Arabic recensions of the *Amritakunda* translation are two recensions in Ottoman Turkish, which were clearly translated directly from their Arabic counterparts. The name of the translator of the first recension, based on family *a*, is not known; there are three manuscripts, and the oldest of all the Turkish manuscripts (Tur^{1}A, dated 1151/1738–39) belongs to this group. The translator of the second recension (from family *b*) was a well-known Ottoman scholar of the eighteenth century, `Abd Allah Salah al-Din al-`Ushshaqi (d. 1196/1782), known as Salahi. He was the author of numerous translations and commentaries, written in Arabic, Turkish, and Persian, on classical works

---

[11] Corbin, *Avicenna*, p.45, n. 51.

[12] Henry Corbin, "Pour une morphologie de la spiritualité Shî`ite," *En islam iranien: Aspects spirituels et philosophiques*, Bibliothèque des Idées (Paris: Gallimard, 1972), 2:325–34; Yusuf Husain, "Haud al-hayat, la version arabe de l'Amratkund," *Journal Asiatique* 213 (1928): 291–344

[13] For Ghazali's *Treatise of the Bird*, see Corbin, *Avicenna*, pp. 196–97.

by Ibn 'Arabi, Rumi, and others.[14] His recension, represented by four manuscripts, also has the distinction of having been printed at Istanbul in 1328/1910–11, and at least two printed copies are preserved (Tur²E). Especially prominent among readers of the Turkish text are members of the Mevlevi order (the so-called "whirling dervishes"), who also owned copies of the Arabic text. Common to both Turkish recensions is that they invariably identify the text as the product of Ibn 'Arabi's pen. The Turkish translations do not offer any major transformation of the text, aside from repetitions for the sake of clarity, plus a few inserted phrases that mostly reinforce the Sufi character of the text.[15] They appear to extend the Arabic textual tradition with little change, except for insisting on the importance of the text as part of the canon of Ibn 'Arabi's writings.

The tradition of *The Pool of Nectar* in Persian is considerably more complicated, with three separate translations having been made from the Arabic by Indian authors; two of these translations contain the "Hymn of the Pearl" in a fragmentary fashion. One of these was the translation of a certain Muhammad ibn 'Abd al-Razzaq (Per²A), which two dissatisfied anonymous readers later revised in distinct recensions (Per²B, Per²C). The main text of the "Hymn of the Pearl" story is missing altogether from these manuscripts, but in one recension, the conclusion of the yoga text inexplicably contains the brief ending of the story.

The best known of the Persian translations of *The Pool of Nectar* was made by Muhammad Ghawth Gwaliyari (d. 1563), an eminent leader of the Shattari Sufi order in India, under the title *The Ocean of Life* (*Bahr al-hayat*). This text is relatively widespread, with at least 24 known manuscripts (several of which were accompanied by miniature illustrations of yoga postures) plus two separate lithograph editions. Remarkably, Muhammad Ghawth's version of the "Hymn of the Pearl" alludes to two passages of the Syriac original that are not found in the Arabic translation, referring to the narrator's royal parents, and to the jeweled garment of his celestial self; this strongly suggests that

---

[14] For Salahi, see Mahmud Erol Kılıç, "'The Ibn al-'Arabi of the Ottomans,' 'Abdullah Ṣalahuddin al-'Ushshaqi (1705–82)," *Journal of the Muhyiddin Ibn 'Arabi Society* 26 (1999): 110–20.

[15] The Ottoman translations also feature misreadings, which in two cases (T20, T24) seriously distort the text.

Muhammad Ghawth worked from a recension of the Arabic text that no longer exists, representing an earlier and fuller stage in the transmission of the text. The Persian translations are all related to the Arabic of family *a*. The Arabic version of the "Hymn" seems to have been very freely translated by Muhammad Ghawth, and he omitted the concluding paragraph altogether from his translation. Since this conclusion can be recovered from the version of Muhammad ibn `Abd al-Razzaq, we can restore the most complete Islamicate version of the "Hymn of the Pearl" by combining these two Persian translations.

Finally, in the middle of the nineteenth century, a scholar in the Indian Deccan made a partial translation of Muhammad Ghawth's Persian *Bahr al-hayat* into Deccani Urdu. The Urdu translation, which in this unique manuscript has several orthographic curiosities, follows the Persian of Muhammad Ghawth fairly closely.[16] As with Muhammad Ghawth, the Urdu lacks the conclusion to the "Hymn of the Pearl." Only one manuscript copy is known.[17] Shah `Ali, a member of the Qadiri Sufi order residing in Imtiyazgarh or Adoni, entitled his Urdu translation *The Sea of Life* (*Hayat Samandar*), and he reportedly dedicated it to his spiritual guide, Hajji `Abd al-Karim, in 1250/1834–35. He did this with some trepidation, and his lack of confidence initially led him to translate only the two introductory frame stories and the first two chapters of the yoga text (fols. 1–47b).

TRANSFORMATION AND INTERPRETATION OF THE "HYMN OF THE PEARL"

From the foregoing remarks, it is evident that all four Islamicate versions of the "Hymn of the Pearl" are fragmentary at best. The Persian, Turkish, and Urdu translators evidently did not even recognize that the story had a conclusion that came after the main body of the text on hatha yoga. In the tabular arrangement of these texts and translations below, it is also clear

---

[16] The very clear script has frequent double . in one-syllable words, uses four dots to indicate retroflex consonants, drops aspiration from the postposition *sath*, and is inconsistent with the spelling of *do-chashmi he* and *ya-i majhul*.

[17] Andhra Pradesh Oriental Manuscript Research Library (Asafiyya) 1997/1-47 Tasawwuf Urdu, Asafiyya catalogue, II, 275. I am grateful to Dr. Omar Khalidi of MIT for obtaining a photocopy of this manuscript.

that only a small fraction of the Syriac original has been referenced in these Islamicate versions, no more than one sixth (16 of 105 lines). Can one really say, then, that these translations truly represent the narrative of the "Hymn of the Pearl"? I would argue that these new versions contain distinctive elements that cannot easily be explained without reference to the "Hymn." Furthermore, despite the elimination of other salient features of the tale (including the pearl itself), these versions retain core themes of the original story, which justify our retaining this title. Clearly, however, there are transformations and new interpretations of the story, which will be briefly explored here.

The Arabic version in *The Pool of Nectar* simplifies the original "Hymn" story considerably, and it dispenses altogether with many of the more colorful details.[18] The same is true of the other Islamicate versions, which is why they must be considered fragmentary. Quite demythologized, it has now become a much more abstract psychological allegory, in which the soul descends into the world and then finds itself by attaining union with God. The supplies and treasures for the journey, the removal of the jeweled garment, and the archetypal figure of the serpent in the sea, which guards the mysterious pearl that forms the object of the narrator's quest—all these elements have simply disappeared. The dangerous journey from Mesopotamia to Egypt, a typical gnostic allegory for the descent of the soul into the body, has become an explicitly psychocosmic itinerary to the "City of Life," a Suhrawardian symbol for the human body as microcosm. Of the complex sojourn in Egypt, all that remains is the motif of forgetfulness and recollection. The striking image of the letter from the king and queen of the East, which flies like a bird to the narrator and awakens him, is likewise absent. The various anonymous companions, courtiers, and treasurers who appear in the original "Hymn" have been replaced by two figures: a royal minister, who regulates entry to the "City of Life" and informs the hero of all the dangers on the way; and the "master of the City," an initiatic figure who reveals himself as the narrator's true self. The lengthy passage describing the return to the kingdom in the East is almost entirely missing. The existing Arabic version of *The Pool of Nectar* even dispenses with the

---

[18] Poirier, *L'Hymne de la perle*, p. 204, has summarized the plan of the "Hymn of the Pearl."

symbolism of the jeweled royal garment, though it surfaces again in the Persian and Urdu translations. The principal aspects of the original story that remain in these fragmentary versions are the narrator's journey to an unknown land to fulfill his covenant with the king, his forgetfulness and remembrance, and his reunion with the heavenly self.

While the Ottoman version for the most part sticks closely to the Arabic, it nevertheless adds interpretive glosses and atmospheric touches that accentuate the solemnity of the tale by more or less overt theological identifications. One of these gestures occurs when the narrator speaks to the minister (T8); in recension *a*, he adds a phrase redolent of courtly rhetoric, "There is no doubt of my lord's glory (*farr*) and authority (*himma*)." Another such incident takes place at the climax of the story (T20), where the narrator dives into the Water of Life; he now learns that the master of the City of Life is the Supreme Creator (*Cenâb–ı Bârî*), language that can only mean God. In the next passage (T21), the Ottoman version follows a reading from recension *b*, which drastically changes the annunciation that the master gives to the narrator; instead of saying soberly, "Welcome. You are one of us," he takes a more ecstatic tone: "I am longing for you, I am longing for you." This seems to substitute more of a Sufi tone of divine love in place of the flat philosophical proclamation of unity. In the concluding paragraph (T24), the Ottoman version of Salahi takes a considerable liberty in changing the monistic overtones of the final revelation. Where the Arabic reads, "So I understood his allusion and found that my self was he (*nafsi hiya huwa*)," the Ottoman has, "my self was itself (*nefsimi ... hiye hiye*)." The altered text preserves a much more respectable distance between Creator and creature.

As mentioned previously, the Persian translation of Muhammad Ghawth preserves features of "Hymn of the Soul" that do not survive in any copy of the Arabic version. The opening of the Persian translation, which refers separately to the king and queen who are the parents of the protagonist, preserves in this way a fuller evocation of the royal setting of the text than what is found in the Arabic version. More importantly, the Persian text contains a description of the jeweled and golden garment which comes to meet the narrator as he returns home, reflecting him and becoming one with him. This feature is entirely absent from both existing Arabic recensions. From the appearance of this feature, it may be concluded that the translation by Muhammad Ghawth presupposes a no longer extant Arabic recension predating the older recension of the Arabic text. Nevertheless, it is surprising that the Persian translation omits the key passage (A20, P16) in which the narrator dives into the Water of Life. This passage has instead become a characteristically Sufi account of esoteric self-knowledge. The plasticity of the story, and the freedom with which different interpreters have treated it, seem to be regular features of the transmission of the tale.

The marginal jottings on the best copy of the Persian translation of Muhammad Ghawth (included here in the notes) also indicate the application of a characteristically Sufi interpretive strategy to what was originally a philosophical allegory. This commentator employed the metaphysical terminology of the school of Ibn `Arabi to explicate the story as a cosmogonic unfolding, in which the divine qualities are manifested in existence through the primordial human, Adam, with frequent reference to the pre-creational covenant of Qur'an 7:172. Such an interpretation would have found ready acceptance among a readership drawn primarily from members of Indian Sufi orders.

The Urdu translator omits (U1) the Quranic references to the divine fiat of Qur'an 2:117 introduced in the Persian of Muhammad Ghawth (P1), and he makes a number of other changes in vocabulary and emphasis. Most of these changes are of a scribal character, although one interesting addition is the passage in which the narrator completes his journey. The Persian (P13) reads, "I approached a venerable man (*piri*) seated on the king's throne, who was the master (*shaykh*) of that City." In contrast, the Urdu (U13) has, "Traveling gradually I came to the City. I saw a young man (*ek javan*) who was upon the seat of the king; he is the master (*shaykh*) of that City." While the transformation of the old man into a youth could invite further speculation, the Urdu translation in itself is valuable mainly as a witness to the reception of the Persian.

Overall, the chief new elements introduced in the Islamicate versions are mainly theophanic encounters with apparitional figures of authority who represent the true self. First is the king's minister, who controls all coming and going at the gate of the kingdom, and who provides a description of all the perils of the journey. He repeatedly warns the protagonist to pay attention and not to forget his covenant with the king. Second is the mysterious "master seated on the throne of a king," whom the narrator finds in the City of Life after forgetting his mission. This master is clearly both a stand-in for the king and at the same time the narrator's true self, literally mirroring the latter's every word and action; this encounter prompts the narrator to remember his covenants. Next, the minister reappears and makes the hero dive into the Water of Life, which simultaneously bestows mystical knowledge and reveals the king, the goal of the story. The conclusion is reserved, however, for the appendix that is placed at the end of the yoga text (A23–A24). The narrator finds himself in a "web" and lifts up his head, evidently a metaphor for being enmeshed in the world of bodies yet striving to ascend to the spiritual level (the translators seem to have struggled with this image). Once again he sees the king's minister as his own reflection, and he realizes that he and the king are one. The king drives the symbolic point further by "taking a spider's thread; first he split it into halves, then he made them one. Then he said, 'One times one is one.'" Taking the spider's web for the warp and weft of creation, this signals once again that unity with the true self is found in the union of body and spirit that is the City of Life.

More nuances are hidden in the enigmatic image of the sage splitting a spider's thread in half, restoring it to unity, and then uttering the phrase "One times one is one" in explanation. The basic message here, at first sight, appears to be the underlying unity of the creator and the creation, of God and the self, which is further emphasized as a continuation of the imagery of reflection: "So I understood his allusion and found that my self was he, and I was his reflection." Corbin understands this arithmetical symbol in terms of Sufi and Shi`i concepts of multiple theophanies, in which God is manifest in multiple forms (Imams or beautiful faces).[19] Corbin actually cites only one parallel passage in which the arithmetical phrase "one times one" occurs (without the conclusion "is one"), drawing upon the *Risalat al-quds* or *Treatise on Sanctity* by the Persian Sufi Ruzbihan Baqli (d. 1209): "As long as it is not 'one times one,' the wayfarer does not reach the essence of the vision of unification."[20]

---

[19] Corbin, *En islam iranien*, 1:290; 2:24; 3:195.

[20] Ruzbihan Baqli, *Risalat al-quds wa risala-i ghalatat al-salikin*, ed. Javad Nurbakhsh, Intisharat-i Khaniqah-i Ni`mat Allahi 48 (Tehran: Chapkhana-yi Firdawsi, 1351/1972), p. 12. This text is cited differently by Corbin (*En islam iranien*, 3:43, n. 1; 3:63, n. 50; 3:81) from a Paris MS, which reads `iyan-i `iyan instead of `ayn-i `iyan; thus, Corbin translates, "To the extent that 1 x 1 is not produced, the mystical pilgrim does not arrive at the vision of the vision of *tawhid*."

Corbin appears to have gone astray, however, in applying this example to the symbolic arithmetic of *The Pool of Nectar*. In this passage from Ruzbihan, as well as in parallel expressions in other works by the same Sufi, the phrase "one times one" is used to emphasize the transcendence of the divine unity and the distance between creator and creation; the divine unity multiplies itself endlessly without detracting from that unity, while creation by implication adds up to multiplicity.[21]

The probable source for the symbolism of "one times one is one" in *The Pool of Nectar* is rather to be sought in the Illuminationist tradition, from the well-known emanationist adage that "from the one only one proceeds." In Avicennan metaphysics, the First Cause only produces a unitary effect, the First Intellect. The corollary to this point is that the philosopher or mystic must put away plurality and become pure unity in order to contemplate and return to the source of being. As Suhrawardi put it, "The One is not comprehended except by a unitary being, for it is a unitary being, as al-Hallaj said at the time of his crucifixion: 'It is sufficient for the One that the One be isolated in itself.'"[22] The placement of this symbol of unity at the end of the treatise means that it must be considered not as a general and univocal formulation about the unity of the creator and the creation, but as the final (and typically Neoplatonic) insight of the microcosmic pilgrim in the return to the source of being. The frame story itself is introduced as "the answer to someone asking about the source and the goal" (Int.7), invoking by the Arabic phrase "the source and the goal" (*al-mabda' wa-'l-ma`ad*) an array of cosmological and soteriological doctrines pertaining to the final destination of the soul.[23] The splitting of the spider's thread and its restoration is an

---

[21] Ruzbihan Baqli, *Sharh-i shathiyyat*, ed. Henry Corbin, Bibliothéque Iranienne 12 (Tehran: Departement d'Iranologie de l'Institut Franco-Iranien, 1966), pp. 281, 446, 453, 533.

[22] Suhrawardi, *Risalat fi i`tiqad al-hukama'*, in *Oeuvres philosophiques*, ed. Corbin, 2: 266–67. Suhrawardi's reading of al-Hallaj's saying is typically philosophical. Sufi versions of this saying read *al-wajid* ("the ecstatic") for the first instance of *al-wahid* ("the One") so that the saying would now mean, "All that matters to the ecstatic is the increasing solitude of his Only One, in himself"; cf. Louis Massignon, *The Passion of al-Hallaj, Mystic and Martyr of Islam*, trans. and ed. Herbert Mason, abridged ed., Bollingen Series 98 (Princeton: Princeton University Press, 1994), p. 289.

[23] R. Arnaldez, "Ma`ad," EI², 5:893–94.

allusion to the evanescent and illusory status of multiplicity, the web of creation, when viewed from the perspective of the return to the One.

The Islamicate versions of the frame story stress the importance of finding the king, that is, God, in the human world, but this is primarily a philosophical and mystical metaphor for attaining union with God. It is the king that is to be found, since the pearl no longer forms a part of the story. In the Persian translation, the Sufi mystical approach colors the narrative more emphatically than the Arabic, insisting that there is no existence but God and that all transformation takes place through the divine unity (although one of the Ottoman versions is more cautious on this point). The goal in the Syriac original of the "Hymn of the Pearl" is heavily cloaked with symbols; it only occasionally provides an allegorical key, as when the royal garment is explicitly identified as knowledge (gnosis). There the narrator is only told that successful completion of his mission will ensure his appointment as court herald, and toward the end, the story barely hints at his attainment of greater intimacy with the king, when the narrator hopes to stand next to the king by the royal gate. The Islamicate authors are generally not so reticent. In the Arabic version, the narrator's multiple encounters with his higher self in the forms of the king and his minister reinforce the notion that one must seek the theophanic true self. Meeting the spiritual double who is a perfect reflection of oneself is a motif that reverberates throughout early Gnostic and Manichean literature. As Corbin repeatedly pointed out, the symbolism of the spiritual twin can be used to argue for continuity between these earlier Near Eastern traditions and the philosophical mysticism of Suhrawardi.

The significance of the Pearl story for the Arabic version and its translations hinges upon the narrator's mystical relationship with the king, formulated as a covenant. The instruction to remember this covenant is important enough to be repeated in the Arabic version (A3–A4, A9–A10), first in relation to finding the king in the City of Life and, later, to finding both the royal minister and the king there. Some manuscripts insert a gloss, which takes the covenant beyond the boundaries of the story, identifying it as the primordial relationship between the souls of humanity and God, alluded to in a famous verse of the Qur'an (7:172). In this covenant, made in pre-eternity, God asked the souls, "Am I not your Lord?", and they replied, "Yes." This exchange forms the basis for monotheism, but in the Avicennan version, it is mystically interpreted along the lines of the Socratic saying attributed to the Prophet Muhammad: "He who knows himself already knows his Lord." In the same way, the Persian translation connects the symbolism of the garment as an image of the soul to the notion of the soul as an image of God, as formulated in both Hermetic alchemy and in a Prophetic saying:

> When you reach the end of the wayfaring, and you see the ornamented and golden heavenly garment (khirqa), put it on. That is the form of the 'Father of Bodies (abu al-ajsad)' [i.e., alchemical sulphur]; for '[God] created man in his own form' is the essence of this information.

What is the significance of the changes that have taken place in the story of the "Hymn of the Pearl"? The metaphors of clothing and disguise in the original narrative suggest a Manichean disdain or contempt for the body itself, which is simply to be replaced by a spiritual or astral body. The disguise that the narrator adopts in Egypt is the physical body needed in the dark material world, and it is eating the food of Egypt that induces the narrator's forgetfulness. This earthly body contrasts with the royal garment that flies to him and becomes one with him, for it is the gnosis of his otherworldly origin. All this has been abandoned in The Pool of Nectar and replaced with theophanies of divine authority combined with announcements that these figures represent the narrator's true self. The cautious and pessimistic allegories of the "Hymn" have been replaced by bold declarations that God is to be found in the world. These declarations have the additional effect of eliminating all the dramatic tension of the story, but that is the price to be paid for the change of emphasis.

The locus where this divine-human encounter takes place is the City of Life (al-balad al-ma'mura), a distinctively Suhrawardian allegory for the psycho-physical totality of the human being. This phrase is the Arabic translator's rendition of Suhrawardi's Persian term "Citadel of Life" or "Citadel of the Soul" (shahristan-i jan). Although we are told that the journey to this abode is a dangerous one, it is a microcosmic journey, which replaces the journey from Parthia to Egypt with a luxuriant allegory of the external and internal senses and faculties. This allegory (omitted from the translations below), taken directly from a Persian philosophical fable by Suhrawardi, is pure Aristotelian psychology in the Avicennan mold. Its insertion here shifts the mood away from the Gnostic sense of tragedy over the soul's descent into matter, replacing it with a distinctively upbeat confidence in the ability of the soul to recognize God through its natural faculties.

The two distinctive characteristics of the Islamicate versions, then, are the mystical unity between the soul and God in the cosmos (as symbolized by the narrator and the king) and the detailed exploration of the microcosm through an allegorical Aristotelian psychology according to Suhrawardi. Since the key to the now simplified plot is to seek the king in the world, it is clear that the addition of the Suhrawardian psychological allegory was no afterthought. This philosophical gnosis of the microcosm is the very means by which one may know God. And the yogic treatise that follows this introduction is precisely the same sort of psychocosmic analysis, presented to a Muslim audience with many overt invocations of both Aristotelian and Qur'anic vocabulary. The Arabic translator was clearly steeped in the Suhrawardian universe where being is equated with light. The hatha yoga emphasis on the body as the locus of salvation must have greatly appealed to the Arabic translator, who saw yoga as fulfilling the objectives of Islamic Neoplatonism, a tradition that was not averse to incorporating symbols and practices from unconventional sources. The most common title of the Arabic version was *The Pool of the Water of Life*, and the gnostic fount into which the narrator then fell was nothing less than the Water of Life itself. The Water of Life has numerous symbolic associations in Near Eastern lore, in the Qur'an, and in Islamicate philosophy. As part of the frame for the translated yoga text, the invocation of this symbol is a broad enough hint that we may conclude that the yoga teaching is itself the immortality-inducing gnosis which was (or should have been) the object of the original narrator's quest. This suspicion is borne out by further references to the Water of Life in the yoga text, which all have to do with yogic practices such as drinking the "nectar" of saliva (II.7), breath control (V.4), and urethral suction (VI.5). In the *Acts of Thomas*, the "Hymn of the Pearl" was the apostle's lament while he languished imprisoned in India. Now India is no longer a land of exile. The fragmentary versions of the "Hymn of the Pearl" have now become an ode to Indian ascetic practice, though set in an Islamic key.

APPENDIX: TABULAR COMPARISON AND TRANSLATION OF THE ARABIC, TURKISH, PERSIAN, AND URDU VERSIONS OF THE "HYMN OF THE SOUL"

Paragraph numbers are given for each language (A for Arabic, T for Turkish, P for Persian, and U for Urdu); when preceded by S at the left margin of the English translations of the Arabic and Persian, this refers to the numbering of verses of the Syriac version in Poirier's edition.[24] Correspondences between paragraph numbers are indicated by the following Table 14A.1.

TABLE 14A.1

Correspondences between the various versions of the "Hymn of the Pearl"

Syriac	Arabic	Turkish	Persian	Urdu
S1	A1	T1	P8	U8
	A2	T2	P1–P2	U1–U2
S11	A3	T3	P4	U4
S12	A4	T4		
	A5	T5		
S17	A6	T6	P3, P9	U3, U9
	A7	T7	P4	U4
	A8	T8	P8–P9	U8–U9
S11	A9	T9		
S12	A10	T10		
	A11	T11	P10	U10
	A12	T12	P11	U11
	A13	T13		
	A14	T14		
S18–S20	A15	T15		
S33–S34	A16	T16		
	A17	T17	P13	U13
S76	A18	T18	P14	U14
S56–S57	A19	T19	P15	U15
	A20	T20	P16	U16
S99–S102	A21	T21		
	A22	T22		
	A23	T23	P17	
	A24	T24	P18	

---

[24] See Poirier, *L'Hymne de la perle*, 343–48.

Passages of the Persian and Turkish corresponding to the Arabic version are underlined, as are passages of the Urdu corresponding to the Persian; Arabic quotations in the other language texts are in bold, as are Persian quotations in the Urdu version. The Arabic text follows recension *a*, while the Ottoman text (accompanied by transcription in modern Turkish) is based on the more popular recension *b*, translated by Salahi, with notes on significant variants. The Persian text is drawn from the best manuscript of the translation of Muhammad Ghawth (Per¹U, with marginal commentary), except for the concluding paragraphs (P17–P19), which only occur in one manuscript of the translation of ʿAbd al-Razzaq (Per²B). The Urdu text is drawn from the unique manuscript.[25,26]

TABLE 14A.2

The Arabic version of the "Hymn of the Soul"

A1	كنت في قديم البلاد، و هي مسكن أباي وأجدادي.	S1. I was in the olden country, which was the dwelling of my parents and grandparents.
A2	وطلبني صاحب البلاد، وقال، لا يصلح السكنى في بلدي إلا بعد السفر الى البلد المعمورة، و هي منتهى بلادي.	The master of the country summoned me and said, "It is not proper to dwell in this land of mine except after journeying to the City of Life,[25] which is the farthest extreme of my country.
A3	فلا تنس عهدي،	S11. "So do not forget my covenant,[26]
A4	فإنك تجدني في ذلك البلد.	S12. "For you will find me in that City.
A5	واسأل وصفها من وزيري الذي هو قاعد في بابي. ولا يدخل أحد إلا بعلمه و لا بخرج أحد إلا بإذنه. فلمّا وصلت الباب، وجدته وسلمت عليه، فردّ علىّ السلام ورحب بي. وقلت، أمر سيدي أن أسافر الى البلد المعمورة، فصفها. فقال لي.	"Ask its description of my minister, who is seated at my gate. None enters without his knowledge and none leaves without his permission." When I reached the gate, I found him and greeted him, and he returned my greeting and welcomed me. I said, "My lord has ordered me to journey to the City of Life, so describe it for me." He said to me,

(Continued)

---

[25] One MS (K) adds a gloss here, "the spiritual world."

[26] Several MSS (BEFI) add a gloss here, "which is 'Am I not your Lord?'" The phrase is taken from Qur. 7:172, identifying the covenant of this story with the pre-creational covenant between God and the souls of humanity (cf. Annemarie Schimmel, *Mystical Dimensions of Islam* (Chapel Hill, NC: University of North Carolina Press, 1975; New Delhi: Yoda Press, , index, s.v. "Covenant, primordial").

(Continued)

A6	دون وصالك اليه شدائد وعقبات،	S17. "There are hardships and difficulties before you reach him,
A7	وفي رجوعك الينا أعظم من ذلك. فأخاف أن تنس العهود للبعد والشدائد، وتبق الى الأبد أليماً من الفراق وبعيداً من الوصول.	"And in your return to us are others even greater than those. I fear that you will forget the covenants, because of the distance and the hardships, and that you will remain forever suffering from separation and far from returning."
A8	فقلت، لا بدّ من السفر اليها، فصف لي صفاتها وطريقتها. فقال، اسمع وعِ قولي،	I said, "I must travel there, so describe for me its qualities and the path to it." Then he said, "Listen and pay attention to what I say,
A9	ولا تنس عهدي،	S11 (*bis*). "and do not forget my covenant,
A10	فإنك تجدني و سيدي في تلك البلاد.	S12 (*bis*). "for you will find me and my master in this country.
A11	فأوّل ما تقطع من الشدائد بحرين عظيمين، وسبع جبال وأربع عقبات وثلاث منازل محشوة بالبلايا والآفات.	"The first of the hardships that you will encounter is the two great seas,[27] and then there are seven mountains and four passes. Then after that, there are three stations filled with calamities and evils.
A12	ثم تصل من ذلك الى طريق أضيق من عين النملة بحيث لا تقدر على المشي فيها بالرجلين إلا بالرأس ممحّقاً منكساً.	"Then from there you will reach a path narrower than the eye of an ant, so that you will not be able to go upon it on foot; rather, you will go upon it annihilated, upside down, on your head.
A13	فإذا قطعت تلك الشدائد، اطّلعت رأسك في البلد المعمورة.	"And if you pass these difficulties, you will lift up your head in the City of Life."
	[Suhrawardian microcosmic journey interpolated here]	[Suhrawardian microcosmic journey interpolated here]

---

[27] Several MSS insert a gloss, "which are the soul (*nafs*) and nature (*tab`*)." Others (BCDGJ) add, regarding the two seas, that "that first one is the upright heaven (*al-falak al-mustaqim*), and by them is meant the soul and nature." Astronomers define "the upright heaven" (Latin *sphaera recta*) as the celestial sphere as seen from the terrestrial equator, with the celestial equator passing through the zenith (Hartner, "Falak," EI², 2:762b).

A14	فأنت تشاهد هذه العلامات والصفات كلّها، وفحينئذ تنساها العهود كلّها ولا تذكر منها شئاً. فإذا دخلتها فاحذر الغفلة، وإلا، تبق أليماً أبد الأبدين.	"You will observe these signs and all these descriptions, and at that time you will forget all the covenants and not remember anything about them. So when you enter into it, beware of heedlessness, lest you remain suffering for ever and ever."
A15	قال، فسافرت وقطعت البحرين والجبال والعقبات و المنازل ووصلت الى ذلك الطريق الذي ذكرها. فبقيت فيه زماناً طويلاً حتى دنيت ودخلت المقصد،	S18–20. He said, so I traveled and traversed the two oceans, the mountains, the passes, and the stations, and I reached that path which he had mentioned. I remained in it for a long time, until I descended and reached the goal,
A16	لا أذكر منها شئاً.	S33–34. But I remembered nothing of it.
A17	فبينما أنا أدور في كثائفها ولطائفها، وصلت الى شيخ جالس في كرسي الملك وهو شيخها. فسلمت عليه وهو أيضاً سلّم عليّ، فكلّمته وهو أيضاً يتكلّم معي. فكل شئ أعمل وأقول هو يعمل ويقول.	While I was roaming about its grossnesses and subtleties, I reached a master seated on the throne of the king, and he was the master of [the City]. I greeted him and he also greeted me, and I spoke to him and he also spoke to me. Everything I did and said, he did and said.
A18	فمعنت النظر فإذا هو أنا والشيخ عكسي.	S76. Then I looked closely, and [saw that] he was I, and the master was my reflection.
A19	فنبهتني هذه الحالة وذكرتني العهود.	S56–57. This situation awakened me and reminded me of the covenants.
A20	فبينما أنا في هذه الحيرة إذ لقيت وزير سيدي الذي أوصاني وعاهدني.. فأخذ بيدي وقال، اغطس في هذا الماء فإنه ماء الحياة. فلما غطست فيه فهمت جميع رموزه ووجدت سيدي بعد معرفة الإعلامات وترك إستعمالها.	While I was in this astonishment, I suddenly faced the minister of my master, who had advised me and made the covenant with me. He took me by the hand and said, "Dive into this water," and it was the Water of Life. When I dived into it, I understood all its mysteries and found my master, after gaining gnosis of the signs, but abandoning their use.
A21	فقال لي، أهلاً وسهلاً أنت منّا. وبشّرني بالوصول اليه والمراجعة الى بلادي الأصلي عالماً سالماً.	S99–102. He said to me, "Welcome. You are one of us."[28] And he gave me the joyous news of attaining him and returning to my original country, safe and sound.

(Continued)

(Continued)

A22	فإذا كلّها إشارات ورموز لنيل النجاة وسعادة الأبد، وذلك لا يحصل إلا بمعرفة النفس الناطقة المميّزة المتفكّرة لتدبير الأحوال، وبها فاق الإنسان الحيوان.	All these were allusions and symbols for the attainment of salvation and eternal happiness, which cannot be attained except by gnosis of the cognizing and distinguishing rational soul for the managing of states.[29] In this way man is superior to animals.
	[Yoga text comes here]	[Yoga text comes here]
A23	قال، فلما اطّلعت رأسي في هذا الشبّاك، وجدت وزير سيدي الى هو أنا والوزير عكسي. فبقيت حائراً، ففي تلك الحيرة لقيت سيدي.	He said, And when I lifted up my head in this web,[30] I found the minister of my master; he was I, and the minister was my reflection. I remained astonished, and in this astonishment, I beheld my master.
A24	وأشار بأخذ خيط من خيوط العنكبوت. ثم شقّه نصفين، ثم جعله واحداً، ثم قال، الواحد في الواحد واحد. ففهمت إشارته، ووجدت نفسي هي هو وأنا عكسه. والسلام.	He made an allusion by taking a spider's thread; first he split it into halves, then he made them one. Then he said, "One times one is one." So I understood his allusion and found that my self was he, and I was his reflection. Farewell.

---

[28] Several MSS of recension b read instead, "He said to me, 'I am longing, longing [for you]' (*ana mushtaq, mushtaq*)."

[29] The vocabulary here is distinctively Avicennan—everywhere else in the book it is written as Avicenn—?ok and Suhrawardian; the rational soul (*al-nafs al-natiqa*) is characterized as cognizing (*mutafakkira*) and managing (*mudabbira*) the body while distinguishing (*mumayyiza*) between individuals and universals. See John Walbridge, *The Science of Mystic Lights, Qutb al-Din Shirazi and the Illuminationist Tradition in Islamic Philosophy*, Harvard Middle Eastern Monographs 26 (Cambridge, MA: Harvard University Press, 1992), pp. 67–69, 93–94, 195.

[30] Some MSS read, "He saw me in this web." "Web" (*shubbak*) can also mean "net" or "lattice," but it appears to be connected to the mention of the spider's thread a few lines later, and it may also serve as a metaphor for the narrator's predicament as being trapped in the world; in the treatise on "The Simurgh's Shrill Cry," Suhrawardi refers to "those who wish to tear down the spider's web" by expelling the nineteen "pincers" of the internal and external senses and the vegetal and animal faculties (Thackston, *Mystical & Visionary Treatises*, p. 98). Lifting up the head, also mentioned in Int. 8, seems to be a metaphor for departing the cosmic realm and reaching the world of the soul, the City of Life.

TABLE 14A.3

The Turkish translation

T1	ديديكه قديم البلاد ده ايدم اول بنم آبا و اجدادمك مسكنيدر	Dedi ki kadîmü'l-bilâdda idim ol benim âbâ ve ecdâdımın meskenidir.	He said, <u>I was in the olden country, which was the dwelling of my parents and grandparents.</u>
T2	بلاد صاحبى بنى طلب ايلدى و ديديكه بزم بلده مزده ساكن اولمقلق صالح اولمز الا بلدة معموره يه سفردن صكره اولور كه اول بلاد معموره بزم منتها بلادمزدر	Bilâd sahibi beni taleb eyledi ve dedi ki bizim beldemizde sakin olmaklık salih olmaz illâ belde-i mâ'mureye seferden sonra olur ki ol bilâd-ı mâ'mure bizim müntehâ bilâdımızdır.	<u>The master of the country summoned me and said, "It is not proper to dwell in this land of mine except after journeying to the City of Life, which is the farthest extreme of my country.</u>
T3	و سفر ايتدكده عهدمزى اونتمه كه اول عهد **الست بربكم**در	Ve sefer ettikte ahdimizi unutma ki ol ahd "elest-i bi-rabbiküm"dür.	"And on the journey, <u>do not forget</u> our <u>covenant</u>, which is '**Am I not your Lord**' (Qur. 7:172).
T4	تحقيقا سن اول بلاد معموره ده بنى بولورسون	Tahkikan sen ol bilâd-ı mâ'murede beni bulursun.	<u>"You will certainly find me in that Land of Life.</u>
T5	و اول بلاد معموره نك وصفنى قپومزده دوران وزيرمدن سؤال ايله زيرا اول بلاده بر كمسه داخل اولماز الا انك علمى ايله اولور و بر كمسه آندن چقماز الا انك اذنيله چيقار وقتاكه بلاد معموره يه سفر ايدوب اول قپويه واصل اولدم وزيرى بولدم و اكا سلام ويردم اول دخى عليك الوب پس اكا ديدم كه بلدة معموريه سفر ايتمكلكه افندمز بكا امر ايلدى وزير ديديكه	Ve ol bilâd-ı mâ'murenin vasfını kapımızda duran vezirimden sual eyle zira ol bilâda bir kimse dahil olmaz illâ onun ilmi ile olur ve bir kimse ondan çıkmaz illâ onun izniyle çıkar vakta ki bilâd-ı mâ'mureye sefer edip ol kapıya vasıl oldum veziri buldum ve ona selâm verdim ol dahi aleyk alıp pes ona dedim ki belde-i mâ'mureye sefer etmekliğe efendimiz bana emreyledi. Vezir dedi ki;	<u>"And ask the description of that Land of Life from my minister who is standing at our gate. None enters this Land without his knowledge and none leaves without his permission. When</u> I traveled to the Land of Life and <u>reached that gate and found</u> that minister <u>and greeted him, he returned my greeting. I said "My lord has ordered me to travel to the City of Life." The minister</u>[31] said,
T6	تحقيقا سنك سفرنده شدايد و عقبات واردر	Tahkikan senin seferinde şedâid ve 'ukubât vardır.	"There are hardships and difficulties in your journey,

(Continued)

---

[31] Recension *a* calls him "the prime minister" (*vezir-i 'azam*).

(Continued)

T7	و بزه رجو عنده اندن دخي زياده جه شدتلر واردر پس ايمدى خوف ايدرمكي سفر ايتدكده عهدى اونودوب و ابده دك فراقك المنده باقى و وصالدن بعيد اولورسون	Ve bize rücuunda ondan dahi ziyadeler şiddetler vardır. Pes imdi havf ederim ki sefer ettikte ahdi unutup ve ebede dek fırakın eleminde bâkî ve visalden baîd olursun.	"and in your return to us are others even greater than those. I fear that you will forget the covenants on the journey, and that you will remain forever suffering from separation and far from returning."
T8	بن وزيره ديدمكه البتده بو بلدة معموره نك سفرى بزه لابددر پس ايمدى اول بلدة معموره نك صفتنى بكا وصف ايله و طريقنى بكا بيان ايله وزير ديديكه قولمزى دكله	Ben vezire dedim ki elbette bu belde-i mâ'murenin seferi bize lâbüdd'dür. Pes imdi ol belde-i mâ'murenin sıfatını bana vasf eyle ve tarikini bana beyân eyle. Vezir dedi ki; kavlimizi dinle	I said to the minister,[32] "Of course I must travel to the City of Life. So describe for me its quali-ties and the path to it." He said, "Listen to our word,
T9	و عهدى اونتمه	Ve ahdi unutma	"And do not forget the covenant,
T10	تحقيقا سن بنى و افندمزى اول بلده ده بولورسن	Tahkikan sen beni ve efendimizi ol beldede bulursun.	"For you will truly find our lord and me in that City.
T11	پس ايمدى اولا قطع ايده جك شدايددن ايكى دريا واردر برى نفس و برى طبيعت ديدى و يدى طاغ و دورت عقبه و اوچ منزل كه بلا و افات ايله مملودر	Pes imdi evvelâ kat' edecek şedâidden iki derya vardır biri nefs ve biri tabiat dedi ve yedi dağ ve dört akabe ve üç menzil ki belâ ve âfât ile memlûdur.	"The first of the hardships that you will encounter is the two seas, which are the soul and nature, and seven mountains, and four passes, and three stations filled with calamities and evils.
T12	اندنصكره سفرنده بر يوله كله سنكه قرنجه كوزندن دخى ضيقدر و باشك اوزره منكاساً يوررسون	Ondan sonra seferinde bir yola gelesin ki karınca gözünden dahi zaykdır ve başın üzere münekkesen yürürsün.	"Then from there you will reach a path nar-rower than the eye of an ant, so that you will go upon it upside down, on your head[33].
T13	پس ايمدى وقتا كه بو ذكر اولنان شدايدى قطع ايدرسك نفسكى بلدة معموره ده بولورسون و بلدة معموره ده	Pes imdi vakta ki bu zikr olunan şedâidi kat' edersen nefsini belde-i mâ'murede bulursun ve belde-i mâ'murede.	"And when you pass these difficulties, you will find yourself in the City of Life.[34]

---

[32] Recension *a* adds, "There is no doubt of my lord's glory (*farr*) and authority (*himma*)."

[33] Recension *a* adds, "and on your breast (*sadr*)."

[34] Recension *a* reads, "you will save your head and you will be in the City."

	[Suhrawardian micro-cosmic journey interpolated here]	[Suhrawardian micro-cosmic journey interpolated here]	[Suhrawardian micro-cosmic journey interpolated here]
T14	پس ایمدی بو ذكر اولنان علامات و صفاتی مشاهده ایدرسك اول وقتده جمله عهودی اونودرسون و عهدلرندن بر شیء ذكر ایتمزسین پس ایمدی قچان اول بلده یه داخل اوله سن غفلتدن خذر ایله و الا انده ابد الابد باقی قالورسون دیو وصف و تنبیه ایلدی	Pes imdi bu zikr olunan alâmat ve sıfatı müşahede edersen ol vakitte cümle uhudu unutursun ve ahidlerinden bir şey zikr etmezsin. Pes imdi kaçan ol beldeye dahil olasın, gafletten hazer eyle ve illâ onda ebedü'l-ebed bâkî kalırsın diye vasf ve tenbih eyledi.	"You will observe these mentioned signs and all these descriptions, and at that time you will forget all the covenants and not remember anything about them. So when you enter into it, beware of heedlessness, lest you remain suffering for ever and ever."
T15	مصنف دیدی پس ایمدی سفر اتدم و ایكی دریایی و جبال و عقبات و منازلی كچدم و اول ذكر اولنان طریقه واصل اولدم و اول یولده زمان طویل قالدمكه	Musannif dedi: Pes imdi, sefer ettim ve iki deryayı ve cibâl ve ukubât ve menâzili geçtim ve ol zikr olunan tarike vâsıl oldum. Ve ol yolda zaman-ı tavîl kaldım ki;	The author said, So I traveled and traversed the two oceans, the mountains, the passes, and the stations, and I reached that path which he had mentioned.[35] I remained in that mentioned path and stayed there for a long time,
T16	عهودمدن بر شیء ذكر اتمدم اوندم	uhudumdan bir şey zikr etmedim, unuttum.	But I remembered nothing of it.
T17	بو ارالقده ولایتک كثایف و لطایفنی دور ایدركن بر شخصه واصل اولدمكه پادشاهك كرسیسی اوزرینه حلوس ایتمش كه اول بلده نك شیخیدر اول شیخه سلام ویردم اول دخی علیك الدی بن اكا سویلدم بكا سویلدی و هر بر شیكه بن انی ایشلرم و سویلرم اول دخی انی ایشلر و سویلر	Bu aralıkta vilâyetin kesâyîf ve letâyifini devr ederken bir şahsa vâsıl oldum ki; padişahın kürsüsü üzerine cülûs etmiş, ki ol beldenin şeyhidir. Ol şeyhe selâm verdim, ol dahi 'aleyk aldı. Ben ona söyledim bana söyledi. Ve her bir şey ki ben anı işlerim ve söylerim, ol dahi onu işler ve söyler.	While I was roaming about the grossnesses and subtleties of this realm, I reached a person seated on the throne of a king, and he was the master of that City. I greeted him and he also greeted me, and I spoke to him and he also spoke to me. Everything I did and said, he did and said.
T18	پس ایمدی امعان نظر اتدم اول شیخ بن ایمشم و شیخ بنم عكسم ایمش	Pes imdi im'ân nazar ettim ol şeyh ben imişim ve şeyh benim aksim imiş.	Then I looked closely, and saw that he was I, and the master was my reflection.

(Continued)

---

[35] Recension *a* reads, "I reached that place which is narrower than the eye of an ant."

(Continued)

T19	بو حالت بنی مبهوت قلدی و سبقت ایدن عهودی خاطریمه كتوردی	Bu hâlet beni mebhût kıldı ve sebkat eden uhudu hatırıma getirdi.	This situation bewildered[36] me and reminded me of the covenants.
T20	پس ایمدی بو حیرتده ایكن افندمك بكا وصیت و عهد ایتدیكی وزیره ملاقی اولدم و المی الدی و بو صویه دال كه تحقیقا ماء الحیات بودر دیدی وقتا كه دالدم جمیع مرموزاتنی فهم اتدم و افندم اولان جناب باریی بولدم بو علاماتی بیلوب و استعمالنی تركدنصكره	Pes imdi bu hayrette iken efendimin bana vasiyyet ve ahd ettiği vezire mülâkî oldum ve elimi aldı ve bu suya dal ki tahkikan mâ'i'l-hayat budur dedi. Vakta ki daldım, cemîi mermûzatını fehm ettim ve efendim olan Cenâb-ı Bârîyi buldum. Bu alâmatı bilip ve isti'malini terkden sonra,	While I was in this astonishment, I faced the minister of my master, who had advised me and made the covenant with me. He took me by the hand and said, "Dive into this water," and he said, "Truly it is the Water of Life."[37] When I dived into it, I understood all its mysteries and found my master the Supreme Creator, after gaining gnosis of the signs, but abandoning their use.
T21	افندم بكا دیدی بن سكا مشتاقم مشتاقم و كندینه وصلت ایله و بلدة اصله سالما و عالما رجعت ایتمكلك ایله بكا مژده ایلدی	efendim bana dedi, ben sana müştâkım, müştâkım. Ve kendine vuslat ile ve belde-i asla salimen ve 'âlimen ric'at etmeklik ile bana müjde eyledi.	My master said to me, "I am longing for you, I am longing for you!"[38] And he gave me the joyous news of my attaining him and returning to my original country, safe and sound.
T22	پس ایمدی بو مذكوراتك كلیسی نجاته و معاد الابده نیل ایچون اشارات و رموزاتدر و بو دیدیكمز نجات تمام حاصل اولمز الا نفس ناطقه یی بلدكدن صكره كه اول ناطقه دیدیكمز تدبیر افعال ایچون مفكره و ممیزه دركه انك ایله انسان حیوان اوزرینه فاءق اولمشدر	Pes imdi bu mezkûratın küllîsi necâta ve ma'âdü'l-ebede neyl için işârat ve rumûzâttır ve bu dediğimiz necât tamam hasıl olmaz illâ nefs-i nâtıkayı bildikten sonra; ki ol nâtıka dediğimiz tedbir-i	All these were allusions and symbols for the attainment of salvation and eternal return,[39] which cannot be attained except by gnosis of the cognizing and distinguishing rational soul for the managing of

---

[36] "Bewildered" (*mebhût*) seems to be a mistake for "awakened" (Ar. *nabahat*); another Arabic MS (X) in a marginal comment clearly glosses *nabahat* with Ottoman "awareness" (*agahlık*).

[37] Recension *a* has a ludicrous misreading here, caused by dropping a dot; thus "dive" (*ightis*) becomes "sneeze" (Ar. *i'tis*), so the narrator is told, "Sneeze, because to sneeze is the Water of Life (*bu aksırmak âb-ı hayattır*).

[38] See note 27 above.

[39] "Return" (*ma'ad*) seems to be a mistake for "happiness" (*sa'ada*).

	ef'âl için müfekkire ve mümeyyizedir ki, onun ile insan hayvan üzerine fâik olmuştur.

states. In this way man is superior to animals.

[Yoga text comes here] — [Yoga text comes here] — [Yoga text comes here]

T23

مصنف ديدى وقتا كه بو ذكرى
سبقت ايدن
سؤاله مطلع اولدم افندمك بكا
اولان وزيرنى بولدم كه اول بنم
و بو وزير بنم عكسمدر پس
ايمدى حيران قالدم و بو حيرتده
افندمه ملاقى اولدم

Musannif dedi vakta ki bu zikri sebkat eden suale muttali' oldum, efendimin bana olan vezirini buldum, ki ol benim ve bu vezir benim aksimdir. Pes imdi hayran kaldım ve bu hayrette efendime mülâki oldum.

The author <u>said</u>, when I became aware of the preceding question,[40] <u>I found the minister of my master; he was I, and the minister was my reflection. I remained astonished, and in this astonishment, I beheld my master.</u>

T24

و حبوط عنكبوتدن بر ايپلك
اخذ ايله بكا اشارت ايلدى و اول
ايليكى ايكى شق ايلدى اندن
صكره ينه بر ايلدى اندن صكره
ديدى "الواحد فى الواحد واحد"
پس ايمدى فهم اتدم و نفسمى
بولدم هى هى و بن افندمك
عكسى ايمشم

Ve hubut-u ankebûttan bir iplik ahz ile bana işaret eyledi ve ol ipliği iki şakk eyledi. Ondan sonra yine bir eyledi. Ondan sonra dedi, "el-Vahif fi'l-Vahid Vahid". Pes imdi fehm ettim ve nefsimi buldum hiye hiye ve ben efendimin aksi imişim.

He signaled me by taking a spider's futility;[41] <u>first he split it into halves, then he made them one. Then he said, "One times one is one." So I understood and found that my self was itself, and I was my master's reflection.</u>

---

[40] The translator appears to have understood "lifted up" (Ar. *ittila`tu*) metaphorically as gaining awareness or information, instead of its literal meaning.

[41] A misreading of "a thread" (*hayt min huyut*) as "futility" (*hubut*) may have been facilitated by an idiomatic expression in Ottoman. "*hubut-u ankebut*: to come to nothing, fail, miscarry, go wrong, to be futile, be of no avail, be lost."

TABLE 14A.4

The Persian translation

P1	مالک مملکت عدم ملکه را در خور قابلیت در عالم امر اشارت کُن کرد. بر حسب استعداد فیکون گشت, و حکم فرمود: هر چه وزیر من می گوید, بر آن اطاعت باید کرد. و از سرایچه لاهوت و منزل جبروت وحدت صرف تصرف خاص هر اشخاص را بیان کرد	S1. <u>The master of the kingdom</u> of non-existence made to the queen[42] an allusion to "**Be!**", to the extent possible in the world of command; "**And it is**" (Qur. 2:117) came to pass in accord with capacity. He gave the order, "Whatever my minister says is to be obeyed." He explained the special transformation of every entity, from the palace of divinity and the station of the might of pure unity.[43]
P2	و باز نمود که ترا در اینجا قرار گرفتن صواب نیست مگر بعد از سفر کردن بحانب بیت المعمور.	Then he stated, "<u>It is not right for you to dwell here except after traveling to the</u> House of Life (*bayt al-maʿmūr*).[44]
P3	بیا که این مسکن من الازل الی الابد قرارگاه تست. و خبر ماهیت از دریا تا صحرا سرّاً وعلانیةً داد, که در این راه بیست و هشت منزل است, و در هر منزلی عقبه. و در هر عقبه شداید بسیار و مشقهای بیشمار است.	"Come, for this land is your dwelling place **from pre-eternity to post-eternity**." He gave information of the essence, from the sea to the desert, **both openly and secretly**. He said, "In this path there are twenty-eight stations, and in every station there is a pass, and in every pass <u>there are many hardships and numberless troubles.</u>[45]

---

[42] Per¹A and Per¹J only, but confirmed by Urdu translation; Per¹I has "to himself."

[43] A marginal gloss in Per¹J reads, "The divinity that he summoned from his place of seclusion made a journey, and comes into manifestation. He mentioned the palace, and descended to the world of attributes. In relation to the first expression, he made use of the word 'palace,' and the explanation of the word 'station' is the sublime." On "might": "That is, the first specification and manifestation. Another meaning conveys appropriate perfection, i.e., something that once was, the form of which is perfected. That is, might is the essence of divinity. That is, palace has been explained as meaning that the divine and transcendent presence is in the veil of the isthmus. Were it not for that veil, creatures would have seen God visually. Listen to a subtle point: were it not for that veil, creation would never have manifested from God at all. Let one compare by understanding both aspects." On "unity": "That is, every known existence that is stored in pure unity is contained in Adam. This was given to every person. He explains that after the journey, the City becomes inhabited and supported."

[44] For the Arabic text's "the City of Life" (*al-balad al-maʿmūra*)," the translator has substituted the Qur'anic phrase "the House of Life" (*al-bayt al-maʿmur*, Qur. 52:4), commonly identified with the heavenly archetype of the Kaʿba which the angels circumambulate. A marginal gloss in Per1J reads, "The House of Life is in the fourth heaven. Like the image of Adam, that image becomes visible in the form of an image; this becomes an explanation of the Essence and Attributes. This House of Life is one of the subtle compounds, and it is made of the four elements of the Presence."

[45] See Arabic, A6.

P4	باید که بواسطة تشویشات عهد قدیم فراموش نکنی, بفراق ابد مبتلا مانی.	S11. "<u>You should not forget the ancient covenant because of these confusions, and if you do forget, you shall be afflicted by eternal separation</u>".[46]
P5	بیچاره گی را چاره ناچاره اختیار کرد.	In helplessness, willingly or not, he chose.
P6	باز فرمود, وقتی که بأخیر سلوک رسی, خرقة مکلل مرصّع بهشت پیوند بینی. آنرا در بر کنی. آن صورت ابو الاجساد است, که خلق آدم علی صورته عین اخبار است. فتبارک الله أحسن الخالقین (المؤمنین, ۲۳:۱٤) عجب نمودار است.	S14. Then he said, "When you reach the end of the journey, and you see the ornamented and golden heavenly garment,[47] put it on.[48] That is the form of the '**Father of Bodies**' (*abū al-ajsad*);[49] for '**He created man in His own form**' is the essence of this information.[50] '**Blessed be God, the most beautiful of creators!**' (Qur. 23.14) is the marvelous sign of this."[51]

(Continued)

---

[46] Cf. Arabic, A7. A marginal gloss in Per¹J reads, "That is, utterly distant from the ancient gnosis, which you had spoken as 'they said yes' (Qur. 7:172), and which you should not forget; otherwise you will remain in the unbelief of eternal error." This connects the covenant to the same Qur'anic verse cited in some copies of the Arabic version.

[47] *Mukallal* has the sense of adorned with gems or jewels, and can also mean crowned; *murassa'* means set in gold or studded with gems, used mostly with reference to a crown or sword. The terms are often used together in royal contexts in Persian (Dihkhuda, *Lughat nama*).

[48] This sentence preserves a feature of the "Hymn of the Soul" that does not survive in any copy of the Arabic version: the jeweled and golden garment which comes to meet the narrator as he returns home, reflecting him and becoming one with him. From the appearance of this feature, it appears that the translation by Muhammad Ghawth predates the existing recension of the Arabic text.

[49] "Father of Bodies" in alchemical parlance means sulphur, just as "Father of Spirits" (*abu al-arwah*) means mercury (Dihkhuda, *Lughat nama*). A marginal gloss in Per1J reads, "Whatever the revered Father of Spirits commands must be obeyed, for that is the substance of inner things, just as its own state is good. 'I was a prophet when Adam was between water and clay' [hadith]."

[50] "God created man in his own form" is a hadith attributed to the Prophet Muhammad; cf. Badi' al-Zaman Furūzanfar, *Ahadith-i mathnawi* (Tehran: Intisharat-i Daneshgah-i Tehran, 1334/1956), p. 114, no. 346.

[51] A marginal gloss in Per1J reads, "That is, the other creation of humanity was established within Adam, peace be upon him."

(Continued)

P7	و چون وجود قدرت بهمه صنع صانع استظهار یافت, وجود حکمت در ضمن او بتّمام مراتب مهیّا و موجود ساخت. حکما ترتیب و ترکیب تنزل هر فردی از افراد معلوم کند, هر چه در آن بنیاد است و در این نهاد است.	Since the existence of power sought manifestation in all the creation of the Creator, the existence of wisdom became ready and existent within it [creation] at every level. Philosophers teach about the order and composition of the descent of every individual being, whatever is in that foundation and is in this structure.[52]
P8	حقیقت انسانی, وزیر ثانی, که وجود عالم و بحضرت ارتسام تمام است, بأمثال عیان کرد و بیان فرمود که ترا لازم است بجانب شهر معمور سفر کردن, که مسکن ابا و اجداد تست.	The human reality, the second minister, who is cosmic existence and is perfectly imprinted by that presence, clarified through parables, and explained, "It is necessary for you to travel toward the City of Life, for that is the dwelling place of your parents and grandparents."[53]
P9	او باز عرض کرد که تعریف آن شهر و راه آن چنانچه حق تفصیل است.	The minister said further, "The description of that City and the path to it is just as follows."
P10	بیان فرمای گفت, نخست آن عالم عالم نفس است, و از آن شداید بحرین و هفت کوه و سه منزل و چهار طبق است.	He explained: "The first of that world is the world of the soul, and from that are the hardships[54] of the two seas,[55] the seven mountains, the three stations,[56] and the four levels.[57]

---

[52] A marginal gloss in Per¹J reads, "That is, every existent atom that existed in the loins of Adam, according to its capability, comes into manifestation by [divine] power. They are required according to the dictates of wisdom. That is, every member became manifest, and occurred according to capacity. In this there is no excess or defect. 'And when your lord took their seed from their backs and made them testify to themselves, he said, "Am I not your Lord?" They said yes' (Qur. 7:172). The meaning is this."

[53] Cf. Arabic, A1. The change from "House of Life" to "City of Life," although providing a different verbal nuance, is in effect a return toward Suhrawardi's original term "citadel of the soul" (*shahristan-i jan*).

[54] A marginal gloss in Per1J reads, "That is, the hardship of the glory of greatness is (? illegible) the fixed essences, which are the realities of the divine names. They have become adorned by the form of the existential names. In general and in particular, he established nothing but necessity and possibility."

[55] A marginal gloss in Per¹J reads, "That is, the loins of the father and the womb of the mother."

[56] A marginal gloss in Per¹J reads, "That is, the three births, i.e., minerals, vegetables, and animals."

[57] Here Arabic `aqabat, "passes," has become Persian *tabaqa*, "level." A marginal gloss in Per1J reads, "That is, first of all it is without knowledge of the world of command; it is the collective soul. When it becomes limited by a form, it is called the rational soul. When it is connected with the elements, it is called the constituted spirit."

P11	و راه باریکتر از چشم مور است. و آفات بسیار و منازل بیشمار, و آن بهای قطع کردن دشوار, بدل قطع باید کرد.	"The road is narrower than the eye of an ant, and there are many evils and numberless stations. It is difficult to traverse that on foot; one must traverse it with the heart.
P12	چرا که آمدن سالک از راه اسمای کونی بود, و رفتنش براه اسمای الهی, چنانچه بزرگی فرموده است. بیت. طریقش بی قدم می پو خیالش بی بصر می بین کلامش بی زبان می خوان شرابش بی دهن در کش	"Why? The wayfarer's coming is by the path of the existential names, and his going is by the path of the divine names." As a saint has said, "Go his way footless, see his form without eye, recite his word without tongue, and drink his wine without mouth."
	[Suhrawardian microcosmic journey interpolated here]	[Suhrawardian microcosmic journey interpolated here]
P13	و گفت: هر عقبات و منازل که شنیده بودم چون تمام یکیک راه بحرین و عقبات و منازل قطع کردم و بیکی جمله بریدم تا رسیدم سوی پیری که او بر کرسی ملک نشسته و او شیخ آن شهر است. سلام گفتم. بعد از جواب بمکالمت در آمد. من نیز باو بتکلّم در آمدم و هر کاری که کردم او کرده بود.	When I traversed and crossed all at once each of the hardships and stations that I had heard from the minister – including the seas, passes, and stations -- I approached a venerable man (piri) seated on the king's throne, who was the master (shaykh) of that City. I greeted him, and after he returned my greeting, he began to converse, and I began speaking to him. Whatever I did, he did.
P14	چون نیکو نگریستم او من بودم شیح عکس من بود.	S76. When I looked well, [I saw that] he was I, and the master was my reflection.
P15	پس مرا از:ای حاصل شد و از عهود گذشته یاد آمد.	S56-57. Then I awakened and remembered my former covenants.
P16	چون این حال بدیدم سرا حالی پدید آمد و در ان حال وزیررا دیدم. گفت نیکو رسیدی, بیا تا ترا با مالک الملک اعظم و وزیر معظّم برسانم و به	When this state became clear, a state came upon me, and in that state I saw the minister.[58] He said, "You have

(Continued)

---

[58] A marginal gloss in Per1J reads, "That is, when I traversed this realm and stations, and I arrived at the measure of divinity that is the reality of humanity, he said, 'Congratulations!' And he said, 'What you have seen, understood, and passed through is all (? illegible).' By hearing these words, I found a new life, and was qualified by all the attributes. I became the master of knowledge and wisdom for all eternity. I saw one existence; when I began to observe, I comprehended the beauty of witnessing. When I disengaged, I forgot no one; with sign or without is according to what you say. With a subtle understanding, another comprehends the subtle."

(Continued)

	وزیر معظم آشنا سازم. چون بطفیل وزیر در تفحّص در آمدم, شاه و وزیر را در خود یافتم. آنچه وعدة موعود بود تمامی بخود معاینه کردم, بعد از شناختن علامات و اشارات و رموزات سر بسته از اسرار. فهم من فهم, و من یؤت الحكمة فقد اوتی خیراً کثیراً (البقرة، 2:269).	indeed arrived. Come, that I may convey you to the master of the greatest kingdom, and acquaint you with the chief minister." When I began to seek by following the minister, <u>I found the king</u> and minister in myself. <u>That which had been promised I witnessed entirely in myself, after recognizing the signs, allusions, and cyphers wrapped in secrets.</u> **"Let them understand who understand. 'Those given wisdom have been given a great good (Qur. 2:269).'"**
	[Yoga text comes here]	[Yoga text comes here]
P17	چون این سلوک بر آوردم، رسید. او من بودم وزیر عکس او. باقی شدم، ببقا رسیدم.	When I completed this journey, <u>he arrived. I became him, and the minister [became] his reflection.</u> I became subsistent; I reached subsistence.
P18	و این اشارت: بر گرفتن ریسمان عنکبوت دو پاره کردن و باز یکجا کردن او است. چون حس کند بگوید یکی در یکی [یکی] باشد بر این اشارت معلوم شد که اوست و من عکس اویم وباقی. والله أعلم بالصواب.	<u>This was his allusion: to take apart a spider's thread in two pieces and put them together again.</u> When he perceived, <u>he said, "One times one is [one]." By this allusion it was known that [my self]</u> <u>was he, and I am his reflection</u> and subsistent. **And God knows best what is right.**

TABLE 14A.5

The Urdu translation

U1	مالک ملک عدم کا ملکہ کو بیچ لائق قابلیت کے عالم امر میں اشارت کیا وہ موافق استعداد کے نیک ہوا. تب حکم فرمایا کہ جو کچھ وزیر میرا کہے، اس پر عمل کر. وہ کہ لابوت اور منزل جبروت وحدت صرف تصرف خاص ہر اشخاص کا بیان کیا	<u>The master of the</u> realm <u>of nonexistence</u> <u>made to the queen an allusion</u> suitable <u>to possibility in the world of command;</u> it was good, in agreement <u>with its capacity. He gave the order,</u> "Whatever my minister <u>says is to be done." He explained the special transformation of every entity: divinity and the station of the might of pure unity.</u>
U2	اور پھر کہا کہ تیرے تئیں بیچ اس جگہ کے قرار لینا صواب نہیں ہے. لیکن بیت المعمور کا سفر کنے.	<u>Then he stated, "It is not right for you to dwell here,</u> but you must <u>travel to the House of Life."</u>

U3	بعد آ کــه یہ ٹھکانہ ابتدا ســے انتہا تک تیری رہنے کی جائے ہے۔یہ کـه کر۔ے، خبر پہچانت ظاہر باطن کے دروازے سے جنگل تک کی دیا کـه بیچ اس راہ کے بیت المعمور ہے اور آٹ منزل ہیں ہر منزل میں سختیاں بہت اور محنتاں بے شمار ہیں	Then [he said], "<u>Come, for this land is your dwelling place</u> from the beginning to the end." He gave information of the knowledge from the door of the outer and inner to the jungle.[59] He said, "<u>In this path</u> is the House of Life, and <u>there are eight stations, and in every station</u> there are many difficulties and <u>numberless</u> trials.
U4	۔ تجھکو چاہئے کـه راہ کے پریشانیوں کے باعث شرط قدیم فراموش نہ کر۔ے۔ تو اور اگر فراموش کر۔ےگا تو ہمیشہ جدائی کے آفتوں میں پریشان اور سرگردان رہےگا۔	"You should not forget the ancient condition[60] <u>because of</u> the disturbances of the path, <u>and if you do forget, you shall be</u> disturbed and upset by the misfortunes of <u>separation</u>"
U5	بےچارگی کو کچھ علاج نہیں۔ ناچار اختیار کیا	<u>For helplessness</u> there is no cure; <u>unwillingly he chose.</u>
U6	تب فرمایا جسوقت کـه آخری سلوک کو پہنچےگا تو خرقۂ مکلّل بہبشت کے پیوند کا دیکھےگا تو اس کو پہن لے کـه وہ صورت ابو الاجساد کی ہے۔ کـه خلق آدم علی صورت<ہ> عین ظاہر ہے۔ فتبارک الله احسن الخالقین عجیب نمودار ہے۔	Then he said, "When you reach the end of the journey, and you see the ornamented heavenly garment, put it on. That is the form of the '**Father of Bodies**' (*abū al-ajsad*); for '**He created man in [His] own form**' is the essence of outward appearance. '**Blessed be God, the most beautiful of creators!**' (Qur. 23:14) is the marvelous sign of this."
U7	جیسا کـه بہ نسبت قدرت کے ہر صنعت کو صانع ہے ظاہر کیا یافت وجود کا حکمت در میاں اس کے ساتھ تمامیت مراتب کے موجود کیا۔ حکمت ترتیب اور ترکیب منزل ہر منزل فرد ایک کی فردوں سے معلوم کر ے ہو کچھ کـه بیچ اس بنیاد ک ے ہے۔ بیچ اس ذات کے ہے۔	Since it is in relationship to <u>power</u> that <u>every</u> creation has a <u>Creator, the wisdom of</u> the profit of <u>existence</u> made <u>existent the totality of levels within</u> it. Wisdom <u>teaches about the order and composition of the</u> station <u>of every individual station; whatever is in that foundation is in this</u> essence.[61]

(Continued)

---

[59] The Persian expression "from the sea to the desert" (*az darya ta sahra*), signifying all of creation, has been transformed here as *darya* becomes *darvaza*, "door" while *sahra* becomes *jangal* (jungle).

[60] Somehow the key term "covenant" (`*ahd*) has become "condition" (*shart*) both here and in U13, though it mysteriously reappears in U16.

[61] The syntax and vocabulary of the Urdu differ substantially from the Persian here, treating *yaft* as a noun ("profit") rather than an auxiliary verb, and making numerous other changes.

(Continued)

U8	حقیقت انسانی وزیر ثانی کی کہ وجود عام اور ساتھ حضرت کے پیوستگی تمام ہے۔ ساتھ مثال کے ظاہر کیا۔ اور فرمایا کہ تیرے تئیں لازم ہے کہ طرف شہر معمور کے سفر کرنا کہ اور ٹھکانہ تیرے باپ دادے کا ہے۔	The human reality, belonging to the second minister, who is common existence and is perfectly connected to that presence, made it evident by a metaphor, and said, "It is necessary for you to travel toward the City of Life, for that is the dwelling place of your parents and grandparents."
U9	یہ پھر عرض کیا کہ تعریف اس شہر اور راہ کی مفصل بیان فرماوے	The minister said further, "Let me give the description of that City and the detailed explanation of the path."
U10	تب وہ کہا کہ پہلے اس کے عالم انفس ہے جو وہ جانے سختیوں سے آمادہ یعنی دو دریا اور سات پہاڑ اور تین منزل اور چار طبقہ ہیں	He explained: "The first of that world is the world of the souls, which is the place of difficulties, that is, the two seas, the seven mountains, the three stations, and the four levels.
U11	اور وہ راہ باریک زیادہ آنکھ سے چمٹی کے ہے اور آفتان بہت اور منزلاں ہے شمار ہیں اور منزلاں اس کے پاؤں سے قطع چاہنے کرنا	"The road is narrower than the eye of an ant, and there are many evils and numberless stations. One must traverse its stations on foot.
U12	کس واسطے کہ آنا سالک کا راہ سے اسمائی کونی کے ہے اور جانا اس کا راہ سے اسمائی الٰہی کے جیسا کہ ایک بزرگ نے فرمائے ہیں۔ فرد: طریقش بی قدم می رو خیالش بی بصر می بین کلامش بی زبان می خوان شرابش بی دہن می کش	"Why? The wayfarer's coming is by the path of the existential names, and his going is by the path of the divine names. As a saint has said, **'Go his way footless, see his form without eye, recite his word without tongue, and drink his wine without mouth.'"**
	[Suhrawardian microcosmic journey interpolated here]	[Suhrawardian microcosmic journey interpolated here]
U13	جسوقت کہ میں وزیر سے یہ سنا اور نشان پایا تو سفر کیا اور راہ عقبات اور منزلاں کو اس کے جیسا کہ سنا تھا میں ویسا ہے قطع کیا جب تمام تدریجا قطع کر کر شہر کو آیا تو ایک جوان کو دیکھا کہ اوپر ملک کے بیٹھا ہوا وہ شیخ اس شہر کا ہے میں اسکو سلام کہا وہ جواب میرے سلام کا کہکر کلام کرنے میں آیا میں بھی اس کے ساتھ باتاں کرنا شروع کیا جو کام کہ میں کیا تھا سو وہ بھی کیا	When I heard this from the minister and found the sign, I made the journey and traversed the hardships and stations in it as they were. Since all this was as I had heard, traveling gradually I came to the City. I saw a young man who was upon the seat of the king; he is the master (*shaykh*) of that City. I greeted him, and after he returned my greeting, he began to converse, and I began speaking to him. Whatever I did, he did.

U14	جب خوب دیکھا اور تامل کیا تو معلوم ہوا کہ وہ شخص خود میں تھا اور وہ شیخ عکس میرا تھا	When I looked well and made an effort, it became clear that that person was I, and the master was my reflection.
U15	پس میرے تئیں انتہا حاصل ہوئی اور شرطان گذرے ہوئے یاد آئی	Then I attained the goal and remembered my former conditions.
U16	جب یہ حال کو دیکھتے ہے میرے تئیں حیا آئی اس حال میں میں وزیر کو دیکھا وزیر کہا خوب پہنچا تو آ تیرے تئیں ساتھ مالک الملک اعظم وزیر معظم سے آشنا کراؤں جب طفیل سے وزیر کے بیچ تفحص کے آیا میں شاہ اور وزیر کو اپنے میں پایا میں اور جو کچھ کہ وعدہ عہد کیا گیا تھا سو اپنے میں دیکھنا کیا میں بعد از پہچان نے علاقہ اور اشارے اور بھیدان مشکل اور سر بستہ اسرار سے میرے اور فہم سے میرے یؤت الحکمۃ فقد أوتی خیراً کثیراً (البقرۃ، 2:269).	When he saw this state, I became shy, and in that state I saw the minister. The minister said, "You have indeed arrived. Come, that I may convey you to the master of the greatest kingdom, [and] acquaint you with the chief minister." When I began to seek by following the minister, I found the king and minister in myself. That which had been promised by the covenant I witnessed in myself, after recognizing the relationship, allusions, difficult mysteries, and involved secrets. And from my understanding, "[Those] **given wisdom have been given a great good** (Qur'an 2:269)."

15

Accounts of Yogis in Arabic and Persian Historical and Travel Texts

India has long figured in accounts of the marvelous and the fantastic. Travelers and historians for centuries have commented on the wonders of India, from the time of Alexander onward. Ascetics and austere religious figures have always been popular subjects for comment, but there was no guarantee that foreign visitors could gain any real understanding of the spiritual objectives of these Indian recluses.

Megasthenes' account of Alexander's interview with the ascetic Mandanis is a telling example of the limitations that foreigners experienced in communicating with gymnosophists or yogis, particularly through the medium of translation.

> Mandanis . . . said that he commended the king because, although busied with the government of so great an empire, he was desirous of wisdom; for the king was the only philosopher in arms that he ever saw, and that it was the most useful thing in the world if those men were wise who have the power of persuading the willing, and forcing the unwilling to learn self-control; but that he might be pardoned if, conversing through three interpreters, who, with the exception of language, knew no more than the masses, he should be unable to set forth anything in his philosophy that would be useful; for that, he added, would be like expecting water to flow pure through mud![1]

---

[1] Strabo, *Geography*, ed. and trans. Horace Leonard Jones and J. R. Sitlington Sterrett (London: Heinemann, 1917), 15.1.64.

Modern critics have also pointed out how European travelers especially carried with them their own baggage of Orientalist prejudice when attempting to describe their encounters with the Indian other. While historians of religion have attempted to mine travelers' accounts and historical texts for information about the religions of India, there are admittedly limitations with how far one can take this kind of material.[2] Whether the traveler is a European Christian or a Middle Eastern Muslim, such sources often tell us more about the mentality of the narrator than about the subject nominally under discussion.[3]

These strictures on the usefulness of outsiders' reports of Indian religions, one assumes, apply equally to the accounts provided by Muslim travelers as well as Indo-Muslim rulers and their historians. Their descriptions of Indian religions often exhibit a "curious mixture of fear and admiration, and familiarity and loathing."[4] How much can such sources tell us about the teachings of yoga in the South Asian subcontinent?[5] Although Vedantic metaphysics may have fascinated a few Muslim philosophers and yogic practices drew the keen interest of some Sufi mystics, from an ordinary perspective, the yogi himself was one of the most visible—and exotic—signs of Indian spirituality. Having undergone a ritual separation from Brahmanic society through a symbolic death, the yogi was free of

---

[2] For a brief selection of European comments on yogis, see Henry Yule and A. C. Burnell, *Hobson-Jobson, A Glossary of Colloquial Anglo-Indian Words and Phrases*, ed. William Crooke (1903; repr., New Delhi: Munshiram Manoharial, 1979), pp. 461–62, s.v. "Jogee." A number of accounts of yogis by European travelers are reproduced by Richard Schmidt, *Fakire und Fakirtum im alten und modernen Indien: Yoga-lehre und Yoga-praxis* (Berlin: Verlag von hermann Barsdorf, 1908).

[3] Juan Cole, "Mirror of the World: Iranian 'Orientalism' and Early 19th-Century India," *Critique: Journal of Critical Studies of Iran and the Middle East* (Spring 1996): 41–60; Seyyidi 'Ali Re'is, *Le miroir des pays: Une anabase ottomane a travers l'inde et l'asie centrale*, trans. Jean-Louis Bacqué-Grammont (Arles: Sindbad-Actes Sud, 1999), pp. 92–94.

[4] Muzaffar Alam and Sanjay Subrahmanyam, "Empiricism of the Heart: Close Encounters in an 18th-Century Indo-Persian Text," *Studies in History*, n.s., 15, no. 2 (1999): 291.

[5] For the general problem of Muslim interpreters of Indian religion, see Carl W. Ernst, "Situating Sufism and Yoga," *Journal of the Royal Asiatic Society*, Series 3, 15, no. 1 (2005): 15–43, and Chapter 12 in the present volume; id., "The Islamization of Yoga in the Amrtakunda Translations," *Journal of the Royal Asiatic Society*, Series 3, 13, no. 2 (2003): 199–226, and Chapter 10 in the present volume; id., "Muslim Studies of Hinduism? A Reconsideration of Persian and Arabic Translations from Sanskrit," *Iranian Studies* 36 (2003): 173–95, and Chapter 11 in the present volume; id., "Admiring the Works of the Ancients: The Ellora Temples as viewed by Indo-Muslim Authors," in *Beyond Turk and Hindu: Rethinking Religious Identities in Islamicate South Asia*, ed. David Gilmartin and Bruce B. Lawrence (Gainesville, FL: University Press of Florida, 2000): 198–220, and Chapter 9 in the present volume.

the constraints of purity that restricted the social interactions of Brahmins and other high-caste Hindus with foreigners. During Turkish and Mughal rule over India, these naked ash-smeared ascetics attracted the curiosity of Muslim rulers, officials, and travelers.[6] Their reputed magical powers were no doubt responsible for some of the attention the yogis received. A brief survey of accounts in Indo-Muslim historical texts and travel accounts shows that the Nath or Kanphata ("split-ear") yogis, in northern India generally pronounced "jogis," came to occupy an accepted if unusual position in the cosmos of Muslim South Asia. At the same time, it appears that a number of powerful Muslim rulers were relatively familiar with certain yogic practices that they found useful, to an extent that parallels the textual transmission of yoga in Arabic and Persian translation in the different versions of *The Pool of Nectar*.[7]

Jogis have long had a standard place in "believe it or not" accounts of the strange and marvelous in India. One of the earliest Arabic travel accounts of India, an anonymous text written in 851AH (sometimes attributed to a merchant named Sulayman), has a typical portrait of the bizarre Indian ascetic, with characteristics that (like the jogi described here) are made to seem changeless:

> And in the land of India there are those dedicated to wandering in the jungles and the mountains, meeting few other people, and subsisting on herbs and fruits of the jungles. They place around the penis a ring of iron, in order to prevent interaction with women. Some of them are naked, and others expose themselves to the sun, facing it with no other covering than a tiger skin. I once saw one of these men, just as I have described, and I departed. I returned after sixteen years, and I saw him in the same condition. So I marveled how his eyes were not ruined from the heat of the sun.[8]

---

[6] See R. Foltz, "Two Seventeenth-century Central Asian Travellers to Mughal India," *Journal of the Royal Asiatic Society* 6 (1997): 367–77; Nile Green, "A Persian Sufi in British India: The Travels of Mîrzâ Hasan Safî 'Alî Shâh (1251/1835–1316/1899)," *Iran: Journal of Persian Studies* 42 (2004): 210–11; Iqbal Husain, "Hindu Shrines and Practices as Described by a Central Asian Traveller in the First Half of the 17th Century," in *Medieval India 1: Researches in the History of India 1200–1750*, ed. Irfan Habib (Delhi, Oxford University Press, 1992), pp. 141–53.

[7] George Weston Briggs, *Gorakhnath and the Kanphata Yogis* (1938; repr., Delhi: Motilal Banarsidass, 1980); Ernst, "Islamization of Yoga", Chapter 10 in the present volume.

[8] Sulayman (attr.), *'Ahbar as-Sin wa l-Hind, Relation de la Chine et de l'Inde rédigé en [237]/851*, ed. Jean Sauvaget (Paris: Belles Letres, 1948), pp. 22–23 §52.

Several themes are joined together here that will later be associated with the jogi, including solitude, vegetarian diet, unusual attitudes to sex, nakedness, and gazing at the sun.

To the extent that we find it mentioned in Muslim historical sources, yoga, like divination, was regarded as a practical subject that as such attracted the interest of Indo-Muslim kings. Since interest in yoga did not form a normal part of the portrait of the ideal Indo-Muslim king, detailed accounts of jogis only rarely figure in court histories. Nonetheless, evidence survives to indicate a long-standing connection between the courts and the jogis, who seem to have occupied a place similar to that held by astrologers and magicians. During the heyday of the Delhi Sultanate in the fourteenth century, charismatic figures from non-Brahmanical circles attained particular celebrity at court. The poet Amir Khusraw (d. 1325) paid tribute to the supernatural powers of Indian ascetics in his lengthy accolade to the virtues of India in the third chapter of his Persian epic, *Nuh sipihr* (*The Nine Heavens*). Khusraw stressed particularly the Brahmins' skill in divination and the jogis' breathing control.[9] According to Jain sources, Sultan Muhammad ibn Tughluq paid special favor to the celebrated Jain scholar Jinaprabhu Suri, at his urging restoring Jain shrines and ensuring their protection. The sultan obtained a protective amulet from Suri in the form of a yantra diagram and witnessed Suri's mastery over the 64 yoginis (female yogic divinities), a practice also found in *The Pool of Nectar*.[10] The famous traveler Ibn Battutah also confirmed Muhammad ibn Tughluq's interest in jogis, and Ibn Battutah himself was quite intrigued with jogis and their reported miraculous powers. In an account of "yogic magic," he relates,

This group is the source of wonders, among which is that one of them remains for months without eating or drinking. Many of them have caves dug out for them under ground. It is built over him, leaving only a hole through which air enters, and he remains there for months. I have heard that one of them remains thus for a year. I saw in the city of Mangalore

[9] Amir Khusraw, *Nuh sipihr*, ed. Wahid Mirza, (London: Oxford University Press, 1950), pp. 192–94; trans. R. Nath and Faiyaz 'Gwaliari,' in *India as Seen by Amir Khusrau (in 1318 A.D.)* (Jaipur: Historical Research Documentation Programme, 1981), pp. 98–99.
[10] Mohanlal Bhagwandas Jhavery, *Comparative and Critical Study of Mantrasastra (with Special Treatment of Jain Mantravada)*, Sri Jain Kala Sahitya Samsodhak Series 1 (Ahmedabad: Sarabhai Manilal Nawals, n.d.), pp. 230–34.

a man among the Muslims who had studied with them. A platform was erected for him, and he remained on top of it without eating or drinking for a period of twenty-five days. I left him so, and I do not know how long he remained after my departure. The people say that they fashion balls that they eat for a certain number of days or months, during which period they need neither food nor drink. They tell of hidden affairs [i.e., predict the future]. The Sultan reveres them, and admits them to his presence. Some among them restrict food to vegetables, while others refrain from eating meat, and they are the majority. The obvious aspect of their condition is that they subject themselves to discipline (*riyada*). They need nothing from the world and its delights. Some among them can kill a man with a mere look. The people say that if a man is killed by a look, and the chest of the corpse is split open, it is found to lack a heart. They say that his heart has been eaten. This is prevalent among women, and the woman who does that is called a hyena.[11]

Ibn Battutah was astounded one day to witness a jogi levitating before the sultan in his private apartments. He was also accompanied by four jogis on his pilgrimage to Adam's Peak in Ceylon.[12] Evidently some members of the Khalji aristocracy of Malwa were interested in the longevity promised by yoga, as they are said to have lived with jogis to acquire yogic techniques and drugs used for mastering the health of the body as well as sexual practices.[13] Knowledge of divination and access to the female spirits called *joginis* (yoginis) was considered useful by Muslim rulers on military expeditions in Gujarat in the late sixteenth century.[14]

It will not be surprising also to see that the Mughal emperor Akbar was keenly interested in yoga, in view of his well-known penchant for

---

[11] Ibn Battutah, *Voyages d'Ibn Battuta*, ed. and trans. C. Defremery and Beniamino Raffaello Sanguinetti (Paris: Anthropos, 1968–1969), 4:35–36.

[12] Id., *Travels in Asia and Africa 1325–1354*, trans. H. A. R. Gibb, ed. E. Denison Ross and Eileen Power (1929; repr., Karachi: Indus Publications, 1986), pp. 225–26, 255, 257, 259.

[13] Rizq Allah Mushtaqi, *Waqi`at-i Mushtaqi*, MS Add. 11,633, British Museum, fols. 91b–92a, cited by I. H. Siddiqui, "Resurgence of Chishti Silsila in the Sultanate of Delhi," in *Islam in India: Studies and Commentaries*, Vol. 2, *Religion and Religious Education*, ed. Christian W. Troll (New Delhi: Vikas, 1985), p. 71.

[14] Abdullah Muhammad al-Makki al-Asafi al-Ulughkhani Hajji ad-Dabir, *Zafar ul Walih bi Muzaffar wa Alih: An Arabic History of Gujarat*, trans. M. F. Lokhandwala, 2 vols. (Baroda: University of Baroda Press, 1970–74), 1:333 (Arabic text, p. 417) and 1:377 (Arabic text, p. 470), where a Deccani Muslim named Hasan, a specialist in these arts, is called in.

inquiry into different religions. In what is meant to be a hostile account, the courtier Bada'uni tells us that Akbar in 1583 constructed buildings near Agra for feeding the poor, both Hindus and Muslims. Since many jogis flocked to the place, Abu al-Fazl's staff built them a separate temporary abode called Jogipura ("city of jogis"). Akbar discussed with them the effects of meditation, departing the body, alchemy, and magic (referring to the latter two practices by the rhyming Arabic terms *kimiya, simiya, rimiya*), and they in turn prognosticated long life for him. They recommended that he limit his indulgence in sex and consumption of meat. Bada'uni felt that they wielded a fatal influence over Akbar in this respect, and he further asserted that Akbar began to call his disciples *chelah* after the term used by jogis.[15] Abu al-Fazl has noticed in passing the necromantic art attributed to certain brahmins, similar to that described in Chapter VII of *The Pool of Nectar*, which permitted the summoning of disembodied spirits to animate corpses for purposes of predicting the future; a divination of this kind performed nine centuries previously was held to have foretold Akbar's conquest of Kashmir in 1586.[16] Bada'uni also drew attention to Akbar's apparent adoption of yogic mantras, possibly with purposes of control of planetary deities similar to what is described in *The Pool of Nectar*: "He began also, at midnight and early dawn, to mutter the spells, which Hindus taught him, for the purpose of subduing the sun to his wishes."[17] Abu al-Fazl himself in his survey of the empire, the *A'in-i Akbari* (*The Institutes of Akbar*), says nothing about contemporary jogis, though he gives a summary of Patañjali's classical text on yoga.[18]

Akbar's son Jahangir in his memoirs reported that, in 1607, he had been curious enough to seek out some jogis in their retreat at Ghorakh Hatari (variously spelled Gorkhatri or Ghorakhtari) near Peshawar, a site previously visited by his great-grandfather Babur in 1519; although

---

[15] `Abd al-Qadir ibn Muluk Shah Bada'uni, *Muntakhab ut-tawarikh*, trans. George S. A. Ranking, W. H. Lowe, and Wolseley Haig, 3 vols. (Calcutta: The Asiatic Society of Bengal, 1898–1925), 2:324–25; trans., 2:334–35.

[16] Abu al-Fazl `Allami, *The Akbar nama of Abu-l-Fazl: History of the Reign of Akbar including an Account of His Predecessors*, trans. Henry Beveridge (Delhi: Ess Ess Publications, 1977 [1902]), 1:507; trans., 1:772–73.

[17] *Ibid.*, 2:261; trans., 2:268.

[18] Abu al-Fazl `Allami, *The A'in-i Akbari*, trans. H. S. Jarrett, ed. Jadunath Sarkar, rev. 2nd ed. (1948; repr., New Delhi: Oriental Books Reprint Corporation, 1978), pp. 187–98.

Babur had not been much impressed with the place, illustrated copies of his memoirs depict his encounter with the jogis there.[19] Jahangir's visit was equally disappointing: "Such a person proved to be as rare as a phoenix or the philosopher's stone. All I saw was a herd of miserable ignoramuses, from seeing whom I got nothing but confusion of mind."[20] Jahangir also admitted having an unfriendly encounter with jogis. In 1613, shortly after visiting the Chishti shrine at Ajmer on pilgrimage, he stopped in Pushkar. Being in an iconoclastic mood, he had an idol of the boar avatar of Vishnu destroyed, and he then ran out of town a jogi whom he suspected of deceiving people.[21] In spite of this incident, it seems that Jahangir like his father was interested in maintaining contacts with leading jogis.[22] A collection of revenue documents at the jogi shrine at Jakhbar in the Indian Punjab details the official patronage of this establishment by Mughal emperors over a period extending from 1581 to 1741. Like a number of other non-Muslim religious centers, this jogi shrine received land revenue through grants sanctioned by the department of charitable trusts, and this was confirmed in particular by Akbar and Jahangir, who seem to have had a high personal regard for the jogi leaders. It is noteworthy that the emperor Awrangzib in 1661 addressed

---

[19] Zahiru'd-din Muhammad Babur Padshah Ghazi, *Babur-nama (Memoirs of Babur)*, trans. Annette Susannah Beveridge (New Delhi: Oriental Books Reprint Corporation, 1979 [1922]), p. 230, where the place is referred to as Gur-khattri; Saiyid Athar Abbas Rizvi, *A History of Sufism in India*, Vol. 1, *Early Sufism and its History in India to 1600 AD* (New Delhi: Munshiram Manoharlal Publishers Pvt. Ltd. 1975), plate facing p. 369, from the British Museum copy of *Babur-nama*. For the vocalization of the place name as Gorakh Hatari, based on Sikh sources, see Simon Digby, "Encounters with Jogis in Indian Sufi Hagiography" (Unpublished paper presented at the Seminar on Aspects of Religion in South Asia, University of London, January 1970), pp. 29–30. Briggs (*Gorakhnath*, p. 98) calls Gorkhatri a derivation from Gorakhsetra. Thackston (Zahiru'd-din Muhammad Babur Padshah Ghazi, *The Baburnama: Memoirs of Babur, Prince and Emperor*, trans. W. M. Thackston, Jr. [Washington, D.C.: Freer Gallery of Art, 1996], fol. 232b, p. 285) spells it Gurh Kattri. See also Husain, "Hindu Shrines and Practices," p. 142, n. 1.

[20] Jahangir, *The Jahangirnama: Memoirs of Jahangir, Emperor of India*, trans. W. M. Thackston, Jr. (Washington, D.C.: Freer Gallery of Art, 1999) p. 74; id., *The Tuzuk-i-Jahangiri or Memoirs of Jahangir*, trans. Alexander Rogers, ed. Henry Beveridge, 2 vols. (Lahore: Sang-e-Meel Publications, 1974 [1909]), I:102.

[21] Jahangir, *The Jahangirnama*, p. 153; id., *The Tuzuk-i-Jahangiri*, 1:254–55.

[22] For further incidents of Jahangir with yogis and ascetics, see the reports in Mobad Shah [Muhsin Fani, attr.], *Dabistan al-madhahib* (Bombay, 1262/1846), pp. 146 (Akamnath), 155 (Chatur Vapa), 162 (Sri Kant); id., *The Dabistán: or, School of Manners: The Religious Beliefs, Observances, Philosophic Opinions and Social Customs of the Nations of the East*, trans. David Shea (Washington: M. Walter Dunne, 1901), pp. 234, 247, 255.

a personal letter to the chief jogi at the shrine, requesting alchemical medicine.[23] There are indications as well that opportunistic jogis took advantage of the Mughal administrative system, if we are to believe the charge of the English traveler John Fryer; he maintained that "Fakiers" would extort donations from the "Gentiles" (Hindus) by threatening to accuse them of blaspheming against the Prophet in the qadi courts.[24] The hagiographical traditions of the Nath jogis also made much of their patronage by the Delhi sultans and Mughal emperors, viewing this relationship as both edifying and profitable.[25]

Geographical works written in Persian continued to mention jogis in passing as an unusual feature of India. Amin ibn Ahmad Razi, in his florid *Haft iqlim* (*The Seven Climes*), written in 1594, has cited from a lost earlier source an account of the wonders of India, including the always popular stories of self immolation as well as the breathing techniques of jogis.

Muhammad Yusuf Harawi, who was one of the competent people of his age, wrote a treatise on the wonders and rarities of the people of India. There he relates the following:

> I was in one of the districts of India and heard that a jogi had appeared who wanted to immolate himself in view of the king of that place. The king of that district passed three days in feasting and mirth, and on the fourth day at dawn, when the orb of the sun had arisen from the citadel of the orient and became fixed above the tablecloth of dust, a great crowd of the idolaters gathered. That jogi fled from impermanent existence and was suspended in imperishable nothingness, with the cloak of annihilation on his breast and the cap of renunciation on his head. He came before the king and performed the customs of reverence and the necessary salutations. Like a rosebud, his lip was sealed from speech, and in the manner of a narcissus, he kept his gaze directed at his feet as he stood. At his direction, attendants softened goat and cow manure and piled it around him until it came up to his head and shoulders. Then fire was struck on

---

[23] B. N. Goswamy and J. S. Grewal, *The Mughals and the Jogis of Jakhbar: Some Madad-i-Ma'ash and Other Documents* (Simla: Indian Institute of Advanced Study, 1967).

[24] John Fryer, *New Account of East India and Persia* (London, 1698), p. 95, cited by Schmidt, *Fakire und Fakirtum*, p. 164.

[25] Véronique Bouillier, *Ascètes et rois: Un monastère de Kanphata Yogis au Népal* (Paris : CNRS, 1997), pp. 68–75, 116–18; Briggs, *Gorakhnath*, pp. 70, 92, 94–95, 105, 144; David Gordon White, "The Wonders of Sri Mastnath," in *The Religions of India in Practice*, ed. Donald S. Lopez, Jr. (Princeton: Princeton University Press, 1995), pp. 399–411.

the left and right, and it began to catch fire until flames arose from all sides, and the moment became hot. At the moment when, candle-like, the flame reached to the throat of that burned one, he turned toward the king and spoke a few words. He bowed his head like a supplicant and laid his forehead on the very face of the flame, and closing his eyes, he expired. (Verse:)

> His hot-headed lover put a brick beneath his head;
>
> he burned so much that finally he put his head on ashes.

After searching for the parts of his body for an hour, they saw nothing there except an ashen residue. (Verse:)

> You are raw as long as a remnant of yourself is out of place;
>
> burn wholly like a candle, so you may become perfect.

Furthermore, in India there is a group of jogis who practice breath control. They carry their unremitting persistence to the point that they take but a single breath every few days, and they consider this skill the height of perfection and the greatest achievement. Among them was a jogi in Benares who had this quality, such that once Khan-i Zaman kept him buried underground for over ten days. Another time he had him spend nearly twelve days under water, like an anchor, but he experienced no harm or injury at all. Also in the region of Punjab there was a madman, freed from the trammels of the world, who had cast the wealth of the two worlds to one side, having neither connection to the world nor inclination to worldlings. (Verse:)

> From every eyelash a lily sprang up on his eye,
>
> sewing up his vision from the bad and good of time.

For his whole life, there is a piece of land where there is a crevice, and he has wedged his left breast, which is the treasury of the jewel of the heart, into that crevice. He has restrained his hand from taking food, and he has kept his eye veiled from slumber. [The said Muhammad Yusuf has written], I have seen that person, and I heard from the people who were close to him that it is twenty-two years that he has followed this regime. During this time he has not stirred foot or stretched out his hand, and for nourishment he has been satisfied with the smell of food. And God is the lord of assistance![26]

---

[26] Amín Ahmad Rází, *Haft Iqlím: The Geographical and Biographical Encyclopaedia*, ed. M. Ishaque, Bibliotheca Indica 287 (Calcutta: Royal Asiatic Society of Bengal, 1963), 2:509–11. This critical edition of the Persian text is considerably superior to the Tehran edition published in the 1950s.

Here the marvelous figure of the jogi burning himself alive, and performing superhuman acts of asceticism to rival the desert anchorites of early Christianity, is presented in terms derived from the highly refined esthetic of Persian poetry.

One account of yogic breath control techniques as used by Muslims found its way into a literary anthology, the *Mir'at al-khayal* (*Mirror of Imagination*) of Shir Khan Lodi, composed in 1690 in Bengal. In a digression attached to the notice of his teacher Nazim (d. 1657), Shir Khan described how the latter had become not only a poet but also a geomancer, skilled in the art of using the breath for divination. This skill, he observes, is unknown to the traditions of Greece, Iraq, and Khurasan, being instead derived from the jogis of India. His short treatise gives details on the solar and lunar breaths associated with the right and left nostrils, and how to employ them for success in battle, in combatting illness, and for predicting the future. Shir Khan attributes the origin of this science to the teachings of Mahadev (Śiva) to his consort Parvati, but he does not appear to be aware of a strong Bengali tradition in yoga, regarding instead the jogis of Kashmir as the most accomplished. He concludes by postulating (almost as an afterthought) that it may be that the jogis also derive their teaching from Adam, since that was acknowledged by them in the Arabic work known as *The Pool of Nectar*; that still preserves the Indian character of yoga because it is well known that Adam descended to heaven in Ceylon.[27] Shir Khan's oblique reference to *The Pool of Nectar* Int.3, substituting Adam for Abraham as the Islamic counterpart to a divine Indian teacher, may indicate an alternate version of the text (or possibly a slip of memory).

Another such traveler who reported on his journeys through India was Mahmud ibn Amir Wali Balkhi, who wrote a Persian narrative of a journey from Balkh to India and Ceylon and back, completed after seven

---

[27] Ch. Virolleaud, "Sur un épitomé de la science du souffle rédigé en person," *Journal Asiatique* 235 (1946–47): 113–21. The poet Nazim (d. 1068/1657), though originally from Herat, lived most of his life in Islamabad (Dhaka); he is not to be confused with his compatriot Nazim Harawi (d. 1082/1671), author of a popular *masnavi* on the theme of Yusuf and Zulaykha (C. A. Storey, *Persian Literature: a Bio-bibliographical Survey* [London: The Royal Asiatic Society, 1970], 1:823, n. 3). Shir Khan Lodi only studied briefly with Nazim in his youth.

years' travel in 1631.[28] Balkhi, who seems to have traveled for his own diversion, recounted visits to a number of important religious shrines in India, such as Raja Man Singh's temple at Mathura, the tomb of Mu`in al-Din Chishti at Ajmer, and the Konark and Jagannath temples in Orissa. At the beginning of his journey, near Peshawar, he made a side trip to the same hermitage of jogis also briefly visited by the Mughal emperors Babur and Jahangir, though his visit was similarly disappointing and uninformative. Referring to the jogis as "ascetics" (*murtad*) who practice breath control, Balkhi described their lofty stone and brick retreats as sustaining a thousand followers of the principal master. Somewhat disparagingly he noted that this "erring sect" holds the greatest sign of perfection to be the ability to hold the breath for an entire day; a jogi who could attain this feat was enthroned as master of the hermitage, while the previous master was imprisoned, so that "in a few days he certainly went to hell and became the prisoner of eternal torment." It was assumed that the spirit of the deceased master would soon take another and better body to suit its state of perfection. Balkhi observed that the kings and people of that region supported the jogis' establishment with revenue. He conversed with the new master "without any semblance of enmity or prejudice," though he also claimed to have refuted him theologically with proofs of the divine unity, utterly embarrassing the jogi. Balkhi reported another jogi with enormous moustaches whose practice of wearing heavy chains won him a large following. In this case as well, the jogis are primarily interesting to the traveler as curiosities to be viewed with some disdain.

A comparable description of jogis is found in the travel narrative of Mir `Abd al-Latif Khan Shushtari, a Persian merchant who first came to India in 1788, eventually finding employment in the British-run government of Bengal and later traveling widely in north India and the Deccan for health and family reasons. His Persian memoirs, completed in 1804, contain generally favorable comments on Indian culture. His skeptical reflections on jogis testify to the widespread tales that were current about

---

[28] Mahmud ibn Amir Wali Balkhi, *Bahr al-asrar fi manaqib al-akhyar*, ed. Riazul Islam (Karachi: Institute of Central and West Asian Studies, University of Karachi, 1980), pp. 4–6 of Persian text, pp. 31–32 of English introduction. Cf. Storey, *Persian Literature*, 1:375. This passage is translated in full by Husain, "Hindu Shrines and Practices," pp. 142–144; see also Foltz, "Two Seventeenth-century Central Asian Travellers."

their practices. In particular, he related stories about jogis committing suicide, either by casting themselves into a furious mountain stream in the Himalayas that is lined with swords and knives or by drenching themselves with oil and throwing themselves into bonfires.

> In general, historians exaggerate much in praise of the realm of India, its ascetics (*murtadin*), and so forth. . . . They say that the ascetics of India practice asceticism in this manner, where there is an extremely large and powerful river that springs from the mountains of Sind, in which one encounters much water, very rough, passing over rocks and peaks, the sight of which causes overpowering fear. Near the source of that is a place, behind the mountain that looms over the river, which they call "*kund*." "*Kund*" rhymes with "*tund*" [Persian for "rough"], and it means the source of a spring. From the mountain's peak to the water's edge is an expanse filled with great trees, from the top of the mountain to the bank of the water. On those trees and rocky outcroppings they have placed knives, swords, and cutting tools. In order to attain the reward of having their spirit incarnate again in the body of a king, men cast themselves into it so that on the way their limbs are cut to pieces and they are drowned in the water.
>
> Otherwise they burn themselves in a fire in this fashion, first asking permission of the emperor, kindling a great fire outside town, and proclaiming that such and such a person on a certain day to gain eternal reward will cast himself in the fire in a given place. And people gather at the door of his house and around it, and a great commotion occurs in the town. Coming out of his house, he dons splendid clothes and drenches his clothes and body in oil, sulphur, and red juniper gum. He puts a censer of iron or copper full of blazing flame on his bare head and casts a handful of herbs on one side of his head, and the people and his relatives inhale the sulphur and red juniper gum incense. Gradually, they form a group, singing and dancing. He eats betel with happiness and joy and goes through the streets and the market, and to every one of the spectators who formerly knew him, he gives as a portion a branch of those herbs and prays for him. They say that his prayer is given the power of being answered. In this state, he goes out of the town and casts himself into the fire. Some stand near the fire and cut their limbs off with a knife, throwing them in one by one. Some of them stand close to the fire and cut open their bellies and pull out the liver, cutting it to pieces and putting it in the fire. Then they themselves run into the fire, and if they roll out, the others throw them back.[29]

---

[29] Mir ʿAbd al-Latif Khan Shushtari, *Tuhfat al-ʿalam wa dhayl al-tuhfa*, ed. Samad Muwahhid (Tehran: Kitabkhanah-ʾi Tahuri, 1363/1984), pp. 349–51.

Both stories contain gruesome references to jogis cutting off their limbs, reflecting the initiatic symbolism of dismemberment that is characteristic of yogic scenarios such as the rope trick.[30]

Shushtari also told of yogic feats of breath retention, which in popular lore included jogis buried underground for centuries and then revived at a time specified on a copper plate. At this point he comments, "Although previous historians have all related this kind of story about the ascetics of India, and they are current on the lips of the people (I myself have heard much of this), still the sound intellect and firm mind utterly rejects the correctness and truth of this kind of story. . . . They are pure lies and falsehood."[31] Despite his rejection of the immortal jogis, Shushtari acknowledged that there are practitioners of breath control, particularly those he has seen in the Deccan, who have the power of levitation. When he interrogated one such jogi in Hyderabad about the reasons for his success, he was told that behind all the legends is the practice of retention of semen as a means to perfect breath control. The jogi recommended that Shushtari try practising breath control during sexual intercourse to prevent ejaculation, since loss of semen is the primary cause of aging. The jogi also claimed to have such control over breath as to be able to empty a cup of milk through vasicular suction. On reflection, Shushtari decided that breath control and retention of semen should be understood in terms of Greco-Arabic medical theory, "which I saw in the *Canon* of Ibn Sina or in another book that I do not remember." He further concluded that the yogic technique was no better than the sexual tricks of pleasure lovers, and he wished to insult his readers no further by dwelling on the matter.[32]

Being a prominent part of the Indian scene, jogis were regularly described in the official gazetteers of the Mughal empire as an accepted feature of Hindu society. One such official account of jogis was contained in Sujan Ray Bhandari's Persian *Khulasat al-tawarikh* (*The Essence of Histories*), completed in 1695–96. In addition to containing a comprehensive history of India and statistical descriptions of the Mughal empire's provinces, it provided accounts of the climate, customs, and inhabitants of India. A century later, the British in India found this text so useful

---

[30] Mircea Eliade, *Yoga; Immortality and Freedom*, trans. Willard R. Trask, 2nd ed., Bollingen Series 56 (Princeton, NJ: Princeton University Press, 1969), pp. 322–23, 336, 347.

[31] Shushtari, *Tuhfat al-`alam*, p. 449.

[32] Ibid., pp. 450–51.

that they commissioned the chief Hindustani instructor at Fort William in Calcutta, Shir `Ali Khan Afsus (d. 1809), to write an Urdu translation of it entitled *Arayish-i mahfil* (*The Adornment of the Assembly*). This became a standard text for officials of the East India Company studying Hindustani, and at least seven translations were made into English or French. The chapter on Indian *faqir*s describes Sannyasis, Jogis, Beragis, Nanak Panthis, Jatis Seoras, the four ashramas, and the four castes. The section on the jogis says that they...

> spend their time day and night in recalling their God to memory, and, by holding in their breath (*habs-i dam*) for a long time, live for hundreds of years; by reason of their strict austerities (*riyadat*, i.e., yoga), their earthly garment (i.e., their body) is so light, that they fly in the air and float on the water, and by the power of their actions, they can cause their souls to flee away whenever they please, assume whatever form they like, enter the body of another person, and tell all the news of the hidden world; from putting copper in ashes, they can turn it into gold, and by the power of their magic, fascinate the hearts of the whole world; they can make a sick man, on the point of death, well in one moment, and can instantaneously understand the hearts of other people, and their custom is to have no cares or acquaintances; it is true that "the jogi is no man's friend;" and although, in magic and sorcery, alchemy and chemistry, "Sannyasis" have great skill, still the art of the jogis in these matter is more widely famous.[33]

It is presumably from Persian and Urdu sources such as this that the Arabic word *faqir* ("poor man"), originally a term for a Muslim Sufi who has renounced the world, came to be current in English as "fakeer" to describe any ascetic, whether nominally considered Hindu or Muslim. By the seventeenth century, as this source indicates, the term *faqir* was commonly in use in India to describe jogis, and Europeans quickly picked up this usage.[34] The account just quoted adverts to the practices

---

[33] Shir `Ali Khan Afsus, *The Araish-i-mahfil; or, The Ornament of the Assembly*, trans. Henry Court, 2nd ed. (Calcutta: Baptist Mission, 1882), p. 39–40, slightly modified according to the Urdu text in Shir `Ali Khan Afsus, *Arayish-i mahfil*, ed. Kalb `Ali Khan Fa'iq, Urdu ka Klasiki Adab 31 (Lahore: Majlis Tarraqi Adab, 1963), p. 53. For the Persian original and the various translations, see Storey, *Persian Literature*, 1:454–58.

[34] Yule and Burnell, *Hobson-Jobson*, pp. 347b–48a, s.v. "fakeer"; William Crooke, *Things Indian, Being Discursive Notes on Various Subjects Connected with India* (London: J. Murray, 1906), pp. 199–204 (quoting Barbosa, Bernier, Fryer, and Colebrooke); Eliade, *Yoga*, pp. 423–25.

of breath control and yogic discipline, but it primarily shows the popular fascination with the miraculous powers and magic attributed to the jogis. Similar descriptions of jogis are found in other Mughal gazetteers, frequently in parallel with Sufi orders, as in the *Chahar gulshan* or *The Four Gardens* of Ray Chaturman (ca. 1759), which enumerates 12 pan-Islamic Sufi *silsila* orders, 14 Sufi *khanwada*s ("families") peculiar to India, and six *darshan*s or schools of Indian ascetics.[35]

The official gazetteers of the Mughal empire anticipated and probably provided a model for the later British colonial surveys that detailed different caste, craft, and religious groups in India. As I have discussed elsewhere, the British commissioned a number of Persian texts describing the religious sects and customs of India.[36] Another text from the early British period is the anonymous *Silsila-i jogiyan* or *The Order of Jogis* (commissioned in 1800), an illustrated survey of jogis written in Persian, containing tiny cartoon-like miniature paintings showing the different kinds of ascetic orders. English transliterations have been added in pencil as captions to the illustrations, and the text includes an appendix with revenue statistics concerning the population of Benares. It is divided into three sections: Vaisnava (with 16 orders), Śaiva (with 19) and "Shaktik" (i.e., Śakti, with five main orders each having further subdivisions, oddly including both Sants and Sikhs). The word *jogi* or yogi is used in the title of this work in a generic sense to designate any organized ascetic group in India. In a specific sense, *jogi* is also the term reserved for the Nath or Kanphata ("split-ear") jogis, here rightly included among the Śaiva orders:

The first person who was the originator of this path was Mahadeva [Siva], and after him Gorakhnath and Machhindirnath [Matsyendranath]; they established and made current the rules of yoga. The leaders of this sect were people who lived in ancient times with revelations and miracles, powerful ones who held the choices of life and death, old age and youth. They had the power to fly to heaven, to disappear from sight, and similar wonders and marvels. Those who may be found in our day practice the following external religious path: whenever a jogi takes a disciple, he cuts open the side of the disciple's ear and inserts a ring of whalebone (Hindi

---

[35] Ray Chaturman, *Chahar gulshan*, MS 542, H.L. 92, Khudabakhsh Library, Patna, fols. 127a–141.

[36] Ernst, "Muslim Studies."

kachkara) or crystal or something else of this type, because with this sign of splitting the ear (Arabic *shaqq al-udhn*), he can never again become worldly. They practice ordering of the heart, restraint of breath, and bodily discipline. Smearing their bodies with ash, they wear a hat, patchwork cloak, colorful clothes, and an iron bar (Hindi *sabbal*) on the neck. They spend their youth in servitude. Some are attendants of Bhairoñ [Bhairava, a form of Śiva] and Hanuman, and these do not refrain from consuming meat and wine; their retreats (*kharabatiyan*) are mostly devoted to immorality and debauchery.[37]

This too is a fairly superficial account, joining the founding mythology of the jogis to their wonder-working abilities and current rituals. The depiction of the colorful appearance and sensational reputation of the jogis is a fitting conclusion to the official attitude toward the "sect."

Both the historical and travel accounts illustrate the difficulties that the outsider would have in gaining access to yogic teaching. There is first of all a tremendous layer of colorful legend surrounding jogis, in which they are the heroes of magical tales of the "believe it or not" variety. Then there is the possibility that the individual jogi that one meets may very well be an impostor or at best partially informed about the tradition. Beyond that is the probability that a jogi would only tell bits and pieces to outsiders, calculating what would be of interest to them or explaining in a way that would be likely to fit the interlocutor's perspective. Finally, the Persian-educated outsider (later on, the English-educated outsider) cannot help interpreting the jogi's explanation in terms of an entirely different cosmological system deriving from non-Indian sources. Islamic theological biases played a certain role in the attitudes of Muslim travelers towards jogis, but the yogic practice itself tended to be interpreted as a freakish achievement to be wondered at or explained scientifically. Indo-Muslim exoticism of the Mughal period would find its natural continuation in the anthropological literature of the British colonial period. Somewhat surprisingly, the most knowledgeable Muslim observers of yoga tended to be the kings, not because they were particularly interested in esoteric spirituality, but because they found the occult powers of jogis to be useful adjuncts to their political ambitions.

---

[37] *Silsila-i jugiyan*, MS 2974 Ethé, India Office Library, London (McKenzie MS 3087), fols. 19a–20a. The Christian year 1800 is given on fol. 61a, and the revenue statistics are contained on fols. 60a–71a.

16

Fayzi's Illuminationist Interpretation of Vedanta

The *Shariq al-ma`rifa*

In the history of Indo-Persian culture, the Mughal era stands out as a time characterized by a remarkable number of inventive intellectuals who engaged with Indian thought through the medium of Persian. One of the outstanding representatives of this movement was Abu al-Fayz "Fayzi," later known as Fayyazi (1547–95), poet-laureate at the court of Akbar, who has been somewhat eclipsed historically by his more famous brother, Akbar's chief minister, Abu al-Fazl `Allami.[1] Fayzi was a trusted courtier, serving as a tutor to Akbar's three sons, working as a close adviser on religious affairs, and acting as ambassador to the kingdom of Khandesh in 1591.

Fayzi's literary accomplishments were considerable. In addition to an extensive collection of Persian odes and lyrics, he attempted to compose a quintet of romantic epics in the fashion of the poet Nizami, though he only completed two: *Markaz al-adwar* on moral and mystical ideas, and *Nal-Daman*, a romance based on characters from the *Mahabharata*.[2] Fayzi was also noted for composing two learned works in Arabic using

[1] Munibur Rahman, "Fayzi, Abu'l-Fayz," *Encyclopaedia Iranica*, http://www.iranica.com/newsite/articles/unicode/v9f5/v9f509.html (accessed 20 February 2010); Ziyaud-Din A. Desai, "Life and Works of Faidi," *Indo-Iranica* 16 (1963): 1–35.

[2] For a detailed study of the latter text of Fayzi, see Muzaffar Alam and Sanjay Subrahmanyam, "Love, Passion and Reason: The Poet Fayzi and his *Nal-Daman*," *Studies on Persianate Societies* 2 (2004): 42–80.

only undotted letters: a lengthy Qur'an commentary entitled *Sawati ̓ al-ilham* and an explanation of Prophetic sayings called *Mawarid al-kalim*. When challenged on the grounds of having produced a regrettable innovation (*bid ̓ a*) with these works, he ingeniously responded by quoting the Muslim profession of faith: "There is no god but God, and Muhammad is the Messenger of God" (*la ilaha illa allah, Muhammadun rasul allah*), a phrase that contains only undotted letters. In addition, Fayzi is responsible for a Persian translation of a Sanskrit work on mathematics, the *Lilavati*. He was, in short, a leading intellectual representative of the cosmopolitan tendencies of the Mughal Empire. Fayzi has described his eclectic propensities in a Persian ode of autobiographical character composed to relate the fortunes of his embassy to the Deccan.[3] This lengthy poem has been analyzed, along with his quatrains, in a recent German dissertation by Gerald Grobbel.[4]

A striking interpretation of the philosophical traditions of India is offered by a Persian treatise attributed to Fayzi, entitled *Shariq al-ma ̓ rifa* (*The Illuminator of Gnosis*). This text can be found in a couple of manuscripts, of which I have scrutinized one from the India Office collection, written in a hasty and careless version of the Persian cursive hand known as *nasta ̓ liq*.[5] Fortunately, there is also a much more legible lithograph edition, published in 1877 in a collection of four Indo-Persian texts.[6] This work, which has not to date been the subject of scholarly analysis, is the

---

[3] Shaykh Abu al-Fayz Fayzi, *Kulliyyat-i Fayzi* (*The Complete Works of Fayzi*), ed. A. D. Arshad (Lahore: Idara-i Tahqiqat-i Pakistan, Danishgah-i Punjab, 1967), 74 84. Fayzi has written another poem of self-description, beginning with the line, "Thank God that love of idols is my guide, and that I am in the Brahmin faith and idolatry" (ibid., 53–59).
[4] Gerald Grobbel, *Der Dichter Faidi und die Religion Akbars* (Berlin: Klaus Schwarz Verlag, 2001), 21–28.
[5] Hermann Ethé, *Catalogue of Persian Manuscripts in the Library of the India Office*, 2 vols. (1903–37; repr., London: India Office Library & Records, 1980), 1:1101, no. 1975. Another copy of *Shariq al-ma ̓ rifa*, also attributed to Fayzi, is listed in E. G. Browne, *Catalogue of the Persian Manuscripts in the Library of the University of Cambridge* (Cambridge: At the University Press, 1896), 94–96, no. 35 (Add. 778).
[6] *Majmu ̓ a-i rasa'il* (Lucknow, India: Newal Kishore, 1294/1877). This edition contains *Risala-i shariq al-ma ̓ rifa* (*The Treatise of the Illuminator of Gnosis*); *Risala-i atwar dar hall-i asrar* (*The Treatise of the Modes of Resolving Secrets*); *Risala-i Ram gita* (*The Treatise of the Song of Ram*); *Mathnawi-i Ray Chandar Bhan Barahman* (*The Couplets of Ray Chandar Bhan Barah-man*). Many thanks to University of Chicago's South Asia librarian, James Nye, for making this copy available. A reprint by the same publisher, dated 1303/1885, also exists.

basis of the following remarks on Fayzi's approach to Indian religious thought in this text. Fayzi exhibits here a stimulating example of a mystical and philosophical interpretation of two principal topics, the significance of Krishna in Indian religious thought and the importance of yoga as a spiritual path. Fayzi interprets these Indian traditions very much in terms of Sufism and a generalized form of Illuminationist (*ishraqi*) philosophy, in so doing naturalizing and familiarizing these "Hindu" themes along lines familiar to Muslim intellectuals; in this respect, he follows a number of other cosmopolitan Mughal thinkers who drew upon Illuminationist Neoplatonism to provide an overarching framework to understand Indian religious thought.[7] It is somewhat more difficult to locate the particular school of Vedanta upon which he draws, though it could be described as philosophical rather than devotional. But it would be an exaggeration to characterize Fayzi's approach either to Illuminationism or Vedanta as specialized philosophy; this work plays the part of the popularization.[8]

The *Shariq al-ma`rifa* is a text of medium length, 46 pages in the Lucknow lithograph and 28 folios in the India Office manuscript. It is divided into 12 sections, each of which is entitled a "flash" (*lam`a*), a term with a long history in Arabic and Persian Sufi texts such as the *Kitab al-luma`* (*Book of Glimmerings*) of Abu Nasr al-Sarraj (d. 988) and the *Lama`at* (*Divine Flashes*) of `Iraqi (d. 1289).[9] These 12 "flashes" are described in the preface as follows:

1. On the description of the greatness of Krishna Dev and the application of the practice of yoga.
2. On the explanation of the fact that all the lights of the world are darkness in relation to that illuminated one, which comprehends all lights.

[7] Carl W. Ernst, "Situating Sufism and Yoga," *Journal of the Royal Asiatic Society*, Series 3, 15, no. 1 (2005): 15–43.

[8] For an overview of Illuminationist philosophy, see Roxanne Marcotte, "Suhrawardi," *Stanford Encyclopedia of Philosophy* (2007), http://plato.stanford.edu/entries/suhrawardi/ (accessed 20 February 2010). But as Grobbel points out (*Der Dichter Faidi*, 68), it was light symbolism rather than a technical engagement with Illuminationism that was characteristic of the court of Akbar.

[9] Abu Nasr `Abdallah B. `Ali al-Sarraj al-Tusi, *The Kitab al-Luma` fi 'l-Tasawwuf*, ed. Reynold Alleyne Nicholson, E. J. W. Gibb Memorial Series 22 (1914; repr., London: Luzac & Company Ltd., 1963); Fakhruddin Iraqi, *Divine Flashes*, trans. William Chittick and Peter Wilson, *Classics of Western Spirituality* (Mahwah, NJ: Paulist Press, 1982).

3. On the explanation of the essence of the human form.
4. On the explanation of how the disciple becomes a wayfarer on the path of yoga.
5. On the gnosis of the Essence and the explanation of the substance of His attributes.
6. On the explanation of the wisdom of the gnosis of the Essence.
7. On the explanation of the description of the pure Essence, and the practice of yoga.
8. On the explanation of the composition of the human being, which is known as the microcosm.
9. On the explanation of how a seeker at first performs exercises observing the breath and can obtain knowledge of the internal substance.
10. On passing beyond desire for the things of origination, attachment, and action, and their result, so that perfect asceticism is attained.
11. On the explanation of the fact that everything impermanent is action, because its body is pure action, having come about from action, while the soul, which is the actor, is imperishable and eternal.
12. On the explanation of the fact that the worshiper of the true divinity finally reaches perfection and never suffers any diminution.

As a glance at the contents indicates, there is a fair amount of overlap and repetition in this text. In the remarks that follow, I explore Fayzi's method and approach in the interpretation of Indian philosophical and religious themes, concentrating primarily on the introduction and the first "flash" as examples.

The presentation of the text in its lithograph and manuscript versions has interesting variations. The manuscript begins with an epigraph containing the typical Islamic formula "in the name of God, the Merciful, the Compassionate" (*bismillah al-rahman al-rahim*), but it contains no opening praise of God or the Prophet. Conversely, the lithograph begins strikingly with a Sanskrit epigraph in Urdu script, *sat-chid-anand* (*sic*; "existence-consciousness-bliss"), which is then followed by a page and a half of praise of God and prayers for forgiveness for sin—though the name of the Prophet Muhammad is strikingly absent from both versions. Likewise, it is notable that the famous Lucknow publishing firm of Nawal Kishore highlights on the front and back inside covers its lengthy list of "books on the religion of the Hindus in Urdu" (*kutub-i madhhab-i hunud Urdu bhasha*). The ornate cover uses a vocabulary of Islamic mysticism to proclaim the contents of the anthology as follows: "Four gardens of the enduring spring of Sufism and wayfaring (*tasawwuf o suluk*), that is, a collection of four treatises translated from the *Vedanta-sara* (*badant-sar*), transmitted from Sanskrit to the Persian language." It then goes on to describe the treatise in question primarily as a translation directly from authoritative Sanskrit texts: "the Persian translation of the *Gita*, the *Jog-Bishist* [*Yoga-vasista*], the *Bhagavata*, and the *Vedanta*, a useful translation of the words of Sri Swami Vyasa-ji." Thus, the lithograph edition omits the name of Fayzi altogether, whether as author or translator, while the manuscript clearly gives the name of Fayzi Fayyazi in the colophon.[10] Whether or not the treatise may be securely attributed to Fayzi may still be an open question, since it is not claimed as such in his biographies, and indeed one could assume instead that the author of this work was a Hindu scholar trained in Persianate learning. Regardless, the ultimate authorship of the work may have been irrelevant for the publisher's placement of the text in an anthology of translations from Sanskrit. In this article, by way of convenience I provisionally accept the *Shariq al-maʿrifa* as a product of Fayzi's ingenious pen.

The introduction to the text makes a strong argument for the importance of Indian philosophy, by placing it into a direct and even superior relationship with Greek philosophy. This intricately written passage, with long clauses composed of rhyming prose, touches on themes of universality and cosmopolitanism characteristic of the Mughal imperial ideology as expounded by Abu al-Fazl and others.

> The explanation of the cause of the composition of this treatise is as follows.[11] Since this seeker of the gnosis of God, according to the aspiration centered in his consciousness, by the cherished positions of those from every religion who have realized truth by way of universal peace (P. *sulh-i kull*), having extended the glance of knowledge of universal and particular order, became occupied with the universal, which by certain knowledge is congenial to the reception of peace—in general, [he became occupied with] the explanation of the words inducing peace, based on truth, knowing reality, the gnosis without peer, and the complete unity,

---

[10] The copyist evidently meant to add the date, but the space after the phrase "with the date of" (*bi-tarikh*) is left blank.

[11] This sentence does not occur in the manuscript, which begins with the following sentence.

belonging to the confidant of secrets, and the elite of the elite, Swami Vyasa, who is beyond the description of everything said about him, and is outside and beyond everything that they write about him—just like the first sage, Plato, who attained fame throughout the realms and was renowned among the philosophers of the Arabs and the non-Arabs. Despite the different types of wisdom, he [Plato] was distinguished by the Illuminationist wisdom (P. *hikmat-i ishraqiyya*). He was in the service of discipleship to Tumtum the Indian, who was a philosopher of great stature. Plato in his writings described his [Tumtum's] perfections in a degree of such perfection; he was the master of his age, and this master of his was a student of the chain of the disciples of Swami Vyasa. His rank of greatness cannot be imagined, in terms of the rank that it would have. As soon as one hears it, such influence is exerted that the heart enters into the condition of the perception of the ecstatics.[12]

It is noteworthy that Fayzi places his search for wisdom in the context of "universal peace" (*sulh-i kull*), a formula often used to encode the ecumenic policies of Akbar with respect to non-Muslims.[13] Further, he establishes a genealogy of wisdom, which invokes Plato as well as his Muslim Neoplatonic successors known as the Illuminationists. Yet, in a move reminiscent of early European romantics like Georg Friedrich Creuzer, Fayzi makes the Greek philosophers into students of the ancient sages of India, in this instance linking them to Vyasa through the mysterious sage Tumtum the Indian, a well-known figure in the history of Arabic magical literature such as *Picatrix*.[14]

Fayzi then goes on to proclaim the central importance of Vyasa as the source of Indian wisdom, with respect to both the principal divine personalities and the primary sacred texts. He further explains that in writing this text he has provided the gist of all of this ancient Indian teaching (rather than direct translations, as the cover of the lithograph would have it) in a way that will be suitable for the spiritual goals of his readers.

---

[12] *Shariq*, 3 (citing the 1877 lithograph edition unless otherwise indicated). The source languages for terms in parentheses are indicated by the abbreviations A. (Arabic), H. (Hindi), and P. (Persian). All translations are mine unless otherwise indicated.

[13] Khaliq Ahmad Nizami, *Akbar and Religion* (Delhi: Idarah-i Adabiyat-i Delli, 1989), 19, 230

[14] Manfred Ullmann, *Die Natur und Geheimwissenschaften im Islam* (*The Natural and Occult Sciences in Islam*), Handbuch der Orientalistik, Section 1, Supplemental Volume 6, Part 2 (Leiden: E. J. Brill, 1972), 298–99, 381.

Swami Vyasa, in terms of the conversations he has had about the gnosis of reality in relation to the utmost elite manifestation of divine lordship and the knowledge of the internal secret of Krishna, Arjuna, Ramchandra, Vasista, Vishnu, and Brahma, in the books of the *Gita*, the *Yoga Vasista*, the *Bhagavata*, and the *Vedanta*, has expanded them, and has put them into the form of verses in the Sanskrit language. Among those, he [the author, i.e., Fayzi] has brought one out of a thousand, and a few from many, according to his own understanding, into black on white. For the luminous black point of the heart, when from excessive worldly preoccupations it reaches reduced comprehension and insight, and from the waywardness of heedlessness it reaches injustice, in meeting that exposition and illumination it becomes clear that the path to gnosis is not beyond reach. God Most High speaks to these seekers who are attuned to this action, and since the world-illuminating sun bestows light on the macrocosm, by the same principle of twelve "flashes," this epistle has been composed in twelve flashes, since it is the bestower of light on the microcosm, and it is known by the name of *The Illuminator of Gnosis* (p. 4).

Thus, Fayzi presents this treatise as a compendium of Indian philosophy, which will be of the utmost value to readers. It scarcely needs to be pointed out that the title makes a strong gesture toward Illuminationist (*ishraqi*) wisdom by its use of the agent noun from the same root, i.e., *shariq* or Illuminator.

As he opens the text, Fayzi begins the first section with praise of Krishna as the manifestation of divinity, with a direct allusion to a celebrated incident in the *Mahabharata*, in which Krishna punishes the arrogance of Sisupala (who has objected to the recognition of Krishna as the divine Narayana) by executing him with his discus or chakra. Since Fayzi is believed to have been involved with the revision of the first two books of the Persian translation of the *Mahabharata* sponsored by Akbar, the latter text may have been the initial source of his information on this particular incident.[15]

---

[15] *Mahabharat, buzurgtarin manzuma-i kuhna-i mawjud-i jahan* (*Mahabharata, The Largest Ancient Poem Found in the World*), Persian trans. from Sanskrit by Mir Ghiyath al-Din ʿAli Qazwini Naqib Khan et al., ed. Muhammad Rida Jalali Naʾini and Narayan Shankar Shukla, 4 vols., Hindshinasi 15–18 (Tehran: Kitabfurushi Tuhuri, 1358–59/1979–81), 1:240–45. This passage corresponds (with some abridgement) to *The Mahabharata*, trans. J. A. B. van Buitenen, Books 2 and 3 (Chicago: The University of Chicago Press, 1975), 96–106.

First Flash: On the greatness of Krishna the divine, and the performance of the practice of yoga, and the fact that Krishna the Divine was the essence of God. His definition, description, grace, and generosity cannot be described. His wrath and anger render lofty degrees into lowly states. Such was the case with Sisupala, the king of Chanderi, who was a complete master of might, power, majesty, and pomp, and most of the kings of the earth obeyed him. From extreme stupidity and ignorance, when he did not recognize the praiseworthy power and influence of that unique one of the age, he was continually insulting Krishna the divine, and he was casting the latter's goodness into evil. That day when the assembly of all the kingdoms on earth was held, and Krishna the divine was honored there, in the presence of all of them he made himself an insulter by his own insults. Because Krishna was [characterized by the hadith saying,] "anoint yourself with the qualities of God Most High, the most generous of the generous" (A. *takhallaqu bi-akhlaq allah akram al-mukarrimin*), as much as he shielded his eyes, he did not hold back from the most hateful of his qualities (pp. 4–5).

Krishna then cast the discus and beheaded Sisupala, but because the execution came at his divine hand, Sisupala achieved one of the superior types of salvation (Persian-Arabic *najat*), which "in the Indian language (*hindawi*) is called *sajuj*," a term that Fayzi glosses as "the joining of light to that which is lit" (P. *payvastan-i nur bi-munawwar*); this circumstance allowed Sisupala to "become effaced (A. *mahw*) by gazing on the pure light of Krishna." The term *sajuj* can be restored as Hindi *san-yuj*, or Sanskrit *sayujya*, which in classical Vedantic texts is indeed a type of impersonal liberation (*mukti*) consisting of union with the formless Brahman.[16] In the more devotional forms of Vedanta, as displayed for instance in the teachings of Chaitanya, *sajuj* is rejected as an erroneous deviation from the four types of union with the personal form of the deity.[17] Thus, Fayzi, by introducing the concept of *sayujya*, draws upon a more intellectual aspect of Indian religious thought, of the kind exemplified by Vaishnava philosophers such as Venkatanatha (1595–1671) and

---

[16] For the terms *san-yuj* / *sayujya*, see John T. Platts, *A Dictionary of Urdu, Classical Hindi, and English* (London: W. H. Allen & Co., 1884), 631, 689.

[17] *The "Caitanya Caritamrta" of Krsnadasa Kaviraja*, trans. Edward C. Dimock, Jr., ed. Tony K. Stewart, Harvard Oriental Series no. 56 (Cambridge, MA: Harvard University Press, 1999), pp. 178, 205, 421.

Nimbarka (fourteenth century).[18] This passage illustrates the complexity of Fayzi's approach. He applies theological formulas including an Arabic hadith, much cited by the Sufis, that denotes the process of taking on the qualities of God by meditative practice, and he joins that with a technical term for a Sanskritic formulation for the most abstract form of liberation, redefined with Illuminationist imagery.

Fayzi goes on to remark, drawing on a very typical Sufi vocabulary that the apparent wrath of Krishna is in reality compassion.

> Thus he is called "the most merciful of the merciful" (A. *akram al-mukar-rimin*), and in the Indian language he is named *patit-pavan adham-dharan*, or "the forgiver of the sins of the greatest sinners" (P. *bakhshanda-i gunah-i gunah-karan-i a`zam*), to such a degree that he knows that all of creation (A. *khalq*) is from him, and he knows that no one is separate from him, since no one is apart from him and all are attached to his reality (p. 5).[19]

Likewise, with regard to Sisupala, he observes that,

> Having torn that veil of duality and non-recognition of him, he [Krishna] brought him into the recognition of unity. When the drop fell into the ocean, duality departed and unity took its place. And Krishna Dev, whom they call in the Indian language "abounding in compassion" (H. *karuna-may*), in the same fashion, giving compassion for the pain of all who suffer, he gives peace for their suffering (p. 6).[20]

At this point, Fayzi halts to comment once again on the process of translation, which is fundamental to the entire project of this text:

> Having praised his qualities and recited his signs (Ar. *ayat*), which Swami Vyasa arranged on the thread of mystical poetry (P. *nazm-i suluk*), the translation of that was put into pure Persian by means of that content, since not everyone has command over the Sanskrit language. For once,

---

[18] Surendranath N. Dasgupta, *A History of Indian Philosophy* (Cambridge: At the University Press, 1969), 3:161 (regarding Venkatanatha, where the term *sayujya* is glossed as "same-ness of quality" with the deity), 3:442–43, n. 4 (Nimbarka).
[19] For the Hindi expressions *patit-pavan* ("purifying the guilty") and *adham-dharan* ("he who affords support to the lowest and most unworthy"), see Platts, *Dictionary*, 35, 224.
[20] For *karuna-may*, see ibid., 828.

those who know the language of Persian, which is common to the time, are not excluded and have a share (p. 6).

Fayzi's translation enterprise has a dramatic salvific aim that is enlarged by the process of rendering his topic from Sanskrit into Persian.

Enough has been seen of Fayzi's approach to translation to require a methodological digression on the problem of representing Sanskrit terms in Persian script. While this might seem like a minor technical problem, close examination of the examples cited already reveals a number of serious difficulties. In the many Persian texts that have been written on Indological topics, there is no consistent system of transliteration, and one finds multiple spellings of well-known words, particularly due to the lack of short vowels in the Persian script. In addition, there is the likelihood that Persianate writers were dealing with vernacularized forms and pronunciations, which they vaguely ascribed to "the Indian language" (Hindawi), at a time much prior to the distinct emergence of the modern languages of South Asia such as Hindi and Urdu. Moreover, there is a confusing inconsistency between several commonly used systems for the Roman transliteration of Perso-Arabic script (e.g., Library of Congress, *Encyclopaedia of Islam*, *International Journal of Middle East Studies*, etc.), depending especially on whether the written or spoken forms of the words take priority. Finally, the existence of a reasonably consistent Roman transliteration for Sanskrit runs into the problem that similar transliterations (underdots, for example) are used for entirely different purposes to represent letters of the Perso-Arabic script. Thus, it becomes a problem to decide which system to use to represent letters such as the Indic retroflex consonants. Because of the academic tendency to privilege "classical" Sanskritic forms over vernacular variations, one also has to consider whether it is preferable to demonstrate the spelling of a name or term in Persian script (e.g., Byas) or its more familiar Sanskrit form (Vyasa); frequently, it is simpler to use common forms (e.g., Krishna) without diacriticals, as has been done in this essay. Moreover, as will be seen shortly, it is often extraordinarily difficult to recognize which Indic term lies concealed in Persian script.

While this chaotic situation might be enough to drive Orientalists to despair, there are a number of resources that may be called upon to deepen scholarly access to Indo-Persian texts, beyond what is available in standard dictionaries. One of these is Albrecht Weber's 1887 critical edition, in Roman script, of a short Sanskrit-Persian dictionary composed by a certain Krishnadasa during the reign of Akbar.[21] Another is the 80-page Persian dictionary of Sanskrit terms appended by Tara Chand and S. A. H. Abidi to their critical edition of an important Persian translation of the *Yoga-vasista*.[22] Finally, there are several Sanskrit-Persian dictionaries compiled by the indefatigable Muhammad Reza Jalali-Na'ini.[23] It would be especially useful for future research on Indo-Persian texts if these compendia could serve as a baseline for an expanding collaborative lexicon of Persian and Sanskrit, which could be facilitated by the use of Internet-based software. Likewise, there is a serious need for a reliable and comprehensive inventory of Persian translations of Indic texts, as well as independent Persian writings on Indological subjects. I hope that interested scholars will begin to consider such projects as ways of advancing our knowledge of this significant but neglected area of cultural exchange.[24]

To resume consideration of the text at hand, I would like to go through the remaining portion of the first chapter in order to elucidate further the

---

[21] Albrecht Weber, *Über den Pârasîprakâça des Krishnadâsa* (*On the "Pârasîprakâça" of Krishnadâsa*) (Berlin: Königliche Akademie der Wissenschaften, 1887). Several other such Persian-Sanskrit dictionaries exist: "The *Parasiprakasa* of Viharikrsnadasa gives Persian equivalents of Sanskrit expressions. *Yavanaparipatianukrama* of Dalapatiraya gives Persian words together with Sanskrit equivalents. *Parasiprakasa* of Vedangaraya gives Persian and Arabic terms used in Indian astronomy and astrology and *Rajavyavaharakosa* of Raghunatha gives Persian and Arabic terms with Sanskrit equivalents." See H. L. N. Bharati, "Sanskrit Lexicography: Theory and Practice" (PhD diss., University of Mysore, 1991), chapter 2, 42, http://dspace.vidyanidhi.org.in:8080/dspace/handle/2009/1324 (accessed 20 February 2010). One of these has recently been published, *Rajavyavaharakosha of Raghunatha Pandit: Persian-Sanskrit phraseology* (Delhi: Vidyanidhi Prakashan, 2007).

[22] *Jog bishist/Yogavasistha*, Persian trans. from Sanskrit, ed. Tara Chand and Amir Hasan 'Abidi (Aligarh: Aligarh Muslim University, 1967), 261–340.

[23] Muhammad Reza Jalali Na'ini and Narayan Shanker Shukla, *Lugat-i sanskrit madhkur dar kitab ma lil-Hind-i 'Allama Biruni* (*The Sanskrit Vocabulary Used in the "Indica" of the Scholar, Biruni*) (Tehran: Chapkhana-i Khurrami, 1353/1975); Muhammad Reza Jalali Na'ini, *Farhang-i Sanskrit-Farsi* (Tehran: Pizhuhishgah-i 'Ulum-i Insani wa Mutala'at-i Farhangi, 1996).

[24] Since writing these lines, I have been delighted to learn that a team of scholars led by Fabrizio Speziale and Svevo Onofrio are proposing to establish a database of texts partly along these lines, entitled, "Perso-Indica: A Bibliographic Survey of Persian Works on Indian Learned Traditions," with sponsorship from IFRI (Institut Français de Recherche en Iran).

key terms and concepts that are of primary interest to Fayzi. The next topic to claim his attention is breath control:

> In arranging to lose heart and soul in the essence of God (P. *dhat-i haqq*), who is the beloved (P. *janan*), the spiritual wayfarer (Ar. *salik*) should realize that sight is provided for the eye, smell for the nose, hearing for the ear, speech for the tongue, and the perception of hot, cold, soft, and hard for the enjoyment of physical pleasure, by the exercise of holding the breath, which in the Indian language is called *adhatm* and *pranayam* (p. 6).

This fascination with breath control is well attested among Muslim writers conversant with the practices of yoga.[25] Yet, the Hindi terminology here is anomalous; although the second term, *pranayam,* is well known in yogic literature, the word *adhatm* looks like a version of *adhyatma* or "supreme self," with no obvious connection to breath control.

Nevertheless, our author continues exploring the topic of breath control and its luminous effects:

> Having brought together all one's perception and comprehension of the intelligible qualities (A. *ma`qulat*) of one's essence, one meditates (*muraqaba*) on oneself. That is, one engages in the consciousness of recognizing the breaths, which they call *atha pran* and *apan*. At the moment when this *apan* breath rises, and then goes down from the inhaling of *pran*, he becomes aware of where it comes from, and when it descends [he knows] where it goes. When he grasps the place of their entry and exit, that is the flash (*lam`a*) of the pure light, which they call comprehension and external knowledge (p. 6).

While the linkage of meditative technique and breathing is emphatic, again, the terminology is in part obscure. The terms *pran* and *apan* refer normally to inhalation and exhalation, and they are extensively used in yoga texts. The Hindi term which precedes them is unclear,[26] but the author is quite confident and even masterful in his use of Persian terminology.

---

[25] Ernst, "Situating Sufism and Yoga", Chapter in the present volume.
[26] *Atha* (with retroflex T).

Fayzi continues to explore meditative techniques in the passage that follows, and he considers equivalent the silent recitation of divine names, regardless of their origin:

> This [is] knowledge of the part, which is an expression of fancy (A. *wahm*). For as long as a person practices holding the breath and reciting the name of the essence (P. *dhikr-i ism-i dhat*), which in the Indian language they term "silent recitation" (*ajap*), and does not correct the lotus (*nilufar*) of his breast, which is open in quality, the heart of the matter will never be understood by the intellect, and he will be in a fancy of twisted understanding (p. 6).

By referring to "reciting the name of the essence (P. *dhikr-i ism-i dhat*)," Fayzi appears to be invoking the well-known Sufi practice of recitation of the name "Allah," but he equates it with the silent recitation (*ajap*, the negation of *jap* or recitation) of yoga and demands the correct ordering of the psychic faculty symbolized by the lotus flower, elsewhere correlated with the psychic centers known as cakras.

Fayzi endows these practices with theological and metaphysical properties that would be quite familiar to readers steeped in Islamicate literature. The following extended passage is a rich example of his hermeneutic:

> If by the aforementioned practice he becomes purified, to the contrary, he reaches the level of the universal intellect (P. `aql-i kull*) and universal knowledge, which comprehends God, the mighty and powerful (*haqq `azza wa jalla*). Fanciful knowledge is effaced in that. Afterward, while he meditates on the universal knowledge in himself, since this knowledge is a flash of the generous pure light, when he persists in this thought for a while, he realizes that what comprehends all (*muhit*) is the heart, and the manifestation (*zuhur*) of this knowledge comes from the heart. Knowledge is the clarity of the light of the heart. Thus by that clarity of the light of the heart, like a full moon, it is clear; he has a display of beauty by sixteen perfect rays (A. *shu`a`*) (pp. 6–7).[27]

---

[27] "Sixteen perfect rays" appears to refer to Hindi *kala,* the 16th-part of the moon's diameter, hence 16 rays as the equivalent of completeness.

Successive passages employ the full rhetorical resources of rhyming prose, which is a treasured tool in the tradition of Indo-Persian literature:

He beholds, and he faces this knowledge there. And by the light of the heart, by meditation in the heart, with complete forthrightness (*istiqamat-i tamam*) and unspeakable control (*istihkam-i la kalam*), he practices *pranayam* of concentration (*samadhi*), i.e., peace (*aram*). When he has passed some time in this concentration and never becomes restless, remaining in the state of stability and peace, he beholds in the heart the pure light of the soul, which is refined and incomparable; there is nothing that resembles it. He does this to such an extent that the heart becomes lost in that. When the heart is effaced, he remains one in the attribute of unity, and he realizes his soul by an attribute which is the special attribute of the Most Holy Essence (*sifat-i khass-i dhat-i aqdas*). He knows the existence of the attribute the soul of the essence as his own description, which is the beloved in the kernel of kernels (*lubb-i lubab*); it is Most Holy and most subtle, for it became that by all lights and encompassed all existing things, like the air, which in the Indian language they call *akas* (p. 7).

Now Fayzi has introduced another critical term of Yogi origin, *samadhi* or concentration, which he nevertheless links with the experience of divine light expressed through technical terms from the vocabulary of Islamic theology. Yet in the end, he adroitly reverts to the Indic term *akas* as a cosmic reference for the all-encompassing air.

As Fayzi proceeds to describe a theophany of divine qualities, he again postulates theological equivalences from Muslim and Hindu sources alongside psychological terms:

Possible beings all are from that attribute, for they come into existence from it and they are annihilated (*fani*) in it, and that everlasting eternal essence (*dhat-i baqi-i la yuzal*) is the absolute unity; it has no limit, end, beginning, or term. It is undoubted and without peer. This world fits into the attribute of the essence of God – glory be to Him (*dhat-i haqq subhanahu*), which in the Indian language they call *paramatman*. So that in the human heart the desire that comes from the heart, and again is lost in the heart, which in the Indian language they call purpose (H. *sankalp*) and indecision (H. *vikalp*), even so this varied world that appears so wide comes into manifestation from the attribute of the absolute essence, and it vanishes into it (pp. 7–8).

The main goal of Fayzi's exposition is to demonstrate the illumination of the soul through the meditative techniques just outlined. In a very Neoplatonic mode, he contrasts the degrees of light to such an extent that the lower realms of existence appear to be darkness in relation to the higher sources of light.

> This light of the soul, before that illuminated one, is darkness, but since the darkness of that illumined one is subtler, it is a life full of bliss, and the heart became the darkness of that life full of bliss. Although before this life full of bliss it resembles darkness, yet the flash of that light is full of manifestation, which is the locus of the manifestation of the whole world. That is, the spark of the attribute came to be in the absolute essence, which they call soul, and in the soul the spark of the heart came to be, and in the heart the spark of the body came to be. And this world, which is the appearance of body and form, is dark before the flash of the manifestation of the heart, and the heart is the darkness of the light of the soul. The soul, with the existence of the display (*tajalli*) that accompanies it, before the beloved, resembles darkness. To such an extent it is clear and obvious that darkness, before the light, has no existence at all, just as the darkness of the world has no existence in the flash of the heart. In the same way, the heart and the soul, and the soul in the beloved, have no existence or being. That is that same single pure, eternal essence, which comprehends all (p. 8).

While Fayzi's focus remains the experience of illumination, he concludes his survey of this process with an offhand summary of spiritual practice under the term "asceticism" (*riyadat*), the standard Persian-Arabic equivalent for yoga. All this is enhanced by standard theological language that would be acceptable within any Islamic context.

> Therefore, if the person effaces himself, by the practice of the aforementioned asceticism, in the transcendent essence of God, who is ever eternal, he will hasten from annihilation to eternity, passing beyond humanity, and is honored with divinity, by His generosity and grace (p. 8).

This concludes Fayzi's chapter on Krishna and yoga.

How may we understand Fayzi's method of interpreting his Indian sources in this text? It would be an exaggeration to say that Fayzi here has translated a particular Sanskrit text, nor does he pretend to do so.

The amount of data that is clearly Indic is relatively sparse—perhaps a dozen Hindi terms or phrases are introduced, generally with translations that qualify the subject in terms familiar to the vocabularies of Islamic theology, Sufism, and Illuminationist philosophy. Fayzi's enthusiasm for Krishna is certainly intense, and he is equally fascinated with the powerful effects of breath control and the techniques of meditation. But the bulk of this treatise is so thoroughly defined by the terms of Sufism and Illuminationism that it would be easy to quote whole paragraphs without suspecting the presence of any distinctively Indian topics or themes. The closing lines in particular display a typical Illuminationist argument, rigorously expressed in terms of emanation and the metaphysics of light, but infused with the flavor of Islamic devotion conveyed by pious formulas in Arabic.

These critical observations would doubtless leave Fayzi, if one may pardon the expression, unfazed. He has ingeniously announced the legitimacy of both Indian thought and its Illuminationist interpretation by revealing that Plato was a student of the sages of India. Nevertheless, the ecumenic strategy of this cosmopolitan intellectual succeeded on its own terms precisely to the degree that it subordinated Indian themes to his own enlightened Persianate tradition.

17

Being Careful with the Goddess

Yoginis in Persian and Arabic Texts

When the Italian traveler Pietro della Valle stopped at the western Indian city of Cambay in 1624, he took the opportunity to visit a temple outside of town which was the resort of many yogis. He was fascinated with their appearance and practices, and he continually sought them out during his tour of western and southern India. After describing them in detail in his memoirs, he added a long account of their practices:

They have spiritual Exercises after their way, and also some exercise of Learning, but (by what I gather from a Book of theirs translated into *Persian*, and intitl'd, *Damerdbigiaska*, and, as the Translator saith, a rare piece) both their exercises of wit and their Learning consist onely in Arts of Divination, Secrets of Herbs, and other natural things, and also in Magick and Inchantments, whereunto they are much addicted, and boast of doing great wonders. I include their spiritual exercises herein because, according to the aforesaid Book, they think that by the means of those exercises, Prayers, Fastings and the like superstitious things, they come to Revelations; which indeed are nothing else but correspondence with the Devil, who appears to and deludes them in sundry shapes, forewarning them sometimes of things to come. Yea sometimes they have carnal commerce with him, not believing, or at least not professing, that 'tis the Devil; but that there are certain Immortal, Spiritual, Invisible Women, to the number of forty [*sic*], known to them and distinguisht by various forms, names and operations, whom they reverence as Deities, and

adore in many places with strange worship. . . . And of the Sciences of the
Gioghi [jogi or yogi], and their spiritual exercises, especially of a curious
way, rather superstitious than natural, of Divining by the breathing of a
Man, wherein they have indeed many curious and subtle observations,
which I upon tryal have found true, if any would know more, I refer him
to the Book above mention'd, which I intend to carry with me for a Rarity
into *Italy*; and, if I shall find convenience, I shall one day gratifie the
Curious with a sight of it in a Translation.[1]

Della Valle's account of a Persian text on yoga, containing techniques
for summoning feminine deities, and for divination by observation of
breathing, is a striking curiosity. What Indian traditions of yoga does
this book represent? Under what circumstances would books have been
written in Persian on yogic techniques that include summoning female
spirits? How would a translator prepare a Persian-reading audience for
this kind of subject, and what kind of Islamicate categories would be
used to present material such as yoga and feminine deities?

Della Valle was fluent in Turkish, Arabic, and Persian, so his plan
to translate the work from Persian into his native Italian might have
yielded the first European study of an Islamic interpretation of yoga.
It is remarkable that, despite his theological criticism of the yogis, he
found their divination and breathing practices to be effective; in this
respect his ambivalence matches that of several Muslim students of
yoga. Unfortunately della Valle seems not to have fulfilled this translation project, for he only briefly discussed his collection of Oriental
manuscripts in correspondence with European savants.[2] The Persian text
just described was among the codices that he brought back with him to
Italy; in the list of his oriental manuscripts, donated to the Vatican in
1718 by della Valle's heir, Rinaldo de Bufalo, it was described as "a book
on magic, translated from the Indian into the Persian language."[3] This
work is still preserved in the Vatican library.[4]

---

[1] *The Travels of Pietro della Valle in India*, from the Old English Translation of 1664 by
G. Havers, ed. Edward Grey (London: Hakluyt Society, 1892), 1:106–8.
[2] C. Micocci, "Della Valle, Pietro," *Dizionario Biografico degli Itiliani* (Rome: Istituto
della Enciclopedia Italiana, 1989), 39:764–68.
[3] Ignazio Ciampi, *Della vita e delle opere de Pietro Della Valle il pellegrino* (Rome:
Tipografia Berbèra, 1880), p. 181, no. 52.
[4] Ettore Rossi, *Elenco dei manoscritti persiani della biblioteca Vaticana*, Studi e Testi 136
(Vatican City: Biblioteca Apostolica Vaticana, 1948), pp. 47–49.

What was the origin of della Valle's text? The title that he gave appears to be quite garbled.[5] Nevertheless, it is possible to reconstruct the title of this text, from comparison of the six occurrences of the title in the manuscript with the description of another copy preserved in Islamabad: the original name must have been *Kamaru Pancasika*, or *The Fifty Verses of Kamarupa*.[6] What is especially striking is that della Valle's copy appears to have been copied for his personal use in June 1622, two years **before** he arrived in India. This copy was made in the southern Persian city of Lar, where della Valle lingered for some months, engaging in scientific discussion and theological polemics with Persian Shi'i scholars.[7] In other words, this Persian treatise on yogic breathing and divination techniques was circulating independently in intellectual circles in Iran, from which della Valle learned of it and acquired a copy for himself. He was ready for the yogis before he arrived in India.

On the basis of content, it is more than tempting to connect this treatise to the yogic text most widely known in Islamicate circles, the *Amrtakunda* or *The Pool of Nectar*, a lost hatha yoga text known from an Arabic version which was twice translated into Persian, as well as into Ottoman Turkish and Urdu.[8] In fact, *The Fifty Verses of Kamarupa* was circulating independently in Iran, prior to the translation of *The Pool of*

---

[5] The title *Damerdbigiaska* given in the passage above is elsewhere transliterated as *Kamardinjaska*. The Italian edition of della Valle gives an alternate reading of the title as *Kamerdbigiaska*, "for thus the Persian copy has it, not being accurate in consonants or vowels" (*The Travels of Pietro della Valle*, 1:108, n. 2). The valiant effort of Lach and van Kley to see in della Valle's text a Jain treatise (*Damerdbigiaska* as a corruption of *Digambara*) is not convincing, though I am indebted to them for this reference to della Valle; see Donald F. Lach and Edwin J. van Kley, *Asia in the Making of Europe*, vol. 3, *A Century of Advance* (Chicago: University of Chicago Press, 1993), p. 658.

[6] Kamak Dev, *Kamar deni maka* [*sic*], MS 1957-1060/18-1, National Museum, Islamabad, containing six chapters, so cited by Munzawi, IV, 2178, title no. 3944, MS no. 11777. Kazuyo Sasaki, "Yogico-tantric Traditions in the Hawd al-Hayat," *Journal of the Japanese Association for South Asian* Studies 17 (2005), pp. 135–56. Sasaki's reading of this title is more convincing than my earlier suggestion, *Kamrubijaksa* or *The Kamarupa Seed Syllables*.

[7] See Rossi, *Elenco dei manoscritti persiani*, pp. 33–38, 44, 67–68, for della Valle's Persian texts on astronomy and religious disputation. These include (pp. 35–36) della Valle's own Persian translation of a Latin work on the astronomical theories of Tycho Brahe, composed by him in Goa in 1624.

[8] See my articles "The Islamization of Yoga in the *Amrtakunda* Translations," *Journal of the Royal Asiatic Society*, Series 3, 13, no. 2 (2003): 199–226; and "Situating Sufism and Yoga," *Journal of the Royal Asiatic Society*, Series 3, 15, no. 1 (2005): 15–43.

Nectar, since it was quoted in a fourteenth-century Persian encyclopedia (the *Nafa'is al-funun* of Amuli).[9] The practices described in della Valle's book, particularly divination by breath control, and the 40-odd female deities (clearly an inaccurate recollection of the 64 Yoginis) overlap significantly in content with chapters II and IX of *The Pool of Nectar*. An examination of della Valle's Persian manuscript bears out some of these assumptions. The text in fact contains a description of 64 female magicians (not 40, as he recalled in his memoirs) corresponding to the cult of 64 yoginis; their leader is called Kamak Dev, in whom we can recognize Kamakhya (Sanskrit Kamaksa) Devi, the fierce Tantric goddess of Assam, who is mentioned by Muhammad Ghawth Gwaliyari as a source of yogic teaching in his Persian translation of *The Pool of Nectar*. Other similarities include frequent reference to the water of life (8b, 18b, 19a, 20b, 23a, 28a), the rituals of oblation (*homa*) and mantra recitation (*japa*) (37b, 38a, 41b), the use of mandalas (38a, 40b), visualization of diagrams associated with the cakras, the sun and moon breaths (10b), five kinds of breath associated with the elements (11a), and the summoning of the yoginis, some of whose names are the same as those found in *The Pool of Nectar*. The main difference is that *The Fifty Verses of Kamarupa* provides at least 10 times the number of examples, making it something like a large recipe-book for occultists.

An explicit link with *The Pool of Nectar* is suggested by a partial, though untitled, version of *The Fifty Verses of Kamarupa*, found in a single manuscript.[10] This copy contains only material on divination by breath, corresponding to Chapter 11 of the Arabic text of *The Pool of Nectar*, and it closely matches a section in della Valle's manuscript (11a–14a). It differs in being further subdivided into six sections: 1) incantations, 2) answering questioners, 3) predicting good outcomes, 4) the signs of death, 5) love and hate, and 6) breath and positions. The first line of the manuscript begins abruptly by stating, "This is a copy of *The Ocean of Life* from the Indian (*hindawi*) language, and it was put into Persian. In the Indian language they call it *Ahrat* [i.e., *Amrtakunda*]." This comment suggests that the editor of this version recognized that *The Fifty Verses of Kamarupa*

---

[9] References are provided in Ernst, "Islamization of Yoga."
[10] India Office, Ashburner 258, fols. 7a–10b. See E. Denison Ross and Edward G. Browne, *Catalogue of Two Collections of Persian and Arabic Manuscripts Preserved in the India Office Library* (London: Eyre and Spottiswode, 1902), p. 157.

was closely related to *The Ocean of Life*, which was the title of the Persian translation of *The Pool of Nectar* by Muhammad Ghawth. While it is not possible at this point to be any firmer about the historical relationship between the different Persian translations, it seems likely that *The Fifty Verses of Kamarupa* represents some of the same yogic and divination traditions that are found in *The Pool of Nectar*, but here they are presented with considerable elaboration.

We do not, however, know the origin of this *The Fifty Verses of Kamarupa*. The title suggests a focus on the seed syllables, the fundamental units of the mantra, which play such an important part in yogic and tantric traditions. The allusion to Kamarupa in the title solidifies its connection with the mythical origin of esoteric knowledge, nominally associated with the region of Assam. Little information is provided by the author, except a constant refrain on the book's great importance.

> Thus says the translator of the book: In India I saw many books with complete information about every science. Most of their books are in verse, because they memorize verse better, and one's nature inclines to it more. I found a book which they call *Kamaru Pancasika*, which is one of their choicest books; they have great faith in this. It contains two types of science. One is the science of magical imagination (*wahm*) and discipline (*riyadat*); they have no kind of science that is greater or more powerful than this. On the basis of this science they affirm things that intellect does not accept, but they believe in it, and among them it is customary. For each of these things they adduce and show a thousand proofs and demonstrations. Regarding the subject of this science, this is a summary, which they have affirmed.

> The other is a science that they call *s[v]aroda* [i.e., divination]. Their scholars and sages observe their breath; if their breath goes well, they perform their tasks, but if the breath goes ill, they do no work, but strenuously avoid it. They have taken this subject to the height of perfection. The common people of India know nothing of this, and they are not privy to this secret, nor do they know anything. They call this the science of [reading] thought (Arabic *damir*) (fols. 2a–2b).

As with *The Pool of Nectar*, here we are confronted with a powerful book, alleged to be of the highest authority in India, though in the same breath we are told that it is secret and known only to a few. The translator frequently returns to both the themes of the book's scriptural authority and its hidden esoteric character throughout the work. Thus in another passage he writes,

This book is known throughout India, and among the Hindus no book is nobler than this. Whoever learns this book and knows its explanation is counted as a great scholar and wise man. They serve him, and whoever is occupied with the theory and practice of this they call a jogi and respect him greatly. They serve him just like we respect the saints and the masters of struggle and discipline (15b).

The translator speaks of information gathered from Brahmin informants, regarding practices such as employing the "greatest name (Persian *ism-i a`zam*)" of God (40b) and summoning the goddess Lakshmi for sexual relations (43b), and he testifies to his own success in employing these techniques. In addition, on several occasions the translator cites another text, which he refers to as "the thirty-two verses of Kamak Dev," which may have been a separately circulating text with similar contents.[11]

The translator frequently emphasizes the verse character of the original, and several Hindi *doha* verses are quoted in Persian script (26b, 27a, 29a). He stresses the difficulty of the task of translation. "Then I rendered it from the Indian language to the Persian language, taking many pains, and it was read to a group of brahmins and scholars, and it was compared, corrected, and clarified (16a)." Despite this advertisement of scholarly authority, which makes suspicious use of the terminology of Arabic literary production, on other occasions the translator confesses that the material he is dealing with is more than obscure. After giving a lengthy Hindi passage in Arabic script, he remarks, "I presented these verses to a group of the scholars of India, brahmins, and jogis, and they could not explain it, but were incapable of understanding it, for the words are strange and difficult" (27a). Thus it is not clear to what extent *The Fifty Verses of Kamarupa* represents a single text or a selection from yogic verses available from oral sources but represented as scripture. The organization of the book is not entirely clear. The first part of the book is divided into four sections, on procedures for asking questions

---

[11] In one place (26a), the translator says, "Know that thirty-two verses in the Indian language have been transmitted from the sayings of Kamak. Now Kamak chose a certain kind from those, and added something else to it, and this poem is called *Kamak baray tajanka* (?)." Elsewhere he adds, "This is all a commentary on the thirty-two verses, which someone has written in the Indian language, in which many practices are mentioned, and in which are strange and wonderful sciences which all the practitioners of imagination (*wahm*) and magicians are agreed upon and pleased with" (29a). Once (15b), he says, "Now they put this book into 85 verses, and versified it in the Indian language."

(4a), on reading thoughts (5b), on detecting the signs of death (6b), and on love and hate (8b). Then comes what appears to be a major division or iteration, a heading that reads in large letters "The Book of Magical Imagination, from the Writings of the Sages of India" (14b). Only two other section headings follow: one on breath and magical imagination (16a), and another on the yogini cult (30b), which occupies nearly the last half of the book.

How does this text relate to Islamic themes? *The Pool of Nectar* postulates that famous Indian yogis are the equivalents for Elijah, Jonah, and Khidr. *The Fifty Verses of Kamarupa*, in contrast, merely records the Hindi mantras transmitted by these three Muslim prophets, adding one more from Abraham. This text does, however, provide a new equivalence: the Sanskrit seed mantra *hrim* (invariably represented in Arabic script as *rhin*) now becomes identified with the Arabic name of God *rahim*, "the merciful." This is an interesting esoteric variant on the common pun on the Hindu and Muslim names for God, Rama and Rahim. The minor spiritual beings called "digit of the moon" (*indu-rekha*) in Hindi are rendered by the Persian term for angel (*firishta*) (53b). The text demonstrates an unselfconscious domestication of yogic practices in an Islamicate society. Among the breath prognostications, for instance, one learns to approach "the *qadi* [Islamic judge] or the *amir* [prince]" for judgment or litigation only when the breath from the right nostril is favorable. Casual references mention Muslim magicians or practices that may be performed either in a Muslim or a Hindu graveyard (47b), or else in an empty temple or mosque (49b), and occasionally one is told to recite a Qur'anic passage such as the Throne Verse (Qur. 2:255) or to perform a certain action after the Muslim evening prayer. We even hear of a Muslim from Broach who successfully summoned a yogini and participated in the rites of her devotees (37a). The text is provided with an overall Islamic frame, through a standard invocation of God and praise of the Prophet at the beginning:

> Praise and adoration to that God who brought so many thousands of arts and wonders from the secrecy of non-existence into the courtyard of existence, and who adorned the sublime court with luminous bodies, who made the abodes of spiritual beings, and who commanded the manifestation of the sublunar world with varieties of plants and minerals, and who made the residence and resort of animals, and who chose from all the

animals humanity, creating it in the best of forms, giving the cry: "We have created humanity in the finest of stations" (Qur. 95:4), "so bless God, the finest of creators" (Qur. 23:14). Many blessings and countless salutations on the pure and holy essence of the leader of the world, the best of the children of Adam, the blessings of God and peace be upon him, and upon them all.

Likewise, at the end, a quotation of a hadith saying and some mystical allusions furnish a religious coloring for the magical practices (55a). These practices remain fundamentally ambiguous, however. "If one to whom this door is opened makes the claim, he will be a prophet; if he is good, he will be a saint; and if he is evil, he will be a magician" (55a). As a generalization I would like to observe that for the average Persian reader, the contents of *The Fifty Verses of Kamarupa* fell into the category of the occult sciences, and its Indic origin would have only enhanced its esoteric allure. The text employs standard Arabic terms for astral magic (*tanjim*), the summoning of spirits (*ihdar*) (30b, 37b), and the subjugation (*taskhir*) of demons, fairies, and magicians.[12] Thus, there would be a familiar quality about the text, even when these techniques are employed for summoning the spirits known in India as yoginis. The chants or mantras of the yogis are repeatedly referred to as spells (*afsun*), a term of magical significance. We also read of recognizably magical techniques, such as one using a nail made from bone (51a) that is employed nefariously with a voodoo-type doll (51b). Another recipe uses a comb made from the right paw of a mad dog killed with iron in rituals performed at a cremation ground (48b–49a).

The portrait of Indian wisdom or religion that emerges from the pages of this manuscript is eccentric. It rests, first of all, on the authority of Kamakhya, a goddess from Assam (Kamarupa) who is the stuff of legend. Here is an account of her:

> Kamak is a spiritual woman who is long-lived, and the Hindus call spiritual beings *dev*. This Kamak Dev is in the city of Kamru, in a cave which is in the middle of the mountains. Her followers go into that cave, and some of them see her. Every day they send much food from that city, and they

---

[12] Prior to the twelfth century, the terms *yogin* and *yogini* primarily designated sorcerers, according to David Gordon White, *Kiss of the Yogini. "Tantric Sex" in Its South Asian Contexts* (Chicago: The University of Chicago Press, 2003), p. 221.

leave it by the door of the cave and go back. Another time when they go, they see nothing [remaining]. They say that the servants of Kamak have taken it, and this is true. I have seen many people who have gone to that place, and heard them confirm this. This much explanation is sufficient, so that this science will not be deemed worthless and viewed with contempt, because this is a great science. Now I, the expert, am engaged in clarifying it, and I will explain this whole science (10a).

Elsewhere he describes this cave as only accessible to magicians, and he gives its dimensions as one *farsang* by one *farsang*. "When someone enters that cave, he goes in darkness until he reaches the end of that cave. He sees lamps and a clean, fragrant, beautiful place (15a)." Kamru is described as a faraway land, "in an island at the end of India and in the midst of the China Sea," and it is the source of many exotic items of trade. The cave of Kamakhya is said to have a stone nearby that emits a white fluid (34b–35a).[13] Kamakhya herself is cited as a source for various details of yogic practice. But the real point of her narrative is to get to the 64 yoginis.

The worship of the female deities known as yoginis seems to have been at its height in India from the ninth to the twelfth centuries, but it continued in various places until at least the eighteenth century.[14] Vidya Dehejia has described at length the open-air yogini temples found at remote sites where these deities were honored.[15] *The Fifty Verses of Kamarupa* describes the yoginis as the key to knowledge of all things. At the beginning of the section on breath, we are told,

> So say those sixty-four women, "By the command of God (who is great and majestic), who one day gave us this science, we shall not speak of this science. By the God by whose command the 18,000 worlds exist, this is an oath, that this is the science of magical imagination, for whatever is in the earth and heaven is in the grasp of the children of Adam. We tell everything, for everything that goes on in all the world is all known and clear by the science of magical imagination" (16a).

---

[13] In actuality, the shrine of Kamakhya in Assam is characterized by a red arsenic flow that is identified in tantric thought with the menstrual blood of the goddess; see David Gordon White, *The Alchemical Body: Siddha Traditions in Medieval India* (Chicago: The University of Chicago Press, 1996) pp. 195–96.

[14] White, *Kiss of the Yogini*, p. 8.

[15] Vidya Dehejia, *Yogini Cult and Temples: A Tantric Tradition* (New Delhi: National Museum, 1986).

Furthermore, they say,

> By the command of God most high, and the masterful teaching they have
> taught us, between the moon and the sun one can know whatever goes on
> in all the world. We teach a science of who comes, and from where, and
> what he asks. Also know that this science lengthens life and makes one
> near immortal (17a).

The knowledge the yoginis confer makes poison harmless, cures the
sick, removes desire, and enables one to control all persons and things
in the world. These "spiritual beings" (Persian *ruhaniyan*) are invulnerable to injury by sword or fire, their hair and nails cannot be cut, they
hear from a distance and travel anywhere in an instant (23b). Each of
the 64 yoginis has a particular spot in India, and they go to delightful
places to enjoy themselves at feasts, dressed in gold and jewels, wearing
crowns and wreaths, revered by the *dev*s; they will never die, grow old,
or get sick before the day of judgment, but all appear to be 20 years of
age (30b–31a). These beings are in fact the principal objects of worship
among the Hindus, who carve idols of them. "Just as we have prophets,
saints, and miracle workers, so the Hindus have faith in them" (31a).
Many of their names are given, though the Persian script leaves many
ambiguities: Tutla, Karkala, Tera, Tara, Chalab, Kamak, Kalika, Diba,
Darbu (31b), Antarakati (44b, 46b), Chitraki (56a), Ganga Mati (45a),
Sri Manohar (45a), Katiri (30a), Parvati (49b), Suramati (44b), Susandari
(44b), Talu (30a). Of course, as Vidya Dehejia has pointed out, no two
lists of names of yoginis are the same. The essential thing is the canonical number of the groupings of yoginis into 7, 8, 9, or 64.[16] Sometimes
adepts may have sexual relations with the yoginis (39a), at other times
they regard them as sister and mother (46b). "She is the yogini and you
are the yogi" (48a). Benefits of association with them include money
(44b) and food (48b).

As a comprehensive description of Indian religious practices, a
narrative limited to Kamakhya and the yoginis might seem a bit eccentric. Brahmins are mentioned, but only as occasional sources about *The
Fifty Verses of Kamarupa* and its interpretation. This is clearly a narrow
sample, but what is it based on? In terms of the categories that are available today, we could probably say that this text reflects practices of

---

[16] White, *Kiss of the Yogini*, p. 60.

the yogini temple cult that are associated with Kaula tantrism.[17] There is also some connection with the Nath or Kanphata yogis, as indeed Matsyendranath is usually considered the introducer of the yogini cult among the Kaulas and the name of Gorakhnath is invoked once (51a) in the text.[18] Beyond that general indication, we find multiple strands of Hindu tradition popping up in an incidental fashion. The text assumes a system of nine cakras (yogic subtle centers) rather than the seven cakras current in many Nath yoga writings (19b, 20a, 25a).[19] Meditative exercises are given that concentrate on raising the *shakti* from the navel up the spinal column (17b, 18a, 28a). A standard list of supernormal powers (*siddhis*) is provided (54a).[20] Occasional mantras appear to contain the phrase "Krishna avatar" (48b, 53a). We are told of the temple of Mahakala in Ujjain where many *siddhas* or magicians are said to live (24b, 37a). The story of Shiva (Mahadev) and the churning of the ocean is related at length (31b–32b). Nothing is said about the animal sacrifices associated with the Assamese shrine of Kamakhya today. The basic teachings of *The Fifty Verses of Kamarupa*, however, are use of breath for divination and the summoning of yoginis to obtain various goals; hatha yoga meditation is certainly linked to these practices.

From the point of view of the study of yoga, one of the most striking aspects of the text is the presence of numerous apparent representations of the Sanskrit alphabet, evidently made by a Persian copyist who attempted to draw these unfamiliar characters. Some of these are words and phrases that appear to be marginal notes incorporated into the main text, and by default they tend to resemble Arabic numerals in style. Others are Sanskrit letters intended for visualization, and these are painstakingly drawn in a large format. Instructions for visualization are as follows:

> One takes this letter in the middle, and you draw this other letter, which they call *shakti*, up from the navel with magical imagination and thought, and bring it up, in such as a way that this letter and the first letter are in the same place. Imagine them in the center of the head and gaze at them with the heart (16b).

---

[17] Dehejia, *Yogini Cult*, pp. 30, 36; White, *Kiss of the Yogini*, p. 22.
[18] Dehejia, *Yogini Cult*, pp. 74–75.
[19] It should be emphasized that there was no universal standard system of numbered cakras; see White, *Kiss of the Yogini*, p. 222.
[20] See Mircea Eliade, *Yoga; Immortality and Freedom*, trans. Willard R. Trask, 2nd ed., Bollingen Series 56 (Princeton, NJ: Princeton University Press, 1969), p. 88.

The copying of Indic script here stands in contrast with *The Pool of Nectar* tradition, in which Sanskrit mantras are only transliterated (with varying degrees of success) in Arabic script.

The Fifty Verses of Kamarupa is certainly rich in the use of Indian terminology, but one term in particular presents a riddle. This is the Arabic-Persian term *wahm*, usually rendered as "imagination," which I have here translated as "magical imagination." This term is also crucial in *The Pool of Nectar*, where "magical imagination" forms the main topic of Chapter VII. There it becomes a generic term for mental and magical powers.

> It is called belief, certainty, opinion, magical imagination, thought, fantasy, and fancy, as a single thing is named by various words. . . Answered prayer, the influence of charms, talismans, the [divine] names, enchantment, soothsaying, and sainthood, all are [activated] by magical imagination, and that is the work of the heart (VII.1).

Normal Islamic discourse gives *wahm* the pejorative meaning of "illusion" or "prejudice," and *wahm* also has various technical meanings in Aristotelian philosophy as the "estimative faculty" (Lat. *aestimatio*, Gk. *sunesis, phronesis*) and "compositive imagination" (Gk. *phantasia logistike*). But *wahm* in the sense of "magical imagination" seems to presuppose a correspondence with some unstated Indic term, possibly *bhavana, dharana*, or *kalpana*. It is defined in *The Fifty Verses of Kamarupa* as "the knowledge of breaths" (16a), and in the translator's introduction, magical imagination is also linked with the term "discipline" (*riyadat*), which is the standard Arabic-Persian translation for yoga.

As for the larger question of the religious significance of *The Fifty Verses of Kamarupa*, this remains ambiguous. The presence of Hindu goddesses in a text circulating in Muslim circles confounds one's expectations. Any acquaintance with the history of Islamic theology would lead one to conclude that spiritual practices involving goddesses would be anathema to Sufis whose religious loyalties lie with Islam. The celebrated incident of the so-called "Satanic verses," memorialized in the Salman Rushdie novel of the same name, refers to a reported incident where the Prophet Muhammad mistakenly allowed an invocation of the three principal goddesses of the Meccan pagans into the text of the Qur'an, although in the report this was later expunged. Regardless of the veracity of that account, it remains clear that multiple deities are not tolerable in any standard Islamic theology. Yet, the sophisticated Neoplatonism of the Muslim Illuminationists in Iran (comparable to that of, say, the Christian Platonist Marsilio Ficino in Renaissance Italy) permitted the translation and assimilation of "pagan" themes, deities, and practices, without a sense of radical difference.[21] The same process of translation evidently took place among Muslims in India as well, with practical considerations being uppermost. Knowledge of divination and access to the female spirits called *joginis* (yoginis) was considered useful by Muslim rulers on military expeditions in Gujarat in the late sixteenth century.[22] In fact, there was probably more interest and engagement with yoga and divination on the part of Muslim rulers than in any other sector of society, and in this respect, the cultivation of feminine spirits held a place alongside astrology and other occult arts that might prove useful on the political and military scene.[23]

It is extremely difficult to make a firm line to divide religious practice from magic. The translator of *The Fifty Verses of Kamarupa* drew freely upon Islamicate vocabularies related to magic, but for him there was no clear division between the status of the sorcerer and the saint. It is equally difficult to resolve the text into separate Hindu and Muslim elements. In this respect, it may be compared with a Devanagari text on omens that Simon Digby has discussed; in his view, the text circulated in Muslim circles in western India and was based on a Persian original, which was in turn derived from an earlier Jain work on omens. Based on the character of the omen predictions, Digby relates the text to

> a non-courtly environment in which men were worried about questions
> of cultivation and undertaking improvements, about entering into

---

[21] The Persian scholar Mulla Zayn al-Din of Lar, from whom Pietro della Valle obtained his manuscript of *The Kamarupa Seed Syllables* in 1622, belonged to a sect "which attributed intelligences to the sun, moon and stars, and venerated them as angels of a superior order who would intercede with God and seek his protection" (J. D. Gurney, "Pietro della Valle: The Limits of Perception," *Bulletin of the School of Asian and African Studies* 49 [1986], p. 113).

[22] al-Ulughkhani, *Zafar ul Walih*, trans. Lokhandwala, 1:333 (Arabic text, p. 417), and 1:377 (Arabic text, p. 470), where a Deccani Muslim named Hasan, a specialist in these arts, is called in.

[23] See my article, "Accounts of Yogis in Arabic and Persian Historical and Travel Texts," forthcoming in *Jerusalem Studies in Arabic and Islam*, vol. 32, Yohanon Friedmann Festschrift Volume (2007).

business partnerships and circumventing the wiles of their rivals, about the pursuing of legal claims and the outcome of journeys, about whether they should enter into marriages and whether their sons would grow up and turn out well.[24]

The Fifty Verses of Kamarupa has an equally complicated ancestry, but there is a certain overlap in terms of the kinds of concerns that it addresses. The translator of the text clearly had long experience with this ensemble of practices, which he regarded as being of great practical benefit. The divination practices by breath given here are just as terse and unpoetic as the omens in Digby's texts, e.g., "If someone comes and says, 'I'm going to war,' or 'I'm going on a journey,' if his breath goes [from] the left [nostril], tell him to go, it is good" (4a). These practically oriented questions relate to sickness, death, war, social status, and the perennial uncertainties of life, and the text also provides practical methods to influence people and events, particularly in the first sections of the work. The methods of concentration and visualization provided particularly in the second half of the text imperceptibly move beyond generic magic to link with highly specialized esoteric traditions related to the yogini cult and hatha yoga. In this respect, it could also be compared with the numerous handbooks of Arabic prayers compiled by Sufi masters and circulated among their disciples in seventeenth- and eighteenth-century India, which contained a similarly mixed array of objectives, ranging from the alleviation of illness to the attainment of advanced spiritual states. In both the yogic texts and the Sufi works, the mantric repetition of certain formulas a specific number of times is linked with the attainment of results. It would be worthwhile to translate some of these manuals, to bring out the range of practices and the particular sets of goals in different instances. In some cases, the large number of repetitions required of the practitioner indicates that one needed to make a serious commitment of long periods of time to perform these exercises. One might even suggest that this kind of meditative practice functioned for these readers much as computers and the Internet do for us today.

---

[24] Simon Digby, "Illustrated Muslim Books of Omens from Gujarat or Rajasthan," in *Indian Art and Connoisseurship: Essays in Honour of Douglas Barrett*, ed. John Guy (Middleton NJ: Indira Gandhi National Centre for the Arts and Mapin Publishing Pvt. Ltd., 1995), pp. 342–60.

The translator of *The Fifty Verses of Kamarupa* surrounded this presentation with repeated impressive announcements about the secrecy and the supreme authority of the text. He did not, however, find that the content of the text in any way prevented him from writing in the Islamic religious conventions that permeate Persian literature. Nor, we may suppose, did the text present any ideological problems to the Shi`i scholars in southern Persia who had *The Fifty Verses of Kamarupa* copied out for their Christian interlocutor Pietro della Valle. A text of this kind eludes the standard categories, perhaps because the religious concept that underlies it is practical and not concerned with doctrinal purity. The translator observed the parallelism between the function of "spiritual beings" such as the yoginis on the one hand and Sufi saints on the other. As his preface indicates, it is a larger natural theology that makes possible the science of yoga and "magical imagination" as a special revelation from God to the yoginis, for "whatever is in the earth and heaven is in the grasp of the children of Adam."

18

The Limits of Universalism in Islamic Thought

The Case of Indian Religions*

Every religious tradition is claimed by its followers in a range of identifications, from exclusivist—holding that we alone are correct and all others are condemned— to more pluralistic perspectives, recognizing some legitimacy and worth in other traditions, and even universalist positions, such as the notion that all humans are destined for salvation.[1] To what extent have Muslims regarded followers of other religions and faiths as to some extent acceptable? In this essay, I propose to gauge the extent to which certain Muslim writers (especially from the philosophical and Sufi traditions) were drawn to apply universalist understandings to the religions of India. The reason for this choice of Indian religions is simple. While classical Islamic theology, on the basis of Qur'anic texts, explicitly recognizes only Jews and Christians as "peoples of the book," the extension of this category of recognized religious groups to other traditions (such as Zoroastrians in Persia) was and is, in practice, a matter

---

* An earlier version of this essay was presented at the Levi Della Vida Conference on "Universality in Islamic Thought" at the University of California at Los Angeles, 10–13 May 2007. The article was completed while the author was in residence as visiting scholar at the Centre for Civilisational Dialogue, University of Malaya (Fall 2010). It was published in *The Muslim World* 101 (January 2011), pp. 1–19, and is reproduced here with their kind permission.

[1] See the articles "pluralisme" and "universalisme" in André Lalande, *Vocabulaire technique et critique de la philosophie* (Paris: Presses Universitaires de France, 1972).

of negotiation in local contexts, requiring the use of analogy with Jews and Christians or other forms of argumentation.[2] Pragmatically speaking, Muslim rulers in India had to face the fact that they were a minority in charge of a vast non-Muslim majority, and on the political level, they generally dealt with the situation realistically.[3] So what sort of conceptual accommodations were employed by Muslim thinkers commenting on the Indian religions?

In pursuing this inquiry, my aim is to employ an analysis of religion that takes account of difference without essentialism; I assume that we cannot make generalized and abstract assumptions about the nature of religions but should instead problematize the concept of religion by taking account of historical acts of interpretation, appropriation, and resistance.[4] Paradoxically, Muslim philosophers and mystics have been most ready to confer universalistic recognition on the Indian religions to the extent that Indian doctrines and practices could be assimilated to Islamic categories. They employed familiarizing techniques of translation and interpretation with standard Islamic taxonomies to assimilate Indian religions to norms of monotheism and prophecy, as well as more basic concepts of magic, although the issue of idolatry remained a stubborn problem. The examples here are illustrative rather than exhaustive, and they reveal a spectrum of approaches and conclusions indicative of the difficulty of this problem of interpretation.

AL-BIRUNI AND INDIAN RELIGION

The first Arab Muslim authors to describe religion in India never used a single term such as Hinduism; they referred instead to the multiple religions of India, usually numbered as 42, some of which were considered to be monotheistic and prophetic and hence compatible with Islam, while others

---

[2] Irene Schneider, "Pluralism: Legal and Ethical-Religious"; Gudrun Krämer, "Pluralism: Political," in *Encyclopedia of Islam and the Muslim World*, ed. Richard Martin (New York: Macmillan Reference USA, 2004), 2:533–36.

[3] While Indian Brahmins and others seem to have been assimilated to the category of *dhimmi* early after the Arab conquest of Sind, with a couple of exceptions (notably under the Mughal emperor Aurangzeb), there was hardly ever any systematic attempt by Muslim rulers to apply the *jizya* tax on non-Muslims to the Indian population; see Peter Hardy, "Djizya. In India," EI[2].

[4] Carl W. Ernst, "Situating Sufism and Yoga," *Journal of the Royal Asiatic Society*, Series 3, 15, no. 1 (2005): 15–43, Chapter 12 in this volume.

were not. Early Muslim authors had no clear picture of religion in India, and in fact, the term *Hindu* was initially a geographic and ethnic designation.[5] The concept of a unitary Indian religion (although without the word *Hindu*) seems first to have been proposed in the Arabic description of India by al-Biruni (d. 1048), who studied Sanskrit texts on science and religion while in the service of the Turkish conqueror Mahmud of Ghazna (d. 1030); curiously, al-Biruni's notion of Indian religion in the singular seems to have been forgotten until his great work on India was rediscovered by European Orientalists in the nineteenth century. Al-Biruni is of interest in this discussion, not because he extended a universalizing recognition to Indian religions as such, but because of his typical method of using categories of Islamic thought as templates for understanding the Indian data.

Al-Biruni translated a number of Sanskrit works into Arabic (including selections from Patañjali's *Yogasutras* and the *Bhagavad Gita*) in connection with his encyclopedic treatise on India.[6] Although authors of Arabic books on sects and heresies, such as al-Shahrastani (d. 1153), generally devoted a section or a few pages to the religions of India, no other Arabic writer followed in al-Biruni's footsteps as a specialist on Indian religion and philosophy.[7] Wilhelm Halbfass has attempted an assessment of al-Biruni's contribution, praising him for his fair and objective approach to India:

---

[5] Carl W. Ernst, *Eternal Garden: Mysticism, History, and Politics at a South Asian Sufi Center* (Albany: State University of New York Press, 1992), pp. 22–37.

[6] Eduard Sachau, trans., *Alberuni's India* (1888; repr., Delhi: S. Chand & Co., 1964); Hellmut Ritter, ed., "Al-Biruni's Übersetzung des Yoga-sutra des Patañjali," *Oriens* 9 (1956): 165–200; Bruce B. Lawrence, "The Use of Hindu Religious Texts in al-Biruni's *India* with Special Reference to Patanjali's Yoga-Sutras," in *The Scholar and the Saint: Studies in Commemoration of Abu'l Rayhan al-Biruni and Jalal al-Din al-Rumi*, ed. Peter J. Chelkowski (New York: New York University Press, 1975), pp. 29–48; Shlomo Pines and Tuvia Gelblum, "Al-Biruni's Arabic Version of Patañjali's *Yogasutra*: A Translation of his First Chapter and a Comparison with Related Sanskrit Texts," *Bulletin of the School of Oriental and African Studies* 29 (1966), pp. 302–25; id., "Al-Biruni's Arabic Version of Patañjali's *Yogasutra*: A Translation of the Second Chapter and a Comparison with Related Texts," *Bulletin of the School of Oriental and African Studies* 40 (1977), pp. 522–49; id., "Al-Biruni's Arabic Version of Patañjali's *Yogasutra*: A Translation of the Third Chapter and a Comparison with Related Texts," *Bulletin of the School of Oriental and African Studies* 46 (1983), pp. 258–304.

[7] Bruce B. Lawrence, *Shahrastani on the Indian Religions* (The Hague: Mouton, 1976); id., "al-Biruni and Islamic Mysticism," in *Al-Biruni Commemorative Volume*, ed. Hakim Mohammed Said (Karachi: Hamdard Academy, 1979), p. 372; id., "Biruni, Abu Rayhan. viii. Indology," *Encyclopaedia Iranica* (1990), 4:285–87.

A clear awareness of his *own* religious horizon as a particular context of thought led him to perceive the "otherness" of the Indian religious philosophical context and horizon with remarkable clarity . . . Unlike Megasthenes, Biruni did not "translate" the names of foreign deities, nor did he incorporate them into his own pantheon, and of course he did not possess the amorphous "openness" of syncretism and the search for "common denominators." That is why he could comprehend and appreciate the other, the foreign as such, thematizing and explicating in an essentially new manner the problems of intercultural understanding and the challenge of "objectivity" when shifting from one tradition to another, from one context to another.[8]

Halbfass's admiration for al-Biruni's scholarly achievement is certainly justified, but these remarks call for some qualification. First of all, as stated earlier, al-Biruni's perception of the "otherness" of Indian thought was not just hermeneutical clarity with regard to a pre-existing division; it was effectively the invention of the concept of a unitary Indian religion and philosophy. Furthermore, Halbfass's praise of al-Biruni's bold proclamation of "otherness" obscures the fact that he had to engage in a remarkably complex interpretation of his sources with many "Islamizing" touches. His translation of Patañjali's *Yogasutras* was based on a combination of the original text with a commentary that is still not identified, all rephrased by al-Biruni into a question-and-answer format. Like the translators of pre-Islamic Greek texts (e.g., Plotinus) into Arabic, al-Biruni rendered the Sanskrit "gods" (*deva*) with the Arabic terms for "angels" (*mala'ikah*) or "spiritual beings" (*ruhaniyyat*), surely a theological shift amounting to "translation." He was, moreover, convinced on a deep level that Sanskrit texts were saturated with recognizable philosophical doctrines of reincarnation and union with God, which required comparative treatment: "For this reason their [the Indians'] talk, when it is heard, has a flavour composed of the beliefs (`aqa'id) of the ancient Greeks, of the Christian sects, and of the Sufi leaders."[9] Consequently, al-Biruni made deliberate and selective use of terms derived from Greek philosophy, heresiography, and Sufism to render the Sanskrit technical terms of yoga. But al-Biruni's rationalistic approach to Indian religions

---

[8] Wilhelm Halbfass, *India and Europe: An Essay in Understanding* (Albany: State University of New York Press, 1988), pp. 26–27.

[9] Ritter, "Al-Biruni's Übersetzung," p. 167; Pines and Gelblum, "Arabic Version," pp. 309–10.

remained isolated and almost forgotten, while his Arabic version of Patañjali was described by at least one reader as incomprehensible.[10] There is some superficial reference to al-Biruni's work on India and the Patañjali translation in the Persian *Bayan al-adyan* or *The Explanation of Religions* of Abu al-Ma'ali, written in Ghazna in 1092.[11] It appears, however, that the principal readers of al-Biruni's work on India were interested mainly from a historical and administrative point of view; the world-historian and Mongol minister Rashid al-Din (d. 1318) drew extensively on al-Biruni's geographical information, while the Mughal wazir Abu al-Fazl 'Allami (d. 1602) apparently had al-Biruni's work in mind when he compiled a detailed but uncritical survey of Indian thought in his Persian gazetteer of Akbar's Indian empire.[12] Today, both al-Biruni's work on India and his translation of Patañjali exist in unique manuscripts, suggesting an extremely limited circulation. I would like to suggest that al-Biruni's concept of a unified Indian religion, as a polar opposite to Islam, lay forgotten until it was resurrected in a more radical form by European scholarship a century ago; the growth of the Muslim concept of Indian religions took place largely without reference to al-Biruni. Since Sachau's edition (1886) and translation (1888) of al-Biruni's work on India was undertaken at the suggestion of the board of the Oriental Translation Fund and was entirely subsidized by Her Majesty's India Office, it is tempting to locate this work's historical importance primarily within the larger political concerns of colonial Orientalism.[13] Al-Biruni's rationalistic and reifying approach to religion, which had practically

---

[10] Pines and Gelblum, "Arabic Version," p. 302, n. 1, quoting the incomprehension of Ibrahim ibn Muhammad al-Ghazanfar al-Tibrizi; Fathullah Mujtabai, "Al Biruni and India: The First Attempt to Understand,", in his *Aspects of Hindu Muslim Cultural Relations* (New Delhi: National Book Bureau, 1978), p. 51, n. 52, cites reactions to the Patañjali translation by Persian authors Abu al-Ma'ali in his *Bayan al-adyan*, and Mir Findiriski in his translation of the *Yoga Vasistha*.

[11] Abu al-Ma'ali Muhammad al-Husayni al-'Alawi, *Bayan al-adyan dar sharh-i adyan wa mazahib-i jahili wa islami*, ed. 'Abbas Iqbal Ashtiyani, Muhammad Taqi Danish Puzhuh, and Sayyid Muhammad Dabir Siyaqi (Tehran: 1376/1998), pp. 23–24, 98; H. Massé, trans., "L'Exposé des religions," *Revue de l'Histoire des Religions* 94 (1926) : 17–75; A. Christensen, "Remarques critiques sur le *Kitab bayani-l-adyan* d'Abu'l-Ma'ali," *Le Monde Oriental* 5–6 (1911–12): 205–16; Lawrence, *Shahrastani*, pp. 89–90.

[12] Halbfass, *India and Europe*, pp. 29–30 (Rashid al-Din), 32–33 (Abu al-Fazl); Abu 'l-Fazl 'Allami, *The A'in-i Akbari*, trans. H. S. Jarrett, ed. Jadunath Sarkar, 2nd ed. (1948; repr., New Delhi: Oriental Books Reprint Corporation, 1970), 3.vii in, 141 358

[13] Sachau, *Alberuni's India*, Preface, p. l.

no impact on medieval Islamic thought, is much more palatable to the modern taste, and this helps explain his popularity today.

ILLUMINATIONIST PHILOSOPHY AND MONOTHEISTIC INDIANS

One of the notable philosophical frameworks in the Islamic tradition for understanding religion was the Illuminationist (*ishraqi*) school associated with Shihab al-Din Suhrawardi, which is strongly engaged with Aristotelian, Avicennan, and Neoplatonic philosophy. While it has been frequently suggested that this philosophical school played a significant role among Muslim intellectuals in India, the details have not been well established.[14] The first important Illuminationist author to be widely known in India was Jalal al-Din Davani (d. 1502), a prominent Persian scholar from Shiraz, who was known for his writings on Illuminationism and the Sufi metaphysics of Ibn `Arabi.[15] Davani was also a chief minister to the Aq-Qoyunlu rulers Uzun Hasan and Ya`qub, and his political writings, particularly the *Jalalian Ethics*, were doubtless partly responsible for his fame in India.[16] A number of scattered indications attest to Davani's popularity in India during his own lifetime and in subsequent years, and since Davani and his school are not widely known, I will summarize the evidence here.[17] The Naqshbandi shaykh Khawand Mahmud reportedly studied with Davani before coming to

---

[14] For a recent survey, see Akbar Sobut, "Suhrawardi dar Hind," in *`Irfan, Islam, Iran, va Insan-i Mu`asir: Nikudasht-i Shaykh Shihab al-Din Suhrawardi*, ed. Shahram Pazouki (Tehran: Intisharat-i Haqiqat, 1385/2007), pp. 125–60.

[15] See Carl W. Ernst, "Controversy over Ibn `Arabi's *Fusus*: The Faith of Pharaoh," *Islamic Culture* 59 (1985): 259–66.

[16] The *Akhlaq-i Jalali* or *Jalalian Ethics* has been particularly popular in India, and it has been repeatedly lithographed there in modern times, though never printed in Iran. This text was one of the first Persian texts translated into English during the early colonial period, as *The Practical Philosophy of the Muhammadan People*, by W. T. Thompson (London, 1839); cf. my translation of chapter 5 of this Persian text, in *From the School of Illumination to Philosophical Mysticism*, vol. 4, *An Anthology of Philosophy in Persia*, ed. S. H. Nasr and Mehdi Aminrazavi (London: I. B. Tauris, 2012), 121–35.

[17] Copies of Davani's works preserved in Pakistan include an anthology copied in 1518 and another work copied in 1554 in Tatta (Sind). Cf. Muhammad Bashir Husayn, *Fihrist-i makhtutat-i Sherani*, 3 vols. (Lahore: Danishgah-i Panjab, 1969), 2:207, no. 1127; 2:209, no. 1138; 2:235, no. 1302; 2:266, no. 1475.

India to see Babur.[18] Davani dedicated a political treatise to Sultan Mahmud of Gujarat (r. 1458–1511).[19] One of Davani's foremost pupils, Abu al-Fazl Astarabadi, came to Gujarat and taught there.[20] Another Davani student, `Imad al-Din Tarimi, went to Gujarat where he taught rational sciences to Wajih al-Din `Alawi (1504–89), who later became an important Shattari Sufi master.[21] Davani was also invited to Sind by its ruler, Jam Nizam al-Din (d. 1508), and was evidently planning to go there himself just prior to his death. His disciples Shams al-Din and Mu`in al-Din went in his place and settled in the town of Thatta.[22] Another pupil, `Ala' al-Din Lari, acted as tutor to the emperor Akbar and to his courtier Khan-i Zaman.[23] But in terms of Illuminationism, the most important connection of Davani to India came even earlier through the able minister of the Bahmani kingdom, Mahmud Gawan (d. 1481), who corresponded with many eminent scholars of Iran and Central Asia, such as the Naqshbandi Sufis `Abd al-Rahman Jami and `Ubayd Allah Ahrar.[24] It was to Mahmud Gawan that Davani dedicated one of his

---

[18] Haydar Mirza, *Tarikh-i Rashidi*, in *Classical Writings of the Medieval Islamic World: Persian Histories of the Mongol Dynasties*, trans. Wheeler M. Thackston, Jr. (London: I. B. Tauris, 2012), 1:176 (fol. 217).

[19] Ahmad Munzavi, *Fihrist-i mushtarak nuskhh-ha-yi khatti-i Farsi-i Pakistan* (Islamabad : Markaz-i Tahqiqat-i Farsi-i Iran va Pakistan, 1983–), 4:2385.

[20] `Abdullah Muhammad ibn `Umar al-Makki al-Asafi, "Hajji Dabir" Ulughkhani, *Zafar al-walih bi-Muzaffar wa alih, An Arabic History of Gujarat*, ed. E. Denison Ross, 3 vols , Indian Texts Series (London: John Murray, for the Government of India, 1910–28), 1:337; trans. M. F. Lokhandwala, Gaekwad's Oriental Series 152, 157 (Baroda: Oriental Institute, 1970–74), 1:278.

[21] Wajih al-Din `Alawi, *al-Risala al-musamma bi-l-haqiqat al-Muhammadiyya*, ed. with Urdu trans. Muhammad Zubayr Ghulam Nabi Qurayshi (Ahmedabad: Sarkhej Rawda Committee, 1385/1966), introduction, pp. 9–10.

[22] U. M. Daudpota, "Sind and Multan," in *The Delhi Sultanat (A.D. 1206–1526)*, ed. Mohammed Habib and Khaliq Ahmad Nizami, vol. 5, *A Comprehensive History of India* (1970; repr., New Delhi: People's Publishing House, 1982), p. 1127, quoting *Tarikh-i Ma`sumi*, p. 75.

[23] `Abdu-'l-Qadir ibn-i-Mulukshah al-Badaoni, *Muntakhabu-'t-tawarikh*, trans. Wolseley Haig, Biblioteca Indica 97 (Calcutta: The Asiatic Society of Bengal, 1925), 3:329, n. 1.

[24] Nazir Ahmad, "Language and Literature--Persian," in *History of Medieval Deccan (1295–1724)*, ed. H. K. Sherwani and P. M. Joshi, 2 vols. (Hyderabad: The Government of Andhra Pradesh, 1973–74), 2:79.

chief works of Illuminationist philosophy, his Arabic commentary on Suhrawardi's *Temples of Light*, completed in 1468.[25]

There are further indications of the ongoing popularity of Illuminationism in the Mughal period, frequently in connection with the study of Indian thought. In the formulations of the chief minister Abu al-Fazl, Illuminationism had become one of the underpinnings of the political theory of the empire, so it is not surprising to see that literary works of an Illuminationist bent were composed at this time. As an example, Shahrazuri's thirteenth-century Arabic history of philosophy from the ancient Greeks up through Suhrawardi was translated into Persian and dedicated to Jahangir (then Prince Salim) in 1602.[26] Abu al-Fazl's brother Fayzi composed a treatise on Vedantic metaphysics entitled *The Illuminator of Gnosis (Shariq al-ma`rifa)*, and its vocabulary and style strongly suggests that Illuminationism furnished the base for this explanation of Indian philosophy.[27] And there is a strong Illuminationist underpinning to the Arabic version of the hatha yoga text known as *The Pool of Nectar*, which contains in its preface an Arabic translation of some key Persian texts by Suhrawardi.[28] While Persian and Indian students of philosophy continued to write commentaries on Suhrawardi's works, traces of interest in the Illuminationist philosophy among later

---

[25] Jalal al-Din Muhammad ibn Sa`d al-Din As`ad al-Siddiqi al-Davani, *Shawakil al-hur fi sharh hayakil al-nur*, ed. Muhammad `Abd al-Haqq and Muhammad Yusuf Kukan (Madras: Government Oriental Manuscripts Library, 1373/1953), Arabic introduction, p. xxvi; this edition is based on a manuscript in the Oriental Manuscripts Library in Madras that is contemporary with Davani. Cf. Shihâboddîn Yahyâ Sohravardî Shaykh al-Ishrâq, *L'Archange empourpré*, *Quinze traités et récits mystiques*, trans. Henry Corbin (Paris: Fayard, 1976), pp. 33–66, with extracts from the commentaries of Davani and Ghiyath al-Din Shirazi on pp. 67–73; and my translation of chapter 5 of this Persian text, in *From the School of Illumination to Philosophical Mysticism*, vol. 4, *An Anthology of Philosophy in Persia*, ed. S. H. Nasr and Mehdi Aminrazavi (London: I. B. Tauris, 2012), 121–35.

[26] Shams al-Din Muhammad ibn Mahmud Shahrazuri, *Nuzhat al-arwah va rawzat al-afrah: tarikh al-hukama*, Persian trans. Maqsud `Ali Tabrizi, ed. Muhammad Taqi Danishpazhuh et al. ([Tehran]: Shirkat-i Intisharat-i `Ilmi va Farhangi, 1987). The original Arabic text is Shams al-Din Muhammad ibn Mahmud al-Shahrazuri (d. 1288), *Nuzhat al-arwah wa rawdat al-afrah fi ta'rikh al-hukama' wal-falasifa*, ed. Khurshid Ahmad, 2 vols. (Hyderabad: Da'irat al-Ma`arif al-`Uthmaniyya, 1396/1976).

[27] Carl W. Ernst, "Fayzi's Illuminationist Interpretation of Vedanta: The *Shariq al-Ma`rifa*," *Comparative Studies of South Asia, Africa, and the Middle East* 30, no. 3(2010): 156–64, chapter 16 in this volume.

[28] Carl W. Ernst, "The Islamization of Yoga in the Amrtakunda Translations," *Journal of the Royal Asiatic Society*, Series 3, 13, no. 2 (2003):199–226, Chapter 10 in this volume.

Indian Sufi authors are rare. Yet, one Indian Sufi author, `Abd al-Nabi Shattari (active 1601–30), wrote a commentary on Suhrawardi's *Wisdom of Illumination*, though his interest in Suhrawardi was probably a result of his immersion in scholastic philosophy rather than a product of his Shattari Sufi training.[29]

Another Illuminationist author of the Mughal era, Muhammad Sharif [ibn] Nizam al-Din Ahmad ibn al-Harawi, made significant comments on Indian religions in his Persian translation and commentary on Suhrawardi's *Wisdom of Illumination* under the title *Anwariyya* or *The Luminous Treatise*.[30] Indian sources indicate that Muhammad Sharif was the son of the well-known Mughal courtier and historian Nizam al-Din Ahmad, author of the *Tabaqat-i Akbari* or *The Generations of Akbar*.[31] Muhammad Sharif comments on a number of aspects of Hindu religious thought and practice.[32] Like al-Biruni, he distinguishes between the ordinary Hindu worshipper and the philosopher. "The teaching of the philosophers of Persia is not in agreement with anything that contributes to idolatry, such as the teaching of the Qadariyya and the Sharafiyya [two Muslim sects accused of dualism] or the idolaters of India, contrary to the philosophers

---

[29] This commentary was entitled *Ruh al-arwah fi sharh al-hikmat al-ishraqiyya*. A list of nearly 50 writings by `Abd al-Nabi Shattari (mostly commentaries on Sufi classics, Shattari works, standard philosophical texts, and wujudi writings) is given by Munzavi, *Fihrist*, 2:999–1000, and also in `Abd al-Hayy ibn Fakhr al-Din al- Hasani, *Nuzhat al-khawatir wa bahjat al-masami` wa al-nawazir*, ed. Sharaf al-Din Ahmad, 2nd ed., 9 vols. (Hyderabad: Da'irat al-Ma`arif al-`Uthmaniyya), 5:269–70.

[30] Muhammad Sharif Nizam al-Din Ahmad ibn al-Hirawi, *Anwariyya*, ed. Hossein Ziai, Majmu`a-i Mutala`at-i Islami (Tehran· Markaz-i Irani-i Mutala`a-i Farhang-ha, 1358/1979–80).

[31] See C. A. Storey, *Persian Literature: A Bio-bibliographical Survey* (London: The Royal Asiatic Society, 1970), 1:433–35. Bada'oni (2:363) mentions Muhammad Sharif as having revised his father's history after the latter's death. This same author (or possibly a brother) under the name of Sayf Allah ibn Khwaja Nizam al-Din Ahmad Muqim-i Harawi produced several other works of a philosophical bent, including *Jawahar al-asrar* or *The Jewels of the Secrets*, as well as *Mir'at al-wahdat* or *The Mirror of Oneness*, completed in 1617 in Lahore. Both works were written in the form of questions and answers on difficult metaphysical questions. Cf. Munzavi, 2:951, no. 1611; 2:984, no. 1661. Another MS by the same author, also under the title *Mir'at al-wahdat* (collection of Bruce Lawrence, Duke University), has an extensive discussion of religious pluralism in terms of Sufism and *wahdat al-wujud* (pp. 244 ff.).

[32] Muhammad Sharif mentions unusual natural sites in India where perpetual fire and wind occur, which were the object of pilgrimage (*Anwariyya*, pp. 105–6), cosmological theories of the four ages and the god Brahma (pp. 68–69), and incidents from the life of Krishna taken from the *Mahabharata* (p. 212).

of India, who, like the philosophers of Persia, are unitarians rather than idolaters."[33] In this sense, Muhammad Sharif shared the elitist perspective of the Mughal prince Dara Shikuh, who disdained the ordinary believers among both the Hindus and the Muslims. Muhammad Sharif also comments on the Indian philosophers' view that perfected ascetics (*murtazan*) and scholars may become connected to the planetary spirits, in an apparent allusion to the yogic practices outlined in Chapter IX of *The Pool of Nectar*; these experiences he compares to the ascensions of Idris, Jesus, and Muhammad.[34] Muhammad Sharif makes additional comparisons between the Avicennan theory of multiple separate angelic intellects and the deities (*devata*) whose power the Indian sages recognized in natural phenomena; in both cases, he argues, there is a recognition of a single light or source for these separate manifestations. This insight, he remarked, has unfortunately given way over time to blind worship of bodies in the form of Indian idolatry.[35] This text furnishes an example of how the Illuminationist philosophy, with its basis in the Avicennan critique of religion, provided a means for recognizing the validity of certain aspects of Indian religious thought, although the concept of idolatry acted as a screen for excluding a large sector of Indian religious practices. The Illuminationist school was certainly Islamicate, but since it did not attempt to derive its teachings exclusively from Islamic sources, it was open to reading new teachings, such as those found in India, as part of the same body of material for philosophical analysis. Yet at the same time, Muhammad Sharif employs the standard categories of unitarian monotheism and philosophical angelology to conform Indian teachings to Islamic norms.

ECUMENIC EMPIRE: ABU AL-FAZL'S POLITICAL VIEW OF THE INDIAN EPIC

An oft-cited example of Muslim Indology is the study and translation into Persian of Sanskrit texts (particularly the epics) in an extensive program carried out under Mughal sponsorship; although this enterprise

---

[33] Ibid., p. 10.
[34] Ibid., p. 186.
[35] Ibid., pp. 34–35, where the editor's speculative emendation *advaita* should be restored to the original manuscript reading *devata*, "deity." There is no discussion of Advaita Vedanta in this text.

has often been characterized as religious in intent, I would argue that its primary significance is political. The context for the Mughal interest in Sanskrit lies in the imperial program devised by Akbar and followed in varying degrees by his successors. Although earlier writers on the Mughals have treated this interest primarily as an indication of liberal personal religious inclinations on the part of Akbar, this romantic conception should yield to a more realistic analysis of policy aspects in terms of the Mughal ecumenic empire.[36] It is anachronistic to read an Enlightenment virtue of "tolerance" into the religious politics of the Mughal era. The original precedent for Akbar's policies of patronage of multiple religions is probably best sought in the Mongol era, when the prudent insurance policy of the "pagan" Mongols gave generous treatment to Buddhists, Christians, Taoists, and Muslims. Akbar's family conceived of their regime as a continuation of the neo-Mongol empire of Timur (Tamerlane); like Timur, Akbar was furnished with a genealogy that included Chingiz Khan, but in his case, it was extended to include the Mongol sun-goddess Alanquwa. The symbolism of world-domination inherent in the Mongol political tradition was given an ingenious philosophical and mystical twist in the writings of Akbar's minister Abu al-Fazl, who interpreted Akbar's role in terms of the Neoplatonic metaphysics of Ishraqi Illuminationism and the Sufi doctrine of the Perfect Human. This metaphysical apparatus was invoked not merely for its own philosophical consistency, but essentially to undergird the authority of Akbar in an eclectic fashion.[37]

While coinage with Sanskrit formulas and patronage of different religious institutions (including "Hindu" ones) was a feature of most Indo-Muslim regimes, what distinguished the Mughals under Akbar was their attempt to refocus all religious enthusiasm of whatever

[36] See John F. Richards, *The Mughal Empire*, vol. 1.5, *The New Cambridge History of India* (Cambridge: Cambridge University Press, 1993), pp. 36–40, 44–47. For the general concept of ecumenic empire, see Eric Voegelin, *Order and History*, vol. 4, *The Ecumenic Age* (Baton Rouge: Louisiana State University Press, 1974).

[37] See the stimulating essay of Peter Hardy, "Abul Fazl's Portrait of the Perfect Padshah: A Political Philosophy for Mughal India—or a Personal Puff for a Pal?", in *Islam in India, Studies and Commentaries*, vol. 2, *Religion and Religious Education*, ed. Christian W. Troll (New Delhi: Vikas Publishing House Pvt Ltd, 1985), pp. 114–37.

background onto the person of the emperor.[38] Akbar's sponsorship of the translation of Sanskrit works was part of the overall literary phase of his reign, which included the regular reading aloud of works from the canon of Persian court literature, history, and Sufism. He assigned to the task a number of courtiers who were scholars of Persian but presumably ignorant of Sanskrit; they were assisted, however, by Sanskrit pandits so that, from a literary point of view, the translation process probably involved a considerable amount of oral explication in vernacular Hindi prior to the composition of the Persian "translation." Some translators, like Bada'uni, assisted in this project much against their own inclinations. The extent of the sustained translation enterprise can be judged from the numerous manuscript copies, some lavishly illustrated, and the repeated revisions and new translations (in both poetry and prose) of particularly valued texts.[39] In political terms, the inclusion and translation of Sanskrit works was designed to reduce intellectual provincialism and linguistic divisiveness within the empire.[40] Sanskrit and Hindi romances, such as the story of Nala and Damayanti, seem to have been integrated into a literary continuum along with Near Eastern fables like the story of Majnun and Layla or the tales of Amir Hamza. Abu al-Fazl appears to regard the epic *Mahabharata* and *Ramayana* primarily as histories of ancient India with biographical and philosophical overtones. This even holds true of Puranic extensions of the epic, such as the *Harivamsa*, which Abu al-Fazl describes only as a biography of Krishna. Akbar himself entitled the Persian translation of the *Mahabharata* as the *Razmnamah* or *The Book of War*, underlining its character as a martial epic.

---

[38] For coinage with Sanskrit and patronage of non-Muslim religious institutions, see *Eternal Garden*, pp. 47–53. See also Finbarr Barry Flood, *Objects of Translation: Material Culture and Medieval "Hindu-Muslim" Encounter* (Princeton: Princeton University Press, 2009). On Akbar as the center of all religions, see Harbans Mukhia, *Historians and Historiography During the Reign of Akbar* (New Delhi: Vikas Publishing House Pvt Ltd, 1976), p. 70.

[39] John Seyller, *Workshop and Patron in Mughal India: The Freer Ramayana and other Illustrated Manuscripts of `Abd al-Rahim* (Zurich: Artibus Asiae, 1999).

[40] Khaliq Ahmad Nizami, *Akbar & Religion* (Delhi: Idarah-i-Adabiyat-i Delli, 1989), pp. 180–81.

Abu al-Fazl's complicated vision of the purpose of the *Mahabharata* translation is worth examining in detail. On the one hand, he observes that the epic does contain remarkable philosophical and cosmological perspectives of great complexity. Abu al-Fazl notes that at least 13 different Indian schools of thought are mentioned in the text.[41] On the other hand, he points out that a quarter of its 100,000 verses are devoted to the martial epic of the war between the Kauravas and the Pandavas, making it a *vade mecum* for the conduct of war and battle, and much of the remainder is "advice, sermons, stories, and explanations of past romance and battle (*bazm o razm*)."[42] In one long passage in his introduction to the Persian translation of the Mahabharata, Abu al-Fazl recounts a series of justifications for the translation project, all couched as an expansion of his encomium to his patron Akbar, who is eulogized in the most hyperbolic of terms. Abu al-Fazl outlines five major objectives: reducing sectarian fighting among both Muslims and Hindus; eroding the authority of all religious specialists over the masses; deflating Hindu bigotry towards Muslims by revealing questionable Hindu doctrines; curing Muslim provincialism by exposing Muslims to cosmologies much vaster than official sacred history; and providing access to a major history of the past for the edification and guidance of rulers (the traditional ethical justification for history).[43]

Abu al-Fazl was interested in the philosophical and religious content of the epic, from the perspective of an enlightened intellectual whose cosmopolitan vision had moved him out of a strictly defined Islamic theological perspective. But I think it is fair to say that this intellectual project was thoroughly subordinated to the political aim of making Akbar's authority supreme over all possible rivals in India, including all religious authorities. The translation of the Sanskrit epics was not an academic enterprise comparable to the modern study of religion; it was instead part of an imperial effort to bring both Indic and Persianate culture into the service of Akbar.

---

[41] Abu al-Fazl, in Muhammad Riza Jalali Na'ini and Narayan Shankar Shukla, ed., *Mahabharat, buzurgtarin manzuma-i kukhna-yi mawjud-i jahan*, Persian trans. from Sanskrit by Mir Ghiyath al-Din `Ali Qazwini Naqib Khan et al., 4 vols., Hindshinasi 15–18, (Tehran: Kitabfurushi Tuhuri, 1358–59/1979–81), 1:xx.

[42] Ibid., 1:xl–xli.

[43] Ibid., 1:xviii–xx

PRAGMATIC APPROPRIATIONS OF
INDIAN RELIGIOUS PRACTICES

On a very different level, one can see pragmatic and even enthusiastic appropriations of aspects of Indian practices that were seen as practically beneficial and which could be assimilated to familiar categories. This strategy was applied to the meditative practices of the Nath jogis, known to Indologists as hatha yoga, which became very popular in some Sufi circles. One example of the Sufi adoption of these practices is a short Persian text on yoga and meditation that is pseudonymously attributed to the famous founder of the Indian Chishti Sufi order, Shaykh Mu`in al-Din Chishti (d. 1236). A number of different versions of this treatise are found in manuscripts held in different libraries, often with different titles, though there is a fair amount of overlap in the contents. The fictitious attribution to Mu`in al-Din Chishti is both an indication of the seriousness with which Indian Sufis approached the practices of yoga and a hermeneutic in itself.[44] In other words, these teachings were important enough that they should have been part of the teaching of the greatest Sufi master in the Chishti tradition. This attribution is paralleled by the phenomenon we see in the circulation of the most important Arabic work on hatha yoga, *The Pool of Nectar*, which in many manuscripts is attributed to the great Andalusian Sufi master Shaykh Muhyi al-Din Ibn `Arabi (d. 1240).[45] This form of fictitious attribution to Islamic authorities is paralleled by the repeated assertion of equivalence between the most famous Indian masters of yogic lore and esoteric prophets of Islam (Idris, Khidr, and Jonah) or the even more striking identification of the Indian gods Brahma and Vishnu with Abraham and Moses.

Chapter 3 of Mu`in al-Din's treatise has a composite structure, in which the metaphysical levels and archangels of Islamicate cosmology are linked to the breaths of yogic practice (3.1–6). In the "Treatise on the Nature of Yoga," these are accompanied by what are now unintelligible mantras; unfortunately, the inability of the Persian script to represent short vowels inevitably resulted in chaos whenever it was used for the transcription of Sanskritic phrases. Nevertheless, the text asserts that

---

[44] Carl W. Ernst, "Two Versions of a Persian Text on Yoga and Cosmology, Attributed to Shaykh Mu`in al-Din Chishti," *Elixir* 2 (2006), pp. 69–76, 124–5, Chapter 13 in this volume.

[45] See Ernst, "Islamization of Yoga", and Chapter 10 in this volume.

the realization of these levels is closely related to the supreme spiritual states associated with the Prophet Muhammad. Indeed, the text goes on to link these states with knowledge revealed during the ascension of Muhammad to heaven; moreover, it maintains that this knowledge was then conferred on Mu`in al-Din Chishti, either spontaneously by the Prophet Muhammad or (in a second version) through the agency of Mu`in al-Din's master, Shaykh `Uthman Harwani (3:7–8). In other words, the principal teachings of this yogic text are alleged to be the essential import of what the Prophet Muhammad received during his most sublime spiritual experience. At this point, Mu`in al-Din is warned not to transmit this esoteric teaching to just anybody, but the restrictions are generous enough to include all sincere followers of the Chishti order in later generations (3.9).

The strategy of appropriation demonstrated here is hardly tempered by any sense of difference, in its description of yogic practices as the fruit of the supreme spiritual experience in the history of Islam. Yet, in other ways, this text illustrates a failure to synthesize the sources whose alleged unity is its principal contention. This unintentional differentiation between Indic and Islamicate materials is evident in the first two chapters, which present separately and with no attempt at integration an account of yogic physiology and cosmology alongside a Qur'anic and Islamic account of the nature of the world; the only thing that links the two chapters is their emphasis on the equivalence of the microcosm and the macrocosm.[46]

On an even more basic level is the recognition of Indian practices under the highly flexible category of magic. A fourteenth-century Persian anonymous text on yoga called *The Kamarupa Seed Syllables* draws eclectically upon Islamic references to ease the favorable consideration of occult techniques that are valuable because of their practical results.[47] Here one finds that Hindi mantras are transmitted by the prophets Elijah, Jonah, Khidr, and Abraham. This text also identifies the Sanskrit seed mantra *hrim* (invariably represented in Arabic script as *rhin*) with the Arabic name of God *rahim*, "the merciful." This is an interesting esoteric

---

[46] Ernst, "Two Versions of a Persian Text", and Chapter 13 in this volume.
[47] Carl W. Ernst, "Being Careful with the Goddess: Yoginis in Persian and Arabic Texts," in *Performing Ecstasy: The Poetics and Politics of Religion in India*, ed. Pallabi Chakrabarty and Scott Kugle (Delhi: Manohar, 2009), pp. 189–203, and Chapter 17 in this volume.

variant on the common pun on the Hindu and Muslim names for God, Ram and Rahim. The minor spiritual beings called "digit of the moon" (*indu-rekha*) in Hindi are rendered by the Persian term for angel (*firishta*) (53b). The text demonstrates an unselfconscious domestication of yogic practices in an Islamicate society. Among the breath prognostications, for instance, one learns to approach "the *qadi* [Islamic judge] or the *amir* [prince]" for judgment or litigation only when the breath from the right nostril is favorable. Casual references mention Muslim magicians or practices that may be performed either in a Muslim or a Hindu grave-yard (47b), or else in an empty temple or mosque (49b), and occasionally one is told to recite a Qur'anic passage such as the Throne Verse (Qur. 2:255) or to perform a certain action after the Muslim evening prayer. We even hear of a Muslim from Broach who successfully summoned one of the female deities known as yoginis, participating in the rites of her devotees (37a). The text is provided with an overall Islamic frame, through a standard invocation of God and praise of the Prophet at the beginning. Likewise at the end, a quotation of a hadith saying and some mystical allusions furnish a religious coloring for the magical practices (55a). These practices remain fundamentally ambiguous, however. "If one to whom this door is opened makes the claim, he will be a prophet; if he is good, he will be a saint; and if he is evil, he will be a magician" (55a). For the average Persian reader, the contents of *The Kamarupa Seed Syllables* most likely fell into the category of the occult sciences, and its Indic origin would have only enhanced its esoteric allure. The text employs standard Arabic terms for astral magic (*tanjim*), the summoning of spirits (*ihdar*) (30b, 37b), and the subjugation (*taskhir*) of demons, fairies, and magicians.[48] The chants or mantras of the yogis are repeatedly referred to as spells (*afsun*), a term of magical significance. Thus, there would be a familiar quality about the text, even when these techniques are employed for summoning the female spirits known in India as yoginis.

A similar taxonomic approach is seen in the classification of the principal Arabic work on hatha yoga, *The Pool of Nectar*. Several of the

---

[48] Prior to the twelfth century, the terms *yogin* and *yogini* primarily designated sorcerers, according to David Gordon White, *Kiss of the Yogini: "Tantric Sex" in Its South Asian Contexts* (Chicago: The University of Chicago Press, 2003), p. 221.

manuscripts (mostly found in Istanbul) contain descriptions and glosses of the text that stress its character as a work of Indian magic, and bibliographers and catalogers have also classified the text under this category. Copies in Cairo have been variously catalogued under the headings of medicine or cabalism. The seventeenth-century Ottoman bibliographer Hajji Khalifa, listing the text anonymously, described it in terms of its contents as a work "on the science of magic according to the method of India."[49] The description of the book in terms of Indian magic was the natural result of the presence of this category in the Islamicate cultural world since early times. The eleventh-century Arabic magical compendium of Pseudo-Majriti, *Ghayat al-hakim* or *The Goal of the Sage*, which was translated into Latin under the title *Picatrix*, contains several standard descriptions of the magical arts of the Indians. *Picatrix* associated Indian magic with the sciences of letters and magical operations through conjuring. The author of *Picatrix* also treats control (*taskhir*) of planetary spirits as typical of Indian magic.[50] The Ottoman polymath Tashköprüzada (d. 1561) was adapting the text to this category when he said that Indian magic specializes in purifying the soul, and he cited *The Pool of Nectar* as an example.[51] Evidently it was under the attraction of this concept that one manuscript of the Arabic version of *The Pool of Nectar* (Q) was ascribed to Tumtum the Indian, a name also known to the author of *Picatrix*.[52] The same is true of the marginal note in another manuscript (F) connecting *The Pool of Nectar* to Tinkalusha "the Greek" (otherwise known as "the Babylonian," from Babylon near Memphis in Egypt); Tinkalusha was the Arabic version of Teukros, an Egyptian astrologer of the Hellenistic period. Works on talismans and cheiromancy attributed to

---

[49] Mustafa ibn 'Abd Allah al-shahir bi-Hajji Khalifa, *Kashf al-zunun 'an asami al-kutub wal-funun*, ed. Muhammad Sharaf al-Din Yaltqaya (Istanbul: Wikalat al-Ma'arif, 1362/1943), 2, col. 1649.

[50] Pseudo-Magriti, *"Picatrix": Das Ziel des Weisen*, ed. Hellmut Ritter, Studien der Bibliothek Warburg 12 (Leipzig: B. G. Teubner, 1933), pp. 80–83, 138; German trans. Hellmut Ritter and Martin Plessner, Studies of the Warburg Institute 27 (London: University of London, 1962), pp. 83–86, 145.

[51] Manfred Ullmann, *Die Natur- und Geheimwissenschaften im Islam,* Handbuch der Orientalistik I.VI.2 (Leiden: E. J. Brill, 1972), p. 361.

[52] Ibid., pp. 298–99, 381. The name Tumtum is also found in a cabalistic treatise bound with manuscripts C and D.

him mention also Tumtum and another Indian, Sharasim.[53] These fanciful names were manifestations of a kind of esoteric exoticism, in which India is interchangeable with other remote and mysterious locales.

The acceptance of a text on yogic techniques among Muslim readers also drew upon underlying similarities with pre-Islamic spiritual practices of theurgy and cabalistic letter-mysticism, which partook of some of the characteristics of magic. Philosophical doctrines, such as the emphasis on self-knowledge, were given a magical twist in the Greek magical papyri that described how to encounter and master one's inner daimon.[54] From the Chaldaean Oracles to the Neoplatonic meditations of Iamblichus and Proclus, ritual and contemplative practices were used to attain union with the divine. Proclus himself, in addition to writing commentaries on the works of Plato, composed hymns to the planets as the visible representatives of the divine unities, or henads.[55] Invocations of the planetary deities were also practised by the Hellenized pagans of the ancient Syrian city of Harran, who continued to flourish in Islamic times under the pretense of being the monotheistic Sabians of old, and these practices were preserved in Arabic works on magic such as *Picatrix*.[56] Hellenistic invocations to planetary deities were translated into Arabic as late as 1462, when a compendium of the Greek writings of the "pagan" philosopher Gemistos Pletho (including a version of the Chaldean Oracles) was rendered into Arabic at the court of the Ottoman sultan Mehmet the Conqueror.[57] The Persian philosopher Suhrawardi, whose allegories are connected with the frame-story of *The Pool of Nectar*, was following in the tradition of Proclus when he wrote a series of hymns to the planetary and celestial intelligences.[58] So, from this tradition, there existed an analogue in the Islamic world for the practice of summoning

---

[53] Ibid., pp. 279, 329.

[54] Hans Dieter Betz, "The Delphic Maxim 'Know Yourself' in the Greek Magical Papyri," *History of Religions* 21 (1981): 156–71.

[55] Proclus, Philosophi Platonici, *Opera Inedita*, ed. Victor Cousin (1864; repr., Frankfurt am Main: Minerva G.m.B.H., 1962), pp. 1315–23; Anne Sheppard, "Proclus' Attitude to Theurgy," *Classical Quarterly* 32 (1982): 212–24.

[56] David Pingree, "Some of the Sources of the *Ghayat al-hakim*," *Journal of the Warburg & Courtald Institutes* 43 (1980): 1–15.

[57] Jean Nicolet and Michel Tardieu, "Pletho Arabicus: Identification et contenu du manuscrit arabe d'Istanbul, Topkapi Serai, Ahmet II 1896," *Journal Asiatique* 268 (1980): 35–57.

[58] Sohravardi, *L'archange*, pp. 473–512.

planetary spirits with mantras, as recorded in *The Pool of Nectar*, as a kind of overlay on the technique of summoning yogini goddesses. In this way, the practices described in *The Pool of Nectar* join the many other secular magical practices of diverse origins that became Islamicized in Arabic versions.[59]

While the examples just given might seem eccentric, they nevertheless share the characteristic of providing a positive evaluation of exotic Indian religious techniques either by attributing them to an illustrious Islamic source or by more casually classifying them as the lower order of magical phenomena. In either case, the recognition of the other as valid is accomplished by redefining it in terms of the familiar.

THE LIMITS OF THE APPRECIATION OF IDOLATRY

Despite the status of idolatry as a condemned religious practice considered incompatible with monotheism and Islamic belief, many Muslim thinkers toyed with the symbolism of idolatry as a signifier for the transcendence of conventional norms. The topos of "true infidelity" goes back to the deliberately blasphemous Arabic lyrics composed by Umayyad aristocrats as they relaxed in Christian monasteries, where wine could always be obtained and pretty faces might be found. With minor shifts, the same kind of imagery could be applied to Zoroastrians (as with the Magians of Hafiz) or to Hindus. For Persian authors like Sa`di, the symbolism of infidel religions was interchangeable, as he showed in his picaresque account in his *Bustan* on the temple of Somnath, which mixes indiscriminately terminology from various religions. When treated as a mystical inversion of ordinary religion, "true infidelity" from the time of Hallaj onward became a powerful image for transgressing received ideas. Notable masters of this topos in Sufi literature included `Ayn al-Quzat Hamadani, and especially Mahmud Shabistari, whose *Gulshan-i Raz* contains extensive reflections on how idolatry may conceal the essence of monotheism.[60] According to Alessandro Bausani, the symbolism of mystical infidelity was one of the dominant characteristics of

[59] Johan Christoph Bürgel, *The Feather of Simurgh: The "Licit Magic" of the Arts in Medieval Islam*, Hagop Kevorkian Series on Near Eastern Art and Civilization (New York: New York University Press, 1988), pp. 27–52, esp. 37–43.

[60] Leonard Lewisohn, *Beyond Faith and Infidelity: The Sufi Poetry and Teachings of Mahmud Shabistari* (London: RoutledgeCurzon, 1995).

Persian poetry by the seventeenth century.[61] Yet, it was never the case that these raptures on transcending the norms of Islam coincided with cool-headed approval of the ordinary religions of non-Muslims. In terms of the rhetoric of "mystical infidelity," those common non-Muslims were considered counterfeit infidels.

Nevertheless, one can find in Arabic and Persian literature a tradition of positive aesthetic reception of non-Muslim cultures, even including the idolatrous paganism of pre-Islamic times. In the case of India, we are in possession of a number of travel accounts provided by Muslim authors. Their quasi-Orientalist descriptions of Indian religions often exhibit a "curious mixture of fear and admiration, and familiarity and loathing."[62] Sometimes the dedication and self-sacrifice of the widow immolated on her late husband's funeral pure (the ritual of *sati*) drew admiration and respect, as in Nau`i's Persian poem *Suz o Gudaz* (*Burning and Melting*). It was in this vein that Amin ibn Ahmad Razi, in his florid *Haft iqlim* (*The Seven Climes*), written in 1594, cited from a lost earlier source an account of the wonders of India, including the always popular stories of self-immolation as well as the breathing techniques of jogis.[63]

Here, the marvelous figure of the jogi, burning himself alive and performing superhuman acts of asceticism to rival the desert anchorites of early Christianity, is presented in terms derived from the highly refined esthetic of Persian poetry.

Although examples of such aesthetic admiration of Indian ascetics and other marvels could be multiplied, among Indian Muslims there were limits to such positive expressions when idolatry was involved. It may be that theoretical consideration of idolatry in Persia or Anatolia was not nearly as threatening as the question could be in a land (such as India) that was thriving with idolatry. The example I have in mind is the famous

---

[61] Alessandro Bausani, "Letteratura neopersiana," in A. Pagliaro and A. Bausani, *Storia della letteratura persiana* (Milan, 1960), pp. 242–47; id., "Ghazal. II. — In Persian Literature," EI².

[62] Muzaffar Alam and Sanjay Subrahmanyam, "Empiricism of the Heart: Close Encounters in an 18th-Century Indo-Persian Text," *Studies in History*, n.s., 15, no. 2 (1999): 261–291, quoting p. 291.

[63] Rází, *Haft Iqlím*, 2:509–11, quoted in full by Carl W. Ernst, "Accounts of Yogis in Arabic and Persian Historical and Travel Texts," *Jerusalem Studies in Arabic and Islam* 33 (2008): 409–426, chapter 15 in this volume.

story of Moses and the shepherd, memorably told by Jalal al-Din Rumi in his *Masnavi* (2:1750–1815). There, we see the shepherd addressing God in the most naïve and simple fashion, offering to sew God's shoes, comb his hair, and kill his lice, as well as massage his feet and sweep out his little room. Moses, the arch-monotheist, is enraged at this blasphemy and denounces the poor shepherd in a lengthy and devastating diatribe. But after he departs in triumph, leaving the shepherd crushed in repentance, Moses is addressed by God with a stern rebuke. The sincerity and intensity of the shepherd's worship is all that matters, Moses is told, and in present-ing this Rumi even makes an offhand reference to India as the byword for idolatry. God states to Moses,

> I have bestowed on every one a (special) way of acting: I have given to everyone a (peculiar) form of expression.... Among the Indians the idiom of India is praiseworthy; among the Sindis the idiom of Sind is praisewor-thy.... I look not at the tongue and the speech; I look at the inward (spirit) and the state (feeling).... The religion of Love is apart from all religions: for lovers, the (only) religion and creed is—God.[64]

Accordingly, Moses is forced to run after the shepherd to announce his forgiveness in the most liberal acceptance of religious diversity: "Do not seek any rules or method (of worship); say whatsoever your distressful heart desires. Your blasphemy is (the true) religion, and your religion is the light of the spirit: you are saved, and through you a whole (world) is in salvation."[65] It is noteworthy that in contemporary interpretations of Rumi as a figure who transcends all religion, this particular text has been frequently cited as a proof text, though translators have pushed the text a little farther toward universalism than is probably justified.[66]

A Chishti Sufi master in India was not willing to go so far. Shaykh Nasir al-Din Mahmud "Chiragh-i Dihli" (d. 1356) was one of the princi-pal leaders of this important South Asian Sufi tradition in northern India.

---

[64] Jalaluddin Rumi, *The Mathnawi*, trans. R. A. Nicholson (London: Luzac & Co. Ltd., 1977), 2:1753, 1757, 1759, 1770, with slight modifications.

[65] Ibid., 2:1784–85.

[66] Coleman Barks and John Moyne render the previously quoted verses as follows: "I was wrong. God has revealed to me / that there are no rules for worship. Say whatever / and however your Loving tells you. / Your sweet blasphemy is the truest devotion. / Through you a whole world is freed / I loose your tongue and don't worry what / comes out. It's all the Light of the Spirit." See *This Longing* (Boston: Shambhala, 2000).

Although he seems to have been familiar with the writings of Rumi (he is perhaps the first Indian Sufi known to quote from the poetry of Rumi), he tells a tale similar to the story of Moses and the shepherd, but in a quite different fashion. In his recorded conversations, known as *Khayr al-Majalis (The Best of Assemblies)*, Chiragh-i Dihli locates this story unambiguously in India, having the idolater address his idol in Hindi (although the example remains generic, without any identification of the deity). Yet, the lesson here is not that God approves of all forms of worship, but that God will accept repentance from idolatry even after many years of such blasphemous behavior.[67]

The divergence of Chiragh-i Dihli's story from Rumi's narrative reveals a quite different emphasis. The Indian Sufi is not interested in the sincerity and intensity of the idolater's worship, nor does he provide any excuse for it based on universalist notions. Instead, the theological issue of worshipping false idols is front and center, starkly contrasted with the true God known through prophecy as the Creator, and the Hindi language makes the Indian location of this idolatry unmistakable for the Indian Muslim listeners, who would have understood it perfectly in their mother tongue. Thus, the story of the idolater's renunciation of paganism and his forgiving acceptance by God is what brings the audience to tears, not the notion that God welcomes all forms of worship. This is an instance in which a strong theological resistance barred this Indian Sufi from extending universalist recognition to Indian religions.

CONCLUSION

In its most extreme form, universalism extends the recognition of religious validity not just to followers of other religions, but to every sinner, so that Ibn 'Arabi envisioned the salvation of Pharaoh himself; this is paralleled by the Christian philosopher Origen, whose doctrine of *apokatastasis* or restoration included the salvation even of Satan.[68] Short of that position, there were still a number of Muslim thinkers who proposed varying degrees of positive recognition of the merits of the religions of India, and I have not mentioned all of them here by any

---

[67] For the text of this story, see Chapter 2 in this volume.
[68] Ernst, "Controversy over Ibn 'Arabi's Fusus."

means. This they were able to do by employing the categories (such as Sufism, monotheism, political ethics, magic) that were the common currency of pre-modern Islamicate thought. By pointing to the limitations in their concepts of universalism I am perhaps taking advantage of an ambiguity in our notion of the universal, which is inevitably embedded in the language of some local context or tradition even as it strives for a comprehensive meaning. Nevertheless, these examples indicate that Muslim writers trying to conceptualize the beliefs and practices of Indian religions necessarily drew upon frameworks—political, philosophical, theological, or occult—that were well domesticated in their own culture. As Rumi put it, "Everyone became my friend from his own opinion."

19

A 14th-Century Persian Account of Breath Control and Meditation

While it is perhaps contrary to customary expectations, practices associated with hatha yoga were in fact known outside of India in Muslim intellectual circles. The most important example of this phenomenon, as we have seen in previous chapters, is the text known as the *Amritakunda* or *Pool of Nectar*, which circulated in Arabic, Persian, Ottoman Turkish, and Urdu versions from the seventeenth century onwards, in Persia, Turkey, and North Africa as well as in India. The Muslim readers of these texts understood them differently according to their presuppositions. Some were attracted by the occult and magical powers promised by the yogis, who in these texts are invariably called jogis in North Indian pronunciation. Others saw in these writings significant parallels to the philosophical and mystical traditions current in Persia, which were particularly associated with Sufism and Neoplatonism. As has been discussed in previous chapters, over time, accounts of yogic meditation practices were increasingly Islamized so that, eventually, it became difficult to recognize anything particularly Indian or foreign about them. Although descriptions of jogis are relatively common in Islamicate literature, the word "yoga" (*jog*) hardly ever occurs, but it appears to be regularly represented by the term for ascetic practice, Arabic *riyada* or Persian *riyazat*.

The text translated here is the earliest known description of yogic practices found in the writings of Muslim authors. It is a short passage found in a voluminous encyclopedia compiled in Persia by a noted Shiʿi scholar and physician, Shams al-Din Muhammad ibn Mahmud Amuli, who died in Shiraz in 1353. For decades he had taught in the academies established by the Il-Khan Mongol rulers of Iran. While half of this encyclopedia focuses on the Islamic religious sciences, half of it is concerned with the sciences of the ancients, which for all practical purposes included philosophy, science, and the arts. The passage translated below occurs in the section on natural sciences, which includes medicine, alchemy, interpretation of dreams, astronomy, occult sciences, veterinary science, and agriculture.

Amuli focuses on two elements associated with the yogic tradition: the control of breaths, and meditative practices associated with the cakras. The material that he briefly summarizes here is known to exist in longer versions, most notably the Persian text acquired by the Italian traveler Pietro della Valle in southern Persia in 1622, which bears the Hindi title *Kamaru Pancasika*, or *The Fifty Verses of Kamarupa*. As we have seen in earlier chapter, that work seems to have been composed by a Persian intellectual in India who became interested in yogic practices of breath control and the summoning of the female spirits known as yoginis. Amuli directly refers to that text, and he also repeats its emphasis on associating these teachings with the goddess Kamak (also known as Kāmākhyā). Breath control is said to be employed by jogis for prolonging life and for divination, and the breaths are divided into five types corresponding to the physical elements; numerous examples are provided to show how breath coming from the left or right nostril can predict the future or provide answers to questions. The notion of five breaths appears to be connected to the classic Indian division of breaths into *prāṇa*, *apāna*, *vyāna*, *samāna* and *udāna*, as outlined by Kenneth G. Zysk.[1] The use of breath for divination, particularly for predicting death, seems to reflect widespread Hindu and Buddhist tantric practices found in India and Tibet, as Michael Walter has shown.[2]

---

[1] Kenneth G. Zysk "The Science of Respiration and the Doctrine of the Bodily Winds in Ancient India," *Journal of the American Oriental Society* 113, no. 2 (1993): 198–213

[2] Michael Walter, "Cheating Death," in *Tantra in Practice*, ed. David Gordon White, Princeton Readings in Religions (Princeton: Princeton University Press, 2000), pp. 605–23.

The section on breaths is followed by a brief discussion of the "science of imagination (Arabic *wahm*)," which deals with the ascetic lifestyle and the cultivation of the "water of life" (Persian *ab-i hayat*) to overcome death; the latter is a deliberate parallel for the nectar (*amrta*) sought in yogic practices. This passage also includes a description of a method for predicting the time of death by concentrating on the afterimage of one's shadow, and it contains an account of nine psychic centers corresponding to the cakras of hatha yoga, each of which is associated here with a vivid image. Other texts, such as the *Amritakunda*, give more extensive and varied accounts of cakra meditations, and they also associate them with yogini goddesses, but they continue to employ the term "imagination" for the power that animates all of these extraordinary manifestations. The text concludes on a derisory note, dismissing the entire subject as a waste of time. Although at least one nineteenth-century Orientalist scholar (Alfred von Kramer) saw this passage as proof of the Indian origins of all the mystical practices of Muslim Sufis, in retrospect it appears instead to indicate a relative lack of comprehension of the technical and theoretical aspects of yoga.

THE SCIENCE OF BREATH AND
THE SCIENCE OF IMAGINATION[3]

The former is an expression for the knowledge of the breaths and the proofs thereof. The latter is [an expression for] the knowledge of the summoning of imaginations and managing ascetic practice in that. These two sciences are famous among the Indians, and any one who attains perfection in these two they call a jogi; they consider him among the company of spiritual beings. They say that Kamak Dev has established both sciences.

They call spiritual beings (*ruhaniyan*) "*dev*," and they say that Kamak is still living, abiding in the town of Kamru in a cave. To satisfy their needs, they go to the door of that cave, and some claim that they see her. Every day the emperor of that realm sends pure foods and fresh drinks there, which they place at the door of the cave, where they immediately

---

[3] The Persian-language source from which this translation is taken Shams al-Din Muhammad ibn Mahmud Amuli, *Nafa'is al-funun fi `ara'is al-`uyun*, ed. Mirza Abu al-Hasan Sha`rani (Tehran: Kitabfurusi-i Islamiya, 1379/1960), 3:360-5, collated with a seventeenth-century manuscript in the collection of Dr. Taufiq Sobhani (Tehran).

disappear. Many people have witnessed this affair. The explanation of both sciences is exhaustively discussed in the book *Kamaru Pancasika*, which is the most famous of their books. Here, allusion will be made to each of these in a separate section, God willing.

Part One, On the Science of Breath

Know that the breath sometimes comes from the right side, and sometimes from the left side, and sometimes it is from both nostrils. They relate the right nostril to the sun, and the left to the moon, and they say that in one day 21,600 breaths come forth, or 900 every hour, more or less.

As they say, sometimes in one hour 1,600 breaths come forth, and during two hours, the breath comes from a single nostril. Sometimes it happens that over three days the breath goes from one nostril. There are some jogis who take no more than a single breath in a day and night, one in the morning and one in the evening. Thus, they say that when one reaches this stage, in six months it becomes easy. They consider obtaining this stage to be the cause of long life, the cure for all illnesses, and the attainment of complete happiness.

According to them breath is of five kinds:

1. The earthy breath, and they say that that breath goes towards the ground, and they say it is yellow in color.
2. The watery breath, and that is the breath which goes straight. They say that it is white in color.
3. The fiery breath, and that is the breath that goes upward. They say the color of this breath is red.
4. The airy breath, and that is the breath that goes crooked. They say this breath is green.
5. The heavenly breath, and this breath goes inward. They say its color tends towards whiteness.

They say that whenever the breath goes to the right side, it is a good sign for all of the following: the beginning of affairs, seeing kings and sultans and nobles, asking them for one's needs, going to battle, buying horses and beasts of burden, going to warm climates, cutting nails, branding animals, curing the sick, getting bled, farming, companionship and friendship, looking for lost items, and going north and east.

If it comes from the left side, it is a good sign for planning a trip especially to the west, buying and wearing new clothes, making jewelry, taking children to school, making agreements, marriages, construction, and trade.

They say that the earthy and watery breaths are a sign for abundant fortune and happiness. The fiery and airy breaths for depression, trouble, and illness, and the heavenly breath is a sign for confusion and impediment in one's affairs.

They say that when a questioner asks about the nature of a subject, if the earthy breath appears, the subject concerns plants; if it is airy or watery, the subject concerns animals; if it is fiery, the subject concerns minerals; if it is heavenly, it concerns no subject. When someone asks about affairs or a need, if the name of the questioner has an odd number of letters and the breath comes from the right side, that affair will come out right; but if a need arises, and if the name has an even number of letters and the breath comes from the left side, that affair will not come out right and the need will not be fulfilled.

If one asks about a sick person, and the name of the sick person has an odd number of letters, and the breath of the questioner and the person questioned comes from the right side, the sick person will become well; if the name of the sick person has an even number of letters, and the breath of both is from the left side, that sick person is in danger.

If they ask which of two opponents will triumph, [and] if the questioner has come from the side where the breath is increasing, the person whose name he says first will triumph. If the questioner comes from the side where the breath is decreasing, the person whose name he says last will triumph.

If they ask about a pregnant woman, [and] if the questioner has come from the left side, and the breath is increasing from that side, that child will be a girl; if he is coming from the right side, and the breath from that side is increasing, it will be a boy.

If they ask about a foreign army, and the questioner is from the left side, and the breath goes from that side, that army will come; if the breath does not come from that side, or itself decreases, that army will not come.

If they ask about a missing person, whether he is living or dead, [and] if the questioner comes from the side where the breath is decreasing and sits on that side where the breath is increasing, the person is living; if he has come from the side where the breath is increasing and sits where the breath is decreasing, that missing person will not come back. If he comes from the side where the breath is decreasing and also sits on that side, the missing person is dead.

If they ask about someone kidnapped or escaped, and the questioner comes from the side where the breath is increasing, he will come back. If he is from the side where the breath is decreasing, he will come back later.

They say if one's breath is disturbed so that for an entire day and night one cannot tell [from] which [side] the breath comes, it is proof that one will have a strong child. If both breaths for a day and night are equal, it is a sign of madness. If for four hours continuously breath comes from the left side, it is auspicious for him. If it is for eight hours, one of his friends will be injured. If it comes for nine hours, one of his relatives will suffer affliction. If it comes for ten hours, he will be afflicted. If it comes for twelve hours, a powerful enemy will appear. If it comes for a day and a night, death is to be feared.

They say when one person fears another, if, at a time when the breath comes from the left side he goes to a garden and picks 120 colored blossoms and sits by running water, casting them into the water one by one in the name of that person, he will become kind and no dread or fear will remain.

They say that if at a time when the breath comes from the right one has intercourse with a woman, a male child will come. If the breath comes from the left side, the child that will be born is female. May the breath be blest, the step fortunate, and the outcome praised.

Part Two, The Science of Imagination

The basis of this division in their view is ascetic practice. The lowest stage in ascetic practice is that one choose seclusion and abstain from eating meat, drinking intoxicants, and sexual intercourse. One sleeps little, enjoys sweet fragrances, avoids frivolity, eats little, does not dress in clean or perfumed clothes, and does not mix with anyone. If someone gives him the worst possible injury, he does not seek retribution or become concerned about it. The highest stage is that one is satisfied with fish for daily food, sleeps only one hour a week, and only breathes twice a day, so that his state is perfected, he controls the universe, and after that he does as he pleases.

One of the marvelous things told there is that they say if, at the time of weakness and the sign of death, one imagines that the water of life is flowing within oneself, and one becomes firm in this imagination and makes it continuous so that there is no interruption in his concentration, he will be released from that weakness and death will be repelled. He carefully follows this very method so that he lives, but when he grows tired of himself and no longer is busy repelling [death], he will be destroyed.

Some say such-and-such a person will never die; rather, when he becomes pure of all obscurities, he will no longer need food and drink, but will become purely spiritual and hidden from the eyes of men.

They say if one does not know how much of his life remains, when the sun has risen and is high, one goes to the desert and faces west, opposite one's shadow on the ground, standing straight and motionless. One places both hands on the knees, as when one bows [for Islamic ritual prayer], summoning this imagination without permitting any other thought. Then one raises the head and gazes at the shadow. If he sees the shadow whole in body, it is a sign that he has [much] life remaining. If he sees that he lacks a hand, two years remain to him. If he sees that he lacks a foot, one year remains.

They say that the places of the imagination are nine:

1. The first is the skull.
2. The second is between the two eyebrows.
3. The third is the throat.
4. The fourth is the slender hole near the nostrils, which is in the gullet, and which leads to the brain.
5. The fifth is the heart.
6. The sixth is the belly.
7. The seventh is the navel.
8. The eighth is the genitals.
9. The ninth is the seat.

The imagination of the skull is like the moon become full. The imagination of the eyebrow is like the sun. The imagination of the throat is like light. The imagination of the nostrils is like darkness. The imagination of the heart is like a burning lamp. The imagination of the belly is like a burning candle. The imagination of the navel is like the rays of the sun. The imagination of the genitals is like fire. The imagination of the seat is like moonlight.

They have demonstrated every one of these subjects, but since discussion of that cannot conceivably be very useful, this will be sufficient.

20

Traces of Shattari Sufism and Yoga in North Africa

Sufism in South Asia is a broad and diverse tradition, which has not only been configured on the models of Arabic and Persian Sufism, but which also has drawn upon local cultures and practices of Indian origin. In turn, the popularity of these South Asian Sufi formations has been demonstrated by their subsequent export to other regions, both in past centuries and in modern times. One particularly widespread South Asian Sufi group was the Shattari order, which attained considerable promi-nence in India by the sixteenth century, and which subsequently found new extensions in Southeast Asia, the Arabian peninsula, and even North Africa. A distinctive feature of Shattari Sufism in India was the incor-poration of meditation techniques from the hatha yoga tradition. These yogic practices, including breath control, Sanskrit mantras, and medita-tion on the subtle centers called cakras, had been most widely dissemi-nated to Arabic audiences through a text presented as a translation of an important Sanskrit text called "The Pool of Nectar" (*Amritakunda*).[1]

It was probably through the far-flung networks of the Shattari order that certain yogic teachings made their way to North Africa, through the efforts of Mecca-based Shattari masters such as Sibghat Allah of Broach (d. 1606) and Ahmad al-Qushashi (d. 1660–61). It seems that

---

[1] Carl W. Ernst, "Sufism and Yoga according to Muhammad Ghawth," *Sufi* 29 (Spring 1996): 9–13, and Chapter 8 in the present volume.

the modus operandi of the Shattaris when confronted with practices such as the recitation of mantras was to assimilate them to the familiar Sufi category of *dhikr* or recollection of the Arabic names of God. In this way, one particular formula in Hindi (attributed to the famous Chishti master, Baba Farid al-Din Ganj-i Shakkar, as we shall see) was added to the Arabic chants that formed the repertoire of Sufis and dervishes who traded spiritual expertise in the *zawiyas* and *khanqahs* of the Near East.

The text with which we are concerned is a late compendium of Sufi spiritual practices, *The Clear Fountain on the Forty Orders* (*al-Silsabil al-ma`in fil-tara'iq al-arba`in*), written by a prominent modern North African Sufi teacher, Muhammad al-Sanusi (d. 1859), the founder of the Sanusi order in Libya.[2] This work is constructed as a survey of 40 principal Sufi lineages, whose litanies and meditative techniques had been taught to the author through initiations by qualified masters. In it he covers groups that are well-known today, such as the Mevlevis that were so prominent in the Ottoman Empire, as well as less famous traditions with which he was acquainted.[3] In terms of his engagement with South Asian Sufi orders, it is noteworthy that he spends a good deal of time on a multi-part article on the Shattaris (one of the longer sections in the book), regarding them as a complex group. After several pages on the main branch of the Shattaris, he shifts to a sub-branch which he calls the Ghawthiyya, named after the Indian master Muhammad Ghawth. But then al-Sanusi turns his attention to another division of the Shattaris, called al-Jujiyya, by which he evidently refers to Indian yogis (or jogis, in north Indian pronunciation). He concludes his account with the `Ishqiyya, which was indeed a term for Shattaris in Central Asia.[4] In the

---

[2] Muhammad ibn `Ali al-Sanusi al-Khattabi al-Hasani al-Idrisi, *al-Silsabil al-ma`in fil-tara'iq al-arba`in*, in *al-Majmu`a al-mukhtara min mu'allafat al-ustadh al-a`zam al-imam sayyidi Muhammad ibn `Ali al-Sanusi* (Cairo: n.p., 1989). Each treatise in this anthology is separately paginated. See J.-L. Triaud, "al-Sanūsī, Muḥammad b. `Alī," *Encyclopaedia of Islam*, 2nd ed. (Brill Online, 2012, University of North Carolina at Chapel Hill, 12 October 2012), http://referenceworks.brillonline.com.libproxy.lib.unc.edu/entries/encyclopaedia-of-islam-2/al-sanusi-SIM_6612.

[3] See my translation of al-Sanusi's description of the Qadiri, Mevlevi, and Khawatiri orders in Carl W. Ernst, *Teachings of Sufism* (Boston: Shambhala Publications, 1999), pp. 76–81.

[4] The main section on the Shattaris is on pp. 77–81, followed by a subsection on the Ghawthiyya (the disciples of Muhammad Ghawth) on pp. 81–84. The Jujiyya are described on pp. 84–87 and the `Ishqiyya on pp. 87–88.

case of the Jujiyya, it is striking that a term for nominally non-Muslim ascetics here appears to be assimilated into the category of a sub-branch of a regular Sufi order. At any rate, it is worth translating this passage *in extenso* to examine al-Sanusi's full description of these yogis. It is apparent that al-Sanusi drew upon textual materials closely related to the Arabic version of *The Pool of Nectar*. In the following translation of al-Sanusi's text, references in brackets refer to the sections in my unpublished translation of *The Pool of Nectar* (e.g., IV.1 refers to chapter four, paragraph one, of the translation). Passages marked in bold are direct quotations from *The Pool of Nectar*.

Now I have seen one of the gnostics mention paths from the practices of the yogis (*al-jujiyya*), and I want to mention something of that so that the one who understands this miracle should comprehend it with knowledge. Then, he should know, prior to that, that the basis of their path is absolute unity and perfection. This is only the protection of the balance of discrimination between relationships and degrees in the non-absolute. One who averts his gaze from either of these two points is blind.

We say, with the assistance of the powerful Helper: Know that their posture for recollection is like that of others, sitting cross-legged except that in recollection they raise their heads toward heaven and they recite the following recollection ten thousand times, and more, and, through it, they attain levitation. It is "*wahi uhi.*" Then you should know that three things are conditions in the practice of the yogis, which the wayfarer necessarily acquires and then practices, with the imagination belonging to the first of the postures, [IV.2] **for these are divided into eighty-four postures.** The greatest of them is that [IV.4] **one sits with crossed legs, and that the edge of the left foot be beneath the genitals, and the right foot near it.** Then, one closes the sphincter and the mouth and cleaves the tongue to the top of the mouth. Then one practices the imagination and is absorbed in the internal. The second condition is the pursuit of hunger,[5] and the third condition is abandoning sleep in the four directions. If the wayfarer persists in these three, he is capable of the practice, and "opening" (*fath*) and attaining the goal become easy for him.

[V.2] **Know that the breaths are of three kinds: a breath that ascends upward, a breath that [descends] downward, and a breath that continually circles in the body. This is what runs in the blood in all the limbs, and every limb in which the blood runs is free from paralysis, God willing. But if the flow of blood is cut off from all the limbs, one**

---

[5] Reading *ju'*, hunger, in place of *khushu'*, humility.

is paralyzed on this account and is deprived of motion. The increase of breaths is born from food, [V.3] **so if one wishes to decrease the breaths, one should be restricted to foods like rice and milk, and avoid meat and the like.** But it is appropriate that one should preserve the breath that descends below and not exhale it without urgent need. Holding the breath has evident benefits. The first is bodily health, the second is long life, and the third is immunity from old age and senility. In their technical terms, holding the breath is called "the water of life." So if one wants to control breath, it is appropriate to sit in the previously mentioned posture until dawn, without breathing except when unavoidable. And then one observes things that are beyond calculation or description.

[II.5] **And if he wants to witness the hidden world, it is appropriate for him to align his eyes by the sides of his nose, and visualize in his heart the word, "Allah, Allah," without moving his tongue.** And when he reaches perfection[6] in this practice, then magic and poison have no effect on him, and he is not subject to disease. He discloses the hidden worlds, his prayer is answered, and he becomes famous among the people for acts of piety.

[VII.2] Know that the locations of meditation and imagination are seven. The first is the seat. The second is the center of the genitals. The third is the center of the navel. The fourth is the pineal heart. The fifth is the throat. The sixth is the eyes. The seventh is the brain, and it is a hidden sublime opening like a pinhole. If you apply oil to the head and draw that oil to the mouth, the oil descends to the mouth. In the days of childhood, that spot will be moist and soft. This is the noblest of the locations of visualizations and the nearest of them to divine presence and attaining the goal.

If you confirm that, then know that all habits are only according to imagination, which is one of the activities of hearts, and no one is victorious over it. And when one attains one of these meanings, then all of its objectives are attained for him. And if the wayfarer wishes to depart from imagination and witness the hidden world, then it is appropriate for him that he should summon the seven words to which imagination and thought are related. For in the condition of imagination appears the influence of the special properties of that thought.

1) [VII.3] And the first is that it appears with meditation from the seat, and he gathers his thoughts and says this word in the state of meditation, which is *om*, which means the Generous (*al-jawad*), black, Saturn. Its special property is the witnessing of [divine] commands oneself.

---

[6] Reading *rutbat al-kamāl* instead of *rukbat al-kamal*.

2) [VII.4] The second is that one meditates in the genitals and between the testicles, and says in his heart in the state of meditation *awam*, which means the Mighty (*al-qadir*), red, Mars. Its special property is the attainment of truthfulness when one thinks thoughts in the heart; all that one thinks in the heart, whether salvation or destruction, comes to pass in that manner.

3) [VII.5] The third is in the center of the navel, and one says in his heart in a state of meditation, *rhin*, which means the Knower (*'alim*),[7] dusty, Jupiter. Its special property is the attainment of the divine knowledge (*al-'ilm al-ladunni*) and teleportation.

4) [VII.6] The fourth is meditation under the left breast, and one says in his heart, *nasrin*, which means the Living (*al-hayy*), yellow, the sun. Its special property is the attainment of unveiling so that the hidden realm becomes to him like the visible realm. For the master of [this] meditation the world of the hidden becomes like the witnessing of the visible; he attains awareness of the thoughts of people.

5) [VII.7] The fifth is that one meditates in the location of the throat and says in his heart, *ay*, which means the Aspirant (*al-murid*), white, Venus. Its special property is summoning [spirits] so that the sublime and the lowly obey him and submit to him.

6) [VII.8] The sixth is that one meditates between the eyes, or on the forehead, and says in his heart, *barman*, which means the Just (*al-muqsit*), blue, Mercury. To the master of this recollection are opened the realities of things, without learning from anyone.

7) [VII.9] The seventh is that one meditated in the place above the brain, or visualizes his thought there, and says in his heart, *hansa'*, which means the Speaker (*al-kalim*), green, the moon. Its special property is the attainment of unveiling of the realities of things as a pure divine grace, without acquisition, and the master of this meditation attains eternal life like al-Khidr. This meditation is the greatest kind of meditation that is attained by seekers. In it are all their goals. This much is sufficient, so praise be to God, Lord of creation.

As is typical of his approach, al-Sanusi has begun his account with sweeping general terms drawn from the Sufi metaphysical vocabulary ("the basis of their path is absolute unity and perfection"). But then he proceeds to the portion of their "paths" having to do with bodily postures for meditation. He describes the familiar cross-legged posture known to yogis as the lotus position (*padmasana*), though it must be acknowledged that sitting with legs crossed is probably universal in human societies,

---

[7] Reading *'alim* for *'im*.

and al-Sanusi seems to recognize this as common in Sufi practice as well. But this posture is immediately linked with a *dhikr* formula, "*wahi uhi*," which at first sight seems mysterious and distinctly non-Arabic, though it is credited with miraculous powers. This phrase is clearly a variation on a formula well-known to the Shattaris, though it does not occur in *The Pool of Nectar*. The most popular work by Muhammad Ghawth Gwaliyari was undoubtedly the Persian manual of *dhikr* formulas and incantations known as *The Five Jewels (Jawahir-i khamsa)*, which was widely disseminated in an Arabic translation (*al-Jawahir al-khams*).[8] Although this text consists almost entirely of Arabic litanies, it does contain one formula in Hindi, commonly attributed to the Chishti master Farid al-Din Ganj-i Shakkar (d. 1265), which is widely referred to in Sufi manuals.[9] It is this formula that is inserted here, and its association with yogis evidently reflects the recognition that it is non-Quranic (and non-Arabic) in origin and hence unusual.

Al-Sanusi then proceeds abruptly to introduce the yogic postures, with an oblique reference to the standard number of 84 positions that in Indic texts are commonly associated with 84 archetypal yogis. He draws heavily upon the description of the "lotus position" found in the beginning of the fourth chapter of *The Pool of Nectar*, although it is interesting that he adds further conditions, including physical, psychological, and spiritual efforts, employing the characteristic Sufi term "opening" (*fath*) for higher experience. He then turns to the description of the three breaths from the fifth chapter of *The Pool of Nectar*, which are linked to dietary restrictions. To this he adds an explanation of the benefits of breath control, connecting it to the key symbol of immortality, "the water of life." There is indeed a close correspondence between the symbolism of "the water of life" (*ma' al-hayat*) in the Islamic tradition and the Indic notion of a nectar of immortality (*amrit*). The next reference to *The Pool of Nectar* is the description from Chapter 2 of how one can view the hidden world by crossing the eyes, while silently repeating the word "Allah"—except that the original text employs the Sanskrit word *alakh*,

---

[8] Carl W. Ernst, "Jawāher-e Ḵamsa," *Encyclopaedia Iranica* (2008), 14:608–9, http://www.iranicaonline.org/articles/jawaher-e-kamsa.

[9] Regarding the Hindi formula attributed to Farid al-Din, see Carl W. Ernst and Bruce B. Lawrence, *Sufi Martyrs of Love: Chishti Sufism in South Asia and Beyond* (New York: Palgrave Press, 2002), p. 33; Scott Kugle, *Sufi Meditation and Contemplation: Timeless Wisdom from Mughal India* (New Lebanon, NY: Suluk Press/Omega Publications, 2012), p. 75.

"stainless, transcendent," a mantra commonly employed in yogic circles, which by coincidence looks remarkably similar to "Allah" in the Arabic script. This is a clear example of Islamization of the yogic material in a way that familiarizes the underlying Indic practices, eliding their exotic appearance for the Muslim reader.

The remainder of the text consists of a brief but detailed account of the seven cakras or subtle centers of yogic meditative practice, following the outline of *The Pool of Nectar* but with some significant differences in the Arabic divine names that are proposed as equivalents for yogic mantras. Al-Sanusi repeats the emphasis of *The Pool of Nectar* on the faculty of the imagination (*wahm*) as the means for attaining supernatural experience. In other details the two texts track each other closely; they describe the same bodily locations of the seven cakras from the seat to the brain, with the same associations with the seven planets and their corresponding colors. There are some differences in the spelling of the Sanskrit mantras in the Arabic script, which is not surprising. But it is not at all clear why al-Sanusi confidently announces an almost entirely different list of Arabic *dhikr* formulas as counterparts of the yogic mantras (in one case only, the second cakra, the formula is the same; see Chart 20.1).

One can only speculate that different meditative practices arose within the Sufi orders to create this divergence in ritual practice. The Persian *Ocean of Life* by Muhammad Ghawth also has a rather different list of Arabic divine names in this chapter. It is worth noting that

CHART 20.1.
Planets, cakras, mantras, dhikrs, colors

	Planet	Cakra Location	Mantra, Pool of Nectar	Mantra, Silsabil	Dhikr, Pool of Nectar	Dhikr, Silsabil	Color
1	Saturn	seat	*hum*	*om*	**rabb**	**jawad**	black
2	Mars	genitals	*aum*	*aw`am*	**qadir**	**qadir**	red
3	Jupiter	navel	*hrim*	*rhin*	**khaliq**	**`alim**	dusty
4	Sun	heart	*brinsrin*	*nasrin*	**karim**	**hayy**	yellow
5	Venus	throat	*bray*	*ay*	**musakhkhir**	**murid**	white
6	Mercury	eyebrows	*yum*	*barman*	**`alim**	**muqsit**	blue
7	Moon	brain	*hansamansa*	*hansa'*	**muhyi**	**kalim**	green

al-Sanusi claims that his own teacher was not only initiated into the Ghawthi-Shattari order by a living master, but also by direct contact "in certain divine events" with Muhammad Ghawth himself.[10] This remark suggests that a certain amount of spiritual improvisation was to be expected in the deployment of meditative techniques, rather than slavish adherence to written texts. In any case, each of the seven "locations" and corresponding *dhikr* formulas are described as conferring amazing and miraculous results.

The presence of these excerpts from *The Pool of Nectar* in a comprehensive treatise on the Sufi orders of North Africa is an interesting testimony to the adaptation of Indian spiritual techniques into one of the accepted traditions of Sufism. The integration of yogic meditation into the curriculum of Sufi practice offered by the Shattari order meant that it became available as a standard Sufi teaching throughout the lands, from North Africa and Arabia to India and Indonesia, where the Shattari methods were taught. The Indian (and Hindu) antecedents of these practices were obscured by the transformation of Hindu yogis into something that sounded like a normal Sufi order, al-Jujiyya, and by the effortless conversion of the Sanskrit mantra *alakh* into Allah.

Ironically, a recent polemical work in Arabic has attacked these yogic practices in the course of a full-scale refutation of the Sanusi order written by a Libyan named al-Mahmoudy and published on the internet in 2009, in a mocking tone enhanced by the use of multiple exclamation points.[11] The author ridicules the miraculous claims made by al-Sanusi in *The Clear Fountain*, focusing particular sarcasm on the statement that levitation becomes possible by 10,000 repetitions of the phrase *wahi uhi*. Al-Mahmoudy derisively remarks that, if one follows these instructions for flying through the air, for instance on an aerial pilgrimage to Mecca, problems will occur because there is no indication of how one

---

[10] al-Sanusi, *al-Silsabil*, p. 84.

[11] Libyan Writer al-Mahmoudy (sic), *al-Durar al-bahiyya fi bayan dalal `aqa'id al-firqa al-Sanusiyya, wa fihi al-radd `ala `Ali al-Salabi (Shining Pearls in Demonstration of the Corrupt Beliefs of the Sanusi Sect, with a Refutation of `Ali al-Salabi)*, part 20, http://www.libya-watanona.com/adab/mahmoudi/mm01049a.htm. This text, as indicated by the title, was written in response to a biography of Muhammad al-Sanusi by `Ali al-Salabi, entitled *al-Haraka al-Sanusiyya fi Libiya: al-Imam Muhammad ibn `Ali al-Sanusi wa manhajuhu fil-ta'sis (The Sanusi Movement in Libya; Imam Muhammad ibn `Ali al-Sanusi and his Founding Method)*.

can make a safe landing! He likewise casts scorn on the description of meditation on the cakra located by the genitals and the cleaving of the tongue to the roof of the mouth, condemning these practices as satanic and utterly unconnected with Islamic ethical norms. What is remarkable is that this entire polemic is carried out without any awareness that the practices in question are connected to non-Islamic traditions from India. Al-Mahmoudy was not able to take advantage of the wonderful opportunity this would have offered him to attack al-Sanusi as a promoter of pagan practices. In the end, his polemic remains well within the boundaries of the standard critique of Sufi superstition from the perspective of modern Muslim reformism. The familiarization of yoga in this Sufi text has been so successful that even an ardent opponent of Sufism is unable to detect anything of its Indian background. The traces of yoga in North Africa today have become faint indeed.

21

Indian Lovers in Arabic and Persian Guise

Azad Bilgrami's Depiction of *Nayikas**

Although love may be considered universal, local interpretations of it may be defined in very particular fashions. Not many cultures can match the systematic exposition of the different kinds of lovers found in the Indian *nayika-bheda* tradition. With roots going back to early Sanskrit texts such as the *Nātyaśāstra*, this kind of classification of lovers has been remarkably popular for centuries, with definitive literary works emerging in Sanskrit and Hindi in the sixteenth and seventeenth centuries, such as the *Rasikapriyā* of Keshavdās and the *Rasamañjarī* of Bhānudatta.[1] It is less well known that this distinctively Indian approach to love and poetry was also pursued in Persian and Arabic by writers from courtly Mughal circles. The most remarkable of these compositions is the subject of this preliminary analysis.

In a distinctive Arabic treatise entitled *The Coral Rosary of Indian Traditions* (written in 1763–64), Ghulam `Ali "Azad" Bilgrami (d. 1786) provided a snapshot of his concept of the world, seen from the perspective

* Earlier versions of this paper were given at the American Academy of Religion Conference in San Francisco, November 2011, and the Perso-Indica Conference in Paris, June 2012. I would like to thank several commentators for their valuable suggestions, including Allison Busch, Jack Hawley, Françoise Delvoye, and Heidi Pauwels.
[1] Bhānudatta, *"Bouquet of Rasa" & "River of Rasa"*, ed. and trans. Sheldon Pollock, Clay Sanskrit Library 41 (New York: NYU Press, 2009); K P Bahadur, trans., *The Rasikapriya of Keshavadasa* (Delhi: Motilal Banarsidass, 1972).

of a cultivated Indian Muslim.[2] Azad was a member of a learned family from the qasbah of Bilgram in present-day Uttar Pradesh, whose family served the Mughal empire in various administrative positions; he spent a number of years studying Arabic literature and hadith in Arabia and returned to the Deccan, where he wrote an immense amount of Arabic poetry and compiled three anthologies of Persian poetry.[3] The work under discussion is a composite text that Azad wrote separately in four parts, later combined together. The first part is devoted to the hadith statements of the Prophet Muhammad regarding the sanctity of India as the place where Adam landed on Earth after his expulsion from Paradise.[4] The second part is a biographical dictionary containing accounts of 45 Indian Muslim scholars who wrote in Arabic, ranging from the eighth century to the author's own day.[5] The third part is concerned with rhetorical figures from Indian literature, illustrated with specimens of Arabic poetry. The fourth part focuses on the categories of lovers found in Indian literature, again illustrated by Arabic verses, including both classical poems and verses of the author's own composition. Azad subsequently translated the third and fourth parts into Persian in abridged form, under the title *Gazelles of India* (*Ghizlan al-Hind*), substituting examples of Persian poetry to complete this comparative study of Arabic, Persian, and Indic rhetoric and poetics.[6]

Azad was by no means the first Muslim author to be interested in these Indian descriptions of lovers. Not long after the emergence of full-fledged treatises on nayikas in Hindi in the sixteenth century, it appears that rulers

---

[2] Ghulam `Ali Azad al-Bilgrami, *Subhat al-marjan fi athar Hindustan*, ed. Muhammad Fadl al-Rahman al-Nadwi al-Siwani, 2 vols. (Aligarh: Jami`at `Aligarh al-Islamiyya, 1976–80).
[3] Shawkat Toorawa, "Azad Bilgrami," in *Essays in Arabic Literary Biography 1350–1850*, ed. Joseph E. Lowry and Devin J. Stewart (Wiesbaden: Harrassowitz, 2009), 2:91–97.
[4] An abridged translation of this section is available in Carl W. Ernst, "India as a Sacred Islamic Land," in *Religions of India in Practice*, ed. Donald S. Lopez, Jr., Princeton Readings in Religions 1 (Princeton University Press, 1995), pp. 556–64, and in chapter 2 of this volume.
[5] This section is discussed in Carl W. Ernst, "Reconfiguring South Asian Islam: The 18th and 19th centuries," *Comparative Islamic Studies* 5, no. 2 (2009 [published in 2011]), pp. 247–72, chapter 7 in this volume.
[6] Mir Ghulam `Ali Azad Bilgrami, *Ghazalan [sic] al-Hind: mutala`a-i tatbiqi-i balaghat-i hindi va parsi*, ed. Sirus Shamisa (Tehran: Sada-yi Mu`asir, 1382/2004). The title *Ghizlan al-Hind* (misspelled in this edition) is a chronogram for the year of the book's composition (1178/1764–65). See also Sunil Sharma, "Translating Gender: Azad Bilgrami on the Peotics of the Love Lyric and Cultural Synthesis," *The Translator* 15, no. 1 (2009): 87–103.

of the Mughal period, such as Abu al-Hasan Tana Shah of Golconda, and Shah Jahan himself, became interested in this literature and commissioned new works on the subject in Sanskrit, such as the *Sundarasringara* of Sundar Das and the *Srngaramanjari* of Akbar Shah. The latter text, originally written in Telugu, was translated into Sanskrit and Brajbhasha by Chintamani Tripathi. Akbar's prime minister and biographer, Abu al-Fazl, included a brief but thoughtful discussion of the nayikas in Persian (including a translation of a favorite verse from Bhanudatta) in his survey of Indian culture in the *A'in-i Akbari*.[7] A more extensive elaboration of this tradition was found in the wide-ranging seventeenth-century Persian encyclopedia of Indian culture and Braj literature called *The Bounty of India (Tuhfat al-Hind)*, commissioned around 1675 by one of Aurangzeb's sons and written by Mirza Khan ibn Fakhr al-Din Muhammad. This treatise contains a detailed discussion of lovers, under the heading of the Hindi term *sringara-rasa*.[8] Because of the close association of Braj poetry with the musical tradition, nayikas were also discussed by Faqirullah in his Persian treatise on Indian music, *Rag Darpan*, composed in 1666.[9] But no other literary production of this kind by Mughal authors compares in scope with the fourth part of Azad's *Coral Rosary*, which takes up over 200 pages in the printed Arabic edition, and a more compressed 50 pages in the abridged Persian translation.

The classification system contained in Azad's Arabic treatise is complex (see Chart 21.1). The fourth part of this work contains five chapters. The first chapter treats the types of female lovers according to well-known Indian systems. This includes six main divisions (virtue, age, complaint, excitedness, cleverness, and arrogance), followed by a miscellaneous category containing a total of 33 different types. The Arabic text proper does not include the Hindi terminology, although the manuscripts

---

[7] Abū al-Fazl ibn Mubārak, *The A'in-i Akbari*, ed. H. Blochmann, Biblioteca Indica, N.S. 168 (Calcutta: The Baptist Mission Press, 1869), 2:131–34; ibid., trans. H. S. Jarrett, ed. Jadunath Sarkar, 2nd ed. (1948; reprint, New Delhi: Oriental Books Reprint Corp., 1977–78), 3:256–58.

[8] Mirza Khan ibn Fakhr al-Din Muhammad, *Tuhfat al-Hind*, ed. Nur al-Hasan Ansari, Zaban u Adabiyyat-i Farsi 39 (Tehran: Bunyad-i Farhang-i Iran, 1354/1975), 1:297–321. On this text see Allison Busch, "Hidden in Plain View: Brajbhasha Poets at the Mughal Court," *Modern Asian Studies* 44, no. 2 (2010): 267–309, citing p. 297.

[9] Faqirullah, *Tarjamah-yi Man katohal, va Risalah-yi Rag Darpan*, ed. Shahab Sarmadee (New Delhi: Indira Gandhi National Centre for the Arts and Motilal Banarsidass Publishers, 1996).

often list them as marginal notations (in Arabic script). The Persian translation, however, deliberately states the Hindi equivalents for all but six, spelling them according to the rules of Arabic grammar; this nod to the Hindi tradition may be an indication of greater bilinguality between Hindi and Persian. The second chapter offers nine additional types of female lovers discovered by Azad, at least one of which, the Arab or Bedouin girl (*al-a`rābiyya* or *al-badawiyya*) explicitly invokes an Arabic precedent. The third chapter consists of a lengthy Arabic ode on love composed by Azad (*al-qaṣīda al-ghizlāniyya*), illustrating most of the previously articulated categories of Indian lovers in 37 lines, interrupted by numerous lexical and explanatory comments. The fourth chapter is devoted to the classification of male lovers, though Azad finds the Indian material is decidedly less attractive here, satisfying himself with enumerating the two categories of the monogamous and polygamous lovers (*mustafrid* and *mustakthir*), corresponding to the Hindi terms *anukūla*, "faithful," and *dakṣiṇa*, "gallant" or "adroit." He omits two others he does not deign to describe because of their "lack of beauty"; presumably the two omitted categories of husbands are *dhṛṣṭa*, "brazen," and *śaṭha*, "deceptive."[10] While the Indian tradition emphasized the "male gaze" on women and was for the most part satisfied with cursory attention to male lovers, Azad innovatively expands this brief catalogue by adding no fewer than 30 new types of male lovers. The additions, in part, reflect the categories of female lovers (i.e., in six cases), but others are derived from an Arabic treatise on love by an important author of the Mamluk period, Ibn Abi Ḥajala (d. 1375).[11] The fifth chapter consists of another lengthy ode on passion in 35 lines (*al-qaṣīda al-hayamāniyya*), containing descriptions of male lovers, again with numerous interpolated remarks. The Persian translation contains essentially the same material (with the exception of the two Arabic odes), arranged in four sections: the Indian female lovers, the additional lovers discovered by Azad, the two categories of monogamous and polygamous male lovers, and the newly invented types of male lovers, although all of this is illustrated

---

[10] See Bhanudatta, *Bouquet*, pp. 92–93.

[11] Beatrice Gruendler, "Ibn Abi Hajalah," in *Essays in Arabic Literary Biography*, pp. 118–126. Azad is citing this author's text *Bustan al-sultan (The King's Garden)*, but it does not appear to be extant; cf. Carl Brockelmann, *Geschichte der arabische Litteratur* (Leiden: E. J. Brill, 1943), 2:12, Supplementband 2:5.

by Persian verses instead of Arabic. The Persian version closes with an autobiographical notice of the author.

Azad introduces this catalogue of lovers (pp. 323–27) with Islamic references, beginning the treatise with a slightly truncated version of a prophetic hadith: "From your world, perfume and women have been made desirable to me" (more commonly, this hadith includes as a third desirable thing, "prayer, the delight of my eyes," but that religious reference is omitted here). Azad joins this justification with his earlier discussion of Adam's descent from Paradise to earth, landing on India, which then became the source of all perfumes. He then praises the Indians for the "shining art and sublime explanation" that they have devoted to women, acknowledging that they have outdone the Arabs in this respect (the Persian text goes farther in calling this a divine inspiration, *ilhām*). He further maintains that Indian love poetry is distinctive in offering the perspective of the woman, a trait that he links to the religious duty of the Indian woman to join her deceased husband's funeral pyre as a sati or virtuous wife. Indeed, he finds this kind of devotion reminiscent of Zulaykha, whom the Qur'an depicts as hopelessly in love with Joseph. Yet, this divinely arranged love can be mutual so that both man and woman are lover and beloved. Shifting to another "national characteristic" and repeating a trope already affirmed by Abu al-Fazl, Azad maintains that the Indians and Arabs focus their love poetry on women, while the Persians and Turks aim instead at young men, a predilection he condemns by citing the Qur'anic story of Lot.[12] The Indians, he claims, are unacquainted with such tendencies, reserving their discussion for the husband and wife known as nayaka and nayika. Azad's stereotypical claim that Arabic and Indian literature are devoid of homoerotic themes obviously needs to be taken with a grain of salt; just in terms of Arabic literature, it is ironic that one of Azad's sources, Ibn Abī Hajala, devoted a chapter in one of his works to love between bearded old men, though this is commonly censored in modern editions.

After a lengthy digression (pp. 327–31) on the four different kinds of love (by hearing, by dream, by a picture, and by sight), Azad pauses to recount (pp. 331–38) seven different types of love relationship: male lover and female beloved, and the reverse; male lover and female friend, and the reverse, female friend and female lover, and the reverse: and

---

[12] For the trope in Abu al-Fazl, see *A'in-i Akbari*, trans. Jarrett, 3:256.

female friend and female friend.[13] Each of these types is illustrated by extensive quotations of Arabic poems by famous authors including Azad.

> Eventually, Azad turns to the categories of female lovers from the Indian tradition. I name each division with a clear name, and I define it with a comprehensive and final definition. I set forth examples by which the eyes of the literati are refreshed and sayings by which the dispositions of the elegant are excited. The examples that I refer to myself in this essay are mostly from my own compositions, and a few of them are [translated] from the poetry of the Indians. But the meaning that is from their poems I announce in its place, to distinguish my own property from what is borrowed, and to clarify my children from the child of others (p. 338).

The point here is that Azad will primarily explain the Indian tradition in his own terms.

After this bold declaration, Azad makes an uncharacteristically modest claim about the possibility of translation:

> And by the power of God (glory be to him), the sweetness that may be produced for palates from the poems collected according to the categories of women in the language of India is not produced in the language of the Arabs. The only cause for this is the character of the language, and it is obvious that the translation of the character from one language to another is beyond human capacity; the only capacity is for the explanation of scientific principles.

And with this bald apology, Azad proceeds to present the categories of lovers with poetic illustrations.

It is worth pausing a moment to consider this stricture on the limits of translation. When one considers major translation movements of the past, it is indeed the case that "scientific" subjects—ranging from mathematics and medicine to magic and theology—have been the main target of attention. Belles-lettres has rarely been rendered from Greek into Arabic. While the noted Arab translator Hunayn ibn Ishaq was said to have known the poetry of Homer, no significant traces survive of any Arabic version of the Iliad or the Odyssey before modern Arab authors

---

[13] Compare the digressions of love with Bahadur, *Rasikapriya*, ch. 4.

took up the task in the twentieth century. Azad's strategy here is similar to the curious case of Aristotle's *Poetics*, where examples of Greek drama were replaced with Arabic poetry, causing the commentator Ibn Rushd to identify comedy with panegyric and tragedy with satire.[14] In both instances, the translator did not attempt to translate poetic specimens from the source text but substituted instead standard pieces from the Arabic poetic repertoire.

One or two examples will suffice to demonstrate Azad's approach to the different types of nayikas. The virtuous woman (*al-ṣāliḥa*), defined as only inclined toward her husband, modest, and seeking his satisfaction, is portrayed first by a hadith in which the Prophet describes the ideal obedient wife. This is followed by the instance of Umm Rabāb, who married the Prophet's grandson Husayn. After his martyrdom, she announced that she would not marry again, and she died of grief. Azad then adduces eight quotations of poetry; some are anonymous, but others are by the pre-Islamic poet al-A`sha (d. 625), the Andalusian anthologist Ibn `Abd Rabbihi (d. 940), and Azad himself.[15] A sample from Ibn `Abd Rabbihi:

> No, I've never seen or heard anyone like her,
>> a pearl that turns to ruby from bashfulness.

Or from Azad:

> I called out names at night, but she refused,
>> preserving her chastity from the suspicion of a lie.
> She never appeared to nocturnal eyes,
>> so all the people are certain she's a flower.[16]

---

[14] The ironies of this translational dilemma were famously explored by Jorge Luis Borges in his short story, "Averroes' Search," in *Labyrinths: Selected Stories & Other Writings*, ed. Donal A. Yates & James E. Irby (New York: New Directions Books, 1964), pp. 148–55.

[15] Ahmad ibn Muhammad Ibn `Abd Rabbih, *The Unique Necklace (Al-`Iqd al Farid)*, trans. Issa J. Boullata, 3 vols., Great Books of Islamic Civilization (Reading, UK: Garnet Pub., 2006–12). This publication represents a small fraction of the complete Arabic work.

[16] Azad Bilgrami, *Subhat al-marjan*, 2:338–40.

In the Persian text, this category is illustrated by no less than 10 separate verses by the great Safavid-Mughal poet Sa'ib, such as:

> That shyness that we saw from that rosy face—
>
> it's tough that it entered our dream unveiled.

Then follow verses by 11 other Indo-Persian poets, including Azad's pupil, Lakshmi Narayan "Shafiq" Aurangabadi:

> Modesty ever seals the jewelbox of your mouth;
>
> I think it's hard for you to speak to a lover![17]

All these are simply cited, with no further elaboration, as obvious illustrations of the category of lover under consideration.

Given Azad's determination to explain Indian lovers mainly by Arabic and Persian poetry, it is striking that he periodically admits to having translated a number of verses from "the Indian language" into Arabic.[18] While the original Hindi poems are not quoted, the way they are cited in translation raises interesting questions about Azad's relation to Hindi literature. He generally introduces each such verse only as "my composition, from (or in) Indian poetry," leaving it unclear whether he was simply translating or whether he had also written the original Hindi poem.[19] On one occasion, however, he relates,

> During the time of writing this book, my uncle, the prayer direction of my hopes, Sayyid Muhammad (may his shadow lengthen), wrote to me from Bilgram while I was in Aurangabad. It was a Hindi poem, and he tasked me with rendering its meaning from the Indian language into Arabic. So I composed the following verses.[20]

This brief remark indicates that engagement with Hindi poetry, and its transformation into Arabic, was a literary habit among at least some

---

[17] Azad Bilgrami, *Ghizlan al-Hind*, pp. 118–121.
[18] Azad Bilgrami, *Subhat al-marjan*, 2:359, 364–65, 366–67 (three poems), 372, 385, 423.
[19] While some Urdu writings have been attributed to Azad, their authenticity is doubtful (Ibid., 1:15–16).
[20] Ibid., 2:372.

members of the Mughal cultural elite, even if such bilingual relations were much more common between Hindi and Persian.

Another of Azad's verses recalls a famous Persian poem of Amir Khusraw (d. 1325), which itself recreates the longing of the Indian woman for her absent lover during the rainy season. Azad writes,

> The cloud comes, and my love is not present;
>
> who do I have to bring my friend to me?
>
> Tears rain down, reddened, from my eye,
>
> until the tender cloud weeps over me.[21]

While Khusraw's poem goes:

> The cloud rains, and I am apart from my love.
>
> how can I make my heart part from its owner on this day?
>
> The cloud, the rain, I, and my love are standing in farewell;
>
> I cry apart, the cloud's apart, my love's apart.
>
> The eye is bleeding because of you, pupil of my eye;
>
> be a man, don't be apart from the bloody eye.[22]

This juxtaposition of Azad's Arabic verse with a famous Persian line from his illustrious predecessor suggests a need to consider Indo-Arabic literature in its inter-textual connection, both with Indo-Persian and with the relevant Indic equivalents. But several major questions remain.

Who was Azad's audience? It is difficult to be certain, but the technical difficulty of reading the highly ornate Arabic of this work suggests a limited circulation, and a similar conclusion might be drawn from the three manuscripts used by the editor (one autograph, one copied by a student of Azad's; all three from Indian libraries). A fuller inventory indicates eighteen manuscript copies of the Arabic text in Indian and Pakistani libraries, plus three in Europe.[23] At least one manuscript found

---

[21] Ibid., 2:386.

[22] Yamīn al-Dīn Abū al-Ḥasan Khusraw, *Kulliyyāt-i ghazaliyyāt-i Khusraw*, ed. Iqbal Salah al Din (Lahore: Packages Ltd., 1972), 1:1, lines 1, 2, 5.

[23] Sayyid Hasan `Abbas, *Ahwul o athar-i Sayyid Ghulam-`Ali Azad Bilgrami* (Tehran: Bunyad-i Mawqufat-i Duktur Mahmud Afshar Yazdi, 1384/2006), pp. 277 79

its way to Cairo, and the text was published in a lithograph edition from Bombay in 1884; it would be interesting to know what the readership was.[24] Surprisingly, the first two sections of *Subhat al-marjan* (on references to India in prophetic hadith, and on the lives of Arabic scholars of India) were translated into Persian in 1869, under the patronage of "Mahārāj Īsarī Parshād," the Raja of Benares.[25] Perhaps this translation indicates an interest in Azad's work among a Persian-knowing Hindu elite, who sought access in this way to the overtly Islamic portions of his text. Azad's own Persian translation of sections three and four, *Ghizlan al-Hind*, seems to be fairly widely distributed, in comparison with the Arabic; there are at least 10 copies in Indian libraries, four in Iran, several more in Pakistan and Bangladesh, plus additional manuscripts in European libraries.[26]

Ostensibly, the original Arabic work is aimed at an audience that knows nothing of India, since hardly any Indic terms are provided in the text—yet copyists seem to have added the names for the various categories of nayikas in the margins, indicating a de facto readership that was quite knowledgeable. The Persian translation is more explicit about including these terms within the text of the fourth section (although Indic terminology is almost entirely missing from the third section, on rhetorical figures, in both the Arabic and Persian versions). Probably Azad had in mind readers like his uncle Sayyid Muhammad, who were capable of understanding the multiple layers of meaning implicated between an implied but unspoken Indian literary tradition and the Arabic and Persian poems that were proposed as its exemplars.

Another question is the nature of Azad's connection with *nayika-bheda* literature. There are several possibilities. Was he exposed to this

---

[24] Brockelmann, *Geschichte der arabische Litteratur*, Supplementband 2:600–1, citing Cairo² 5:419; Ghulam ʿAli Azad al-Bilgrami, *Subhat al-marjan fi athar Hindustan* (Bombay: Malik al-Kitab, 1303/1884–85), http://babel.hathitrust.org/cgi/pt?id=nnc1. cu58898506.

[25] *Catalogue of Arabic & Persian Manuscripts in Khuda Bakhsh Oriental Public Library, Patna*, Vol. 8 (Patna: Khuda Bakhsh Oriental Public Library, 1994), pp. 7–8, no. 652.

[26] The printed edition of *Ghizlan al-Hind* edited by Shamisa is based on copies from Dhaka and Tehran (p. 20). Additional copies are described by Sayyid Hasan ʿAbbas, "*Ghizlan al-Hind*-i Mir Ghulam-ʿAli Azad Bilgrami," *Tahqīqāt-i Islāmī* 9, no. 1–2 (1373/1995): 189–95, http://www.ensani.ir/storage/Files/20101027155730-107.pdf. See also C. A. Storey, *Persian Literature: A Bio-bibliographical Survey* (London: Luzac & Company, Ltd., 1972), 1:862, and ʿAbbas, *Ahwal o athar*, pp. 340–41.

through reading Sanskrit or Braj treatises on the subject?[27] Would it have been possible to obtain a relatively complete view of the subject through oral sources? As we shall see below, Azad himself observed performance and discussion of these Indian genres of poetry at a Muslim Court. Was he following earlier Persian accounts of the nayika tradition? None of this is indicated in the Arabic text, although closer study of his Arabic versions of Indian poetry may yield some clues.

Fortunately there is external evidence to indicate Azad's thorough acquaintance with Braj poetry. He came from a long line of scholars in Bilgram, many of whom were deeply immersed in Hindi literature. One such was `Abd al-Wahid Bilgrami (1509–1608), a prolific author of Persian Sufi texts who also wrote a Persian treatise called *Haqa'iq-i Hindi* (*Indian Realities*, written in 1566–67) that defended the use of Krishna bhakti poems in Sufi music sessions.[28] Of him the conservative Mughal historian Bada'uni optimistically remarked, "He used formerly to indulge in ecstatic exercises and sing ecstatic songs in Hindi and fall into trances, but he is now past all this."[29] Azad further detailed his own knowledge of Hindi poetry in his biographical anthology of Indo-Persian poets and poets of Hindi, *Sarv-i Azad* (*The Free Cypress/Azad's Cypress*), composed in 1752–53; this is the second volume of *Ma'athir al-kiram tarikh-i Bilgram* (*Traditions of the Eminent, A History of Bilgram*), which was devoted to the saints and scholars of Bilgram. In *Sarv-i Azad*,

---

[27] As was doubtless the case with Abu al-Fazl; see Allison Busch, *Braj beyond Braj: Classical Hindi in the Mughal World*, IIC Occasional Publication 12 (New Delhi: India International Centre, 2009), p. 8.

[28] Heidi Pauwels, "A Sufi Listening to Hindi Religious Poetry: Mir Abdul Wahid Bilgrami's Haqayaq-i Hindi," (rewrite of student paper originally written in 1992 and submitted as field exam towards degree of PhD at University of Washington, Seattle, 2001), http://hdl.handle.net/1773/19592; Francesca Orsini, "'Krishna is the Truth of Man': Mir `Abdul Wahid Bilgrāmī's *Haqā'iq-i Hindi* (*Indian Truths*) and the Circulation of *dhrupad* and *bishnupad*," in *Culture and Circulation*, ed. Allison Busch and Thomas de Brujin (Leiden: Brill, forthcoming) http://eprints.soas.ac.uk/8578/1/Krishna_is_the_Truth_of_Man.pdf. This text has now been published in a critical edition; see `Abd al-Wahid Bilgrami, *Ḥaqāyiq-i hindi*, ed. Muḥammad Iḥtishām al-Din (Aligarh: Center for Persian Studies, Aligarh Muslim University, 2010). Another manuscript of this work is said to be found in the shrine of Shah Barakat Allah (or Barkatullah) in Marehra (near Aligarh); the latter, a poet in both Braj and Persian, was a descendant of Azad's grandfather, `Abd al-Jalil Bilgrami.

[29] `Abd al-Qadir ibn Mulukshah al-Bada'uni, *Muntakhab al-tawarikh*, trans. George S. A. Ranking, W. H. Lowe, and Wolseley Haig, 3 vols. (Calcutta: The Asiatic Society of Bengal, 1898–1925), 3:106–7.

he gives accounts of eight poets of Hindi from the town of Bilgram (two of whom were also known as Persian poets), including an extensive excerpt from the *Rasprabodh* of Sayyid Ghulam Naba Bilgrami, whose pen-name in Hindi was "Raslan."[30] Another of the Hindi poets listed here was Azad's maternal grandfather, `Abd al-Jalil Bilgrami, with whom he studied religious and literary texts for two years.[31] Azad's attention to Hindi poetry in a Persian biographical anthology was not uncommon at the time; at least a dozen other Persian *tazkiras*, either partially or wholly dedicated to Hindi poetry, were produced in the late eighteenth and early nineteenth centuries.[32] Azad portrays literary discussions taking place in the assemblies of local Mughal administrators debating figures of speech in Hindi poetry.[33] He describes how his grandfather `Abd al-Jalil secured an appointment for a Brahmin poet from Bilgram at the court of Husayn `Ali Khan.[34] In short, Azad came from an environment in which Hindi was fully integrated into a literary continuum alongside Persian and Arabic.[35]

As Azad stated in introducing the Hindi poets of Bilgram,

Part Two, on the rhyme-masters of Hindi—may God reward them with the best of prizes! This ignorant one is familiar with the languages of Arabic, Persian, and Hindi, and from each tavern I have measured a cup according to my capacity. I have spent lifetimes in the practice of Arabic and Persian poetry, and I have cherished the fresh blooms of meaning in the embrace of thought. But I have not happened to practice Hindi poetry as much, and the opportunity to master the greenery of this realm has not occurred. But

---

[30] Ghulam `Ali Azad al-Bilgrami, *Ma'āthir al-kirām mawsūm bi-Sarv-i Āzād* (Hyderabad: Kutub Khāna Āsafiyya, 1913), pp. 352–407, http://babel.hathitrust.org/cgi/pt?id=njp.3210 1062276348;page=root;seq=1;view=2up;size=100;orient=0;num=1; Sayyid Ghulam Nabi Raslin Bilgrami, *Ras Prabodh* (Rampur: Rampur Reza Library, 2001), a facsimile of the nasta`liq manuscript with Devanagri transcription.

[31] Azad Bilgrami, *Sarv-i Āzād*, pp. 369–71.

[32] Storey, *Persian Literature*, 1:851, 852, 853, 867, 868 (two), 873, 876 (three), 877, 880, 882 (two), 883, 884.

[33] Allison Busch, *Poetry of Kings: The Classical Hindi Literature of Mughal India* (Oxford: Oxford University Press, 2011), pp. 154–55, quoting *Ma'athir al-kiram* (i.e., *Sarv-i Āzād*), pp. 364–65.

[34] Azad Bilgrami, *Sarv-i Āzād*, pp. 370.

[35] Shailesh Zaidi, *Bilgrām ke musalmān hindī kavi* (Varanasi: Nagari Pracharini Sabha, 1969); Francesca Orsini, "How to do Multilingual Literary History? Lessons from Fifteenth- and Sixteenth-century North India," *Indian Economic and Social History Review* 49, no. 2 (2012): 225–46.

to the ear the call of India's parrots has an encompassing pleasure, and to the taste this rose bower has a plentiful share of the sugar-seller's flavor.

The creators of meaning in Arabic and Persian spill blood from the vein of thought, and they convey the style of subtle imagination to the highest of levels. The fable reciters of Hindi have also made no little progress in this valley, but in the art of *nayika bheda* they have taken a magical step forward. One who uses both Persian and Hindi, and who has a perfect acquaintance with white and black, will confirm the truth of this poor man's poetry, and will adorn the register of this humble one's claim with the seal of witnessing. The versifiers of the Hindi language have displayed exceptional glory in Bilgram, and have increased the freshness and exuberance of intellects with the fragrances of fresh aloes. For this reason the section on this particular group has been written, and the aromatic scents have been conveyed to the hand of the connoisseurs of perfume.[36]

Indeed, it seems clear that Azad was already playing with ways to link India to Islamic religious themes in the conclusion to *Sarv-i Azad*, some 11 years before writing *Subhat al-marjan*, when he drew on works of hadith to argue that the paradisal vocabulary of the Qur'an may come from the Indian language.[37]

Azad's relationship with the existing nayika tradition is complicated by his willingness to engage in creative revision and expansion of the categories of lovers. This is seen in the additional six categories he slips into the list of female lovers in Chapter 1, the nine new categories he introduces in Chapter 2, and the nearly 30 categories of male lovers (unprecedented in the Hindi sources) that he either establishes as parallels of the females or else incorporates from Arabic sources. Indeed, he urges others to be equally creative: "Let whoever wishes add to this, for the field is wide, and the garden is fertile." He finds further scriptural warrant for considering the different types of lover, by citing a well-known hadith that describes the diverse relationships that 11 different women had with their husbands.[38] In this respect, Azad resembled Hindi poets such as Kesavdas and Cintamani, whom Allison Busch describes as "assessing the continuing viability of . . . classificatory distinctions,

---

[36] Azad Bilgrami, *Sarv-i Āzād*, pp. 351–52.
[37] Ibid., p. 406.
[38] Azad Bilgrami, *Subhat al-marjan*, 2:420. This is the hadith of Umm Zara`, from *Ṣaḥīḥ Muslim*, book 31, chapter 14, no. 5998 http://theonlyquran.com/hadith/Sahih-Muslim/?volume=31&chapter=14.

reconfiguring them as necessary, and occasionally proposing new ones."[39] One might consider this Indo-Arabic production as a courtly parallel to the emerging Hindi riti tradition, which was at the time "a fledgling branch of vernacular knowledge as it began to put forward increasingly strong claims to a separate existence from Sanskrit."[40] Azad makes no obvious gestures here either toward devotional bhakti or Sufi interpretations in his approach to love poetry, citing in his Arabic version only classical poetry and Islamic scriptures. There is probably more of a Sufi flavor in the Persian translation, simply because of the pervasive Sufi imagery found in Indo-Persian poetry.

Much more remains to be said about this formidable literary production on the types of lovers. Yet, at the very least it should now be acknowledged that the nayika-bheda tradition can be understood in a new dimension through this intertextual exploration in the medium of Arabic and Persian.

---

[39] Allison Busch, "The Anxiety of Innovation: The Practice of Literary Science in the Hindi/Riti Tradition," *Comparative Studies of South Asia, Africa and the Middle East* 24, no. 2 (2004): 45–59, citing p. 54.

[40] Ibid., p. 56.

CHART. 21.1

Contents of Chapters 1, 2, and 4 of Ghulam ʿAli Azad Bilgrami, *Subhat al-marjan fi athar Hindustan,* book 4 (Arabic)/*Ghizlan al-Hind* (Persian)

Chapter 1. *On the types of female lovers* (ghizlān)

Section	Arabic term	Subsets	More Subsets	Persian Spelling	Standard Hindi	Arabic	Persian
A. According to virtue or depravity	1. *al-ṣāliḥa* (virtuous)			sūkiyā	svakīya, svīya (one's own wife)	337	118
	2. *al-ṭāliḥa* (depraved)	a. *al-bayṭiyyᵉ* (mistress)		parkiyā	parakīyā (another's wife)	341	121
			1. *al-mukhtafiyya* (hidden)	guptā	gupta (hidden)	341	121
			2. *al-mutasattara* (concealed)	lachchhtā	lakshitā (discovered/found out)	345	121
			3. *al-muʿallana* (naked)	kulatā	kulaṭā (harlot)	345	121
		b. *al-sūqiyya* (prostitute)		sāmānyā	sāmānyā (courtesan)	347	123
B. According to age	1. *al-ṣaghīra* (young)			mugdahā	mugdhā (virgin)	348	124
	2. *al-ghāfila* (heedless)			aggiyātjiūbnān	ajñātayauvanā (heedless of her own youth)	348	124
		a. *aʾl-mutaraqqiyya fil-ḥusn* (exceedingly beautiful)				351	126

(Continued)

(Continued)

Chapter 1. On the types of female lovers (ghizlān)

Section	Arabic term	Subsets	More subsets	Persian spelling	Standard Hindi	Arabic	Persian
		b. al-ghayr al-muta-zayyana (unadorned)				352	127
		c. al-bākira (virginal)				—	127
		d. al-thayyiba (divorced)				—	127
		e. al-nāfira 'an al-jimā' (averse to intercourse)				353	128
	3. al-khabīra (knowing)			giyātjūbnān	jñātayauvanā (knowing youth)	356	128
	4. al-mutawassiṭa (adolescent)			maddhyā	madhya (in between)	356	129
	5. al-kabīra (mature)			paridahā	praurha (mature)	359	130
C. Defined by the complainer	1. al-shākiyya (complainer)			ghandītā	khanditā (enraged over a lover's infidelity)	362	131
		a. al-rāmiza (hinting)		dhīrā	dhīrā (constant in the expression of anger)	362	131
		b. al-muṣarriḥa (blatant)		adhirā	adhirā (lashing out in anger)	365	132

D. Defined by the excited one	1. *al-muḍṭaraba* (excited)	*asārikā, absārikā*	*abhisārikā* (eagerly goes out to meet her lover)	367	133
	a. *al-munaḥhira* (by day)			368	133
	b. *al-ṭāriqa* (by night)	*siyām asārikā*	*syām abhisārikā* (eager in the dark)	369	133
E. Defined by the clever one	1. *al-fāṭina qawlan* (clever in speech)	*bachan bidugdahā*	*bacan vidagdhā* (artful in speech)	374	134
	2. *al-fāṭina fiʿlan* (clever in deed)	*kiryā bidugdahā*	*kiryā vidagdhā* (artful in deed)	—	134
F. Defined by the arrogant one	1. *al-mustakbira* (arrogant)			379	137
	a. *al-mustakbira bi-ḥusnihā* (arrogant about her beauty)	*rūp garbatā*	*rūp garvitā* (proud of form)	379	137
	b. *al-mustakbira bi-muwaddat al-ḥubb* (arrogant with the affection of love)	*pēm garbatā*	*pēm garvitā* (proud of love)	380	138

(Continued)

(Continued)

Chapter 1. On the types of female lovers (ghizlān)

Section	Arabic term	Subsets	More subsets	Persian spelling	Standard Hindi	Arabic	Persian
G. Miscellaneous	1. al-ḥāṣira (preventer)			kachap pankā, kahachchat patikā	gacchyata patikā (tries to prevent husband from leaving)	380	138
	2. al-mutarajji-yya (hopeful)			bāsak sajjayā	vāsaka-sajjā (decorates the bed and waits for her lover to come)	385	139
	3. al-mahjūra (abandoned)			barahini	virahinī (woman alone)	385	—
	4. al-nādima (regretful)			kalhantaritā	kalahantarita (quarreling)	386	139
	5. al-mughtarra (deceived)					388	—

Chapter 2. On the types of female lovers (ghizlān) discovered by the author

Arabic term		Arabic	Persian
1.	*al-zā'irat fil-rū'yā* (visiting in a dream)	390	141
2.	*al-nāfira `an al-shīb* (averse to old age)	391	142
3.	*al-`ā'ida* (returning to nurse the sick lover)	394	142
4.	*al-ghayrī* (jealous)	396	142
5.	*al-khā'ifa min al-wushāt* (fearful of informants)	398	142
6.	*al-muṣghiyya lil-wushāt* (attentive to informants)	398	143
7.	*al-mukhallifa al-wa`da* (breaking the promise)	400	143
8.	*al-a`rābiyya or al-badawiyya* (bedouin, nomadic)	405	143
9.	*al-mursila* (messenger)	407	144

Chapter 4. On the types of male lovers

Arabic term		Persian spelling	Standard Hindi	Arabic	Persian
1.	*al-mustafrid* (monogamous)	*anukūl*	*anukūla*	421	147
2.	*al-mustakthir* (polygamous)	*dachchin*	*dakṣiṇa*	422	148
3.	*al-`afīf* (chaste)			423	149
4.	*al-fāṭin* (clever)*			431	150
5.	*al-ṭāriq* (unexpected visitor)				152
6.	*al-wāṣil* (attaining union)			437	152
7.	*al-mahjūr* (abandoned)*			441	153
8.	*al-muwaddi`* (bidding farewell) or *al-jāzi` min al-widā`* (concerned about farewell)			447	155
9.	*al-sāmir bil-layl* (telling night stories by day)			453	156
10.	*al-muta'ādhī bil-riqba* (offended by observation)			461	158
11.	*al-muta'ādhī bil-wushāt* (offended by informants)			462	—
12.	*al-rāḍī `an jūr al-ḥabīb* (pleased with the lover's oppression)			—	156

(Continued)

(Continued)

Chapter 4. On the types of male lovers

Arabic term	Persian spelling	Standard Hindi	Arabic	Persian
13. *al-shākī min jūr al-ḥabīb* (complaining of the lover's oppression)*			467	157
14. *al-shākī min ʿaynayhi* (complaining with his eyes)			467	157
15. *al-ghayūr* (jealous)*			473	159
16. *al-mughtabiṭ* (rejoicing)			478	—
17. *al-ʿāʾid* (returning to nurse the sick lover)*			478	—
18. *al-mutarajjī* (hopeful)*			479	—
19. *al-masʾūl ʿan ḥālihi* (asked about his state)			*480*	—
20. *al-māʾil ilā ashbāh al-ḥabīb* (inclined toward those who resemble the beloved)			481	—
21. *al-muʿaẓẓim li-āthār al-ḥabīb* (praising traces of the beloved)			483	—
22. *al-bākī ʿalā al-aṭlāl wal-āthār* (weeping over ruins and traces)			487	—
23. *ṣāḥib ḥadīth al-nasīm* (teller of the breeze's story)			507	162
24. *ṣāḥib ḥadīth al-qalb* (teller of the heart's story)			513	160
25. *ṣāḥib ḥadīth al-ṭayf* (teller of the phantom's story)			518	—
26. *al-shātim* (scolder)			521	—
27. *al-dhākir li-ayyām al-ḥummā* (recalling days of fever)			525	—
28. *al-shāʾib al-mutaʾassif ʿalā al-shabāb* (old man regretting youth)			528	—
29. *al-nādhir* (avower, who swears an oath in love)			531	—
30. *al-mūṣī* (testator, leaving postmortem orders to a lover)			531	—
31. *al-mutakallim baʿd al-mawt* (speaking after death)			532	—

* Terms paralleling those in Chapter 1.

22

A Persian Philosophical
Defense of Vedanta

One of the key definitional questions surrounding the relation between philosophy and religion has been whether one can define philosophy by one or another religious identity. In the centuries of interaction between Greek philosophy and the prophetic religious traditions, to what extent is it justifiable to speak of Jewish philosophy, Christian philosophy, and Islamic philosophy? Some prefer the notion of "Arabic philosophy," based upon the language of communication established after the translation of Greek philosophical texts into Arabic under the patronage of the `Abbasid Caliphs and their ministers.[1] This terminology was obviously inadequate, however, when one considered the development of philosophical treatises in Persian, by authors no less than Avicenna; and likewise, the concept of Arabic philosophy failed to take account of the transmission of these texts into Hebrew, which in some cases has preserved the only surviving examples of writings by authors such as Averroes.[2] Moreover, the presence of translators and authors who were Christians, Jews, and even Hellenized pagans, alongside Muslims, as well as the establishment of key philosophical themes in the pre-Islamic era, makes it difficult to describe this movement as "Islamic philosophy" without further qualification. Throughout his career, Seyyed Hossein Nasr

---

[1] *Classical Arabic Philosophy: An Anthology of Sources*, ed. Jon McGinnis and David C. Reisman (Indianapolis, IN: Hackett Publishing Co., 2007), pp. xii-xv.

[2] *Averroes on Plato's Republic*, trans. Ralph Lerner (Ithaca. Cornell University Press, 2005); this is a work written originally in Arabic which survives only in the Hebrew translation.

has persuasively argued for the need to understand Islamic philosophy in terms of "its real nature and its significance as a philosophy that remains aware of the realities of prophecy."[3] Following the suggestions of Henry Corbin, Christian Jambet considers Islamic philosophy to have a cultural connotation rather than a strictly religious identification, since in his view these thinkers "were not philosophers despite Islam, but starting from it, with it, and in it."[4] Others prefer to use Marshall Hodgson's term and speak of Islamicate philosophy, specifically opening the door to the participation of non-Muslims in an intellectual tradition largely formed in relation to a dominant Islamic milieu.[5]

Keeping this problem in mind, it is striking to observe the deployment of philosophical argumentation from the post-Avicenna tradition by a Hindu author writing in Persian on the cusp of the transition between the Mughal Empire and the British colonial regime. Sital Singh, a secretary (*munshi*) in the service of the raja of Benares, was commissioned in 1800 by a British magistrate named John Deane to write a treatise describing the different Indian religious groups found in the city at that time. This took the form of a Persian text in three parts: the first part described 47 different types of ascetic groups (divided into five chapters on Vaishnavas, Shaivas, Shaktas, Sikhs, and Jains); the second part consisted of a philosophical defense of Vedanta; and the third part was an early census of the different religious and professional groups to be found in Benares. The text is known by three different titles found in the three known copies: *Silsila-i jogiyān* or *The Order of Yogis; Fuqarā-yi Hind* or *Ascetics of India;* and *Kāshī nāma* or *The Benares Book*.[6] Since the first of these titles seem to

[3] Seyyed Hossein Nasr, *Islamic Philosophy from Its Origin to the Present: Philosophy in the Land of Prophecy*, SUNY series in Islam (Albany: State University of New York Press, 2006), p. 21. It is noteworthy that the *History of Islamic Philosophy* edited by Oliver Leaman and Seyyed Hossein Nasr for the Routledge History of World Philosophies series (New York: Routledge, 2001) included a major section on Jewish philosophy.

[4] Christian Jambet, *Qu'est-ce que la philosophie islamique?* (Paris: Gallimard, 2011), p. 62.

[5] Steven Wasserstrom, "The Islamic Social and Cultural Context," in *History of Jewish Philosophy*, ed. Daniel Frank and Oliver Leaman (New York: Routledge, 1997), p. 80.

[6] *Silsila-i jogiyān*, MS India Office Library Persian, Ethé 2974, British Library (referred to in the edition below as copy A); *Fuqarā-yi Hind*, MS I.O. Islamic 4777, British Library, described in Ursula Sims-Williams, *Handlist of Islamic manuscripts acquired by the India Office Library 1938-85* (London: India Office Library and Records, 1986), p. 20 (=copy B); and Sital Singh Munshi, *Kāshī nāma*, ed Munshi Harbans La'l and Bhairav Parshad (Benares: Matba`-i Mufad-i Hind, 1854), (copy P). The latter text, a lithograph surviving in a single copy at the Bibliotheque Nationale in Paris, may be consulted online at

be marginally better known, I will refer to this work as *Silsila-i jogiyān* or *The Order of Yogis*. It is an important source for the understanding of Indian religious groups, and it was one of two Persian texts on Hinduism, written by Hindu authors, that formed key sources for the first major work in English written about the religions of India, H. H. Wilson's *Sketch of the Religious Sects of the Hindus* (1828-32).[7]

Sital Singh was an outstanding member of the secretarial class of munshis who served the Mughal emperors and lesser sovereigns thanks to their mastery over Persian language and literature. The bureaucratic apparatus that ruled India from the sixteenth to the nineteenth century drew heavily upon Hindu scholars from certain castes, principally Kayasths, Khatris, and Brahmins. These Persianate Hindus were part of the Persian "monopoly on literacy," based on statecraft and literature, that stretched from the Balkans to Bengal.[8] While these secretaries were expected to know accounting as part of the taxation system, their education was saturated with the classics of Persian poetry, epistolography, and ethics. To judge from the curriculum recommended by the famous Chandrabhan "Brahman" in a letter to his son, a successful munshi would possess an encyclopedic knowledge of Persian poetry as well as the ethical writings of Sa`di, Jami, and many others.[9] Sital Singh was clearly well educated in this tradition. He was also the author of a significant body of Persian poetry written in a Sufi vein, under the pen name "Bikhwud" ("selfless" or "egoless"), as well as a collection of mystical aphorisms. His writings included, remarkably, a commentary on the Arabic verses from the signature work on prophetology by the famous Andalusian Sufi, Ibn

---

<http://gallica.bnf.fr/ark:/12148/bpt6k852849n>. In the translation below, parenthetical transliterations of terms are identified by language: A. = Arabic; P. = Persian; H. - Hindi.

[7] Wilson's second Persian source on Indian religions written by a Hindu author was the *Riyaz al-mazahib (Gardens of Religious Teachings)* composed by Mathuranath in 1812. See Ilyse R. Morgenstein Fuerst, "Religions of Empire: Islamicate Texts, Imperial Taxonomies, and South Asian Definitions of Religion," PhD dissertation, University of North Carolina at Chapel Hill, 2012.

[8] Brian Spooner and William L. Hanaway, ed., *Literacy in the Persianate World: Writing and the Social Order* (Philadelphia: University of Pennsylvania Press, 2012).

[9] Muzaffar Alam & Sanjay Subrahmanyam, "The Making of a Munshi," *Comparative Studies of South Asia, Africa and the Middle East,* 24:2 (2004), pp. 61–72. See also S. A. Abidi, "Čandra Bhān (or Čandarbhān Barahman)," *Encyclopaedia Iranica* (New York: Columbia University Press, 1990), 4:755–756, available online at http://www.iranicaonline.org/articles/candra-bhan-or-candarbhan-barahman-indian-poet-and-writer-in-persian-b, accessed 23 February 2015.

`Arabi (d. 1240), *Fusus al-hikam* or *Bezels of Wisdom*. His disciple Ram Sita Singh "Fikrat" evidently wrote a Persian biography of Sital Singh under the title *The Realities of the Selfless (Haqiqat-ha-yi Bi-khwud)*, published in 1848 in Lucknow, but this is unfortunately lost.[10] The collected writings of Sital Singh appeared in 1871 as *The Imagination of Selflessness (Khayal-i Bi-khwudi)*.[11] Moreover, in addition to his immersion in Sufi poetry and metaphysics, Sital Singh's cosmopolitan tendencies also expressed themselves in his close friendship with the Greek scholar Demetrios Galanos, who resided in Benares from 1793 until his death in 1833 (Sital Singh was the executor of Galanos's will, and he composed a Persian quatrain as an epitaph for Galanos, calling him "the Plato of the age"). Galanos had the distinction of having translated numerous Sanskrit texts, including the *Devi Mahatmya* (an important work on the Goddess), into modern Greek.[12]

Sital Singh's engagement with philosophy evidently drew upon the strong intellectual emphasis of the Dars-i Nizami curriculum that was prevalent in India in the eighteenth and early nineteenth century, a field that is only just being explored by modern scholars. Major elements in this curriculum included the philosophical writings of Safavid authors such as Mir Damad and Mulla Sadra, as well as the Sufi teachings of Ibn `Arabi as mediated by his most important Indian commentator, Shah Muhibb

---

[10] Sayyid `Abd Allah, *Adabiyat-i farsi men Hindu'on ka hissa* (2nd ed., New Delhi: Anjuman-i Taraqqi-i Urdu, 1992), p. 241. A copy of *Haqiqat-ha-yi Bi-khwud* was formerly preserved in Calcutta; see Mawlavi Mirza Ashraf Ali, *A Catalogue of the Persian Books and Manuscripts in the Library of the Asiatic Society of Bengal* (Fasciculus I, Calcutta, 1890), p. 92, new no. Na37, old no. 1393, with the following description: Halat-i Munshi Sital Singh Bi-khwud-i Ba-Khuda (The life of Munshi Sital Singh, without self, but with God). No trace of the book can be found in the Asiatic Society library today.

[11] This volume, published in Lucknow in 1871 by Newal Kishor, contains the following: *Nukat-i Bi-khwudi* (mystical aphorisms, pp. 2-11); lyrical poems or ghazals (pp. 12–46), quatrains and rhyming couplets (pp. 47–60), the commentary on the Arabic verses in Ibn `Arabi's *Fusus al-hikam* (pp. 61–78), *Sharh-i Umm al-Asma'* on the Arabic names of God (pp. 79–81), and a postscript on mysticism entitled *Rumuz al-`arifin* (p. 82). The text is available online at http://babel.hathitrust.org/cgi/pt?view=image;size=100;id=njp.321010 76496478;page=root;seq=28;num=28.

[12] Siegfried A. Schulz, "Demetrios Galanos (1760-1833): A Greek Indologist," *Journal of the American Oriental Society*, 89/2 (April–June 1969), pp. 339–56, esp. p. 354; id., "The Devi-Mahatmya in Greek: D. Galanos' Translation," *Purana* 24/1 (1982), pp. 7–40, esp. p. 8. Schulz records that Sital Singh was probably born in 1776 and died on 18 December 1854, though his source for this information is unclear.

Allah Ilahabadi.[13] But from the perspective of a Hindu author, the madrasa tradition also reflected the problematic relationship between Greek and Indian thought over many centuries. Leaving aside the encounters between Alexander the Great and the gymnosophists, it is striking to see that Arab authors such as al-Biruni and al-Shahrastani approached Indian thinkers with the assumption that they were deeply influenced by the Greek philosopher Pythagoras, both in science and in the doctrine of reincarnation.[14] This assumption of a Greek source for Indian philosophy must have irritated the Indians who noticed it. Such seems to be the implication of a Persian text attributed to the Mughal poet Fayzi, *Shariq al-ma`rifa* or *The Illuminator of Gnosis*. There we are told that the situation was quite the reverse; Plato in fact learned illuminationist wisdom (*hikmat-i ishraqiyya*) as a student of Tumtum the Indian, a disciple of Swami Vyasa, the legendary author of the Vedas.[15] This contention over who has precedence in philosophy may help explain the strategy of Sital Singh in employing the resources of post-Avicenna argumentation to defend Indian philosophy.

Sital Singh was not the only Hindu intellectual of his day to draw upon the Persian intellectual tradition to elaborate Hindu philosophical positions. His contemporary, the Bengali reformer Raja Ram Mohan Roy, was also trained in the madrasa tradition, and indeed his first literary production, the *Tuhfat al-muwahhidin (Gift to the Monotheists)*, was written in Persian, with a preface in Arabic. Roy's treatise, which was first published in 1803, employed rationalistic arguments to criticize superstitious practices in Hinduism, so his polemical project of Hindu reform differed from Sital Singh's apologia in defense of a Vedantic monist theology. Yet, it is striking that both thinkers employed some of the same standard phrases from Arabic/Islamic philosophical texts, such as the notion in causality of "a preference without a reason" (*tarjih bi-lā murajjih*), which is considered to be self-contradictory and hence

---

[13] Sajjad H. Rizvi, "Mīr Dāmād in India: Islamic Philosophical Traditions and the Problem of Creation," *Journal of the American Oriental Society* 131/1 (2011), pp. 9–23; G. A. Lipton, *"The Equivalence" (Al-Taswiya) of Muhibb Allah Ilahabadi: Avicennan Neoplatonism and the School of Ibn 'Arabi in South Asia* (Saarbruecken: VDM Verlag, 2009.).

[14] Abu al-Fath ibn `Abd al-Karim al-Shahrastani, *Kitab al-Milal wa al-Nihal*, ed. Muhammad Fath Allah Badran (2 vols, Cairo: Maktaba al-Anglo al-Misriyya, 1366–1375/1947–1955), 2:270.

[15] Carl W. Ernst, "Fayzi's Illuminationist Interpretation of Vedanta: The *Shariq al-Ma`rifa*," *Comparative Studies of South Asia, Africa and the Middle East* 30/3 (2010), pp. 156–64.

impossible.[16] There are numerous other Persian texts on Indian religions, written by Hindu scholars who were educated in the late Mughal intellectual curriculum, but they have yet to be analyzed for their role in the evolution of religious identities in the colonial era.

Indeed, from his other writings it is clear that Sital Singh's immersion in Sufism was also fraught with an unavoidable tension between his Hindu status and the obvious expressions of Islamic loyalty that permeate Sufi literature. While Sital Singh was deeply engaged with the dialectical arguments of Ibn 'Arabi, his Persian poetry is filled with references to mystical idolatry, in a tone that seems more than merely ironic. Consider the following ghazal:

> I have nothing but the beloved's light, by God!
>
> I have no other friend but you, by God!
>
> I'm always drunk on the wine of your beauty,
>
> I have no sober heart, by God!
>
> Love made me sorrowful and sad,
>
> I have no other sufferings, by God!
>
> From the fever of your love comes helplessness;
>
> I cannot deny anyone, by God!
>
> I am the slave of the love of idols, Bi-khwud;
>
> I have nothing to do with God, by God![17]

When Sital Singh calls himself "the slave of the love of idols," the reader who knows the poet is a Hindu inevitably understands this as more than a literary conceit.

Moreover, in a short Persian text on the 7 chief Arabic names of God, Sital Singh comments on what is unmistakably the mystical notion of the Perfect Human (*insan-i kamil*) according to Ibn 'Arabi, but his

---

[16] An extensive discussion of this phrase is found at *Danishnama-i Jahan-i Islam* (Mu'assasa-i Da'irat al-Ma'arif al-Fiqh al-Islami), 1:3442, available online at <http://lib.eshia.ir/23019/1/3442>, accessed 25 May 2015. The phrase is quoted in the text and translation below, 6.4; and also in Raja Rammohun Roy, *Tuhfatu'l-Muwahhidin* (Calcutta, s.n., 1950), pp. 1, 8; English trans., Obaidullah El Obaide, *Rammohun Roy and Tuhfatul Muwahhiddin* (Calcutta: K. P. Bagchi & Company, 1975), pp. 3, 14.

[17] *Khayal-i Bikhwudi*, pp. 12–13.

remarks betray a significant reservation about restricting it to a particular historical manifestation:

> It is not hidden that, however much the manifestation of all these influences and attributes, which exist by reason of the blessed names, is seen in the comprehensive existence, that is, the revered human (*hazrat-i insan*), in a most complete and most perfect aspect, and in the same way in the noblest of creation and the Vicegerent of the Merciful (*khalifat al-rahman*), nevertheless, since the cause of the effects of the blessed names is not in a single time or place, the manifestation of the influences of these names is according to difference in capacity and substratum, so it is evident everywhere.[18]

By insisting that the vicegerency of God is not limited to "a single time or place," i.e., to the Prophet Muhammad, Sital Singh appears to argue that the Sufi concept of the divine names needs to be understood in a universal fashion that is not limited to Islam.

In any case, Sital Singh begins his disquisition on Vedanta in the sixth chapter of the *Silsila-i jogiyan* with an offhand and dismissive remark about superficial religious attachments. After having described 47 varieties of Indian ascetic in the first portion of the text, he then comments that "all these different religious teachings (*madāhib*) and various faiths (*adyān*), which have been written about for the comprehension of seekers and students, only differ and diverge in terms of external correctness, ego-display, and showing off" (6.1). This dismissive comment is indeed matched by the sarcastic and disapproving tone, with which, in earlier sections of the text, Sital Singh regularly criticized the supposed ascetics who find ways to gratify their desires. He then proceeds to assert that Vedanta, which he equates with theology (*ilāhiyyat*), is the basis of all Hindu teachings and beliefs (*mu`taqadāt*).

Sital Singh's account of Vedanta is in fact cursory in the extreme, and he makes only the vaguest gestures toward Hindu traditions, invoking the deities Vishnu, Mahadeva, and Brahma, along with the sage Vyasa. Without making any specific reference to particular schools of Vedantic philosophy, Sital Singh merely asserts that the teaching of "the extensive books of divinity and volumes (*pūthē*) of Vedanta" is clear to everyone. And it basically amounts to a simplified version of Advaita

---

[18] *Khayal-i Bikhwudi*, p. 81.

Vedanta, arguing that the world of appearances is nothing less than the essence of God. Moreover, from his incidental remark that most of these texts have been translated into Persian, one begins to suspect that Sital Singh may have been more comfortable with those Persian translations than with the Sanskrit originals. In addition, the language used in this presentation owes practically nothing to the technical vocabulary of Sanskrit philosophy. All is subsumed under a theological framework expressed entirely through Islamic references.

The argument for demonstrating the unity of the creator and the world (6.4-9) proceeds through examples that would have been familiar to anyone trained in the post-Avicenna tradition of philosophy. Sital Singh first insists on a necessary existence as the cause of possible effects. He handles the old emanationist problem of deriving multiplicity from unity by allowing for intermediate causes that do not negate the ultimate causality of the necessary being. He then summarizes Aristotle's classic example of the making of a clay pot as an illustration of the 4 causes (material, formal, efficient, and final). This section is neatly capped by an anonymous Persian verse using the same imagery of the pot, which has the effect of shifting the whole discussion in a monistic direction.

Sital Singh returns (6.8) to the question of the creation of multiplicity in terms of the celestial spheres which Muslim philosopher-scientists postulated to account for the apparently wayward motion of the planets. Here it is the outermost "encompassing (muḥīṭ)" heaven (introduced by a Qur'anic phrase) that provides motion and hence change for all living beings. By invoking the phrase "substantial changes" (taġayyurāt-i jawhariyya), Sital Singh also effectively alludes to Mulla Sadra's theory of "substantial motion" as another explanation of change. In his view, temporal and eternal are differing forms of the same underlying material elements.

The emanation of the faculties that distinguish the animal from the vegetable and the mineral is explained (6.10) as a necessary effect of the eternal essence, rather than the coming to be of possibilities. This line of reasoning allows Sital Singh to introduce the concept of the indwelling (ḥulūl) of the subtle cause in creation, a term with weighty consequences. This hidden essence, he argues, can only be perceived by the intellect – a point he tries to clinch by quoting a popular Persian verse on how one can only see the overwhelming beauty of the sun through a veil.

Sital Singh's bold and repeated use of the term ḥulūl (6.10-11) is a calculated appropriation of a term largely considered anathema by

Muslim thinkers, and generally equated with the Christian doctrine of incarnation.[19] So when he triumphantly announces that "the essence of the Creator is indwelling in the sun, the moon, and the rest of the manifestation of possibilities," he is in effect proclaiming a pantheism that most readers would see as shocking heresy, at least when stated as a formal proposition. But he cleverly cushions this pronouncement with another line of poetry, this time from the great Sufi poet 'Iraqi, declaring that God "is the essence of all things."

The concluding paragraphs of this treatise drive home the point with further insistence. The unity of water in all its forms is juxtaposed with quotations from the Qur'an and hadith to underline the idea that the Creator becomes imminent in creation through his imagination. While the outcome of this presentation is evidently a univocal assertion of the unity of God and existence, in closing, Sital Singh coyly refers to many other Vedantic teachings "on the affirmation and negation, and the isolation and transcendence, of the essence of the Creator." That final sentence is latent with subtler and more ambiguous possibilities that are unexplored here.

The formal character of Sital Singh's argument begs the question of what his ultimate purpose was in writing this section of *The Order of Yogis*. Although we cannot be sure of the chronology of his writings, this simplistic presentation of Vedantic theology contrasts oddly with his much more sophisticated commentary on the poems of Ibn 'Arabi. There, and also in his own epigrams, Sital Singh exhibited a highly sensitive approach to the problem of describing God, always balancing one assertion with its paradoxical opposite.

It is tempting to see in this manifesto a rhetorical gesture of defiance, by a subaltern participant in the dominant discourse of Persianate culture. Sital Singh as a munshi attained an extraordinary expertise in some of the key intellectual resources of Indo-Islamic thought, and indeed it is difficult to think of another Hindu scholar who was so deeply engaged with both Sufism and Islamic philosophy. Yet, he remained a Hindu, and in his proud declaration of his mastery in Persian, he is fully comparable to those non-Arabs of the Shu'ubiyya who demonstrated their superiority to the Arabs, precisely through their superior control of Arabic. In a similar fashion, Sital Singh produced a philosophical tour de force in

---

[19] Ahmad Pakatchi, "Hulul," *The Great Islamic Encyclopaedia* 21:306–8, http://www.cgie.org.ir/fa/publication/entryview/16164.

Persian, blithely defending what he identified as the foundation of Hindu teachings, by using a key term—indwelling or incarnation—that Muslim thinkers would instinctively reject. In other words, this brief exposition is an explicitly Hindu appropriation of the argumentation of Islamic philosophical theology, spiced with adroitly chosen lines of Sufi poetry to soften the blow. At the same time, it is an undeniable homage both to the intellectual rigor of the philosophical tradition and to the mystical insights of Sufism. To be sure, the way that Sital Singh turns to key Sufi concepts at crucial points reveals his deep connection to the Sufi way.

Yet, there is a deeper irony surrounding this brief philosophical pamphlet. It is not accidental that the work of Sital Singh has lain forgotten for two centuries. After all, the British magistrate, John Deane, had only asked Sital Singh to produce a census, an enumeration of the population of Benares according to profession and religion, which would be helpful to the expanding British colonial regime in India. The census section of *The Order of Yogis* was in fact the only portion of the text that has appeared in an English publication.[20] The description of the 47 kinds of ascetics of Benares, and the defense of Vedanta, were ignored. Sital Singh had mastered a tradition that was soon to become irrelevant.

Much more could be said regarding the distinctive literary contribution of this prodigy of the late Indo-Persian world. There is something poignant about a Hindu munshi demonstrating his proficiency in Islamic philosophy and Sufi thought, just at the moment when new expressions of Hindu identity were being articulated, doubtless drawing on Sanskrit sources but inescapably formed under the sign of British colonialism. Yet fundamentally this philosophical treatise by Sital Singh demonstrates the amplitude of that tradition of Islamic – or Islamicate – philosophy, with which he had the antagonistic attitude of an advanced initiate. It was Sital Singh's goal to press Avicenna and Mulla Sadra into the service of Brahma, Mahesh, and Vishnu, and indeed, for a moment, he succeeded.

* * *

---

[20] George, Viscount Valentia, *Voyages and travels to India, Ceylon, the Red Sea, Abyssinia, and Egypt, in the years 1802, 1803, 1804, 1805, and 1806* (London, Printed for F., C., and J. Rivington, 1811), 4:407–11.

TRANSLATION

6. [Section on the Principles of Vedanta or Theology]

6.1. It is neither hidden nor concealed from the realizers of the mysteries of gnosis and the wayfarers of the path of reality that all these different religious teachings (*maḏāhib*) and various faiths (*adyān*), which have been written about for the comprehension of seekers and students, only differ and diverge in terms of external correctness, ego-display, and showing off. Otherwise in reality the fundamental path (*ṭarīq*) and teaching of truth (*maḏhab-i ḥaqq*) has no difference, and that is Vedanta, i.e., theology (A. *ilāhiyāt*), which is for all the teachings of the Hindus and is accepted by visionaries and experts. One who knows that is called a Vedanti, i.e., a sage and philosopher (P. *ḥakīm o faylasūf*). However much the author deserved to glance first at their greatness and stature, in order to write about the conditions of this teaching and the high praises of its pure jewels, he purified and honored the tongue of his pen. But because immanence after transcendence (P. *tashbīh ba'd-i tanzīh*) is the cause of prolixity and vanity, thus, truth has no end, and its discussion is suspended. So thinking to complete this treatise, he has produced a few lines on their realities.

6.2. Now Vedanta, i.e., the end of the Veda (H. *bed*) is the uttermost divine core (P. *lubb-i lubāb-i albāb-i ilāhī*), and in the beliefs of the Hindus (P. *mu'taqadāt-i Hinduvān*) this is the chosen teaching of Vishnu, Mahadeva, and Brahma, who are the authors of destiny (P. *kārkunān-i taqdīr*). But the manifestation of this treasure in this perishable abode and its composition in fact is this very grace of Vyasa, whom they consider one of the 24 avatars of Vishnu; that is, Vishnu himself, having become embodied in the form of Vyasa, gave instruction and guidance of that delight of all creatures to Brahmins and Rishis. Although the reality of this teaching, in commentary and explanation from the extensive books of divinity and volumes (H. *pūthē*) of Vedanta, which have been mostly translated into the Persian language, is clear and obvious to enlightened observers, yet here is a summary by way of abbreviation and abridgement.

6.3. This world they treat like affairs occurring in a dream. In certainty and proof, whatever is heard and seen they consider the very essence of

God (P. *'ayn-i dāt-i ḥaqq*). They are always happy and carefree. With demonstrated proofs they have well confirmed that the creator of the world, having taken on the form of the world, is manifest in diverse colors and manifold forms, with the following proofs:

6.4. There is a necessary cause for originated effects, and an undoubted creator of possible creations. If the effect were its own cause, it is apparent that the cause precedes the effect, otherwise "a thing preceding itself" (A. *taqaddum al-shay' 'ala nafsihi*) necessarily follows. If the existentiating cause is other than the effect, they say it is temporal, or else eternal. If it is temporal, that is "a preference without a reason" (A. *tarjīḥ bi-lā murajjiḥ*), because when both are in temporality on the same level, why is the existence of one dependent on the other? And if some possible beings are cause and effect of each other, or each is the cause of the other in turn, that assumes circular reasoning (A. *mustalzim al-dawr wal-tasalsul*), which is false. Thus the existentiating cause [as shown] by investigation is eternal. And if they say the creative forms are possible beings and the active cause is effective, they too are possible beings. Then the possible would be the cause of the possible, that is, the temporal is the cause of the temporal. Likewise for multiple effects, one cause cannot be sufficient, because "from the one only one action proceeds."[21]

6.5. The response is that in reality here the eternal is the cause of the temporal through multiplicities, and multiplicities are called the intermediate cause. Thus A is the cause of B, and B is the cause of C, and C is the cause of D, and D is the cause of E.[22] The proximate influence of E is D, but the first cause is A, and the rest that come in between are intermediaries. So in reality A is the cause of E. Likewise a carpenter who carves wood with an axe, for the shape of the wood, if the axe is the proximate cause, but in reality it is the effect of the carpenter on the wood, and the axe is the intermediate cause from the conditions of the influence of the effective cause. Even so, the human is part of the complete cause (P. *'illat-i tāmma*), for the creative forms come into manifestation from the complete cause by human intermediary, motions, and resting. In this

---

[21] This is the famous principle of emanation in Neoplatonic philosophy, that a unitary being (such as an intellect) produces only one sequel.

[22] The Persian text uses letters of the Arabic alphabet as examples, which are replaced here with Latin letters.

there is no insufficiency (P. *iftiqār*) of the complete cause, for it is a single cause that makes its effect the cause for another effect, and it for another, etc. Thus, no insufficiency is implied.

6.6. It is like a particle of fire that falls into a cotton warehouse, and makes its abode like itself and fills it. Then another particle comes into existence, and from that another particle, etc.; many sparks become visible. If a great spark did not at once come to be from that first particle, nevertheless gradually that first particle or numerous multiplicities is a cause for the existence of the spark. But since that first particle went from unity to multiplicity, even so it became overwhelmed in its effects, for its distinction was excused by that great spark.

6.7. By way of comparison, one can make the same analogy, between the essence of the Creator, who is the Real One, and the rest of possible beings. The certain becomes conclusive, for the existentiating cause for the world is one, which is absolutely eternal and omnipotent in truth, and they call that the cause, because the existence of a thing depends upon it. This [cause] is of two types: complete and incomplete. The incomplete [cause] is of 4 kinds: material, formal, efficient, and final. The material [cause] is like the clay of a vessel for the vessel. The formal [cause] is similar to the shape of the vessel. The efficient [cause] is its maker, and the final [cause] is the drinking of water, or whatever purpose for the success of which the vessel was made. The complete cause for the vessel is the totality of these 4 causes. Thus, the pure essence (P. *ḏāt-i baḥt*) is the complete cause for the existentiation of the world.

> "He is the pot, he is the potter, and he is the pot's clay;
>
> He came as the buyer for the sake of that pot."[23]

6.8. If it is said, "The complete cause of the world of the possible is always the necessary essence, which manifests by reason of '[He is] encompassing (*muḥīṭ*) all things' [Qur. 41:54], so how do changes come to pass?" We say, it is the ninth heaven, which moves every day of its own volition, by following which the other heavens also have compulsory motions. From one morning to the next, the diverse positions of the heavens and the planets occur. Thus, the four elements, which are encompassed in the midst of that, therefore undergo change from the

---

[23] This verse, though quite popular, still circulates anonymously.

changes of the encompassing [heaven]. But these changes are accidental; "substantial changes" is an expression for removing one form and putting on another form, which they call "generation and corruption."[24] It is like the spark of a lamp that occasionally becomes air, removing the fiery form and putting on the form of air. But it remains the same one matter on which diverse forms descended. That matter is "now as it was" (A. *al-ān kamā kāna*). In reality, matter is a single element, and when the forms of those 4 [elements] left one form, they found another form. This continuous habit has always happened, happens, and will happen.

6.9. Even so is the human form and other elemental compositions, which after death with the passage of time become earth, that is, the specific form is nonexistent and the generic form, which is earth, is existent. They call these very changes nonexistence and existence, death and life. This removal and putting on, that is, the changes, will never be suspended, because their complete cause is eternal, and their effects undergo no real annihilation. This is because their complete cause is unending and necessary existence (A. *lā zawāl wa wājib al-wujūd*), so existing elemental things on the basis of their own specificity and genericality are eternal, and on the basis of their singularity and individuality they are temporal. The meaning of temporality and eternity is specific forms, not matter and substance.

6.10. From the composition of the four elements, to the degree of capacity and conformity with conditions, the temperaments of different faculties become apparent in composites, that is, in only certain bodies there is a faculty that protects the specific form, such as the mineral. Others have a nutritive (A. *nāmiyya*) faculty, like plants, and to some two faculties are added, such as perception and voluntary motion, and they are called animals. If along with that the faculty of reason (A. *nuṭq*) is added, it becomes human. By this analogy, by adding faculties they call it nobler and more sublime. The emanation of possibilities does not mean that they were before nonexistence, and then afterward emanated, because this is impossible. For the complete cause was existent and the effect was not, so it is established that the emanation of effects is necessary, because its essence is eternal. It is like the ray of the sun, and heat of the fire,

---

[24] "Generation and corruption" (A. *kawn wa fasād*), the title of a work by Aristotle, is synonymous with the world of ordinary existence.

whose separation from their essence is impossible. Inasmuch as the subtle cannot be perceived, that is, the external senses cannot grasp it except by intellect, because the pure essence, like the fire that permeates charcoal by indwelling (A. *ḥulūl*) with such subtlety that it is not seen on its own (A. *bi-ra'sihi*), like fire that is not seen on its own without location. How can one distinguish something from fire that is indwelling in the fire? For example, there is color and quality in fire, and the extinction of the fire is from the charcoal; the loss of color and quality indicates that there is no fire. But something that is colorless and without quality, and altogether more subtle than fire—how then can one perceive it indwelling in all existing things, except by intellection? That is, the intellect can comprehend. Verse:

> "One cannot see your beauty's perfection without a veil,
>
> for without the hand's protection, one cannot see the sun!"[25]

6.11. For its indwelling in possible compositions, lofty and lowly, simple and complex, light and dark, small and great, and other conditions and quantities, indicates that its reality is like the example of a storehouse in which there is wood, straw, stone, gold, silver, and other different things. Fire falls within, and by the influence of heat it makes everything equally hot, but each of these things will be different in quantity, smoothness, roughness, smallness, and greatness, to the measure of its substance, like the light of a lamp and a great torch are in reality similar in heat and light, but different because of greater or lesser capacity. Even so, the essence of the Creator is indwelling in the sun, the moon, and the rest of the manifestation of possibilities. Thus, it is established and verified that he is in all (P. *dar hama ūst*). Verse:

> "His jealousy left no other in the world; surely he is the essence of all things."[26]

6.12. The spirit of ice, which is a metaphor for its internal aspect, which is water, and the existence of ice, which is an expression for its external

---

[25] With slight variations, going back to a quatrain by Abu Sa'id ibn Abi-l Khayr, this verse seems to have circulated anonymously with some popularity. It is sometimes attributed to Gulban-i Afshar, a poet of 18th-century Persia.

[26] This verse is by the famous Persian poet 'Iraqi (d. 1289), and it is taken from one of his stanzaic poems (P, *tarjī'āt*) which carries the refrain, "For all is he, it's certain, all that is – soul, beloved, lover, heart, and faith." The full poem is available at http://ganjoor.net/eraghi/divane/tarjeeate/sh2/ (accessed February 28, 2014).

aspect, are certainly the same water, for in the same ice, that is, in the external and internal ice, there is nothing but water. "He is the outer, he is the inner" (Qur'an 57:3). From water he became manifest, and he is on water, in water, and he is the essence of water. He does not have anything from himself and in himself; it is from his imagination (A. *wahm*) that he brings himself into the middle on the basis of individuation (A. *ta'ayyun*). But his individuation is also the very same he. If one knows, how perfect! And if one does not know, what is lost? Because of the assumptions of "One who has known himself has known his Lord,"[27] the perfection of ice lies in knowing one's own essentiality and locality.

6.13. So it is not concealed that the few lines that have been written on the theories and opinions of the Vedantis, that is, their philosophy, is [only] a handful sample out of a heavy load. Otherwise, there are many examples of this teaching on the affirmation and negation, and the isolation and transcendence, of the essence of the Creator. At this point, so much can be considered sufficient.

---

[27] A well-known Arabic saying attributed to the Prophet Muhammad and very popular among Sufis.

Bibliography of the Publications of Carl W. Ernst

BOOKS

How to Read the Qur'an: A New Guide with Select Translations. Chapel Hill, NC: University of North Carolina Press, 2011.
- UK edition, Edinburgh: University of Edinburgh Press, 2012.

Following Muhammad: Rethinking Islam in the Contemporary World. Chapel Hill, NC: University of North Carolina Press, 2003.
- Excerpt: "Spiritual Life," reprinted in *A Companion to Muslim Cultures*, ed. Amyn B. Sajoo (London: I. B. Tauris, 2011), pp. 57–75.
- Persian translation by Ghasem Kakaie: *Iqtida bi-Muhammad: Nigarishi naw bi-islam dar jahan-i mu`asir*, Tehran: Hermes Press, 2011. Co-Winner of Book of the Year prize from the Iranian Ministry of Culture, 2011.
- Persian translation by Hasan Nura'i Bidukht: *Iqtida bi-Muhammad: Baz andishi-yi islam dar jahan-ı mu`asir*, Tehran: Intishirat-i Haqiqat, 1389/2011. Co-Winner of Book of the Year prize from the Iranian Ministry of Culture, 2011.
- Arabic translation by Hamza Halayqa `Ala nahj Muhammad: I`adat al-tafkir fil-Islam fil-`alam al-mu`asir, Beirut: Arab Scientific Publishers, 2008.
- German translation by Kurt Maier, *Mohammed folgen: Der Islam in der modernen Welt.* Goettingen: Vandenhoeck & Ruprecht GmbH & Co., 2007.
- Turkish translation by Cangüzel Zülfikar: *Hz. Muhammed'in Yolunda: Günümüz Dünyasında İslâmiyeti Yeniden Düşünmek,* Istanbul: Okuyan Us, 2005.
- Korean translation, Seoul: Simsan Munhwa, 2005.
- India edition, New Delhi: Yoda Books, 2005.
- UK edition: *Rethinking Islam In the Contemporary World.* Edinburgh: University of Edinburgh Press, 2004.

Sufi Martyrs of Love: Chishti Sufism in South Asia and Beyond (co-authored with Bruce B. Lawrence). New York: Palgrave Press, 2002.
  • Excerpt: "What is a Sufi Order?", pp. 11–26. In *Sufism*, ed. Lloyd Ridgeon, Critical Concepts in Islamic Studies (London: Routledge, 2008), vol. 1, essay 11.
Teachings of Sufism. Boston: Shambhala Publications, 1999, an anthology of translations from Arabic, Persian, and Urdu.
  • India edition, New Delhi: Rupa & Co., 2005.
  • Turkish translation, Istanbul: Dharma Yayinlari, forthcoming.
Guide to Sufism. Boston: Shambhala Publications, 1997.
  • Russian translation by M. R. Platonov: *Sufizm: Misticheskii Islam.* Moscow: Eksmo/Nashe Slovo, 2012.
  • New edition: *Sufism: An Introduction to Islamic Mysticism.* Boston: Shambhala Publications, 2010.
  • Russian translation by A. Gorkavago: *Sufizm.* Moscow: Fair-Press, 2002.
  • Persian translation of chapter 1 by Ma`suma Amin-Dihqan, "Tarikhche-yi vorud-i mafhum-i tasavvuf ba-gharb," in `Irfan-i Iran* 13 (Tehran: Intisharat-i Haqiqat, 2002), pp. 100–121.
  • Greek translation by Sophia Leibadopolou: *Souphismos.* Athens: Ekdoseis Archetypo, 2001.
  • Italian translation by Laura Franco: *Il grande libro della sapienza sufi.* Milan: Oscar Saggi Mondadori, 2000.
  • India edition, New Delhi: Rupa & Co., 2000.
  • Spanish translation by Joan Carles Guix: *Sufismo*, Guías de Sabiduría Oriental, 4. Barcelona: Oniro, 1999.
Ruzbihan Baqli. *The Unveiling of Secrets: Diary of a Sufi Master.* Translated from the Arabic by Carl W. Ernst. Chapel Hill NC: Parvardigar Press, 1997.
Ruzbihan Baqli: Mysticism and the Rhetoric of Sainthood in Persian Sufism. Curzon Sufi Series, 4. London: Curzon Press, 1996.
  • Revised Persian translation and notes by Kurus Divsalar: *Ruzbihan Baqli, tajriba-i `irfani va shath-i vilayat dar tasavvuf-i irani.* Tehran: Amir Kabir, 2004.
  • Persian translation by Majdoddin Keyvani: *Ruzbihan Baqli, `irfan va shath-i awliya' dar tasavvuf-i islami.* Tehran: Nashr-i Markaz, 1999.
Eternal Garden: Mysticism, History, and Politics at a South Asian Sufi Center. SUNY Series in Muslim Spirituality in South Asia. State University of New York Press, 1992.
  • Excerpt: "The Textual Formation of Oral Teachings in the Early Chishti Order" (pp 62–77), Persian trans. Mas`ud Faryamanish, in *A'ineh-i puzhuhish* 25/4 (1393/2015), pp. 5–14.
  • Excerpt: "The Indian Environment and the Question of Conversion." In Raziuddin Aquil, ed., *Sufism and Society in Medieval India,* Debates in Indian History and Society Series (New Delhi: Oxford University Press, 2010), pp. 82–101.
  • 2nd edition, New Delhi: Oxford University Press, 2004.

Words of Ecstasy in Sufism. SUNY Series in Islam. Albany: State University of New York Press, 1985.
  • Excerpt: "Topics and Forms of Expression," pp. 25–45. In *Sufism*, ed. Lloyd Ridgeon, Critical Concepts in Islamic Studies (London: Routledge, 2008), vol. 1, essay 9.
  • 2nd edition, New Delhi: Yoda Press, forthcoming.
Malay translation, Kuala Lumpur: S. Abdul Majeed & Co, 1994.

EDITED VOLUMES

Co-Editor (with Fabrizio Speziale), *Perso-Indica. An Analytical Survey of Persian Works on Indian Learned Traditions* (Leiden: E. J. Brill, and New Delhi: Oxford University Press, forthcoming in 2017).
Editor, *Islamophobia in America: The Anatomy of Intolerance* (Palgrave-McMillan, 2013).
Co-Editor (with Richard C. Martin), *Rethinking Islamic Studies: From Post-Orientalism to Cosmopolitanism* (Columbia SC: University of South Carolina Press, 2010); co-author of "Introduction: Toward a Post-Orientalist Islamic Approach to Islamic Religious Studies" (pp. 1–22) and author of "The Perils of Civilizational Islam in Malaysia" (pp. 266–80).
Pakistan at the Millennium, edited by Charles Kennedy, Kathleen McNeil, Carl Ernst, and David Gilmartin. Karachi: Oxford University Press, 2003.
Associate editor (with Grace Martin Smith), *Manifestations of Sainthood in Islam.* Istanbul: The Isis Press, 1993; also principal author of "Introduction," pp. xi–xxviii; author of article "An Indo-Persian Guide to Sufi Shrine Pilgrimage," pp. 43–67; abridged version of the latter reprinted in *Tales of God's Friends: Islamic Hagiography in Translation*, ed. John Renard (University of California Press, 2009), pp. 269–85.

ARTICLES IN JOURNALS AND COLLECTIVE VOLUMES

A. General and Critical Issues in Islamic Studies

"Persianate Islamic Studies in American Universities." In *Iranian Studies in America: Looking Back, Looking Ahead*, ed. Franklin Lewis and Erica Ehrenberg (American Institute of Iranian Studies/Eisenbruns, 2017).
"Ten Questions about Islamic Civilization." In *Islam for Journalists*, ed. Lawrence Pintak and Stephen Franklin (Social Science Research Council, 2013), pp. 50–62.
"Changing Approaches to Islamic Studies in North American Universities." In *Islamic Studies and Civilisational Dialogue: A Transdisciplinary Approach for Sustainability*, ed Azizan Baharuddin (Kuala Lumpur: Centre for Civilisational Dialogue, University of Malaya, 2013), pp. 75–92.
"The Global Significance of Arabic Language and Literature." *Religion Compass* 7/6 (2013), pp. 191–200.

"Islamic Studies in U.S. Universities," co-author with Charles Kurzman. *Review of Middle East Studies* 46/1 (Summer 2012), pp. 24–46.

"It's Not Just Academic – Writing Public Scholarship in Middle Eastern and Islamic Studies." *Review of Middle East Studies* 45/2 (Winter 2011 [published 2012]), pp. 164–71.

"'The West and Islam?' Rethinking Orientalism and Occidentalism." *Ishraq: Islamic Philosophy Yearbook* (Moscow/Tehran), vol. 1 (2010), pp. 23–34.

* Persian translation by Ruhollah `Alizada, "Gharb o eslam: baz andi-shi dar sharq-shinasi o gharb-shinasi," *Ittila`at-i hikmat o ma`rifat* 25 (1390/2012), pp. 20–24.

* Spanish translation by Carl Ernst and Luis Xavier López Farjeat, "¿El Occidente y el Islam? Repensar el orientalismo y el occidentalismo," *Istor: revista de historia internacional* 10/38 (2009), pp. 123–39.

"Muhammad as the Pole of Existence." In *The Cambridge Companion to Muhammad*, ed. Jonathan Brockopp (Cambridge: Cambridge University Press, 2010), pp. 123–38.

"Universalism in Islamic Thought." Keynote address for *International Symposium on Religion and World Peace* (Istanbul: Istanbul University, 2008), pp. 8–17.

"Demystifying the Rhetoric of Civilizational Conflict." In *Dialogue of Civilizations and the Construction of Peace*, ed. Thomas W. Simon and Azizan Baharuddin (Kuala Lumpur: Centre for Civilisational Dialogue, 2008), pp. 1–22.

"Reading Strategies for Introducing the Qur'an as Literature in an American Public University." *Islamic Studies* (Islamabad) 45:3 (2006), pp. 333–44. Reprinted as *Islamic Studies Occasional Papers* 77 (Islamabad: Islamic Research Institute, 2007).

"From Philosophy of Religion to History of Religion." In *Problems in the Philosophy of Religion: Critical Studies of the Work of John Hick*, ed. Harold Hewitt, Jr (London: Macmillan, 1991), pp. 46–50.

B. Premodern and Contemporary Sufism

"Wakened by the Dove's Trill: Structure and Meaning in the Arabic Preface of Rumi's *Mathnawi*, Book IV." In *The Philosophy of Ecstasy: Rumi and the Sufi Tradition*, ed. Leonard Lewisohn (London: World Wisdom, 2014).

"'A Little Indicates Much': Structure and Meaning in the Prefaces of Rumi's *Mathnawi* (Books I–III)." *Mawlana Rumi Review* V (2014), pp. 14–25.

"Piety and Devotion." In *Islam in the Modern World*, ed. Jeffrey T. Kenney, Ebrahim Moosa (Routledge, 2013), pp. 107–24.

Translations from the writings of Jalal al-Din Dawani: Commentary on Suhrawardi's "Temples of Light" (*Sharḥ hayākil al-nūr*, Book 5; Arabic), and Flashes of Illumination on Praiseworthy Ethics, or the Jalalian Ethics (*Akhlāq-i Jalālī*, Book 4; Persian), in *An Anthology of Philosophy in Persia*, ed. S. H. Nasr and Mehdi Aminrazavi, vol. 4, *From the School of Illumination to Philosophical Mysticism* (London: I.B. Tauris, 2012), pp. 93–120, 121–35.

"Jalal al-Din Davani's Interpretation of Hafiz." In *Hafiz and the School of Love in Persian Poetry*, ed. Leonard Lewisohn (London: I. B. Tauris, 2010), pp. 197–210.

"Shams-i Tabrizi and the Audacity of Bayazid Bistami." In *Şems: Güneşle Aydinlananlar / Enlightened By The Sun* (Istanbul: Nefes Yayınevi, 2010), pp. 286–95.

"Sufism and the Aesthetics of Penmanship according to Siraj al-Shirazi's *Tuhfat al-Muhibbin* (1454)." *Journal of the American Oriental Society* 129.3 (2009), pp. 431–42.

- Abridged version in *Hadeeth ad-Dar* (Dar al-Athar al-Islamiyyah Museum, Kuwait) 27 (2008), pp. 30–33.

"Beauty and the Feminine Element of Spirituality." In *Women and Tasawwuf* (Istanbul: Nefes, 2008), pp. 147–54.

"Sufism, Islam, and Globalization in the Contemporary World: Methodological Reflections on a Changing Field of Study." In Memoriam: The 4th Victor Danner Memorial Lecture. Bloomington, IN: Department of Near Eastern Languages, 2009.

- Italian translation by Marco Cena of an earlier version: "Il sufismo nel mondo musulmano contemporaneo: la 'divulgazione del segreto.'" In *Sufismo e confraternite nell'islam contemporaneo: Il difficile equilibrio tra mistica e politica*, ed. Marietta Stepanyants (Turin, Italy: Edizioni della Fondazione Giovanni Agnelli, 2003), pp. 301–24.

"On Losing One's Head: Hallajian themes in works attributed to `Attar." In *Attar and the Persian Sufi Tradition: The Art of Spiritual Flight*, ed. Leonard Lewisohn and Christopher Shackle (London: I. B. Tauris, 2006), pp. 330–43.

"Ideological and Technological Transformations of Contemporary Sufism." In *Muslim Networks: Medium, Metaphor, and Method*, ed. miriam cooke and Bruce B. Lawrence. Islamic Civilization and Muslim Networks Series, 2. Chapel Hill: University of North Carolina Press, 2005), pp. 198–207.

"Between Orientalism and Fundamentalism: Problematizing the Teaching of Sufism." In *Teaching Islam*, ed. Brannon Wheeler (Oxford: Oxford University Press, 2002), pp. 108–23.

"Sufism and Philosophy in Mulla Sadra." In *Islam-West Philosophical Dialogue: The Papers presented at the World Congress on Mulla Sadra (May, 1999, Tehran)* (Tehran: Sadra Islamic Philosophy Research Institute, 2001), 1: 173–92; reprinted in *Afkar: Journal of `Aqidah & Islamic Thought* 6 (2005), pp. 143–60.

- Persian translation: "Tasavvuf va falsafa az nazar-i Mulla Sadra." In *Majmu`a-i maqalat-i humayish-i jahani-i Mulla Sadra, avval Khurdad ma 1378 – Tehran, Mulla Sadra va hikmat-i muta`aliya* (Tehran: Bunyad-i Hikmat-i Islami-i Sadra, 2001), 2:51–64.

"Chishti Meditation Practices of the Later Mughal Period." In *The Heritage of Sufism*, Volume 3: *Late Classical Persianate Sufism (1501–1750): The Safavid and Mughal Period*, ed. Leonard Lewisohn and David Morgan (Oxford: Oneworld, 1999), pp. 344–57.

"Persecution and Circumspection in the Shattari Sufi Order." In *Islamic Mysticism Contested: Thirteen Centuries of Controversies & Polemics*, ed. Fred De Jong and Berndt Radtke, Islamic History and Civilization: Studies and Texts, 29 (Leiden: Brill, 1999), pp. 416–35.

"Vertical Pilgrimage and Interior Landscape in the Visionary Diary of Ruzbihan Baqli." *Muslim World* 88/2 (1998), pp. 129–40.

"The Interpretation of the Classical Sufi Tradition in India: The *Shama'il al-atqiya'* of Rukn al-Din Kashani." *Sufi* 22 (1994), pp. 5–10.

- Persian translation by Karim Zayyani: "Tafsiri bar sunnat-i tasavvuf-i klasik-i Hindustan: *Shamayil al-atqiya'*, athar-i Rukn al-Din Kashani," in *Sufi* 24 (1373/1994), pp. 6–12.

"Ruzbihan Baqli on Love as 'Essential Desire.'" In *Gott is schön und Er liebt die Schönheit/God is Beautiful and He Loves Beauty: Festschrift für Annemarie Schimmel*, ed. Alma Giese and J. Christoph Bürgel (Bern: Peter Lang, 1994), pp. 181–89.

"The Man without Attributes: Ibn 'Arabi's Interpretation of Abu Yazid al-Bistami." *Journal of the Muhyiddin Ibn 'Arabi Society* XIII (1993), pp. 1–18. Also in *Muhyiddin: The Revivifier of the Way, Proceedings of the Sixth Annual U.S.A. Symposium of the Muhyiddin Ibn 'Arabi Society* (Oxford: Muhyiddin Ibn 'Arabi Society, 1993), pp. 47–62.

"Mystical Language and the Teaching Context in the Early Sufi Lexicons." In *Mysticism and Language*, ed. Steven T. Katz (Oxford: Oxford University Press, 1992), pp. 181–201.

"The Stages of Love in Persian Sufism, from Rabi'a to Ruzbihan." In *Classical Persian Sufism from its Origins to Rumi*, ed. Leonard Lewisohn (London: Khaniqahi Nimatullahi, 1994), pp. 435–55; also in *Sufi* 14 (1992), pp. 16–23; reprinted in *The Heritage of Sufism*, Volume 1, *Classical Persian Sufism from its Origins to Rumi (700–1300)*, ed. Leonard Lewisohn (Oxford: One World, 1999), pp. 435–55.

- Persian translation by Mojde-i Bayat: "Marahil-i 'ishq dar nakhustin advar-i tasavvuf-i Iran, az Rabi'a ta Ruzbihan," in *Sufi* 16 (1371/1992), pp. 6–17.
- Revised Persian translation: "Marahil-i 'ishq dar tasavvuf-i aghazin-i Irani: az Rabi'a ta Ruzbihan," *Miras-i Tasavvuf*, trans. Majdoddin Keyvani (Tehran: Nashr-i Markaz, 1384/2006), 1:315–37.
- Spanish translation: "Las etapas del amor en el sufismo persa primitivo de Rābea a Ruzbahan," *Revista Sufi*, Número VIII (Otoño / Invierno 2004).

"The Spirit of Islamic Calligraphy: Baba Shah Isfahani's *Adab al-Mashq*." *Journal of the American Oriental Society* 112 (1992), pp. 279–86.

"The Symbolism of Birds and Flight in the Writings of Ruzbihan Baqli." In *The Legacy of Mediaeval Persian Sufism*, ed. Leonard Lewisohn (London: Khaniqahi Nimatullahi, 1992), pp. 353–66; also in *Sufi* 11 (Autumn, 1991), pp. 5–12; reprinted in *The Heritage of Sufism*, vol. 2, *The Legacy of Mediaeval Persian Sufism (1150–1500)*, ed. Leonard Lewisohn (Oxford: One World, 1999), pp. 353–66.

- Persian translation: "Namad-ha-yi parandah o parvaz dar musannafat-i Ruzbihan Baqli," *Miras-i Tasavvuf*, trans. Majdoddin Keyvani (Tehran: Nashr-i Markaz, 1384/2006), 2:231–52.

"The Textual Formation of Oral Teachings in Early Chishti Sufism." In *Texts and Contexts: Traditional Hermeneutics in South Asia*, ed. Jeffrey Timm (Albany: State University of New York Press, 1991), pp. 271–97.

"Ibn al-`Arabi on the Divine Beauty: Some Comparative Considerations." In *Truth and Beauty: Proceedings of the Second Annual U.S.A. Symposium of the Muhyiddin Ibn al-`Arabi Society* (Oxford: Muhyiddin Ibn `Arabi Society, 1989), pp. 59–67.

"Inner Perspectives" (a series of ten weekly newspaper columns on Sufism). *The Nation* (Lahore, Oct.-Dec. 1986).

"Controversy over Ibn `Arabi's *Fusus*: The Faith of Pharaoh." *Islamic Culture* LIX (1985), pp. 259–66.

"From Hagiography to Martyrology: Conflicting Testimonies to a Sufi Martyr of the Delhi Sultanate." *History of Religions* XXIV (May, 1985), pp. 308–27.

"Mystical and Esoteric Aspects of Religious Knowledge in Sufism." *The Journal of Religious Studies* XIII (1984), pp. 93–100; also in *Islam and the Modern Age* XV (1984), pp. 201–8.

C. Indo-Muslim Culture

"Muslim Interpreters of Yoga." In *Yoga: The Art of Transformation*, ed. Debra Diamond (Smithsonian Books, 2013), pp. 59–68.

"Indian Lovers in Arabic and Persian Guise: Azad Bilgrami's Depiction of *nayikas*." *The Journal of Hindu Studies* (2013), pp. 1–15.

"Traces of Šattari Sufism and Yoga in North Africa." *Oriente Moderno* XCII/2 (2013), pp. 361–67.

"The Limits of Universalism in Islamic Thought: The Case of Indian Religions." *Muslim World* 101 (January 2011), pp. 1–19.

- Revised edition in *Universality in Islamic Thought: Rationalism, Science and Religious Belief*, ed. Michael Morony (New York: I. B. Tauris, 2014), pp. 193–222.

"A Fourteenth-Century Persian Account of Breath Control and Meditation." In *Yoga in Practice*, ed. David Gordon White, Princeton Readings in Religions (Princeton: Princeton University Press, 2011), pp. 133–39.

"Fayzi's Illuminationist Interpretation of Vedanta: The *Shariq al-Ma`rifa*." *Comparative Studies of South Asia, Africa and the Middle East* 30/3 (2010), pp. 156–64.

"Reconfiguring South Asian Islam: From the 18th to the 19th Century." *Comparative Islamic Studies* 5/2 (2009 [published 2011]), pp. 247–72.

"Islam and Sufism in Contemporary South Asia." In *Sacred Spaces: A Journey with the Sufis of the Indus*, by Samina Quraeshi (Cambridge, MA: Peabody Museum Press, 2009), pp. 21–40.

"The Daily Life of a Saint, Ahmad Sirhindi (d. 1624), by Badr al-Din Sirhindi," in *Islam in South Asia in Practice*, ed. Barbara D. Metcalf (Princeton: Princeton University Press, 2009), pp. 158–65.

"Being Careful with the Goddess: Yoginis in Persian and Arabic Texts." In *Performing Ecstasy: The Poetics and Politics of Religion in India*, ed. Pallabi Chakrabarty and Scott Kugle (Delhi: Manohar, 2009), pp. 189–203.

"Accounts of Yogis in Arabic and Persian Historical and Travel Texts." *Jerusalem Studies in Arabic and Islam*, vol. 33 (2008), pp. 409–26.

"Two Versions of a Persian Text on Yoga and Cosmology, Attributed to Shaykh Mu`in al-Din Chishti." *Elixir* 2 (2006), pp. 69–76, 124–5.
   • Revised edition by Scott Kugle, "Mu`in al-Din Chishti, Treatise on the Human Body," in *Sufi Meditation and Contemplation: Timeless Wisdom from Mughal India* (New Lebanon, NY: Suluk Press/Omega Publications, 2012), pp. 167–9, 181–92.

"Fragmentary Versions of the Apocryphal 'Hymn of the Pearl' in Arabic, Turkish, Persian, and Urdu." *Jerusalem Studies in Arabic and Islam*, vol. 32 (2006), pp. 144–88.

"Situating Sufism and Yoga." *Journal of the Royal Asiatic Society*, Series 3, 15:1 (2005), pp. 15–43.
   • Reprint, in *Sufism*, ed. Lloyd Ridgeon, Critical Concepts in Islamic Studies (London: Routledge, 2008), vol. 2, essay 24.

"Khuldabad: Dargahs of Shaykh Burhanuddin Gharib and Shaykh Zaynuddin Shirazi." In *Dargahs: Abodes of the Saints*, ed. Mumtaz Currim and George Michell, special issue of *Marg* 56/1 (2004; reprint, 2011), pp. 104–19.

"The Islamization of Yoga in the Amrtakunda Translations." *Journal of the Royal Asiatic Society*, Series 3, 13:2 (2003), pp. 199–226.

"Muslim Studies of Hinduism? A Reconsideration of Persian and Arabic Translations from Sanskrit." *Iranian Studies* 36 (2003), pp. 173–95.
   • Persian translation by Sayyid Mahdi Husayni Isfidvajani, "Tarjuma-i mutun-i dini-i Hind bi-zaban-ha-yi parsi o `arabi," in *Andisha-i Irani o farhang-i hindi* (Tehran: Nashr-i `Ilm, 1391/2013).

"Abu Nasr Muhammad Khalidi (d. 1406/1985): A Brief Memoir." *The Annual of Urdu Studies* 15 (2000), pp. 305–13.

"Admiring the Works of the Ancients: The Ellora Temples as viewed by Indo-Muslim Authors." In *Beyond Turk and Hindu: Rethinking Religious Identities in Islamicate South Asia,* ed. David Gilmartin and Bruce B. Lawrence (Gainseville, FL: University Press of Florida, 2000), pp. 198–220.

"Local Cultural Nationalism as Anti-Fundamentalist Strategy in Pakistan." *Comparative Studies of South Asia, Africa, and the Middle East* 16 (1996), pp. 68–76.

"Sufism and Yoga according to Muhammad Ghawth." *Sufi* 29 (Spring 1996), pp. 9–13.
- Spanish translation by Pedro Soto: "El Sufismo y Yoga según Muhammad Ghawth." *Sarasvati* 9 (2006), pp. 77–85.

"Royal Policy and Patronage of Sufi Shrines in Mughul Revenue Documents from Khuldabad." In *Mediaeval Deccan History, Commemoration Volume in Honour of Purshottam Mahadeo Joshi*, ed. A. R. Kulkarni, M. A. Nayeem, and R. de Souza (Bombay: Popular Prakashan, 1996), pp. 76–93.

Translations for *Religions of India in Practice*, ed. Donald S. Lopez, Jr., Princeton Readings in Religions, 1 (Princeton University Press, 1995): "Lives of Sufi Saints" (Persian; pp. 495–512), "Conversations of Sufi Saints" (Persian; pp. 513–17), and "India as a Sacred Islamic Land" (Arabic; pp. 556–64).

"The Khuldabad-Burhanpur Axis, and Local Sufism in the Deccan." In *Islam and Indian Regions*, ed. Anna Libera Dallapiccola and Stephanie Zingel-Avé Lallemant, Beiträge zur Südasienforschung, Südasien-Institut der Universität Heidelberg, 145 (Stuttgart: Franz Steiner Verlag, 1993), I, pp. 169–83.

ARTICLES FOR REFERENCE WORKS

Encyclopaedia Iranica (Costa Mesa CA: Mazda Publishers): "Deccan I. Political and Literary History," (VII:181–85, 1995); "Ebrahim Shirazi" (VIII:76, 1997); "Faruqi Dynasty of Khandesh" (IX:374–5, 1999); "Jawāher-e Kamsa" (XIV:608–9, 2008); "Ruzbihan Baqli" (forthcoming).

Encyclopaedia of Islam, 2nd edition (Leiden: E. J. Brill): "Ruzbihan Bakli" (VII:651–2, 1995); "Shath" (IX:361–2, 1997); "Shirazi, Rafi` al-Din" (IX:483, 1997); "Tasawwuf (iii): 19th and 20th-century Sufism, in Muslim India" (X:333–7, 1999).

Encyclopaedia of Islam Three (Leiden: E. J. Brill): "Bibi Jamal Khatun" (I:165, 2010).

Encyclopedia of Islam and the Muslim World, ed. Richard Martin (New York: Macmillan Reference USA, 2004): "Tariqa" (2:680–4), "Tasawwuf" (2:684–90).

Encyclopedia of Politics and Religion, ed. Robert Wuthnow (Congressional Quarterly, Inc., 1998): "Iqbal, Muhammad," pp. 375–6; "Sufism," pp. 719–21.

Encyclopedia of Religion, ed. Mircea Eliade et al. (New York: Macmillan Publishing Company, 1987): "Blasphemy (Islamic Concept)," vol. 2, pp. 242–45.

The HarperCollins Dictionary of Religion, ed. Jonathan Z. Smith (San Francisco: Harper San Francisco, 1995): "Brethren of Purity," "Rightly Guided Caliphs," "Sufi," "Sunna," pp. 128, 928–9, 1029, 1035.

The Muslim Almanac: A Reference Work on the History, Faith, Cultures, and Peoples of Islam, ed. Azim A. Nanji (Gale Research, Inc., 1996): "Spiritual Life and Institutions in Muslim Society," pp. 253–59.

South Asian Folklore: An Encyclopedia, ed. Peter J. Claus and Margaret A. Mills (Garland Publishing, Inc., 2003): "Syncretism" (with Tony K. Stewart).

BOOK REVIEWS

Toby Mayer, *Keys to the Arcana: Shahrastani's Esoteric Commentary on the Qur'an. Journal of Shi'a Islamic Studies* 3/1(2009), pp. 237–8.

Anna Suvorova, *Muslim Saints of South Asia: The Eleventh to Fifteenth Centuries. Islamic Studies* 47/4 (Winter 2008), pp. 555–7.

Noorjehan Bilgrami, "Sun, Fire, River: Ajrak Cloth from the Soil of Sindh" (film review). *Middle East Studies Association Bulletin* 34\2 (Winter 2000), pp. 299–300.

John Peter Kenney, *Mystical Monotheism: A Study in Ancient Platonic Theology. Ancient Philosophy* 15 (1995), pp. 300–1.

"Traditionalism, the Perennial Philosophy, and Islamic Studies" (review article of Seyyed Hossein Nasr, ed., *Islamic Spirituality: Manifestations*, Le Gai Eaton, *King of the Castle*, Martin Lings, *Symbol and Archetype*, and Seyyed Hossein Nasr, *Islam in the Modern World*). *Middle East Studies Association Bulletin* 28 (1994), pp. 176–80.

"Embracing the Contradictions of 'Living Islam,' the Film," review of a six-part film series by BBC Enterprises. *Middle East Studies Association Bulletin* 28 (1994), pp. 25–27.

Sachiko Murata, *The Tao of Islam. Journal of the American Oriental Society* 114 (1994), pp. 677–8.

Raymond Lifchez, ed., *The Dervish Lodge. Parabola* XVIII/2 (Summer 1993), pp. 100–3.

Nizam Ad-Din Awliya, *Morals for the Heart*, trans. Bruce B. Lawrence. *Parabola* XVII/4 (Winter 1992), pp. 108–110.

Seyyed Hossein Nasr, *Traditional Islam in the Modern World. Journal of Islamic Studies* III (1992), pp. 260–61.

Proclus' Commentary on Plato's Parmenides, tr. Glenn R. Morrow and John M. Dillon. *Ancient Philosophy* 12 (1992), pp. 237–39.

Yohanan Friedmann, *Prophecy Continuous: Aspects of Ahmadi Religious Thought and Its Medieval Background. Journal of the American Oriental Society* 111 (1991), pp. 162–63.

Miriam Levering, ed., *Rethinking Scripture: Essays from a Comparative Perspective. Journal of Asian Studies* 49 (1990), pp. 106–7.

Seyyed Hossein Nasr, ed., *Islamic Spirituality: Foundations. Journal of the American Oriental Society* 110 (1990), pp. 368–69.

Julian Baldick, *Mystical Islam: An Introduction to Sufism. Iranian Studies* XXII/4 (1989), pp. 102–4.

J. M. S. Baljon, *Religion and Thought of Shah Wali Allah Dihlawi 1703–1762. Journal of the American Oriental Society* 109/2 (1989), pp. 309–11.

Testimonies and Reflections: Essays of Louis Massignon, trans. Herbert Mason. *Parabola* XIV/4 (1989), pp. 125–28.

Ayatullah Murtaza Mutahhari, *Fundamentals of Islamic Thought: God, Man, and the Universe*, trans. R. Campbell. *Muslim World* LXXVIII (1988), p. 286.

Victor Danner, *The Islamic Tradition: An Introduction. Parabola* XIII/3 (1988), pp. 110–12.

Najm al-Din Razi, *The Path of God's Bondsmen from Origin to Return*, trans. Hamid Algar. *Muslim World* LXXVIII (1988), p. 151.

Peter Lamborn Wilson, *Scandal: Essays in Islamic Heresy. Gnosis* 8 (1988), pp. 52–53.

The Drunken Universe: An Anthology of Persian Sufi Poetry, trans. Peter Lamborn Wilson and Nasrollah Pourjavady. *Gnosis* 8 (1988), pp. 52–53.

Khushwant Singh, *A History of the Sikhs. Muslim World.* LXXVIII (1988), p. 99.

Ylana N. Miller, *Government and Society in Rural Palestine, 1920–1948. Los Angeles Times*, Oct. 25, 1985.

Wendy Doniger O'Flaherty, *Dreams, Illusion and Other Realities. Journal of Asian and African Studies* XX (1985), pp. 252–54.

Everett K. Rowson, *A Muslim Philosopher on the Soul and Its Fate. Muslim World*, 82.1–2 (Jan 1992): 164.

BOOK NOTES

Clifford E. Bosworth, *The New Islamic Dynasties, A Chronological and Genealogical Manual. Religious Studies Review* 25/2 (April 1999), p. 216.

Mohammad Ebn-e Munawwar, *The Secrets of God's Mystical Oneness*, trans. John O'Kane. *Middle East Studies Association Bulletin* 27 (1993), p. 245.

Ahmad Saidi, trans. *Ruba'iyat of Omar Khayyam. Middle East Studies Association Bulletin* 27 (1993), pp. 98–99.

Assad Ali, *Happiness Without Death: Desert Hymns*, tr. Camille Adams Helminski, Kabir Helminski, and Ibrahim al-Shihabi. *Choice* (May 1992), p. 216.

Complete Works of Pir-o-Murshid Hazrat Inayat Khan, 1923 I: January-June. Gnosis 20 (1991), p. 76.

Ozay Mehmet, *Islamic Identity and Development. Choice* (March 1991), p. 443.

Paul Jackson, *The Muslims of India: Beliefs and Practices. The Journal of Ecumenical Studies* 27 (1990), pp. 373–74.

H. T. Norris, *Sufis of the Niger Desert. Choice* (July 1990), p. 305.

Abdul Malik Mujahid, *Conversion to Islam: Untouchables' Strategy for Protest in India. Choice* (June 1990), p. 293.

William Chittick, *The Sufi Path of Knowledge: Ibn al-'Arabi's Metaphysics of Imagination. Parabola* XV/2 (1990), pp. 104–6.

Bruce B. Lawrence, *Defenders of God. Gnosis* 15 (1990), p. 74.

Cyril Glassé, *The Concise Encyclopedia of Islam. Gnosis* 15 (1990), pp. 75–76.

Sheikh Muzaffer Ozak al-Jerrahi, *Irshad: Wisdom of a Sufi Master*, trans. Muhtar Holland. *Gnosis* 9 (1989), p. 51.

Daniel Gold, *Comprehending the Guru. Religious Studies Review* 15 (1989), p. 239.

Sheikh Muzaffer Ozak al-Jerrahi al-Halveti, *Love is the Wine: Talks of a Sufi Master in America*, ed. and comp. Sheikh Ragip Frager. *Gnosis* 7 (1988), p. 53.

Shaykh Fadhlalla Haeri, *Beginning's End. Gnosis* 7 (1988), p. 53.

Syed Vahiduddin, *Islam in India. Religious Studies Review* 14 (1988), p. 172.

William Chittick, *The Sufi Path of Love: The Spiritual Teachings of Rumi. Parabola* IX/1 (1984), p. 122.

An-Nawawi's Forty Hadith, trans. Ezzeddin Ibrahim and Denys Johnson-Davies. *Muslim World* LXXI (1981), p. 78.

OTHERS

"Herbert Luther Bodman (obituary)." *Review of Middle East Studies* 45/1 (Summer 2011), p. 154.

"Annemarie Schimmel (obituary)," *Middle East Studies Association Bulletin* 37.2 (2003): 310–12.

Co-author (with Bruce Lawrence, Alan Godlas, Arthur Buehler, and Michael Hillman). "First International Congress of Professors of Persian Language and Literature, Tehran, January 3–5, 1996." *Middle East Studies Association Bulletin* 30.1 (1996): 18–22.

Index

About the Author

Carl W. Ernst is the William R. Kenan, Jr., Distinguished Professor of Islamic studies at the Department of Religious Studies (2005–) and Co-director of the Carolina Center for the Study of the Middle East and Muslim Civilizations at the University of North Carolina at Chapel Hill, USA. He is a specialist in Islamic studies, with a focus on West and South Asia. His published research, based on the study of Arabic, Persian, and Urdu, has been mainly devoted to the study of three areas: general and critical issues of Islamic studies, pre-modern and contemporary Sufism, and Indo-Muslim culture. Professor Ernst has received research fellowships from the Fulbright program, the National Endowment for the Humanities, and the John Simon Guggenheim Foundation, and he has been elected a Fellow of the American Academy of Arts and Sciences. His publications, which have received several international awards, include *Rethinking Islamic Studies: From Orientalism to Cosmopolitanism* (co-edited with Richard Martin, 2010); *Following Muhammad: Rethinking Islam in the Contemporary World* (2003); and *Teachings of Sufism* (1999). Carl Ernst and Bruce Lawrence are co-editors of the Islamic Civilization and Muslim Networks Series at the University of North Carolina Press.